Botulinum Toxin
Therapeutic Clinical Practice and Science

Joseph Jankovic, MD
Chief Editor
Professor of Neurology
Distinguished Chair in Movement Disorders
Director of Parkinson's Disease Center and Movement Disorders Clinic
Department of Neurology
Baylor College of Medicine
Houston, Texas

Alberto Albanese, MD
Professor of Neurology
Center for Neurosciences
Catholic University
Head Neurologist
National Neurological Institute Carlo Besta
Milan, Italy

M. Zouhair Atassi, PhD, DSc
Robert A. Welch Chair of Chemistry
Professor of Biochemistry and Molecular Biology
Professor of Immunology
Baylor College of Medicine
Houston, Texas

J. Oliver Dolly, MSc, PhD, DSc
Science Foundation Ireland Research Professor
Director, International Centre for
    Neurotherapeutics
Dublin City University
Dublin, Ireland

Mark Hallett, MD
Chief, Human Motor Control Section
National Institute of Neurological Disorders and
    Stroke
National Institutes of Health
Bethesda, Maryland

Nathaniel H. Mayer, MD
Emeritus Professor of Physical Medicine and
    Rehabilitation
Temple University School of Medicine
Philadelphia, Pennsylvania
Director, Motor Control Analysis Laboratory
MossRehab
Elkins Park, Pennsylvania

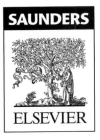

SAUNDERS

ELSEVIER

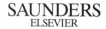

1600 John F. Kennedy Blvd.
Ste 1800
Philadelphia, PA 19103-2899

BOTULINUM TOXIN:
THERAPEUTIC CLINICAL PRACTICE AND SCIENCE

ISBN: 978-1-4160-4928-9

Notice

Knowledge and best practice in this field are constantly changing. As new research and experience broaden our knowledge, changes in practice, treatment and drug therapy may become necessary or appropriate. Readers are advised to check the most current information provided (i) on procedures featured or (ii) by the manufacturer of each product to be administered, to verify the recommended dose or formula, the method and duration of administration, and contraindications. It is the respon-sibility of the practitioner, relying on their own experience and knowledge of the patient, to make diagnoses, to determine dosages and the best treatment for each individual patient, and to take all appropriate safety precautions. To the fullest extent of the law, neither the Publisher nor the Editors assumes any liability for any injury and/or damage to persons or property arising out of or related to any use of the material contained in this book.

The Publisher

Library of Congress Cataloging-in-Publication Data

Botulinum toxin : therapeutic clinical practice and science / [edited by] Joseph Jankovic ... [et al.]. – 1st ed.
    p. ; cm.
Includes bibliographical references.
ISBN 978-1-4160-4928-9
1. Botulinum toxin–Therapeutic use. I. Jankovic, Joseph.
[DNLM: 1. Botulinum Toxins–therapeutic use. QV 140 B751 2008]
RC935.S64B68 2008
615′.329364–dc22   2008043233

Acquisitions Editor: Adrianne Brigido
Developmental Editor: Angela Norton
Project Manager: David Saltzberg
Design Direction: Steven Stave

Printed in United States of America

Last digit is the print number: 9 8 7 6 5 4 3 2 1

Contributors

Giovanni Abbruzzese, MD, PhD
Professor of Neurology, Department of
  Neurosciences, Ophthalmology and
  Genetics, University of Genoa, Genoa, Italy
*Effects of Botulinum Toxin on Central Nervous System
  Function*

Emily J. Adams, BSc (Hons), PhD
Postdoctoral Research Fellow, National Heart
  and Lung Institute, Imperial College
  London, London, United Kingdom
*Understanding Botulinum Neurotoxin Mechanism of
  Action and Structure to Enhance Therapeutics and
  Improve Care*

Alberto Albanese, MD
Professor of Neurology, Center for
  Neurosciences, Catholic University; Head
  Neurologist, National Neurological Institute
  Carlo Besta, Milan, Italy
*Botulinum Neurotoxin in Tremors, Tics, Hemifacial
  Spasm, Spasmodic Dysphonia, and Stuttering;
  Clinical Trials of Botulinum Toxin in Adult Spasticity*

K. Roger Aoki, PhD
Vice President, Neurotoxins, Discovery
  Research, Allergan, Inc., Irvine, California
*Immune Recognition of Botulinum Neurotoxins A and
  B: Molecular Elucidation of Immune Protection
  Against the Toxins*

Debra Elaine Artim, PhD
Research Associate, Department of
  Pharmacology and Chemical Biology,
  University of Pittsburgh School of
  Medicine, Pittsburgh, Pennsylvania
Bungarotoxins

M. Zouhair Atassi, PhD, DSc
Robert A. Welch Chair of Chemistry,
  Professor of Biochemistry and Molecular
  Biology, and Professor of Immunology,
  Baylor College of Medicine, Houston,
  Texas
*Immune Recognition of Botulinum Neurotoxins A and
  B: Molecular Elucidation of Immune Protection
  Against the Toxins*

Anna Rita Bentivoglio, MD, PhD
Confirmed Researcher, Istituto di Neurologia,
  Università Cattolica del Sacro Cuore;
  Assistant Professor of Neurology, Istituto di
  Neurologia, Policlinico Agostino Gemelli,
  Rome, Italy
*Botulinum Neurotoxin in Tremors, Tics, Hemifacial
  Spasm, Spasmodic Dysphonia, and Stuttering*

Alfredo Berardelli, MD, PhD
Professor of Neurology, Department of
  Neurological Sciences and Neuromed
  Institute, "Sapienza" University of Rome,
  Rome, Italy
*Effects of Botulinum Toxin on Central Nervous System
  Function*

Hans Bigalke, MD
Institute of Toxicology, Hannover Medical
  School, Hannover, Germany
*Properties of Pharmaceutical Products of Botulinum
  Neurotoxins*

Andrew Blitzer, MD, DDS
Professor of Clinical Otolaryngology, College
  of Physicians and Surgeons, Columbia
  University; Senior Attending
  Otolaryngologist, St. Luke's/Roosevelt
  Hospital Center; Director, New York Center
  for Voice and Swallowing Disorders, New
  York, New York
*Treatment of Oromandibular Dystonia, Bruxism, and
  Temporomandibular Disorders with Botulinum Toxin*

MacDara Bodeker, PhD
International Centre for Neurotherapeutics,
  Dublin City University, Dublin, Ireland
*Multiple Steps in the Blockade of Exocytosis by
  Botulinum Neurotoxins*

Mark A. Breidenbach, PhD
Postdoctoral Fellow, Department of
  Chemistry, University of California,
  Berkeley, Berkeley, California
*Interactions Between Botulinum Neurotoxins and
  Synaptic Vesicle Proteins*

Axel T. Brunger, PhD
Professor, Stanford University School of
Medicine, Stanford, California
*Interactions Between Botulinum Neurotoxins and
Synaptic Vesicle Proteins*

Michael B. Chancellor, MD
Director of Neurourology Program,
Department of Urology, William Beaumont
Hospital, Royal Oak, Michigan
*Mechanism of Action of Botulinum Neurotoxin in the
Lower Urinary Tract; Application of Botulinum Toxin
in the Prostate*

Martin K. Childers, DO, PhD
Associate Professor, Department of
Neurology, Wake Forest University Health
Sciences, Winston-Salem, North Carolina
*Clinical Application of Botulinum Neurotoxin in the
Treatment of Myofascial Pain Syndromes*

Yao-Chi Chuang, MD
Associate Professor, Department of Urology,
Chang Gung University, Kaohsiung Hsien,
Taiwan
Application of Botulinum Toxin in the Prostate

Cynthia L. Comella, MD
Professor, Department of Neurological
Sciences, Rush University Medical Center,
Chicago, Illinois
Comparative Clinical Trials of Botulinum Toxins

William Chet de Groat, PhD
Professor of Pharmacology, Department of
Pharmacology and Chemical Biology,
University of Pittsburgh School of
Medicine, Pittsburgh, Pennsylvania
Bungarotoxins

J. Oliver Dolly, MSc, PhD, DSc
Science Foundation Ireland Research
Professor, and Director, International
Centre for Neurotherapeutics, Dublin City
University, Dublin, Ireland
*Multiple Steps in the Blockade of Exocytosis by
Botulinum Neurotoxins*

**Wagner Ferreira dos Santos, BsC,
MsC, PhD**
Associate Professor, Faculdade de Filosofia,
Ciências e Letras de Ribeirão Preto,
University of São Paulo, Ribeirão Preto, São
Paulo, Brazil
Spider and Wasp Neurotoxins

Dirk Dressler, MD, PhD
Professor of Neurology, and Head, Movement
Disorders Section, Department of
Neurology, Hannover Medical School,
Hannover, Germany
Comparative Clinical Trials of Botulinum Toxins

Dennis Dykstra, MD, PhD, MHA
Associate Professor, and Chairman,
Department of Physical Medicine and
Rehabilitation, University of Minnesota
Medical School, Minneapolis, Minnesota
*Botulinum Toxin in Overactive Bladder; Botulinum
Toxin for Osteoarticular Pain*

Roberto Eleopra, MD
Chairman of Neurological Department,
Angel's Hospital of Mestre, Venice, Italy
*Biology and Clinical Pharmacology of Botulinum
Neurotoxin Type C and Other Non-A/Non-B
Botulinum Neurotoxins*

Antonio Elia, MD
Department of Neurology, National
Neurological Institute Carlo Besta,
Milan, Italy
Clinical Trials of Botulinum Toxin in Adult Spasticity

Alberto Esquenazi, MD
Professor of Physical Medicine and
Rehabilitation, Jefferson School of
Medicine, Thomas Jefferson University,
Philadelphia; Chair of Physical Medicine
and Rehabilitation, and Director, Gait and
Motion Analysis Laboratory, MossRehab,
Elkins Park, Pennsylvania
*Upper Limb Skin and Musculoskeletal Consequences of
the Upper Motor Neuron Syndrome; Clinical
Experience and Recent Advances in the
Management of Gait Disorders with Botulinum
Neurotoxin*

Alfonso Fasano, MD
Università Cattolica del Sacro Cuore; Istituto
di Neurologia, Policlinico Agostino
Gemelli, Rome, Italy
*Botulinum Neurotoxin in Tremors, Tics, Hemifacial
Spasm, Spasmodic Dysphonia, and Stuttering*

Graziella Filippini, MD
Department of Neuroepidemiology,
National Neurological Institute Carlo Besta,
Milan, Italy
Clinical Trials of Botulinum Toxin in Adult Spasticity

Audrey Fischer, PhD
Postdoctoral Fellow, Harvard Medical School, Boston, Massachusetts
Botulinum Neurotoxin—a Modular Nanomachine

Paul S. Fishman, MD, PhD
Professor and Research Director, Department of Neurology; Chief, Neurology Service, Maryland Veterans Affairs Health Care System, Baltimore, Maryland
Tetanus Toxin

Keith A. Foster, MA, PhD
Founder and Head of Technology Development, Syntaxin Ltd., Abingdon, Oxon, United Kingdom
Understanding Botulinum Neurotoxin Mechanism of Action and Structure to Enhance Therapeutics and Improve Care

Oren Friedman, MD
Assistant Professor of Otolaryngology, Department of Otorhinolaryngology, Mayo Medical School; Director, Facial Plastic and Reconstructive Surgery, Department of Otorhinolaryngology, Mayo Clinic, Rochester, Minnesota
The Role of Botulinum Toxin in Wound Healing

Holger G. Gassner, MD
Fellow, Facial Plastic and Reconstructive Surgery, Department of Otorhinolaryngology, Head and Neck Surgery, University of Washington; Fellow, Facial Plastic and Reconstructive Surgery, The Larrabee Center, Harborview Hospital, and Virginia Mason Hospital, Seattle, Washington
The Role of Botulinum Toxin in Wound Healing

Dee Anna Glaser, MD
Professor, and Director of Cosmetic and Laser Surgery, Department of Dermatology, Associate Professor, Department of Otolaryngology, and Assistant Professor, Department of Internal Medicine, Saint Louis University School of Medicine, St. Louis, Missouri
Botulinum Neurotoxin in the Management of Hyperhidrosis and Other Hypersecretory Disorders; Botulinum Neurotoxin for Dermatologic and Cosmetic Disorders

H. Kerr Graham, MD, FRCS (Ed), FRACS
Professor of Orthopaedic Surgery, The University of Melbourne; Professor of Orthopaedic Surgery, Director, The Hugh Williamson Gait Laboratory, and Honorary Fellow, Murdoch Children's Research Institute, The Royal Children's Hospital, Melbourne, Victoria, Australia
Treatment of Motor Disorders in Cerebral Palsy with Botulinum Neurotoxin

Mark Hallett, MD
Chief, Human Motor Control Section, National Institute of Neurological Disorders and Stroke, National Institutes of Health, Bethesda, Maryland
Potential New Therapeutic Indications for Botulinum Neurotoxins

Joseph Jankovic, MD
Professor of Neurology, Distinguished Chair in Movement Disorders, and Director of Parkinson's Disease Center and Movement Disorders Clinic, Department of Neurology, Baylor College of Medicine, Houston, Texas
Botulinum Neurotoxin Treatment of Cranial-Cervical Dystonia

Elsie C. Jimenez, PhD
Professor of Chemistry, University of the Philippines Baguio, Baguio City, Philippines; Formerly Research Fellow, Department of Biology, University of Utah, Salt Lake City, Utah
Biology and Pharmacology of Conotoxins

Rongsheng Jin, PhD
Assistant Professor, Neuroscience, Aging and Stem Cell Research Center, Burnham Institute for Medical Research, La Jolla, California
Interactions Between Botulinum Neurotoxins and Synaptic Vesicle Proteins

Barbara Illowsky Karp, MD
Chair, Combined Neuroscience Institutional Review Board, National Institute of Neurological Disorders and Stroke, National Institutes of Health, Bethesda, Maryland
Botulinum Neurotoxin Treatment of Limb and Occupational Dystonias

Christopher Kenney, MD
Parkinson's Disease Center and Movement
   Disorders Clinic, Department of Neurology,
   Baylor College of Medicine, Houston, Texas
*Botulinum Neurotoxin Treatment of Cranial-Cervical
   Dystonia*

Lilia Koriazova, PhD
Group Leader, Antibody Production, Kirin
   Pharma USA, Inc., La Jolla, California
Botulinum Neurotoxin—a Modular Nanomachine

Hollis E. Krug, MD
Associate Professor of Medicine, University of
   Minnesota Medical School; Staff
   Rheumatologist, Minneapolis Veterans
   Affairs Medical Center, Minneapolis,
   Minnesota
Botulinum Toxin for Osteoarticular Pain

Florenta Aura Kullmann, PhD
Visiting Research Associate, Department of
   Pharmacology and Chemical Biology,
   University of Pittsburgh School of
   Medicine, Pittsburgh, Pennsylvania
Bungarotoxins

Gary W. Lawrence, BSc, PhD
Senior Research Fellow, International Centre
   for Neurotherapeutics, Dublin City
   University, Dublin, Ireland
*Multiple Steps in the Blockade of Exocytosis by
   Botulinum Neurotoxins*

Jane Leonard, MB, BCh, BAO, MRCPI
Research Fellow in Developmental Medicine,
   The Royal Children's Hospital, Melbourne,
   Victoria, Australia
*Treatment of Motor Disorders in Cerebral Palsy with
   Botulinum Neurotoxin*

Richard L. Lieber, PhD
Professor, Departments of Orthopaedic
   Surgery and Bioengineering, University of
   California, San Diego, San Diego,
   California
*Biological and Mechanical Pathologies in Spastic
   Skeletal Muscle: The Functional Implications of
   Therapeutic Neurotoxins*

Maren Lawson Mahowald, MD
Professor of Medicine, University of
   Minnesota Medical School; Rheumatology
   Section Chief, Minneapolis Veterans Affairs
   Medical Center, Minneapolis, Minnesota
Botulinum Toxin for Osteoarticular Pain

Nathaniel H. Mayer, MD
Emeritus Professor of Physical Medicine and
   Rehabilitation, Temple University School of
   Medicine, Philadelphia; Director, Motor
   Control Analysis Laboratory, MossRehab,
   Elkins Park, Pennsylvania
*Upper Limb Skin and Musculoskeletal Consequences of
   the Upper Motor Neuron Syndrome; Clinical
   Experience and Recent Advances in the
   Management of Gait Disorders with Botulinum
   Neurotoxin*

Jianghui Meng, BSc, MSc, PhD
Post-doctoral Research Associate, International
   Centre for Neurotherapeutics, Dublin City
   University, Dublin, Ireland
*Multiple Steps in the Blockade of Exocytosis by
   Botulinum Neurotoxins*

Kris S. Moe, MD, FACS
Chief, Division of Facial Plastic and
   Reconstructive Surgery, Department of
   Otolaryngology – Head and Neck Surgery,
   University of Washington, Seattle,
   Washington
The Role of Botulinum Toxin in Wound Healing

Mauricio Montal, MD, PhD
Distinguished Professor, Section of
   Neurobiology, Division of Biological
   Sciences, University of California, San
   Diego, La Jolla, California
Botulinum Neurotoxin—a Modular Nanomachine

Cesare Montecucco, PhD
Professor, Department of Biomedical Sciences,
   University of Padova, Padova, Italy
*Biology and Clinical Pharmacology of Botulinum
   Neurotoxin Type C and Other Non-A/Non-B
   Botulinum Neurotoxins*

Rajasekhara Mummadi, MD
Fellow in Gastroenterology, The University of
   Texas Medical Branch, Galveston, Texas
Botulinum Toxin Therapy in Gastrointestinal Disorders

Markus Naumann, MD
Department of Neurology and Clinical
   Neurophysiology, Klinikum Augsburg,
   Augsburg, Germany
*Botulinum Neurotoxin in the Management of
   Hyperhidrosis and Other Hypersecretory Disorders*

Myrta Oblatt-Montal, PhD
Research Associate, Section of Neurobiology, Division of Biological Sciences, University of California, San Diego, La Jolla, California
Botulinum Neurotoxin—a Modular Nanomachine

Baldomero M. Olivera, PhD
Distinguished Professor, Department of Biology, University of Utah, Salt Lake City, Utah
Biology and Pharmacology of Conotoxins

Pankaj J. Pasricha, MD
Chief, Division of Gastroenterology and Hepatology, Department of Medicine, Stanford University School of Medicine; Professor of Medicine, Department of Medicine, Stanford Hospital and Clinics, and Lucile Packard Children's Hospital, Stanford, California
Botulinum Toxin Therapy in Gastrointestinal Disorders

Duncan F. Rogers, BSc (Hons), PhD
Reader in Respiratory Pharmacology, National Heart and Lung Institute, Imperial College London, London, United Kingdom
Understanding Botulinum Neurotoxin Mechanism of Action and Structure to Enhance Therapeutics and Improve Care

Janice M. Rusnak, MD, FACP, FIDSA
Contractor Goldbelt Raven, Inc. as Research Physician in Special Immunizations Program at United States Army Medical Research Institute of Infectious Diseases, Fort Detrick, Maryland
Botulism Vaccines and the Immune Response

Astrid Sasse, PhD
Lecturer, School of Pharmacy and Pharmaceutical Sciences, Trinity College, Dublin, Ireland
Multiple Steps in the Blockade of Exocytosis by Botulinum Neurotoxins

Michael F. Saulino, MD, PhD
Assistant Professor, Department of Rehabilitation Medicine, Thomas Jefferson University, Philadelphia; Adjunct Assistant Professor, Department of Physical Medicine and Rehabilitation, Temple University, Philadelphia; Adjunct Assistant Professor, Department of Occupational Therapy, University of the Sciences in Philadelphia, Philadelphia; Staff Physiatrist, MossRehab, Elkins Park, Pennsylvania
Therapeutic Applications of Conotoxins

Brigitte Schurch, MD
Professor, Swiss Paraplegic Centre, Zürich, Switzerland
Botulinum Toxin in Overactive Bladder

David A. Sherris, MD
Professor and Chairman, Department of Otolaryngology, University at Buffalo; Chief of Service, Department of Otolaryngology, Kaleida Health System, Buffalo, New York
The Role of Botulinum Toxin in Wound Healing

Stephen D. Silberstein, MD
Professor of Neurology, Jefferson Medical College, Thomas Jefferson University; Director, Jefferson Headache Center, Philadelphia, Pennsylvania
Botulinum Toxin in Headache Management

David M. Simpson, MD
Professor, Department of Neurology, Mount Sinai School of Medicine; Director, Clinical Neurophysiology Laboratories, and Neuro-AIDS Program, Mount Sinai Hospital, New York, New York
Unmet Needs and Challenges in the Therapeutic Use of Botulinum Neurotoxins

Jasvinder A. Singh, MBBS, MPH
Assistant Professor, University of Minnesota Medical School, Minneapolis; Visiting Scientist, Mayo Clinic School of Medicine, Rochester; Staff Physician, Minneapolis Veterans Affairs Medical Center, Minneapolis, Minnesota
Botulinum Toxin for Osteoarticular Pain

Christopher P. Smith, MD, MBA
Associate Professor, Scott Department of Urology, Baylor College of Medicine, Houston, Texas
Mechanism of Action of Botulinum Neurotoxin in the Lower Urinary Tract; Botulinum Toxin in the Treatment of Chronic Pelvic Pain Syndromes

Leonard A. Smith, PhD
Senior Research Scientist (ST), Medical Countermeasures Technology, United States Army Medical Research Institute of Infectious Diseases, Fort Detrick, Maryland
Botulism Vaccines and the Immune Response

Phillip P. Smith, MD
Senior Fellow and Clinical Instructor, Scott Department of Urology, Baylor College of Medicine, Houston, Texas
Botulinum Toxin in the Treatment of Chronic Pelvic Pain Syndromes

Yuen T. So, MD, PhD
Professor, Department of Neurology and Neurological Sciences, Stanford University School of Medicine; Director, Neurology Clinics, Department of Neurology and Neurological Sciences, Stanford University Hospital, Stanford, California
Unmet Needs and Challenges in the Therapeutic Use of Botulinum Neurotoxins

George T. Somogyi, MD, PhD
Professor, Scott Department of Urology, Baylor College of Medicine, Houston, Texas
Mechanism of Action of Botulinum Neurotoxin in the Lower Urinary Tract

Antonio Suppa, MD
Research Fellow, Department of Neurological Sciences and Neuromed Institute, "Sapienza" University of Rome, Rome, Italy
Effects of Botulinum Toxin on Central Nervous System Function

Subramanyam Swaminathan, PhD
Biophysicist, Biology Department, Brookhaven National Laboratory, Upton, New York
Molecular Structures and Functional Relationships of Botulinum Neurotoxins

Russell W. Teichert, PhD
Research Assistant Professor, Department of Biology, University of Utah, Salt Lake City, Utah
Biology and Pharmacology of Conotoxins

Carlo Trompetto, MD, PhD
Assistant Professor, Department of Neurosciences, Ophthalmology and Genetics, University of Genoa, Genoa, Italy
Effects of Botulinum Toxin on Central Nervous System Function

Valeria Tugnoli, MD, PhD
Chief of the Neurophysiology Unit, Department of Neuroscience and Rehabilitation, S. Anna Hospital, Ferrara, Italy
Biology and Clinical Pharmacology of Botulinum Neurotoxin Type C and Other Non-A/Non-B Botulinum Neurotoxins

Jiafu Wang, BSc, PhD
Research Fellow, International Centre for Neurotherapeutics, Dublin City University, Dublin, Ireland
Multiple Steps in the Blockade of Exocytosis by Botulinum Neurotoxins

Samuel R. Ward, PT, PhD
Assistant Professor, Departments of Radiology, Orthopaedic Surgery, and Bioengineering, University of California, San Diego, San Diego, California
Biological and Mechanical Pathologies in Spastic Skeletal Muscle: The Functional Implications of Therapeutic Neurotoxins

Nwanmegha Young, MD
Fellow in Laryngology/Neurolaryngology, New York Center for Voice and Swallowing Disorders; Attending Otolaryngologist, St. Luke's/Roosevelt Hospital Center, New York, New York
Treatment of Oromandibular Dystonia, Bruxism, and Temporomandibular Disorders with Botulinum Toxin

Tomas H. Zurawski, MSc, PhD
Post-doctoral Research Associate, International Centre for Neurotherapeutics, Dublin City University, Dublin, Ireland
Multiple Steps in the Blockade of Exocytosis by Botulinum Neurotoxins

Preface

Botulinum and Other Neurotoxins: Translating Science into Therapeutic Applications

Our knowledge about clostridial neurotoxins has increased dramatically since 1817 when Christian Andreas Justinus Kerner, the German physician and poet, provided the earliest account of food borne botulism, correctly recognized that the toxin paralyzed skeletal muscles and blocked parasympathetic function, and proposed that botulinum neurotoxin (BoNT) could be used as a therapeutic agent in St. Vitus dance, hypersalivation, and hyperhidrosis. In 1870, Muller, another German physician, coined the name botulism, after the Latin name for "sausage," a common source of food poisoning. The next milestone in the development of BoNT was the 1895 outbreak of food intoxication from infected sausages consumed after a funeral ceremony in the Belgian village Ellezelle, which led to the first isolation of clostridium botulinum and of botulinum toxin by E. van Ermengem. In 1920, Hermann Sommer (University of California) first purified BoNT and in 1944, Edward Schantz (Fort Detrick, MD) first cultured clostridium botulinum and developed a method for isolation of the toxin. In 1949, A.S. Burgen (Cambridge, England) discovered that BoNT blocks neuromuscular transmission by blocking release of acetylcholine. In 1964, D.B. Drachman (Johns Hopkins University) first showed that botulinum neurotoxin can be used to paralyze the injected muscle and demonstrated the critical role of acetylcholine in "neurotrophic" maintenance. Applying Drachman's observations, Alan Scott published the 1973 seminal paper describing the beneficial effects of BoNT injections into eye muscles of monkeys to correct strabismus, thus starting the therapeutic era of BoNT.

The most potent biologic toxin known (can be lethal even at doses as low as 0.2 ng), BoNT has been feared as a potent biological weapon, but today it is mainly utilized as a therapeutic agent. As a result of the clinical use of BoNT in millions of individuals worldwide, the perception of BoNT as a powerful poison and potential biological weapon has changed dramatically in the past quarter century. In the beginning, BoNT was applied to treat neurological disorders in which an overactivity of distinct neurons caused disabling and painful spasms of striated muscles such as seen in blepharospasm, cervical dystonia, other forms of dystonia, spasticity, and various pain disorders including headaches and post-traumatic muscle spasms. In the next stage, the clinical indications for BoNT expanded to its use in the treatment of hyperhidrosis, other hypersecretory disorders, gastrointenstinal and urological disorders, and various cosmetic indications. Few drugs have been better understood in terms of their mechanism of action before their clinical application. Today, no therapeutic agent in medicine has more clinical indications (although only a few have been officially approved) than BoNT.

The purpose of this book is to review the current knowledge about the basic science and clinical use of BoNT. The idea for the book was conceived during the International Conference on Neurotoxins (ICON), sponsored by the Neurotoxin Institute (www.neurotoxininstitute.com) and held in Hollywood, Florida, November 29-December 2, 2006. One of the major aims of the ICON meeting (and this book) was not only to disseminate current information about BoNT, but to stimulate more scientists and clinicians to learn about this extraordinary molecule and to apply the growing knowledge in improving patients' functioning and favorably impact on the quality of life. The editors hope that the book will draw attention to the expanding knowledge of neurotoxins and will serve to highlight the fruitful progress in this growing field of translational research and stimulate imagination for potential future applications. This book should be of interest to neuroscientists and practicing physicians working in a wide range of specialties including neurology, physiatry and rehabilitation medicine, orthopedics, sports medicine, pediatrics, dermatology, plastic surgery, otolaryngology, urology, gastroenterology, pain medicine, and esthetics.

The book would not be possible without the scholarly contributions by the many authors, all of whom were selected because of their leadership in the field. We also want to thank Susan Pioli, who appreciated the value of the book and brought it to the attention of Elsevier Inc., Adrianne Brigido, the Acquisitions Editor for Elsevier Inc. for her continued guidance, and, most importantly, to Angela Norton, the Associate Developmental Editor, Elsevier Inc., for her tireless effort in coordinating the pre-publication process and her exemplary professionalism.

J.Jankovic(chief editor)
A.Albanese
M.Z.Atassi
J.O.Dolly
M.Hallett
N.H.Mayer

Foreword

DEVELOPMENT OF BOTULINUM TOXIN

Carter Collins and I were exploring the forces and actions of the eye muscles through the 1960s and 1970s. Experienced with placing EMG recording electrodes into muscles, we hit on the idea of injecting local anesthetic into individual muscles through needle electrodes to knock out their function and to tell thereby what they did. As many strabismus procedures acted to weaken over acting muscles, it was a small step to wonder if we might inject something having a longer duration of action and thus practical clinical utility. Botulinum toxin soon came up for consideration, but was moved to the bottom of the list, as it seemed too crazy to really try it–it was too toxic and we would never get to use it anyway with the FDA looking, right? Well, very close to right! We had worked down the list of ineffective substances, when I became aware of Daniel Drachman's work injecting minute amounts of botulinum toxin directly into the hind limb of chicks and achieving local denervation effects. Drachman told us of Edward Schantz who supplied toxin to him. Ed had left the US Army Chemical Corps to work at the University of Wisconsin where he continued to make purified botulinum toxins using techniques worked out earlier at Fort Detrick by Lamanna and Duff. He gave these generously to the academic community, and was kind enough to supply us with crystalline botulinum toxin. Reference to the literature on botulism showed that epidemics caused by type A were characterized by extensive and long lasting motor paralysis (type B tended toward autonomic problems, other types were uncommon), so selecting type A was an easy first choice. Schantz sent his toxin via regular mail; a metal tube within a tube, never a problem. Crone, who had the same idea as us, got freeze-dried toxin in Amsterdam from the Porton Labs in the UK, one shipment leaking powdered toxin out of the damaged paper package, he told me! So much for safety and security in the 1960s and 1970s.

We started with the laboratory steps to dilute the crystalline toxin into small aliquots for practical dosage forms, buffered it with albumin rather than gelatin, learned to freeze-dry it, and worked out the facilities, personnel and protocols to test potency, sterility, safety, and so on. It was remarkably easy to produce long lasting strabismus in a monkey model. This showed that effects were confined to the target muscle, a clear dose-effect relationship, and lack of systemic toxicity, in the amounts used. These results were published in 1973. I then submitted an Investigative Drug Application to the FDA as a Physician/Sponsor, an IND category for drugs that were never expected to go commercial. Years and dozens of letters passed. Finally the FDA issued an IND for the treatment of strabismus in 1977. I injected one patient in 1977; the protocol required it to be done in the hospital and the patient kept in the ICU for 3 days. Three more were done in 1978. The tests with strabismus patients proved successful and the results of 67 injections were published in 1980. I then moved to blepharospasm, and later hemifacial spasm, where it was immediately effective. Rather large doses of 300 units in two patients with thigh adductor spasm showed systemic safety, and we were encouraged that the drug had wide potential, as we had commented in 1973. Three injections for torticollis showed that it was magical for pain, helpful for stiffness and motility, but less so for position and tremor. It was obvious that evaluation of torticollis was going to be complex. Joseph Tsui took my initial data, added his own and developed an original evaluative scale. Joe Jankovic came to Smith-Kettlewell Institute and subsequently performed the first double-blind, placebo-controlled study in patients with blepharospasm. We were thrilled to later learn from Andy Blitzer that it worked also for laryngeal spasms (spasmodic dysphonia).

But now the surprise was that no one in Northern California would try it for anything! Not at Children's hospital for spastic limbs, although we had by then done many childrens' eye muscles, not at the Rehab Center for post stroke spasm, not at the neurology or ophthalmology or rehab departments at UCSF or Stanford. My institution, Smith-Kettlewell Institute, was afraid of liability and wanted all manufacturing moved out. But no manufacturer (we tried 8 including Allergan), would take it on at the time. Much of the problem was lack of patent coverage; as amateurs we had applied late. What to do with this orphan? I was too convinced of its potential to let it die. I incorporated under the name Oculinum® Inc., took out a loan on my house, and, with the invaluable help of Dennis Honeychurch, a pharmacologist, leased space in Berkeley across the street from an animal lab which did our dozens of potency tests. Dennis developed many of the testing and manufacturing techniques later adopted by others. The therapeutic potential and wide safety margin of botulinum toxin, so evident to us, began to leak out during the 1980's. Use increased and broadened as Oculinum® Inc. supplied investigators with varied interests. We chose 100 units vial sizes, enough for all ocular use and a safe dosage even if mishandled. The investigators were encouraged (coerced is perhaps too strong a word), to support the project with the donations that kept us above water financially. At this point, Big Pharma might have defined a tight protocol, used a few manageable sites, and pushed for FDA approval. But we gave it out widely, more interested in what the drug did over a wide spectrum of uses than in commerce.

We relied on Schantz for crystalline toxin and used outsourced freeze-drying capability. It is interesting that the FDA never inspected our facilities and procedures for a decade, but got interested when we applied for licensure. In December 1989, the FDA licensed the manufacturing facilities and clinical product using the lot of toxin produced by Schantz in 1979. The FDA identified it as an orphan drug for the treatment of strabismus, hemifacial spasm, and blepharospasm. For about two years, Oculinum® Inc. was the licensed manufacturer, and Allergan distribtued the product. The facilities and license were turned over to

Allergan in late 1991 and the drug later renamed Botox®. I am not sure if we had all the fun and Allergan got all the money, but it was something like that.

A better and more potent lot of toxin made in 1988 was the basis for European licensing, and subsequent lots of toxin for US sale are much more potent and less liable to elicit antibodies than was the 1979 lot. We developed botulinum toxin type B in 1998 and applied for a trademark for "B-Botox". It showed a bit less effect than type A and we dropped it. The clinical applications for botulinum toxin continued to expand in the 1990s to include hyperhidrosis and gustatory sweating, tremor, overactive bladder, anal fissure, achalasia, hyperfunctional facial lines, and various sorts of pain such as headache. The varied titles of chapters in this volume attest to the continued expansion of uses. Extensive basic investigation of nerve terminal function and of toxin structure and action has been stimulated by the clinical use of toxin. My own early attempts with Sugiama to link the short arm of ricin to the long arm of the toxin to create a poison specific to cholinergic neurons, is the sort of idea being developed by basic scientists as the molecular structures are revealed. Terminal sprouting, vesicle cycling, enzymatic function of the various toxins, their substrate proteins in the terminal, their epitope adhesion areas and similarities are just a few of the areas of early interest now expanded by the new tools of biology and chemistry to whole chapter length in this volume. Blocking of secretion from many sorts of cells beyond the nerve terminal by linking the short arm of botulinum toxins with molecules with affinity for specific cell receptors is moving forward apace. Both the therapeutic uses, the research applications of clostridial toxins, and the adaptations of the molecules appear destined to increase still further in the years to come. It is fun to look back; more fun to look forward!

Alan B. Scott, MD
The Smith-Kettlewell Eye
Research Institute
San Francisco, California

Contents

A

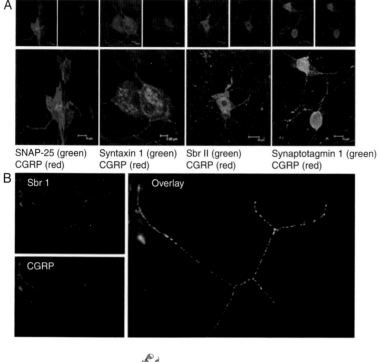

SNAP-25 (green) CGRP (red)   Syntaxin 1 (green) CGRP (red)   Sbr II (green) CGRP (red)   Synaptotagmin 1 (green) CGRP (red)

B

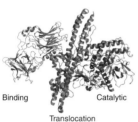

Sbr 1

Overlay

CGRP

FIGURE 1-5. CGRP release from trigeminal ganglionic neurons (TGNs) uses isoform I of synaptobrevin (Sbr), and SNAP-25: lack of susceptibility to BoNT/E is overcome with a novel chimera made by substituting its binding domain with that from /A. **A,** All three SNAREs and synaptotagmin I are largely colocalized in rat TGNs, a good source of sensory neurons. Confocal fluorescent micrographs for CGRP, each SNARE, and synaptotagmin I are displayed in upper panels, with merged views beneath. B, Images showing that Sbr I and CGRP colocalize in neurites of TGNs.

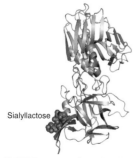

Binding   Catalytic

Translocation

FIGURE 2-1. Ribbons diagram of botulinum neurotoxin type B. The three functional domains are labeled as binding, translocation, and catalytic. The active site residues and the catalytic zinc ion are shown in the catalytic domain. The three-dimensional structure clearly demarcated the three functional domains. The lower half of the binding domain is involved in ganglioside and receptor binding.

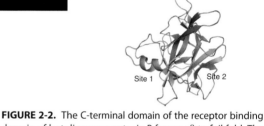

Site 1   Site 2

FIGURE 2-2. The C-terminal domain of the receptor binding domain of botulinum neurotoxin B forms a β-trefoil fold. The trefoil domain forms a subdomain of the binding domain, and both ganglioside and the protein receptor bind to this subdomain. The two binding sites are marked as site 1 and site 2, and will form the binding sites for ganglioside and protein receptor.

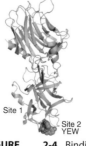

Sialyllactose

Site 1

Site 2 YEW

FIGURE 2-3. The binding domain of BoNT/B with sialyllactose at site 1. Sialyllactose is shown in sphere model. This binding site also validated most of the mutagenesis studies.

FIGURE 2-4. Binding domain of tetanus toxin with a tripeptide (Tyr-Glu-Trp) bound at site 2. The tripeptide is shown in sphere model. The orientation is similar to that shown in Figure 2-3.

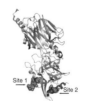

Site 1   Site 2

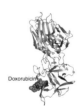

Doxorubicin

FIGURE 2-5. A composite figure of the binding domain of BoNT/B with sialyllactose and the tripeptide as it is bound in tetanus (both shown in sphere model). The helical fragment of Syt II from Chai et al. is superposed.[27] The helical fragment occupies the same place as the tripeptide in tetanus. This strongly supports our earlier prediction that site 2 may be the site where the receptor protein would bind.

FIGURE 2-6. Doxorubicin binding in site 1 of BoNT/B. Sialyllactose, a mimic of GT1b, binds in the same site. Also, doxorubicin has been shown to compete with gangliosides for binding to this site. The fact that it competes with gangliosides or displaces sialyllactose (during crystallization) shows that this site can be blocked and used for drug design.

Color Plate 2

FIGURE 2-7. The catalytic domain of BoNT/E shown in ribbons representation. The active site residues, zinc, and the nucleophilic water are shown in ball and stick model. In BoNT/E, the zinc is coordinated by His211, His215, Glu250, and the nucleophilic water. Glu212, which acts as a base for catalytic action, is hydrogen bonded to the nucleophilic water. This arrangement is similar in all BoNTs.

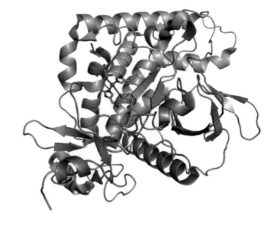

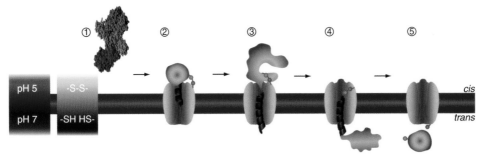

FIGURE 3-1. Sequence of events underlying BoNT LC translocation through the HC channel. (1) BoNT/A holotoxin prior to insertion in the membrane (*gray bar*); BoNT/A is represented by the crystal structure rendered on YASARA (www.YASARA.org) using the Protein Data Bank accession code 3BTA.[10] Then, schematic representation of the membrane inserted BoNT/A during an entry event (2), a series of transfer steps (3, 4), and an exit event (5) under conditions that recapitulate those across endosomes. (Reproduced with permission from Fischer A, Montal ML. Single molecule detection of intermediates during botulinum neurotoxin translocation across membranes. *Proc Natl Acad Sci U S A*. 2007;104:10447-10452. Copyright [2007], National Academy of Sciences, U S A.)

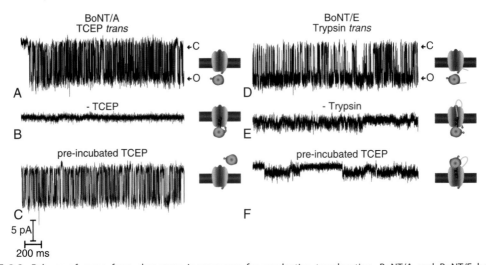

FIGURE 3-2. Release of cargo from chaperone is necessary for productive translocation. BoNT/A and BoNT/E holotoxin channels in excised patches of Neuro 2A cells. Diagrams on the right side of each record depict an interpretation. Top and bottom represent *cis* and *trans* compartments; LC cargo (*purple*), HC (*orange*), disulfide linkage (*green*), and the membrane (*gray bar with magenta boundaries*). **A.** Single-channel currents for holotoxin BoNT/A; the *trans* compartment contained 0.25 mM TCEP. C and O denote the closed and open states. The characteristic fast transitions between the closed and open states are clearly discernible; γ is determined from the amplitude of the fluctuations between the closed and open states. **B.** Nonreduced holotoxin BoNT/A does not form channels; note the absence of current fluctuations. **C.** Single-channel currents of reduced holotoxin BoNT/A by preincubation with reductant TCEP (0.25 mM). **D.** Single-channel currents of holotoxin BoNT/E in the presence of both trypsin and TCEP in the *trans* compartment. **E.** Single-channel currents of holotoxin BoNT/E in the absence of trypsin in the TCEP-containing *trans* compartment. **F.** Single-channel currents of reduced holotoxin BoNT/E by preincubation with 10 mM TCEP and in the presence of 4 mM trypsin in the *trans* compartment. Single-channel currents were recorded at −100 mV in symmetric 0.2 M NaCl; all other conditions were identical to those previously described.[34,35] Other conventions as in Figure 3-1.

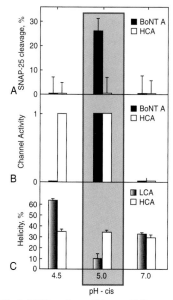

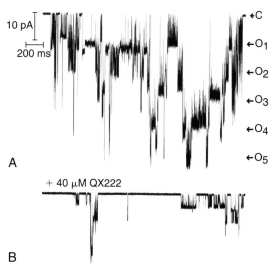

FIGURE 3-3. BoNT/A endopeptidase activity correlates with BoNT/A channel activity and the unfolding of LC/A. **A.** Endopeptidase activity in samples collected from the *trans* chamber of bilayer experiments as function of pH in the *cis* compartment; the *trans* compartment pH was 7.0. **B.** Channel activity of BoNT/A and HC/A as function of pH in the *cis* compartment; the *trans* compartment pH was 7.0. Absence or presence of channel activity is arbitrarily defined as 0 or 1; number of experiments (n) = 6 for HC/A and n = 10 for BoNT/A. **C.** α-Helical content of LC/A and HC/A as function of pH calculated from far UV-CD measurements carried out at 25°C; n = 3. (Modified and reproduced with permission from Koriazova LK, Montal M. Translocation of botulinum neurotoxin light chain protease through the heavy chain channel. *Nat Struct Biol.* 2003;10:13-18.)

FIGURE 3-5. QX-222 blocks the BoNT HC channel. Single-channel recordings of BoNT/A holotoxin reconstituted in planar lipid bilayers in the absence (**A**) and presence (**B**) of 40-μM QX-222. Records obtained at −100 mV in symmetric 0.5 M KCl, 1 mM CaCl$_2$, 2.5 mM citrate pH 5.5. Final protein concentration was 0.5 μg/mL. In the absence of QX-222, the current histogram is fitted with the sum of five Gaussians (excluding the closed state) corresponding to the occurrence of five channels with a γ ≅ 110 pS. In the presence of QX-222, there is a marked reduction in both γ and in the number of openings; the open states are scarcely populated to allow a meaningful fit to the data points, and the histogram is best fitted with a single Gaussian corresponding to the closed state. Other conditions as for Figure 3-3B. (Unpublished data, experimental method from Koriazova and Montal.)

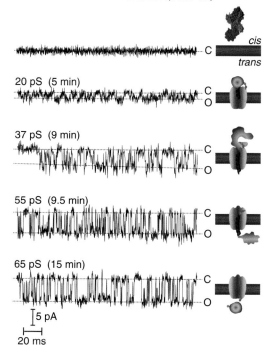

FIGURE 3-4. Single-molecule detection of discrete intermediates during BoNT translocation. High-gain and fast-time resolution of BoNT/A single-channel currents recorded at −100 mV in excised patches of Neuro 2A cells, with schematic representation (*right*). Top panel shows absence of channel currents prior to exposure to BoNT/A. Subsequent panels represent the time course of change of channel conductance. Each segment indicates the representative γ at the recorded time; the dotted lines are traced on the average current for the closed and open states. All other conditions were identical to those previously described[30,32] and other conventions as in Figure 3-1.

Color Plate 4

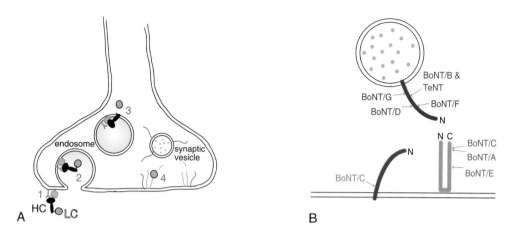

FIGURE 4-1. Synaptic SNAREs are targeted by CNT light chains. **A,** A four-step model for CNT intoxication includes (1) neurospecific cell-surface binding, (2) receptor-mediated endocytosis, (3) translocation of the light chain, and (4) SNARE-specific proteolysis.[16,111,112] The toxin heavy chain (HC, *black*) mediates cell-surface binding with ganglioside and glycoprotein receptors (*orange*). Following endocytosis, the HC also mediates translocation of the light chain (LC, *gray*) if the endosome is acidified. LCs can target the synaptic SNAREs, including vesicle-bound synaptobrevin (*blue*), presynaptic membrane-bound syntaxin (*red*), and SNAP-25 (*green*) before ternary SNARE complex formation. **B,** The relative locations of the peptide bonds hydrolyzed by LCs in the core domains of SNARE proteins are shown. The cut sites of the seven botulinum neurotoxin serotypes (BoNT/A-G) and that of tetanus toxin (TeNT) are indicated by arrows.

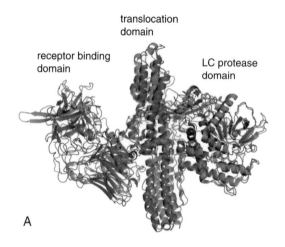

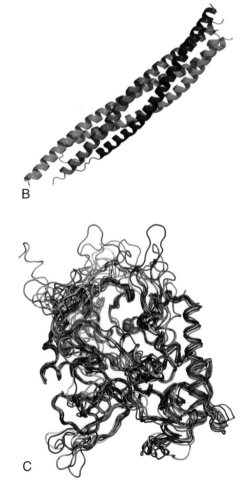

FIGURE 4-2. Structures of apo CNTs and a ternary SNARE complex. **A,** Apo holotoxin structures: BoNT/A (PDB code 3BTA)[20] (*magenta*) and BoNT/B (PDB code 1EPW)[21] (*green*). The LC protease, translocation, and receptor binding domains are indicated. The structures were superimposed using the backbone atoms of the LC protease domain. **B,** Crystal structure of the neuronal SNARE complex[39] consisting of synaptobrevin (*blue*), syntaxin (*red*), and SNAP-25 (*green*) (PDB code 1SFC). This structure represents the post-fusion state of the SNARE complex. **C,** An overall superposition of the LC protease structures from all seven serotypes of BoNTs and TeNT: BoNT/A (PDB code 1XTF, green),[20,74,75] BoNT/B (1EPW, magenta),[21] BoNT/C1 (gold), BoNT/D (2FPQ, blue),[77] BoNT/E (1T3A, cyan),[64] BoNT/F (2A8A, red),[78] BoNT/G (1ZB7, orange),[79] and TeNT (1Z7H, grey).[65] Despite their different substrate specificities, CNT-LCs display high structural similarity. The zinc iron is indicated by a red sphere.

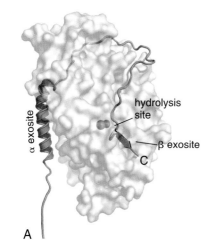

A

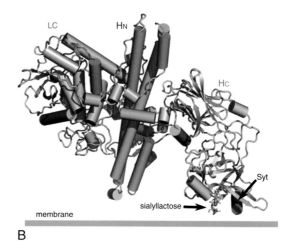

B

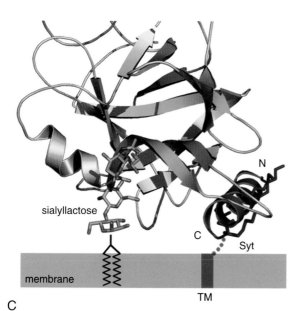

C

FIGURE 4-3. Interactions between BoNTs and synaptic vesicle proteins. **A,** Structure of the BoNT/A·SNAP-25 complex. The protease component of BoNT/A (*gray*) forms an extended interface with the C-terminal core domain of SNAP-25 (*green*). Multiple sites of enzyme-substrate interaction remote from the catalytic Zn^{2+} (*magenta* sphere) and associated nucleophile (*blue* sphere) extend around most of the toxin's circumference, imparting the protease with exquisite specificity. SNAP-25 is unstructured in the absence of a binding partner but adopts a mix of α-helix, β-sheet, and extended conformations when complexed with BoNT/A. **B,** Proposed binding mode of BoNT/B on the membrane surface. The structure of a sialyllactose-bound BoNT/B (PDB code 1F31) was superimposed on the complex of BoNT/B-HC_C and synaptotagmin II by using the coordinates of the HC_C fragment for the alignment. The LC, the amino-terminal part of the heavy chain (HC_N), and the carboxy-terminal domain of the heavy chain (HC_C) are shown. **C,** A close-up view of the proposed interface between BoNT/B and membrane. Four lysine residues that are conserved in synaptotagmins I and II are colored *blue.*

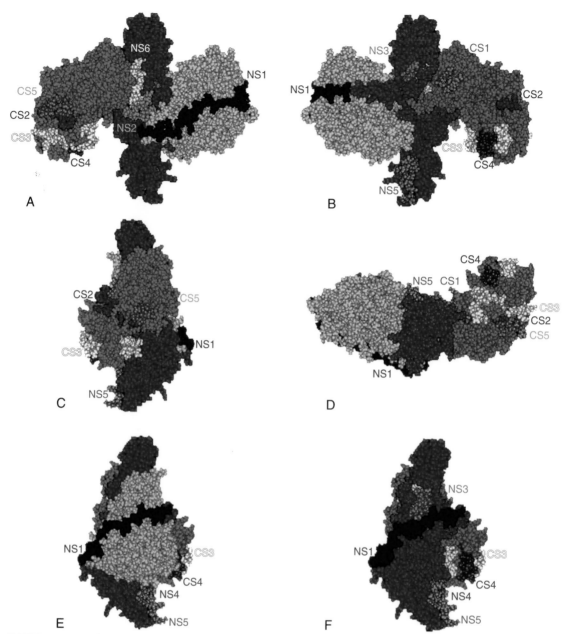

FIGURE 5-1. Space-filling images of botulinum neurotoxin A (BoNT/A) three-dimensional structure with the mouse brain synaptosome (snps)–binding regions (**A**) front view, (**B**) back view (rotated 180 degrees on the Y-axis, relative to [**A**]), (**C**) side view looking through the H_C domain (rotated −90 degrees on the Y-axis, relative to [**A**]), (**D**) bottom view (rotated 90 degrees on the X-axis, relative to [**B**]), (**E**) side view looking through the L chain (rotated 90 degrees on the Y-axis, relative to [**A**]), (**F**) same view as (**E**) but with the L chain removed. The snps-binding regions in the H_N domain are labeled NS1–NS6, and those in the H_C domain are labeled CS1–CS5, corresponding to the designations in Table 5-2. The H_N domain is shown in *red*, the H_C domain is shown in *green*, and the L chain is shown in *yellow*. The images were generated with the x-ray structure coordinates of BoNT/A.[76] (From Maruta T, Dolimbek BZ, Aoki KR, Steward LE, Atassi MZ. Mapping of the synaptosome-binding regions on the heavy chain of botulinum neurotoxin A by synthetic overlapping peptides encompassing the entire chain. *Protein J.* 2004;23:539-552.)

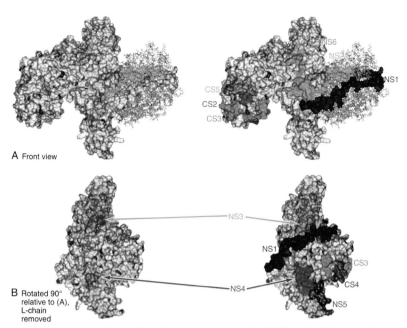

FIGURE 5-2. Electrostatic potential surfaces of botulinum neurotoxin A (BoNT/A), with *(right panel)* and without *(left panel)* mouse brain synaptosome (snps)–binding regions mapped on the surface (**A**) front view with and without snps-binding regions mapped on the structure *(right and left panels,* respectively), (**B**) side view (rotated 90 degrees relative to [**A**] and with the L chain removed), with and without snps-binding regions mapped on the surface *(right and left panels,* respectively). The significant overlap of snps-binding regions NS3 and NS4 with negative electrostatic potential is highlighted with arrows. Positive, negative, and neutral electrostatic potential surfaces are shown in *blue, red,* and *white,* respectively. The L chain is shown in *yellow* stick form. The images were generated with the x-ray structure coordinates of BoNT/A from Lacy et al[76] and the electrostatic potential surfaces were calculated with DelPhi[96-97] and mapped onto a solvent-accessible surface as computed by INSIGHTII. (From Maruta T, Dolimbek BZ, Aoki KR, Steward LE, Atassi MZ. Mapping of the synaptosome-binding regions on the heavy chain of botulinum neurotoxin A by synthetic overlapping peptides encompassing the entire chain. *Protein J.* 2004;23:539-552.)

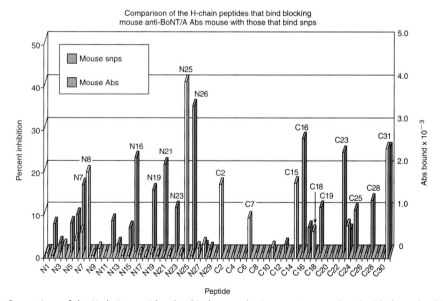

FIGURE 5-3. Comparison of the H-chain peptides that bind mouse brain synaptosomes (snps) with those that bind blocking (i.e., protecting) mouse anti–botulinum neurotoxin A (BoNT/A) antibodies. (From Maruta T, Dolimbek BZ, Aoki KR, Steward LE, Atassi MZ. Mapping of the synaptosome-binding regions on the heavy chain of botulinum neurotoxin A by synthetic overlapping peptides encompassing the entire chain. *Protein J.* 2004;23:539-552.)

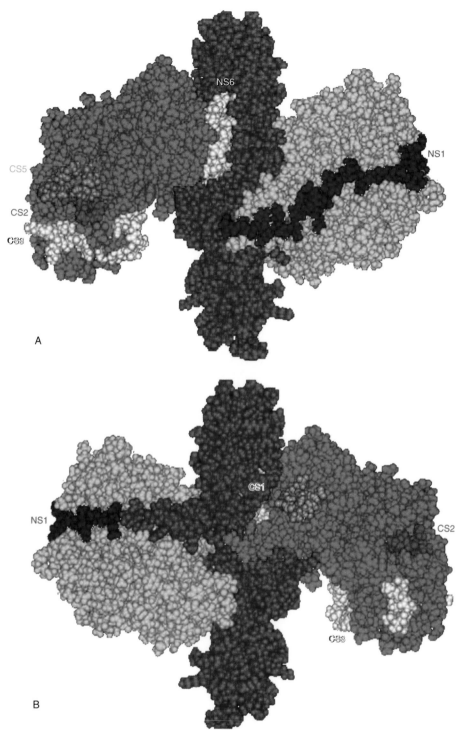

FIGURE 5-4. Space-filling images ([**A**] front view, [**B**] back view rotated 180 degrees on the Y-axis, relative to [**A**]) showing the locations in the three-dimensional structure of botulinum neurotoxin A (BoNT/A) of the limited set of major regions on the H chain that bind to mouse brain synaptosomes and which either coincide or overlap with the regions that bind protective (i.e., blocking) mouse anti-BoNT/A antibodies. The H_N domain is shown in *red* and the HC domain is in *green*, whereas the L chain is shown in *yellow*. The antigenic regions were obtained from Atassi and Dolimbek,[18] and the images were generated with the x-ray structure coordinates of BoNT/A.[76] (From Maruta T, Dolimbek BZ, Aoki KR, Steward LE, Atassi MZ. Mapping of the synaptosome-binding regions on the heavy chain of botulinum neurotoxin A by synthetic overlapping peptides encompassing the entire chain. *Protein J.* 2004;23:539-552.)

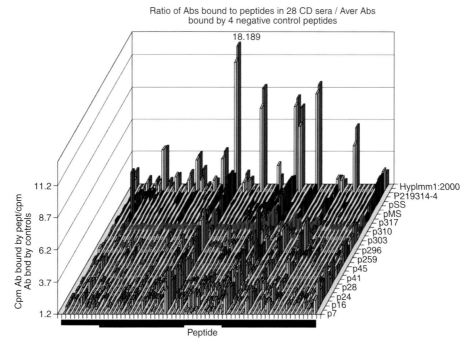

FIGURE 5-5. Mapping of the antibody (Ab)-recognition profiles for the individual 28 mouse protection assy (MPA)–positive cervical dystonia (CD) sera. The results, which represent the average of four experiments that varied ± 5% or less, are expressed in ratio of Abs bound to peptides in the CD serum/Abs bound by the four peptides N2, N12, C17, and C23, which as a rule showed no Ab binding with any of the 28 sera studied and were therefore used as negative control. (From Dolimbek BZ, Aoki KR, Steward LE, Jankovic J, Atassi MZ. Mapping of the regions on the heavy chain of botulinum neurotoxin A (BoNT/A) recognized by antibodies of cervical dystonia patients with immunoresistance to BoNT/A. *Mol Immunol.* 2007;44:1029-1041.)

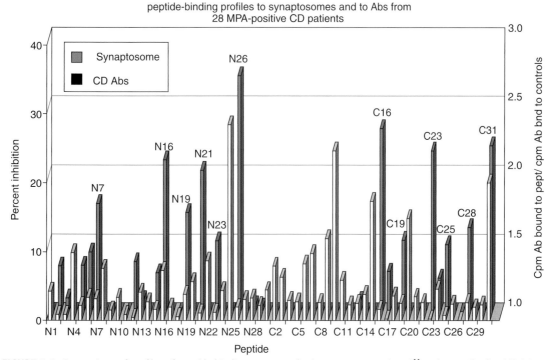

FIGURE 5-6. Comparison of profiles of peptide-binding to mouse brain synaptosomes (snps)[11] and to antibodies (Abs) in an antiserum pool of equal volumes from the 28 mouse protective assay (MPA)–positive patients with cervical dystonia (CD)[20] analyzed in Figure 5-5.

Color Plate 10

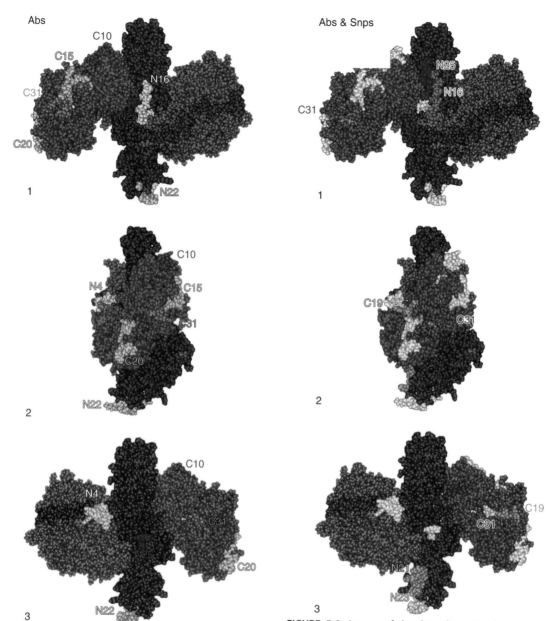

FIGURE 5-7. Images of the three-dimensional structure of botulinum neurotoxin (BoNT/A) showing the locations of the regions that bind anti-BoNT/A antibodies (Abs) in mouse protective assay (MPA)–positive sera from BoNT/A-treated patients with cervical dystonia (CD). The regions are colored *white* (low amounts of Ab binding), *pink* (medium levels of binding), *rose* (high binding) and *red* (very high binding). Image 2 is obtained by rotating the molecule in image 1 90 degrees counterclockwise around the vertical axis, and image 3 is obtained by rotating image 2 again 90 degrees counterclockwise around the vertical axis. (From Dolimbek BZ, Aoki KR, Steward LE, Jankovic J, Atassi MZ. Mapping of the regions on the heavy chain of botulinum neurotoxin A [BoNT/A] recognized by antibodies of cervical dystonia patients with immunoresistance to BoNT/A. *Mol Immunol.* 2007;44:1029-1041.)

FIGURE 5-8. Images of the three-dimensional representations of botulinum neurotoxin A (BoNT/A) showing the antibody (Ab)–binding regions localized with mouse protective assay (MPA)–positive sera[20] from BoNT/A-treated patients with cervical dystonia (CD) and the mouse brain synaptosome (snps)–binding regions on BoNT/A. The Ab-binding regions that do not coincide but might overlap with snps binding regions are colored *white*. The snps-binding regions, two of which (N16 and C31) coincide completely with Ab-binding regions, are colored *rose* or *red*. Images in panels 2 and 3 are obtained by rotating the image in panel 1 90 and 180 degrees, respectively, counterclockwise around the vertical axis. (From Dolimbek BZ, Aoki KR, Steward LE, Jankovic J, Atassi MZ. Mapping of the regions on the heavy chain of botulinum neurotoxin A (BoNT/A) recognized by antibodies of cervical dystonia patients with immunoresistance to BoNT/A. *Mol Immunol.* 2007;44:1029-1041.)

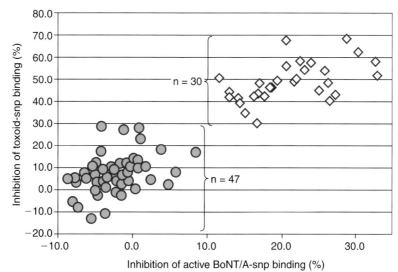

FIGURE 5-9. Comparison of the inhibition levels by human sera of the binding of active botulinum neurotoxin A (BoNT/A) and inactive toxin (toxoid) to mouse brain synaptosomes (snps). The figure compares the results of inhibition by ($\div$) mouse protective assay (MPA)–positive sera (n = 30), ($\square$) MPA-negative sera (n = 28) and control sera (n = 19) of the binding of ^{125}I-labeled active BoNT/A and ^{125}I-labeled toxoid binding to snps. The figure shows that active toxin and toxoid gave comparable results that clearly differentiated the MPA-positive sera from MPA-negative sera and controls. The inhibitions by sera of latter two groups were not distinguishable. (From Maruta T, Dolimbek BZ, Aoki KR, Atassi MZ. Inhibition by human sera of botulinum neurotoxin-A binding to synaptosomes: A new assay for blocking and non-blocking antibodies *J Neurosci Methods*. 2006;151:90-96.)

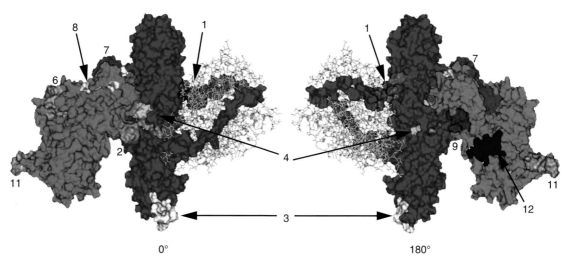

FIGURE 5-11. Three-dimensional images of botulinum neurotoxin B (BoNT/B) showing the locations of antigenic regions that are recognized by human and mouse anti-BoNT/B antibodies (Abs) with overlaps of seven or more residues.[21] The H_C domain of the heavy chain is in *green* and the translocation (H_N) domain is in *red*. The L chain, displayed in wire style, is *yellow*. The right image is obtained by 180 degrees rotation of the left image. The numbers labeling the regions refer to the numbers and sequences.[21] Regions that describe a distinct patch on the surface and may form in each case a single unique antigenic site that binds the polyclonal Abs directed against that site. The three-dimensional coordinates used for these images were from the RCSB Protein Data Bank (PDB), accession code 1EPW.[84] (From Dolimbek BZ, Steward LE, Aoki KR, Atassi MZ. Immune recognition of botulinum neurotoxin B: Antibody-binding regions on the heavy chain of the toxin. *Mol Immunol*. 2007, doi:10.1016/j.molimm.2007.08.007.)

Color Plate 12

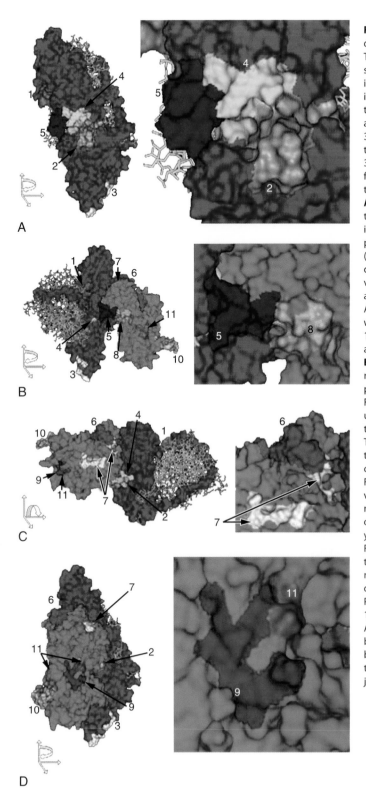

FIGURE 5-12. Contiguous regions that describe distinct patches on the surface. These combinations may each form a single site. Three-dimensional surface-mapped images of botulinum neurotoxin B (BoNT/B) illustrating antigenic regions on the surface that are recognized by human and mouse anti-BoNT/B antibodies (Abs) (see Table 5-3).[21] The numbers correspond with the peptide numbers and sequences listed in Table 5-3.[21] The orientations and close-ups in this figure highlight contiguous surface regions that are formed by discontinuous peptides. **A,** The left panel is a view of the BoNT/B structure with the H$_C$ domain removed. The image is rotated 80 degrees around the y-axis compared with the 0 degree image in Figure 5-11 (see panel D for a similar display with the H$_C$ domain present). The right panel is a close-up view and clearly illustrates that regions 2, 4, and 5 form a contiguous surface patch. Although regions 2 and 5 are accessible when the H$_C$ domain is present (see Fig. 5-11), the solution accessibility of region 4 to antibodies is unknown (see the discussion). **B,** The left panel is a view of the structure rotated 40 degrees around the y-axis compared with the 180-degree structure in Figure 5-11. The right panel shows a close-up view of regions 5 and 8, illustrating that these regions form a contiguous surface. **C,** The left panel is a view of the BoNT/B structure rotated 70 degrees around the x-axis compared with the 0-degree structure in Figure 5-11. The right panel is a close-up view of the contiguous surface between regions 6 and 7. **D,** The left panel is a view of the structure rotated 90 degrees around the y-axis relative to the 0-degree structure in Figure 5-11. The right panel is a close-up of the contiguous surface formed between regions 9 and 11. The three-dimensional coordinates for these images were from the RCSB Protein Data Bank (PDB), accession code 1EPW.[84] (From Dolimbek BZ, Steward LE, Aoki KR, Atassi MZ. Immune recognition of botulinum neurotoxin B: Antibody-binding regions on the heavy chain of the toxin. *Mol Immunol.* 2007, doi:10.1016/j.molimm.2007.08.007)

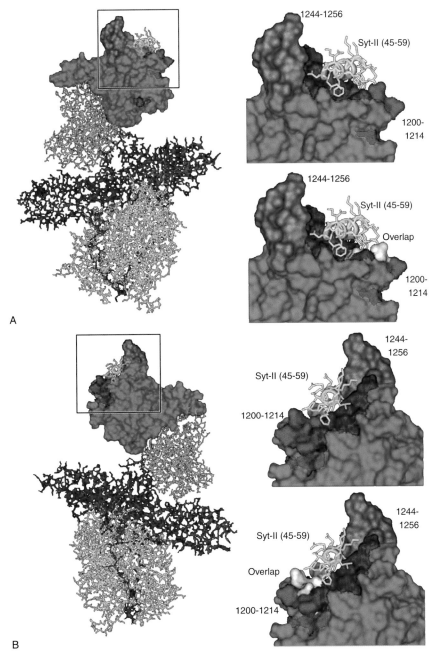

FIGURE 5-13. Proximity of the mouse synaptotagmin II (Syt-II) binding site to mouse Ab-binding epitopes on botulinum neurotoxin B (BoNT/B). **A,** The left panel is a view of the three-dimensional structure of BoNT/B showing the locations on the molecule of the mouse anti-BoNT/B antibody (Ab)-binding epitopes within residues 1200–1214 and 1244–1256 relative to the area to which mouse Syt-II binds. The boxed area is detailed in the right panels. **Upper Panel,** The antigenic sites and Syt-II binding site are independently colored as follows: *Magenta*, Ab-binding region 1200–1214; *blue*, 1244–1256; *dark red*, Syt-II binding pocket. **Lower Panel,** Colors signify the same but in addition the overlap of Syt-II binding site and 1200–1214 is shown in *silver-gray*. **B,** Back view obtained by rotating the BoNT/B structure in A by 180 degrees. The labels and colors connote the same information as described in **A**. Note that there are residues that actually overlap between region 1200-1214 and the Syt-II binding site, whereas region 1244–1256 is immediately adjacent to the Syt-II binding site (see text for details). These images make it clear why binding of Abs to either region 1200–1214 or 1244–1256 would be expected to block the binding of Syt-II to BoNT/B. The three-dimensional coordinates used for these images were from the RCSB Protein Data Bank (PDB), accession code 2NPO.[13] Note that rat Syt-II binds to the same BoNT/B area.[12] (From Dolimbek BZ, Steward LE, Aoki KR, Atassi MZ. Immune recognition of botulinum neurotoxin B: Antibody-binding regions on the heavy chain of the toxin. *Mol Immunol.* 2007, doi:10.1016/j.molimm.2007.08.007)

Color Plate 14

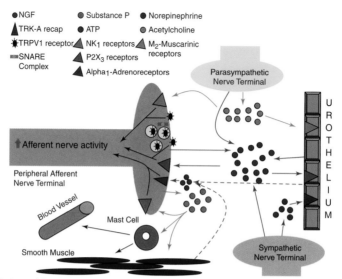

FIGURE 19-4. Potential sites of botulinum neurotoxin type A (BoNT/A) modulation within bladder sensory pathways. By decreasing local pools of transmitters, growth factors, and sensory receptors, BoNT/A could thereby inhibit bladder afferent nerve activity, particularly in conditions of increased excitability (e.g., detrusor overactivity).

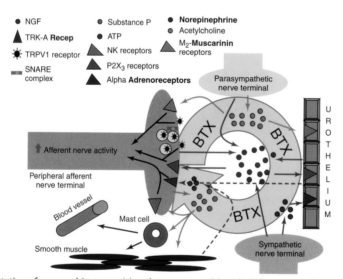

FIGURE 21-1. Representation of neuronal (autonomic) and non-neuronal (urothelial) sources of neurotransmitters modulating bladder afferent nerve activity and the effect of botulinum neurotoxin (BoNT) in the treatment of interstitial cystitis/painful bladder syndrome. BoNT inhibits neurotransmitter release, reducing sensory afferent excitability, thus diminishing or eliminating symptoms.

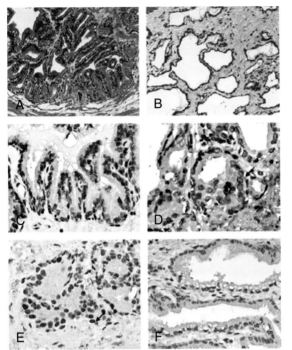

FIGURE 22-2. Representative saline or botulinum neurotoxin type A (BoNT/A) treatment in canine prostate at 3 months for H & E, terminal deoxynucleotidyl-mediated deoxyuridine triphosphate nick end labeling (TUNEL) and proliferative cell nuclear antigen (PCNA) staining. Significant glandular proliferation with papillary infolding in the lumen was seen in the control canine (**A**). Atrophy change of glandular component with flattening of the lining epithelium was seen in the BoNT/A-treated canine (**B**). More TUNEL-stained cells are recognized in the BoNT/A-treated animal (**D**) than the saline-treated animal (**C**). More PCNA-stained cells are recognized in the control animal (**E**) than the BoNT/A-treated animal (**F**). (With permission from BJU International.)

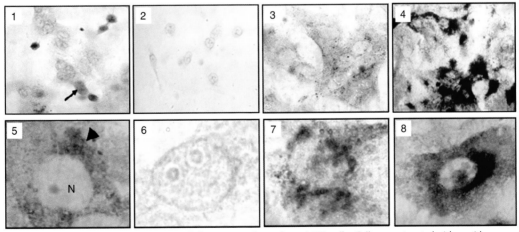

FIGURE 28-3. Effect of EGF-LH$_N$/C on intracellular mucin release from A549 cells. Cells were treated either with serum-free media for 72 hours or serum-free media for 48 hours, followed by stimulation for 24 hours with EGF-TNFα, or were preincubated with EGF-LH$_N$/C for 48 hours, followed by stimulation for 24 hours with EGF-TNFα in the continued presence of EGF-LH$_N$/C. Cells were either fixed and stained with AB-PAS for intracellular mucin or were analysed for MUC5AC mRNA expression. Representative images of stained intracellular mucin (*arrow*) in a control cell (*arrowhead*) (1 and 5), a stimulated cell (2 and 6), and in stimulated cells pretreated with either 0.5 nM (3 and 7) or 1 nM EGF-LH$_N$/C (4 and 8). Panels 1, 2, 3 and 4 = × 40 magnification, panels 5, 6, 7 and 8 = × 100 magnification. N, nucleus.

Color Plate 16

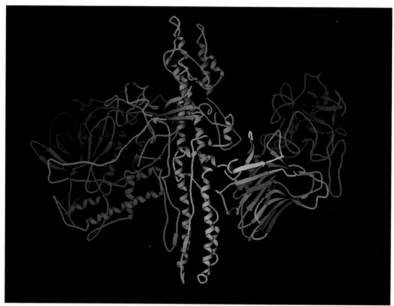

FIGURE 31-1. Botulinum neurotoxin is composed of a ∼50-kDa light chain (LC) and a ∼100-kDa heavy chain linked by a single disulfide bond. The LC functions as a zinc-dependent endopeptidase, whereas the heavy chain contains two functional ∼50-kDa domains: a C-terminal receptor-binding domain (Hc or fragment C) and an N-terminal translocation domain (Hn). The Hc is subdivided into a 25-kDa Hc-C terminal subdomain and an Hc-N amino terminal subdomain. The Hc-C has a single ganglioside-binding site. An amino acid sequence of ∼ 50 amino acid residues (referred to as a belt) makes up the N-terminal region of the Hn and wraps around LC domain. (Rendition of BoNT/A structure was obtained from the Protein Data Base (PDB) website: BoNT/A: *http://www.rcsb.org/pdb/explore/explore.do?structureId=3BTA* Structure for BoNT/A was from Lacy DB, Tepp W, Cohen AC, DasGupta BR, Stevens RC. Crystal structure of botulinum neurotoxin type A and implications for toxicity. *Nat Struct Biol.* 1998;5:898-902.)

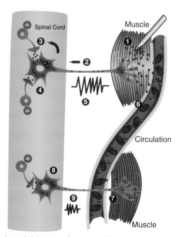

FIGURE 34-1. Tetanus toxin uptake and action. (1) Internalization of toxin at the neuromuscular junction from a nearby wound (or local injection). (2) Retrograde transport to motor neuron cell bodies in the spinal cord. (3) Transsynaptic transfer to presynaptic terminals (inhibitory). (4) Cleavage of vesicle-associated membrane protein with failure of transmitter release. (5) Increased motor neuron excitability, firing rate, and local muscle tetanic contraction. (6) Spread of toxin into the bloodstream. (7) Toxin uptake by ALL motor neurons. (8) Widespread inactivation of spinal motor inhibition. (9) General increase in motor neuron excitability—generalized tetanus.

Multiple Steps in the Blockade of Exocytosis by Botulinum Neurotoxins

J. Oliver Dolly, Jianghui Meng,
Jiafu Wang, Gary W. Lawrence, MacDara Bodeker,
Tomas H. Zurawski, and Astrid Sasse

INTRODUCTION

Early studies established that the seven serotypes (A–G) of botulinum neurotoxin (BoNT) inhibit the release of acetylcholine (ACh) from peripheral motor nerve terminals[1,2] by a complex process involving several steps.[3] Because these measurements were made at mammalian neuromuscular junctions— the prime pharmacologic target tissue—it is important to review this pioneering work in order to assess how these pertinent outcomes relate to recent advances made with various cell types.

MULTIPHASIC MECHANISM OF ACTION OF BOTULINUM NEUROTOXINS

Targeting via binding to neuronal acceptors, followed by endocytosis. Initially, it was proposed that the presynaptic inhibitory action of BoNT on ACh release from rodent nerve-muscle preparations (Fig. 1-1A) entailed binding, internalization, and a lytic step[3,4]; because this was based on pharmacologic experiments, biochemical data were sought to decipher the molecular basis for these different phases. This was achieved by radiolabeling of BoNTs A and B with ^{125}I to high specific activities (450–1700 Ci/mmol) with demonstrated retention of their biologic activities,[5,6] and

injecting a small quantity into mice to induce respiratory paralysis. After dissection of the phrenic nerve hemidiaphragm, sections were subjected to electron microscopic autoradiography.[7] The resultant micrographs revealed remarkably selective targeting to motor nerve endings of ^{125}I-labeled BoNT/A (see Fig. 1-1B) and/B that culminated in significant uptake.[8,9] Saturable interaction with the presynaptic acceptors was found to be essential because binding (and, thus, subsequent uptake) could be abrogated with an excess of either nonradioactive toxin. Furthermore, the internalization step for each toxin was blocked by de-energization with inhibitors of energy production (see Fig. 1-1C) or lowering the temperature to 5°C, such that a halo of silver grains was then observed dispersed on the neuronal plasmalemma. The requirement for acceptor binding, followed by uptake, which was both temperature- and energy-dependent, plus the direct correlation between this molecular/cellular data and the pharmacologic findings, led to the conclusion that neuromuscular paralysis requires acceptor-mediated endocytosis of BoNT.[7-9] Preventing uptake, as noted earlier, afforded quantitation of the acceptors at saturation, giving different densities for BoNT/A and /B of 153 and 630 sites per squared micrometer of plasma membrane (Fig. 1-1C legend).[9] The dissimilar number of binding sites concurs with the observation that three BoNT serotypes tested appear to use acceptors distinct from

The authors of this chapter do not report any conflicts of interest.

Intracellular recordings of
synaptic potentials

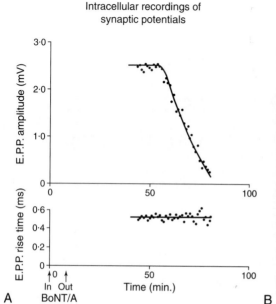

A   In Out
BoNT/A

E.M. autoradiography of
^{125}I-BoNT/A treated diaphragm

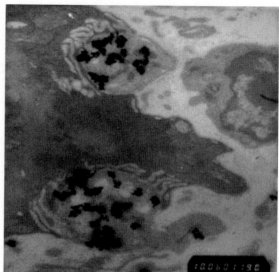

B

Azide blocks endocytotic uptake of
^{125}I-labelled BoNT/A and /B

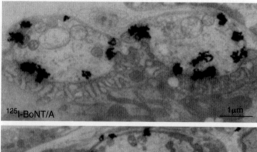

C

Reduced alkylated BoNT/A antagonizes neuromuscular
paralysis by type A but not /B, /E, /F or TeTx

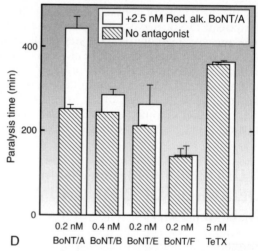

D   0.2 nM   0.4 nM   0.2 nM   0.2 nM   5 nM
BoNT/A BoNT/B BoNT/E BoNT/F TeTX

FIGURE 1-1. BoNT/A and /B target motor nerve endings by binding to distinct ecto-acceptors, entering via acceptor-mediated endocytosis and blocking neuromuscular transmission. **A,** Transient bath application of 10 nM BoNT/A to mouse phrenic nerve–diaphragm blocked quantal release of ACh, as indicated by a complete reduction in the amplitude of endplate potentials without any change in their rise-times. **B** and **C,** Mouse hemidiaphragms were incubated with ^{125}I-labeled BoNT/A at 22°C in the absence (**B**) or presence (**C**) of azide and processed for electron microscope autoradiography. The presence of silver grains in the motor nerve endings demonstrates remarkably specific targeting. Inclusion of azide during the incubation with the radioiodinated toxins prevented uptake and allowed quantification of the binding sites for ^{125}I-BoNT/A and /B to be 153±30 and 630±130/μm^2 of presynaptic membrane. **D,** A reduced alkylated derivative of BoNT/A[10] antagonized the neuroparalytic effect of native/A but not significantly the other serotypes tested. (**A** is from Dolly JO, Lande S, Wray DW. The effects of in vitro application of purified botulinum neurotoxin at mouse motor nerve terminals. *J Physiol.* 1987;386:475-484. **B** and **C** from Black JD, Dolly JO. Interaction of ^{125}I-labeled botulinum neurotoxins with nerve terminals. II. Autoradiographic evidence for its uptake into motor nerves by acceptor-mediated endocytosis. *J Cell Biol.* 1986;103:535-544; and Black JD, Dolly JO. Interaction of ^{125}I-labeled botulinum neurotoxins with nerve terminals. I. Ultrastructural autoradiographic localization and quantitation of distinct membrane acceptors for types A and B on motor nerves. *J Cell Biol.* 1986;103:521-534. **D** is from Dolly JO, et al. Probing the process of transmitter release with botulinum and tetanus neurotoxins. *Semin Neurosci.* 1994;6:149-158.)

those for type A. This was demonstrated initially using a reduced alkylated BoNT/A derivative that retained ability to bind motor nerve endings but was unable to undergo internalization; this nontoxic form of BoNT/A antagonized the neuromuscular paralytic activity of native type A but not /B, /E, /F, or tetanus toxin (see Fig. 1-1D). The same derivative also proved instrumental in establishing that the interchain disulfide bond is essential for toxin translocation leading to neuroparalysis,[10] as was also reported for tetanus toxin.[11,12] It is noteworthy that the aforementioned evidence (from electron microscopic and physiologic measurements) for BoNT serotypes apparently using distinct binding sites was later borne out by the important identification of synaptic vesicle protein 2 (SV2) and synaptotagmin I/II, plus gangliosides, as the neuronal acceptors for BoNT/A and B/G, respectively.[13-17] Notably, proteomic analysis of a heterogeneous population of brain synaptic vesicles demonstrated that synaptotagmins are present in higher copy number per vesicle than SV2[18] (see later), which accords with the greater abundance of binding sites for BoNT/B compared with /A (see earlier).

Neural stimulation promotes BoNT internalization, which involves trafficking through an acidic membrane compartment. Returning to the internalization step, uptake of ^{125}I-BoNT/A was increased by electrical stimulation of the phrenic nerve[7,8] (Fig. 1-2A), consistent with the known ability of neural stimulation to accelerate the blockade of neuromuscular transmission by type A[19] and E (see Fig. 1-2B).[20] Moreover, recycling of the ecto-acceptor for BoNT/A seemed to occur in phrenic nerve endings.[8] These early microscopic data are in general agreement with the elevation in binding of BoNT/A, measured immunologically, seen on neural stimulation of the nerve-diaphragm preparation.[14] However, an adequate quantity of BoNT/A can bind its productive acceptors at mouse motor terminals without nerve stimulation,[4,20] so that paralysis ensues even after removal of toxin. Perhaps, a lower sensitivity of the immunodetection of BoNT/A binding to the same preparation could explain the absence of measurable binding unless stimulation was applied.[14] Interestingly, in cultured neurons, a significant fraction of synaptotagmin (the BoNT/B/G acceptor) forms a cell surface reservoir for restocking this protein into rapid recycling synaptic vesicles, whereas distribution of the /A SV2 acceptor is more skewed toward the synaptic vesicle than the cell surface.[21] A well-known increase in vesicle recycling on neural stimulation readily accords with its acceleration of acceptor recycling, increased BoNT uptake,[7,8] and subsequent paralysis[19]: importantly, these collective and consistent findings reaffirm the involvement of acceptor-mediated endocytosis in the toxins' inhibition of ACh release.[7,22] Notably, the increased toxin binding to active nerve endings is deemed important in the clinical use of this toxin as a muscle relaxant because it ought to be taken up preferentially into abnormally active nerves in dystonic patients.[23-25] The transfer of ^{125}I-BoNT/A into presynaptic terminals was shown to be perturbed by lysosomotropic agents[7,8] (see Fig. 1-2A), which is entirely consistent with pharmacologic data on type A[26] and E (see Fig. 1-2C).[20] In fact, BoNT/E appears to exploit two processes to gain entry and paralyse motor nerves; these can be distinguished by altering the temperature or toxin concentration and, interestingly, both uptake systems are susceptible to an inhibitor of H^+-ATPase, bafilomycin A1 (see Fig. 1-2C). It is tempting to relate these uptake routes to the two endocytotic pathways proposed for recycling of small clear synaptic vesicle (see Fig. 1-2D), which may accord with the different pathways revealed using dynamin I knock-out mice.[27] Details of the actual transfer of an active BoNT moiety across the limiting (endosomal-like) membrane[28] have remained unclear until recent elegant experiments (see Chapter 3).[29] The proton gradient across the vesicle membrane enables BoNT/A to form a channel that allows the light chain to be translocated. Consistent with the evidence cited earlier for the toxin's interchain disulfide being essential for cytosolic transfer leading to neuroparalysis,[10] this bond had to be intact for translocation to occur and its subsequent reduction is reflected in changes in the single channels measured.[30]

BoNTs act intracellularly on ubiquitous targets essential for most Ca^{2+}-regulated exocytosis. The relevance of binding, internalization, and translocation had to be established by demonstrating directly that BoNT or its light chain acts within cells to inhibit exocytosis. Initially, intracellular injection of BoNT/A into large cholinergic neurons of *Aplysia* was found to inhibit synaptic transmission, as measured by electrophysiologic recordings.[31] Moreover, neuromuscular transmission could be blocked in the mouse hemidiaphragm by the light chain alone of BoNT/A,[32] when delivered via liposomes (see Fig. 1-3A). Microinjection of BoNT/A into noncholinergic neurons of

¹²⁵I-BoNT/A	Location relative to the plasmalemma (%)	
	On	Inside
Control (22 °C)	60	40
4 °C	100	0
At 22 °C		
+Azide	100	0
+Methylamine	73	27
+Ammonium chloride	74	26
+Nerve stimulation	41	59

A

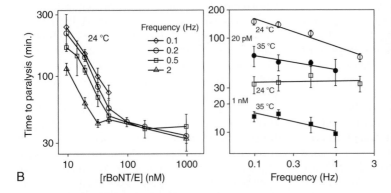

B

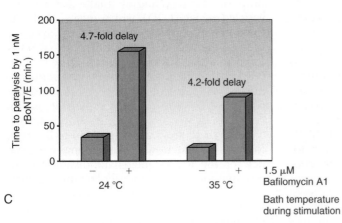

C

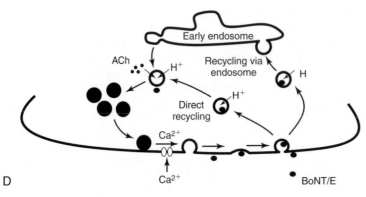

D

FIGURE 1-2. Internalization of BoNT/A and /E at murine nerve terminals is increased on neural stimulation and retarded by low temperature or inhibition of vacuolar H$^+$-ATPases. **A,** Quantitative data from experiments outlined for Figure 1-1 B, C. **B** and **C,** BoNT/E uses two uptake routes that may be related to the endocytotic pathways proposed (**D**) for recycling of synaptic vesicles. (**A-C** from Black JD, Dolly JO. Interaction of ^{125}I-labeled botulinum neurotoxins with nerve terminals. II. Autoradiographic evidence for its uptake into motor nerves by acceptor-mediated endocytosis. *J Cell Biol.* 1986;103:535-644; Lawrence G, Wang J, Chion CK, Aoki KR, Dolly JO. Two protein trafficking processes at motor nerve endings unveiled by botulinum neurotoxin E. *J Pharmacol Exp Ther.* 2007;320:410-418; **D** is adapted from Sudhof TC: The synaptic vesicle cycle. *Annu Rev Neurosci.* 2004;27: 509-547.)

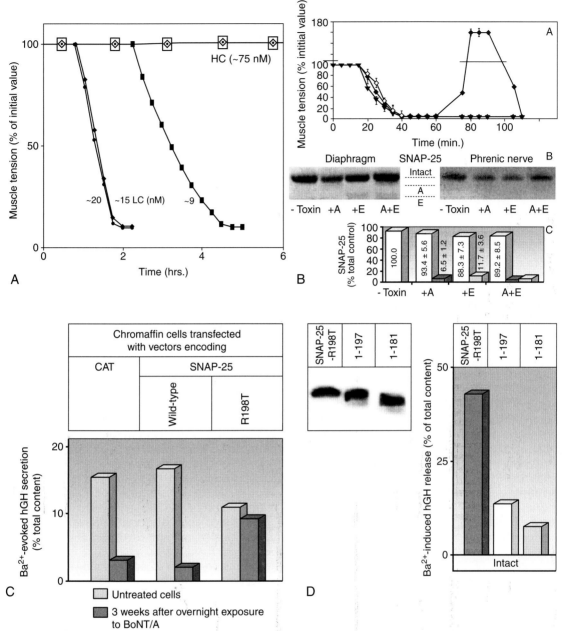

FIGURE 1-3. The separated light chain of BoNT/A acts intracellularly to block neuromuscular transmission by cleaving SNAP-25: BoNT/A protease persists for weeks in chromaffin cells and /A- or /E-truncated SNAP-25 inhibit exocytosis. **A,** The light (but not heavy) chain of BoNT/A causes neuromuscular paralysis when delivered via liposomes. **B,** 4-Aminopyridine (horizontal lines) can transiently reverse the blockade of neuromuscular transmission by BoNT/A (♦) but not /E (○) or both toxins (△); only partial cleavage of SNAP-25 is required for paralysis. **C,** Expression of BoNT/A-resistant, but not wild-type, SNAP-25, in chromaffin cells rescues exocytosis preblocked with BoNT/A 3 weeks previously. **D,** Regulated exocytosis from intact chromaffin cells is diminished by expression of SNAP-25$_{1-197}$ or SNAP-25$_{1-181}$. (**A** is from de Paiva A, Dolly JO. Light chain of botulinum neurotoxin is active in mammalian motor nerve terminals when delivered via liposomes. *FEBS Lett.* 1990;277:171-174; **B** is from Meunier FA, Lisk G, Sesardic D, Dolly JO. Dynamics of motor nerve terminal remodeling unveiled using SNARE-cleaving botulinum toxins: the extent and duration are dictated by the sites of SNAP-25 truncation. *Mol Cell Neurosci.* 2003;22:454-466; **C** is from O'Sullivan GA, Mohammed N, Foran PG, Lawrence GW, Dolly JO. Rescue of exocytosis in botulinum toxin A-poisoned chromaffin cells by expression of cleavage-resistant SNAP-25. Identification of the minimal essential C-terminal residues. *J Biol Chem.* 1999;274:36897-36904; **D** is from O'Sullivan GA, Dolly JO. The two core domains of SNAP-25 are functionally distinct and act inter-dependently in exocytosis. In preparation for publication.)

Aplysia led to blockade of transmitter release.[33] Likewise, inhibition of Ca^{2+}-dependent exocytosis of all transmitters tested (peptides, catecholamines, and other cell mediators) resulted from intracellular delivery of BoNT serotypes into different neuronal preparations, by exposure over several hours to relatively high concentrations[34,35] or via permeablization of chromaffin,[36-38] PC-12,[39,40] or other secretory cells.[41] These collective findings established that the targets for BoNTs are intracellular and ubiquitous, being essential for regulated exocytosis of numerous substances. This led to the deduction that the preferential action of BoNTs on motor and autonomic[42] cholinergic nerves was attributable to the occurrence thereon of productive ecto-acceptors[7,43] that can mediate efficient internalization.[9,44] Because the acceptors identified recently for BoNT/A and /B/G, SV2 and synaptotagmin I/II respectively (see earlier) appear to occur on all neurons as well as on the large granules in non-neuronal chromaffin cells,[45] the greater toxin susceptibilies of cholinergic nerve endings must arise from a larger density or recycling of the binding components, as well as additional determinants, for example, the nature of gangliosides in the presynaptic membrane which have been shown to be intimately involved in the interactions of BoNT/A and /B/G with their acceptors.[46-48]

The light chains of BoNTs proteolytically inactivate SNAREs: blockade of regulated secretion by serotypes show subtle differences exploitable for research purposes. After the discovery in 1992 of the BoNT light chains being Zn^{2+}-dependent endopeptidases[49-52] and the demonstration that type A cleaved off 9 residues from the C-terminus of SNAP-25,[53,54] such truncation and inactivation of this SNARE was more observed[55] in mouse phrenic nerve endings (see Fig. 1-3B). Notably, only a fraction of the total SNAP-25 had been cleaved by BoNT/A under conditions of complete blockade of neuromuscular transmission (see Fig. 1-3B). Incomplete cleavage of SNAP-25 by BoNT/A has also been observed by others in nerve-muscle preparations.[56,57] This contrasts with the more extensive or total cleavage of SNAP-25 seen after application of BoNTs to cultures of chromaffin cells, cerebellar granule, or sensory neurons.[58-60] One reasonable interpretation of these various findings is that BoNT/A acts on a SNAP-25 pool directly involved in ACh release from highly differentiated motor nerve terminals whose cell bodies reside a distance away in the spinal cord.[55] This is likely to result from localized uptake of BoNT/A, which is demonstrated at the unmyelinated presynaptic membrane only and not on the nerve trunk[9] (see Fig. 1-1B, C), presumably due to recycling there of small synaptic clear vesicles at the active zones. Retention of the type A light chain through its special membrane-anchoring motifs[61] would also contribute. Notwithstanding these different extents of SNAP-25 cleavage by BoNT/A in various cell types, there is overwhelming evidence that this selective action underlies its inhibition of exocytosis. For example, transmitter release from a nerve-muscle preparation of the leech is not blocked because SNAP-25 cannot be cleaved by this toxin owing to a mutation at the scissile bond.[62] Further support for this conclusion comes from the rescue of exocytosis from chromaffin cells pre-intoxicated with BoNT/A by the expression only of a SNAP-25 variant rendered toxin resistant (see Fig. 1-3C) by a mutation incorporated (R198T); the wild-type SNAP-25 proved ineffective.[63,64] Exceptionally, the t-SNARE SNAP-25 gets cleaved also by BoNT/C1 (at a bond one residue closer to the C-terminus than that susceptible to /A) and /E, which removes 26 residues.[54,58,65] The addition in vitro of a peptide, complementary to the region deleted by /E from SNAP-25, has been reported to overcome the SNARE complex formation that is, otherwise, prevented by this toxin.[66] Such selective proteolysis by /A and /E underlies inactivation of SNAP-25 because expressing the respective truncated products (SNAP-25_{1-197} and SNAP-25_{1-181}) in chromaffin cells diminished evoked exocytosis (see Fig. 1-3D). Additionally, this unveiled the ability of these SNAP-25 fragments to antagonize functionality of the endogenous intact protein, which is also observed in other cells.[67]

On the other hand, different peptide bonds in the v-SNARE (vesicle-associated membrane protein [VAMP] or synaptobrevin [Sbr]) are susceptible to BoNT/B, /D, /F and /G; only BoNT/B and tetanus toxin cleave at the same site.[49] It is noteworthy that isoform I of rat Sbr has a mutation at the scissile bond for BoNT/B; in this case, its inhibition of Ca^{2+}-dependent neuro-exocytosis can be observed only if another toxin-sensitive isoform is functional[51,60] (see later). Finally, certain isoforms of the t-SNARE, syntaxin, are susceptible to BoNT/C1[68]; regulated exocytosis from cells that contain resistant isoforms would only exhibit sensitivity due to cleavage of the SNAP-25 present. From a research viewpoint, advantages accrue from the availability of an array of BoNT serotypes that cleave one or more of the SNAREs and at different sites because this can dictate the subtle characteristics of the resultant blockade of exocytosis.[69] Hence, use of such discriminating probes for exocytosis can yield insights into this complicated multistage process. For example, BoNT/A-induced inhibition of transmitter release from peripheral and central neurons can be reversed (at least transiently) by elevating intraneuronal Ca^{2+} concentration,[70-72] whereas it is difficult to achieve this when other BoNT serotypes are used. In-depth investigations by Sakaba et al.[73] have revealed that BoNT/A slows down the kinetics of vesicle exocytosis in the large presynaptic terminal of the calyx of Held, whereas syntaxin- or VAMP-cleaving toxins appear to cause an outright blockade. Likewise, cleavage of the three target SNAREs with the different BoNTs has helped to evaluate the contributions of cytosolic moieties to the formation and dissociation/stabilities of SNARE complexes.[74,75]

MOLECULAR BASIS FOR THE THERAPEUTIC EFFECTIVENESS OF BoNT/A

Much of the information acquired to date on the sequential steps in the neuroparalytic action of BoNTs is depicted in Figure 1-4A, although caution is advised in extrapolating observations made in cells cultured in the absence of target organ or different cell types to those measured at nerve-muscle junction. Highly specialized motor nerve endings seem to exhibit properties that underlie their exquisite sensitivities to BoNTs. In addition to the precise nature, density, and location of the respective BoNT ecto-acceptors, plus the rapid recycling of small synaptic clear vesicles that apparently affords efficient internalization, other aspects of their cell biology contribute to the absence of nerve terminal death and eventual reversibility of BoNT-induced neuroparalysis, regardless of the period of muscle weakness. This lack of neurodegeneration, a reassuring safety feature for patients receiving toxin therapy, probably relates to the partial and localized cleavage of SNAP-25 (see earlier), subsequent triggering of the motor nerves to sprout, and over several weeks, formation of functional extrajunctional synapses.[55,76] Signaling for sprouting seems to require that exocytosis is blocked for at least 3 days because shorter-acting BoNTs such as /F and /E

(see later) induced minimal or no outgrowths, in contrast to the extensive remodeling triggered by /A[55,76] and /C.[77] An absence of detectable longer-acting BoNT/A-cleaved SNAP-25 in nerve sprouts (due, presumably, to the toxin's action being restricted to the parent nerve terminals) fits with intact SNAP-25 being essential for neurite outgrowth in rat cortical neurons, PC-12 cells, and chick retinal neurons.[78] In any case, the nerve-muscle communication ensuing sprouting, albeit less efficient than neurotransmission in normal muscle, may aid the survival and rehabilitation of the original paralyzed nerve terminals. Eventually, after 2 to 3 months in murine sternamastoid muscle, full endocytotic activity resumes at the parent nerve endings, and this is accompanied by retraction of the sprouts, with an amazing return of endplates indistinguishable from the original at the light microscope level.[76] This is a striking example of synaptic plasticity in the peripheral nervous system. Another intriguing aspect of BoNT-mediated neuromuscular paralysis is the extraordinarily extended duration seen with type /A or /C1, especially in human muscles, where weakening persists for over 3 months.[79,80] In clinical treatments of dystonias, the beneficial effects of BoNT/A hemagglutinin complex last for similarly long periods.[81] Mice injected with different BoNTs into hind leg muscles showed detectable weakness over a 4-week period with type A but for much shorter times with /F (8 days) and /E (5 days)[55] when assessed using the toe-spread reflex assay.[82] The exceptionally long duration of action of BoNT/A seems largely due to the longevity of its protease activity, demonstrated in bovine chromaffin cells (see Fig. 1-3C), rat cerebellar granule cells,[58] spinal cord neurons,[83] and nerve-muscle preparations[84] to range from greater than 3 weeks up to ~11 weeks. In contrast, the paralytic activity of BoNT/E proved to be short lived (<15 days); note that this value, obtained with the more sensitive electrophysiologic recordings, is longer than that observed (see earlier) with the toe spread reflex assay. Apart from BoNT/C1, which shows a similar time course to/A, other serotypes gave shorter values for $t_{1/2}$ of transmitter inhibition from cultured neurons (>>31, >>25, ~10, ~2 and 0.8 days for /A, /C1, /B, /F and /E, respectively).[58] Despite the long duration of action of BoNT/A-hemagglutinin being a great advantage for therapy, it remains a major scientific challenge to decipher how the protease of BoNT/A and/C1 survives degradation over such extended periods. Motifs

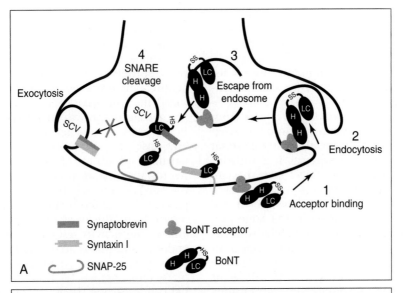

FIGURE 1-4. Current understanding of the sophisticated neuroparalytic action of BoNT. **A,** Schematic of the multistep mechanism for inhibition of transmitter release by BoNTs. **B,** Multiple synergistic activities identified in BoNT/A that underlie its therapeutics usefulness.

have been identified at the N- and C-termini of the light chain from BoNT/A that contribute to its membrane sequestration, whereas these are absent from the /E toxin, explaining a largely cytosolic localization when its light chain was expressed in cultured cells.[61] Although this offers valuable insights into their half-lives, additional factors are likely to be involved because /C1 exhibits a protracted action despite lacking these motifs.[61] In summary, these extensive investigations on BoNT/A or its hemagglutinin complex have defined an impressive array of advantageous functional properties that act synergistically to make this neurotherapeutic agent highly effective (see Fig. 1-4B) for an ever-increasing number of disorders involving overactive muscles (see other chapters herein).

INHIBITION OF PEPTIDE RELEASE FROM SENSORY NEURONS BY CERTAIN BoNTS REFLECT THEIR ANTINOCICEPTIVE POTENTIAL

Sbr I is required for CGRP release from trigeminal ganglionic neurons (TGNs). In addition to a preferential action of BoNT on peripheral cholinergic nerves as outlined earlier, it inhibits regulated exocytosis of many transmitter types including peptides[33-35] (see earlier). Accordingly, BoNT/A complex has been reported to block evoked release of calcitonin gene–related peptide (CGRP) from sensory neurons of rat trigeminal ganglia.[85] CGRP is a potent vasodilator that gets released from large dense-core vesicles and acts as a mediator of inflammatory pain.[86] Because the level of this peptide is elevated in jugular venous blood of migraine sufferers,[87] inhibition of its release from peripheral nerves by BoNT/A complex[88] may provide an explanation for its effectiveness in treating certain types of pain.[89,90] However, a molecular basis for the response of certain migraine sufferers and not others[91] remains to be elucidated. Toward this goal, we characterized the release process for CGRP from cultured TGNs, a convenient model for biochemical investigations of sensory neurons.[92] Confocal fluorescence microscopy revealed that all three SNAREs (SNAP-25, syntaxin, and Sbr) and the putative Ca^{2+} sensor synaptotagmin largely occur together in rat TGNs (Fig. 1-5A). The punctate colocalization of Sbr isoform I and CGRP in neurites of TGNs is particularly striking (see Fig. 1-5B). In fact, Sbr I was found to be essential for evoked Ca^{2+}-dependent CGRP release from TGNs.[60] For example, cleavage of Sbr II and III by BoNT/B in rat TGNs (I is resistant in this species) failed to block release of the peptide, whereas the latter was inhibited in mouse neurons where Sbr I was also proteolyzed (see Fig. 1-5C). In preliminary experiments, knock-down of Sbr I expression led to a substantial reduction of CGRP release from these sensory neurons. This demonstrated requirement for Sbr I in large dense-core vesicle peptide release from sensory neurons contrasts with the ability of Sbr II/III to suffice for exocytosis of several neurotransmitters from small synaptic clear vesicles or, indeed, for secretion from granules in chromaffin cells, cerebrocortical synaptosomes, and PC-12 cells (discussed in reference 60). Such an unusual feature of a dependence on Sbr I for CGRP exocytosis from rat TGNs may be related to this occurring at sites remote from the active zones,[93] enabling this pain mediator to reach blood vessels in the vicinity and activate its receptor thereon.

A novel BoNT EA chimera blocks capsaicin-evoked exocytosis of CGRP from TGNs much more effectively than /A or /E. SNAP-25 present in TGNs also participates in exocytosis[60] because exposure to BoNT/A resulted in cleavage of this SNARE, together with blockade of

CGRP release (see Fig. 1-5D) evoked by K^+-depolarization, or bradykinin to a lesser extent. Interestingly, BoNT/A caused negligible inhibition of CGRP efflux elicited by capsaicin, which binds to the vanilloid receptor (type 1) present on TGNs[60] and produces pain by activating its nonselective cation channel.[94] Another SNAP-25 cleaving BoNT, type E, proved unable to truncate its target in TGNs or affect CGRP release triggered by any of the stimuli (see Fig. 1-5E). To ascertain if this lack of activity in BoNT/E arose from inability to bind or enter the TGNs, a novel chimeric toxin was generated recombinantly by replacing the H_C binding domain in type E with its counterpart from BoNT/A.[95] When expressed in *Escherichi coli*, the resultant purified protein exhibited pronounced neuromuscular paralysis and efficiently cleaved SNAP-25 in TGNs. Most importantly, this EA chimera gave a dose-dependent inhibition of CGRP release from these sensory neurons elicited by capsaicin or bradykinin, displaying higher potency than the parental toxins (/A or /E) (see Fig. 1-5E). These novel observations provide proof of principle for recombinantly endowing BoNT/E with a domain from/A that can productively interact with SV2 acceptors observed on TGNs[60] and, presumably, gangliosides and, thereby, target its protease to allow delivery into neurons that were previously nonsusceptible to BoNT/E. Moreover, the removal of 26 residues from SNAP-25 by chimera EA compared with the 9 amino acids deleted by BoNT/A yields a complete blockade of CGRP release rather than the partial inhibition seen with /A (see Fig. 1-5E).

CONCLUSIONS

Seven homologous but structurally distinct BoNTs (A–G), produced by *Clostridium botulinum*, represent a truly remarkable array of research tools owing to their intriguing multiphasic actions and because each inhibits regulated exocytosis in subtly different ways. Their suspected use of separate acceptors (except for /B and /G; see later) was established by the visualization plus quantitation of membrane binding sites for /A and /B on motor nerve endings. Identification of SV2 and synaptotagmin I/II as their respective acceptors followed later; the anticipated discovery of others should reveal novel (functional) components on presynaptic membranes. Likewise, internalization of BoNTs via acceptor-mediated endocytosis is

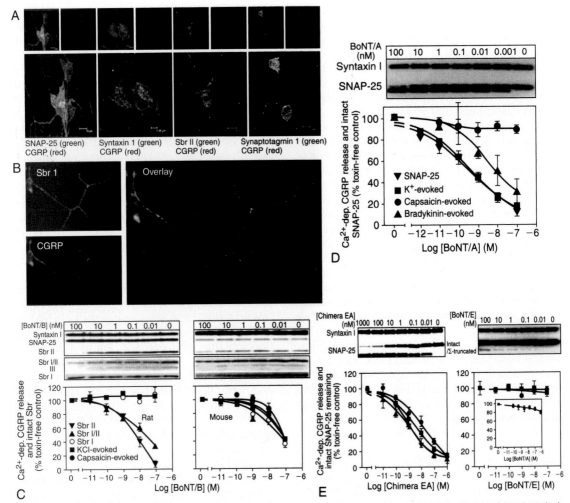

FIGURE 1-5. CGRP release from trigeminal ganglionic neurons (TGNs) uses isoform I of synaptobrevin (Sbr), and SNAP-25: lack of susceptibility to BoNT/E is overcome with a novel chimera made by substituting its binding domain with that from /A. **A,** All three SNAREs and synaptotagmin I are largely colocalized in rat TGNs, a good source of sensory neurons. Confocal fluorescent micrographs for CGRP, each SNARE, and synaptotagmin I are displayed in upper panels, with merged views beneath. **B,** Images showing that Sbr I and CGRP colocalize in neurites of TGNs. **C,** Inability of BoNT/B to cleave Sbr I in the rat sensory neurons is accompanied by a lack of inhibition of evoked CGRP release, whereas cleavage of all Sbr isoforms in mouse TGNs blocks exocytosis of this pain-mediating peptide. **D,** Cleavage of SNAP-25 in TGNs by BoNT/A inhibits CGRP exocytosis evoked by K+ or bradykinin but not capsaicin. **E,** Whereas BoNT/E proved unable to affect exocytosis or cleave SNAP-25, a recombinantly-created chimera of BoNT/E, having the H_C domain replaced by its counterpart from /A, cleaved SNAP-25, and inhibited capsaicin- or bradykinin-elicited CGRP release more potently than the parental toxins (/E and /A). Symbols are the same as in **D**; note that the values for SNAP-25 cleavage (■) and bradykinin-evoked CGRP release (■) overlap. (**A** to **D** are from Meng J, Wang J, Lawrence G, Dolly JO. Synaptobrevin I mediates exocytosis of CGRP from sensory neurons and inhibition by botulinum toxins reflects their anti-nociceptive potential. *J Cell Sci.* 2007;120(Pt 16):2864-2874. Reproduced with permission of the Company of Biologists. **E** is from Meng J, Wang J, Zurawski T, et al. A chimera of botulinum neurotoxin A and E with pronounced anti-nociceptive potential. *J Cell Sci.* 2008; (in press).) *See Color Plate*

allowing new insights to be gained into membrane and protein trafficking in neurons, poorly understood topics but of major scientific (and medical) importance. Already, BoNT/E is known to highjack two endocytotic processes to enter peripheral cholinergic nerves, whereas /A follows one route; clearly,

deciphering possible sharing or use of separate pathways would be aided by finding the identity and/or location of the acceptors for additional serotypes. The elegant data published recently on the mechanism for translocating LC of BoNT/A is likely to be extended by examination of other BoNTs because /E appears to translocate faster than /A. In terms of the toxins' enzymic activities, the LCs represent a family of Zn^{2+}-dependent proteases displaying unique properties; moreover, recent elucidation of their intricate multisite interactions with the SNARE substrates are yielding molecular basis for the toxins' spectacular specificities for a single scissile bond in the respective targets.

In addition to the toxins being instrumental in advancing fundamental research, BoNT/A-hemagglutinin complex, in particular, has proved to a miraculous and versatile therapeutic for numerous disorders involving hyperactivity of various muscles. Even more exciting, it is showing promise as an antinociceptive drug; success in this regard will increase due to progress being made in deciphering the inhibitory actions of BoNTs on the exocytosis of pain mediators from sensory neurons. Further improvements will accrue from recombinantly creating new toxins whose pharmacologic properties can be tailored for particular clinical applications. With proof of principle for this approach already obtained, there is scope for controlling SNARE-dependent secretion in a wide variety of diseased states. Thus, the medical applications of these engineered molecules will become enormous and limited only by the ingenuity of clinical practitioners.

ACKNOWLEDGMENTS

The authors are grateful for support of this research through a Research Professorship grant (to JOD) from Science Foundation Ireland and contracts from Allergan Inc., USAMRIID and DTRA.

References

1. Burgen AS, Dickens F, Zatman LJ. The action of botulinum toxin on the neuro-muscular junction. *J Physiol.* 1949;109:10-24.
2. Sellin LC: The action of botulinum toxin at the neuromuscular junction. *Med Biol.* 1981;59:11-20.
3. Simpson LL. The origin, structure, and pharmacological activity of botulinum toxin. *Pharmacol Rev.* 1981;33:155-188.
4. Simpson LL: Kinetic studies on the interaction between botulinum toxin type A and the cholinergic neuromuscular junction. *J Pharmacol Exp Ther.* 1980;212:16-21.
5. Williams R., Tse CK, Dolly JO, Hambleton P, Melling J. Radioiodination of botulinum neurotoxin type A with retention of biological activity and its binding to brain synaptosomes. *Eur J Biochem.* 1983;131:437-445.
6. Dolly JO, Williams RS, Black JC, Tse CK, Hambleton P, Melling J. Localization of sites for ^{125}I-labelled botulinum neurotoxin at murine neuromuscular junction and its binding to rat brain synaptosomes. *Toxicon.* 1982;20:141-148.
7. Dolly JO, Williams RS, Melling J. Acceptors for botulinum neurotoxin reside on motor nerve terminals and mediate its internalization. *Nature.* 1984;307: 457-460.
8. Black JD, Dolly JO. Interaction of ^{125}I-labeled botulinum neurotoxins with nerve terminals. II. Autoradiographic evidence for its uptake into motor nerves by acceptor-mediated endocytosis. *J Cell Biol.* 1986;103:535-544.
9. Black JD, Dolly JO. Interaction of ^{125}I-labeled botulinum neurotoxins with nerve terminals. I. Ultrastructural autoradiographic localization and quantitation of distinct membrane acceptors for types A and B on motor nerves. *J Cell Biol.* 1986;103:521-534.
10. de Paiva A, Poulain B, Lawrence GW, Shone CC, Tauc L, Dolly JO. A role for the interchain disulfide or its participating thiols in the internalization of botulinum neurotoxin A revealed by a toxin derivative that binds to ecto-acceptors and inhibits transmitter release intracellularly. *J Biol Chem.* 1993;268:20838-20844.
11. Montecucco C, Schiavo G. Mechanism of action of tetanus and botulinum neurotoxins. *Mol Microbiol.* 1994;13:1-8.
12. Schiavo G, Papini E, Genna G, Montecucco C. An intact interchain disulfide bond is required for the neurotoxicity of tetanus toxin. *Infect Immun.* 1990;58:4136-4141.
13. Dong M, Richards DA, Goonough MC, Tepp WH, Johnson EA, Chapman ER. Synaptotagmins I and II mediate entry of botulinum neurotoxin B into cells. *J Cell Biol.* 2003;162:1293-1303.
14. Dong M, Yeh F, Tepp WH, Dean C, Johnson EA, Janz R, et al. SV2 is the protein receptor for botulinum neurotoxin A. *Science.* 2006;312:592-596.
15. Mahrhold S, Rummel A, Bigalke H, Davletov B, Binz T. The synaptic vesicle protein 2C mediates the uptake of botulinum neurotoxin A into phrenic nerves. *FEBS Lett.* 2006;580:2011-2014.
16. Rummel A, Karnath T, Henke T, Bigalke H, Binz T. Synaptotagmins I and II act as nerve cell receptors for botulinum neurotoxin G. *J Biol Chem.* 2004;279:30865-30870.
17. Nishiki T, Ogasawara J, Kamata Y, Kozki S. Solubilization and characterization of the acceptor for Clostridium botulinum type B neurotoxin from rat brain synaptic membranes. *Biochim Biophys Acta.* 1993;1158:333-338.
18. Takamori S, Holt M, Stenius K, Lemke EA, Grønborg M, Riedel D, et al. Molecular anatomy of a trafficking organelle. *Cell.* 2006;127:831-846.
19. Hughes R, Whaler BC. Influence of nerve-ending activity and of drugs on the rate of paralysis of rat diaphragm preparations by Cl. botulinum type A toxin. *J Physiol.* 1962;160:221-233.
20. Lawrence G, Wang J, Chion CK, Aoki KR, Dolly JO. Two protein trafficking processes at motor nerve endings unveiled by botulinum neurotoxin E. *J Pharmacol Exp Ther.* 2007;320:410-418.
21. Fernandez-Alfonso T, Kwan R, Ryan TA. Synaptic vesicles interchange their membrane proteins with a large surface reservoir during recycling. *Neuron.* 2006;51:179-186.
22. Simpson LL. Identification of the major steps in botulinum toxin action. *Annu Rev Pharmacol Toxicol.* 2004;44:167-193.
23. Chen R, Karp BI, Goldstein SR, Bara-Jimenez W, Yaseen Z, Hallett M. Effect of muscle activity immediately after botulinum toxin injection for writer's cramp. *Mov Disord.* 1999;14:307-312.

24. Eleopra R, Tugnoli V, De Grandis D. The variability in the clinical effect induced by botulinum toxin type A: the role of muscle activity in humans. *Mov Disord.* 1997;12:89-94.

25. Hesse S, Jahnke MT, Luecke D, Mauritz KH. Short-term electrical stimulation enhances the effectiveness of botulinum toxin in the treatment of lower limb spasticity in hemiparetic patients. *Neurosci Lett.* 1995;201:37-40.

26. Simpson LL. Ammonium chloride and methylamine hydrochloride antagonize clostridial neurotoxins. *J Pharmacol Exp Ther.* 1983;225:546-552.

27. Ferguson SM, Brasnjo G, Hayashi M, Wölfel M, Collesi C, Giovedi S, et al. A selective activity-dependent requirement for dynamin 1 in synaptic vesicle endocytosis. *Science.* 2007;316:570-574.

28. Dolly JO, de Paiva A, Toran P, Daniels-Holgate P, Ashton A. Probing the process of transmitter release with botulinum and tetanus neurotoxins. *Seminars in the Neurosciences.* 1994;6:149-158.

29. Fischer A, Montal M. Single molecule detection of intermediates during botulinum neurotoxin transloca-tion across membranes. *Proc Natl Acad Sci U S A.* 2007;104:10447-10452.

30. Fischer A, Montal M. Crucial role of the disulfide bridge between botulinum neurotoxin light and heavy chains in protease translocation across mem-branes. *J Biol Chem.* 2007;282:29604-29611.

31. Poulain B, Tauc L, Maisey EA, Wadsworth JD, Mohan PM, Dolly JO. Neurotransmitter release is blocked intracellularly by botulinum neurotoxin, and this requires uptake of both toxin polypeptides by a process mediated by the larger chain. *Proc Natl Acad Sci U S A.* 1988;85:4090-4094.

32. de Paiva A, Dolly JO. Light chain of botulinum neuro-toxin is active in mammalian motor nerve terminals when delivered via liposomes. *FEBS Lett.* 1990;277:171-174.

33. Poulain B, Mochida S, Wadsworth JD, Weller U, Habermann E, Dolly JO, et al. Inhibition of neuro-transmitter release by botulinum neurotoxins and tet-anus toxin at Aplysia synapses: role of the constituent chains. *J Physiol. (Paris)* 1990;84:247-261.

34. Ashton AC, Dolly JO. Characterization of the inhibi-tory action of botulinum neurotoxin type A on the release of several transmitters from rat cerebrocortical synaptosomes. *J Neurochem.* 1988;50:1808-1816.

35. McMahon HT, Foran P, Dolly JO, Verhage M, Wiegant VM, Nicholls DG. Tetanus toxin and botulinum toxins type A and B inhibit glutamate, gamma-aminobutyric acid, aspartate, and met-enkephalin release from synaptosomes. *Clues to the locus of action. J Biol Chem.* 1992;267:21338-21343.

36. Lawrence GW, Weller U, Dolly JO. Botulinum A and the light chain of tetanus toxins inhibit distinct stages of Mg.ATP-dependent catecholamine exocytosis from permeabilized chromaffin cells. *Eur J Biochem.* 1994;222:325-333.

37. Bittner MA, Habig WH, Holz RW. Isolated light chain of tetanus toxin inhibits exocytosis: studies in digitonin-permeabilized cells. *J Neurochem.* 1989;53:966-968.

38. Ahnert-Hilger G, Weller U. Comparison of the intra-cellular effects of clostridial neurotoxins on exocytosis from streptolysin O-permeabilized rat pheochromocy-toma (PC 12) and bovine adrenal chromaffin cells. *Neuroscience.* 1993;53:547-552.

39. McInnes C, Dolly JO. Ca^{2+}-dependent noradrenaline release from permeabilised PC12 cells is blocked by botulinum neurotoxin A or its light chain. *FEBS Lett.* 1990;261:323-326.

40. Lomneth R, Martin TF, DasGupta BR. Botulinum neu-rotoxin light chain inhibits norepinephrine secretion in PC12 cells at an intracellular membranous or cyto-skeletal site. *J Neurochem.* 1991;57:1413-1421.

41. Stecher B, Ahnert-Hilger G, Weller U, Kemmer TP, Gratzl M. Amylase release from streptolysin O-permea-bilized pancreatic acinar cells. Effects of Ca^{2+}, guano-sine 5'-[gamma-thio]triphosphate, cyclic AMP, tetanus toxin and botulinum A toxin. *Biochem J.* 1992;283(Pt 3):899-904.

42. MacKenzie I, Burnstock G, Dolly JO. The effects of purified botulinum neurotoxin type A on cholinergic, adrenergic and non-adrenergic, atropine-resistant auto-nomic neuromuscular transmission. *Neuroscience.* 1982;7:997-1006.

43. Black JD, Dolly JO. Selective location of acceptors for botulinum neurotoxin A in the central and peripheral nervous systems. *Neuroscience.* 1987;23:767-779.

44. Daniels-Holgate PU, Dolly JO. Productive and non-productive binding of botulinum neurotoxin A to motor nerve endings are distinguished by its heavy chain. *J Neurosci Res.* 1996;44:263-271.

45. Lowe AW, Madeddu L, Kelly RB. Endocrine secretory granules and neuronal synaptic vesicles have three integral membrane proteins in common. *J Cell Biol.* 1988;106:51-59.

46. Jin R, Rummel A, Binz T, Brunger AT. Botulinum neu-rotoxin B recognizes its protein receptor with high affinity and specificity. *Nature.* 2006;444:1092-1095.

47. Rummel A, Eichner T, Weil T, Karnath T, Gutcaits A, Mahrhold S, et al. Identification of the protein receptor binding site of botulinum neurotoxins B and G proves the double-receptor concept. *Proc Natl Acad Sci U S A.* 2007;104:359-364.

48. Chai Q, Arndt AW, Dong M, Tepp WH, Johnson EA, Chapman ER, et al. Structural basis of cell surface receptor recognition by botulinum neurotoxin B. *Nature.* 2006;444:1096-1100.

49. Schiavo G, Matteoli M, Montecucco C. Neurotoxins affecting neuroexocytosis. *Physiol Rev.* 2000;80:717-766.

50. Schiavo G, Benfenati F, Poulain B, Rossetto O, Polverino de Laureto P, et al. Tetanus and botuli-num-B neurotoxins block neurotransmitter release by proteolytic cleavage of synaptobrevin. *Nature.* 1992;359:832-835.

51. Schiavo G, Poulain B, Rossetto O, Benfenati F, Tauc L, Montecucco C. Tetanus toxin is a zinc protein and its inhibition of neurotransmitter release and protease activity depend on zinc. *EMBO J.* 1992;11:3577-3583.

52. Wright JF, Pernoller M, Reboul A, Aude C, Colomb MG. Identification and partial characterization of a low affinity metal-binding site in the light chain of tetanus toxin. *J Biol Chem.* 1992;267:9053-9058.

53. Blasi J, Chapman ER, Link E, Binz T, Yamasaki S, De Camilli P, et al. Botulinum neurotoxin A selectively cleaves the synaptic protein SNAP-25. *Nature.* 1993;365:160-163.

54. Schiavo G, Santucci A, Dasgupta BR, Mehta PP, Jontes J, Benfenati F, et al. Botulinum neurotoxins serotypes A and E cleave SNAP-25 at distinct COOH-terminal pep-tide bonds. *FEBS Lett.* 1993;335:99-103.

55. Meunier FA, Lisk G, Sesardic D, Dolly JO. Dynamics of motor nerve terminal remodeling unveiled using SNARE-cleaving botulinum toxins: the extent and duration are dictated by the sites of SNAP-25 trunca-tion. *Mol Cell Neurosci.* 2003;22:454-466.

56. Kalandakanond S, Coffield JA. Cleavage of intracellular substrates of botulinum toxins A, C, and D in a

mammalian target tissue. *J Pharmacol Exp Ther.* 2001;296:749-755.

57. Raciborska DA, Trimble WS, Charlton MP. Presynaptic protein interactions in vivo: evidence from botulinum A, C, D and E action at frog neuromuscular junction. *Eur J Neurosci.* 1998;10:2528-2617.

58. Foran PG, Mohammed N, Lisk GO, Nagwaney S, Lawrence GW, Johnson E, et al. Evaluation of the therapeutic usefulness of botulinum neurotoxin B, C1, E, and F compared with the long lasting type A. Basis for distinct durations of inhibition of exocytosis in central neurons. *J Biol Chem.* 2003;278:1363-1371.

59. Lawrence GW, Foran P, Dolly JO. Distinct exocytotic responses of intact and permeabilised chromaffin cells after cleavage of the 25-kDa synaptosomal-associated protein (SNAP-25) or synaptobrevin by botulinum toxin A or B. *Eur J Biochem.* 1996;236:877-886.

60. Meng J, Wang J, Lawrence G, Dolly JO. Synaptobrevin I mediates exocytosis of CGRP from sensory neurons and inhibition by botulinum toxins reflects their anti-nociceptive potential. *J Cell Sci.* 2007;120(Pt 16):2864-2874.

61. Fernandez-Salas E, Steward LE, Ho H, Garay PE, Sun SW, Gilmore MA, et al. Plasma membrane localization signals in the light chain of botulinum neurotoxin. *Proc Natl Acad Sci U S A.* 2004;101:3208-3213.

62. Bruns D, Engers S, Yang C, Ossig R, Jeromin A, Jahn R. Inhibition of transmitter release correlates with the proteolytic activity of tetanus toxin and botulinus toxin A in individual cultured synapses of Hirudo medicinalis. *J Neurosci.* 1997;17:1898-1910.

63. O'Sullivan GA, Mohammed N, Foran PG, Lawrence GW, Dolly JO. Rescue of exocytosis in botulinum toxin A-poisoned chromaffin cells by expression of cleavage-resistant SNAP-25. Identification of the minimal essential C-terminal residues. *J Biol Chem.* 1999;274:36897-36904.

64. Criado M, Gil A, Viniegra S, Gutierrez LM. A single amino acid near the C terminus of the synaptosome-associated protein of 25 kDa (SNAP-25) is essential for exocytosis in chromaffin cells. *Proc Natl Acad Sci U S A.* 1999;96:7256-7261.

65. Foran P, Lawrence GW, Shone CC, Foster KA, Dolly JO. Botulinum neurotoxin C1 cleaves both syntaxin and SNAP-25 in intact and permeabilized chromaffin cells: correlation with its blockade of catecholamine release. *Biochemistry.* 1996;35:2630-2636.

66. Chen YA, Scales SJ, Patel SM, Doung YC, Scheller RH. SNARE complex formation is triggered by Ca^{2+} and drives membrane fusion. *Cell.* 1999;97:165-174.

67. Huang X, Wheeler MB, Kang YH, Sheu L, Lukacs GL, Trimble WS, et al. Truncated SNAP-25 (1-197), like botulinum neurotoxin A, can inhibit insulin secretion from HIT-T15 insulinoma cells. *Mol Endocrinol.* 1998;12:1060-1070.

68. Blasi J, Chapman ER, Yamasaki S, Binz T, Niemann H, Jahn R. Botulinum neurotoxin C1 blocks neurotransmitter release by means of cleaving HPC-1/syntaxin. *EMBO J.* 1993;12:4821-4828.

69. Humeau Y, Dousseau F, Grant NJ, Poulain B. How botulinum and tetanus neurotoxins block neurotransmitter release. *Biochimie.* 2000;82:427-446.

70. Ashton AC, Dolly JO. Microtubule-dissociating drugs and A23187 reveal differences in the inhibition of synaptosomal transmitter release by botulinum neurotoxins types A and B. *J Neurochem.* 1991;56:827-835.

71. Molgo J, Lemeignan M, Thesleff S. Aminoglycosides and 3,4-diaminopyridine on neuromuscular block caused by botulinum type A toxin. *Muscle Nerve.* 1987;10:464-470.

72. Lundh H, Leander S, Thesleff S. Antagonism of the paralysis produced by botulinum toxin in the rat. The effects of tetraethylammonium, guanidine and 4-aminopyridine. *J Neurol Sci.* 1977;32:29-43.

73. Sakaba T, Stein A, Jahn R, Neher E. Distinct kinetic changes in neurotransmitter release after SNARE protein cleavage. *Science.* 2005;309:491-494.

74. Hayashi T, McMahon H, Yamasaki S, Binz T, Hata Y, Südhof TC, et al. Synaptic vesicle membrane fusion complex: action of clostridial neurotoxins on assembly. *EMBO J.* 1994;13:5051-5561.

75. Pellegrini LL, O'Connor V, Lottspeich F, Betz H. Clostridial neurotoxins compromise the stability of a low energy SNARE complex mediating NSF activation of synaptic vesicle fusion. *EMBO J.* 1995;14:4705-4713.

76. de Paiva A, Meunier FA, Molgó J, Aoki KR, Dolly JO. Functional repair of motor endplates after botulinum neurotoxin type A poisoning: biphasic switch of synaptic activity between nerve sprouts and their parent terminals. *Proc Natl Acad Sci U S A.* 1999;96:3200-3205.

77. Morbiato L, Carli L, Johnson EA, Montecucco C, Molgó J, Rossetto O. Neuromuscular paralysis and recovery in mice injected with botulinum neurotoxins A and C. *Eur J Neurosci.* 2007;25:2697-2704.

78. Osen-Sand A, Catsicas M, Staple JK, Jones KA, Ayala G, Knowles J, et al. Inhibition of axonal growth by SNAP-25 antisense oligonucleotides in vitro and in vivo. *Nature.* 1993;364:445-448.

79. Eleopra R, Tugnoli V, Rossetto O, De Grandis D, Montecucco C. Different time courses of recovery after poisoning with botulinum neurotoxin serotypes A and E in humans. *Neurosci Lett.* 1998;256:135-138.

80. Eleopra R, Tugnoli V, Rossetto O, Montecucco C, De Grandis D. Botulinum neurotoxin serotype C: a novel effective botulinum toxin therapy in human. *Neurosci Lett.* 1997;224:91-94.

81. Ward AB, Barnes MP. *Clinical Uses of Botulinum Toxin.* Cambridge, UK, Cambridge University Press, 2007, p 384.

82. Aoki KR, Guyer B. Botulinum toxin type A and other botulinum toxin serotypes: a comparative review of biochemical and pharmacological actions. *Eur J Neurol.* 2001;8(suppl 5):21-29.

83. Keller JE, Neale EA, Oyler G, Adler M. Persistence of botulinum neurotoxin action in cultured spinal cord cells. *FEBS Lett.* 1999;456:137-142.

84. Adler M, Keller JE, Sheridan RE, Deshpande SS. Persistence of botulinum neurotoxin A demonstrated by sequential administration of serotypes A and E in rat EDL muscle. *Toxicon.* 2001;39:233-243.

85. Durham PL, Cady R. Regulation of calcitonin gene-related peptide secretion from trigeminal nerve cells by botulinum toxin type A: implications for migraine therapy. *Headache.* 2004;44:35-42; discussion 42-43.

86. Kummer W. Ultrastructure of calcitonin gene-related peptide-immunoreactive nerve fibres in guinea-pig peribronchial ganglia. *Regul Pept.* 1992;37:135-142.

87. Edvinsson L, Goadsby PJ. Neuropeptides in the cerebral circulation: relevance to headache. *Cephalalgia.* 1995;15:272-276.

88. Aoki KR. Evidence for antinociceptive activity of botulinum toxin type A in pain management. *Headache.* 2003;43(suppl 1):S9-15.

89. Gazerani P, Staahl C, Drewes AM, Arendt-Nielsen L. The effects of botulinum toxin type A on capsaicin-evoked pain, flare, and secondary hyperalgesia in an

experimental human model of trigeminal sensitization. *Pain*. 2006;122:315-325.

90. Gupta VK. Botulinum toxin type A therapy for chronic tension-type headache: fact versus fiction. *Pain*. 2005;116:166-167; author reply 167.

91. Schulte-Mattler WJ, Martinez-Castrillo JC. Botulinum toxin therapy of migraine and tension-type headache: comparing different botulinum toxin preparations. *Eur J Neurol*. 2006;13(suppl 1):51-54.

92. Eckert SP, Taddese A, McCleskey EW. Isolation and culture of rat sensory neurons having distinct sensory modalities. *J Neurosci Methods*. 1997;77:183-190.

93. Bernardini N, Neuhuber W, Reeh PW, Saurer SK. Morphological evidence for functional capsaicin receptor expression and calcitonin gene-related peptide exocytosis in isolated peripheral nerve axons of the mouse. *Neuroscience*. 2004;126:585-590.

94. Caterina MJ, Schumacher MA, Tominaga M, Rosen TA, Levine JD, Julius D. The capsaicin receptor: a heat-activated ion channel in the pain pathway. *Nature*. 1997;389:816-824.

95. Wang J, Meng J, Lawrence GW, Zurawski TH, Sasse A, Bodeker M, Gilmore MA, Fernandez-Salas E, et al. Novel chimeras of botulinum neurotoxin A and E unveil contributions from the binding, translocation and protease domains to their functional characteristics. *J Biol Chem*. 2008;283:16993-17002.

96. Dolly JO, Lande S, Wray DW. The effects of in vitro application of purified botulinum neurotoxin at mouse motor nerve terminals. *J Physiol*. 1987;386:475-484.

97. Sudhof TC. The synaptic vesicle cycle. *Annu Rev Neurosci*. 2004;27:509-547.

98. O'Sullivan GA, Dolly JO. The two core domains of SNAP-25 are functionally distinct and act interdependently in exocytosis. (In preparation for publication.)

99. Meng J, Wang J, Zurawski T, et al. A chimera of botulinum neurotoxin A and E with pronounced anti-nociceptive potential. *J Cell Sci*. 2008; (in press).

Molecular Structures and Functional Relationships of Botulinum Neurotoxins

2

Subramanyam Swaminathan

INTRODUCTION

Botulinum and tetanus neurotoxins are solely responsible for neuroparalytic syndromes of botulism and tetanus characterized by serious neurologic disorders. Their median lethal dose (LD_{50}) in humans is in the range of 0.1 to 1 ng per kg,[1] which make them the most poisonous substances known to humans. Of the seven serotypes produced by *Clostridium botulinum*, only botulinum neurotoxin (BoNT)/A, B, and E (and possibly C and F) have been implicated in cases of botulism in humans. Other BoNTs primarily affect animals. *Clostridium* neurotoxins are produced as a single inactive polypeptide chain of 150 kDa, which is cleaved by tissue proteinases into an active di-chain molecule: a heavy chain (H) of ~100 kDa and a light chain (L) of ~50 kDa held together by a single disulfide bond. Most of the serotypes of BoNT are released as di-chains by a proteolytic strain, whereas BoNT/E is released as a single chain by a nonproteolytic strain, which is activated into a di-chain by host proteases only after uptake into host organisms.[2,3] In vitro activation can also be achieved by incubation with trypsin. BoNTs are AB toxins with activating (A) and binding (B) protomers. Protomer B is the heavy chain (H) and protomer A, the light chain (L). The H chain can be cleaved into two chains by papain digestion; the C-terminal chain, H_C, acts as the binding domain, whereas the N-terminal domain, H_N, acts as the translocation domain. H_C, H_N, and L form the three functional domains of the neurotoxin, and each is involved in one of the four stages of toxicity, which are binding, internalization, translocation into cytosol, and catalytic activity.[4-8] In spite of different clinical symptoms, both BoNTs and tetanus toxin (TeNT) intoxicate neuronal cells in the same way and have similar functional and structural organizations.[9-12] BoNT/A and other serotypes are now used as therapeutic agents in patients with strabismus, blepharospasm, and other facial nerve disorders.[13,14] Here, we will correlate the three-dimensional structure of each domain with various stages of toxicity and explore the possibility of using these domains as therapeutic targets to counter botulism.

STRUCTURE OF BOTULINUM NEUROTOXINS

A breakthrough in BoNT research happened when the crystal structure of BoNT/A was determined at 3.2 Å resolution, followed by BoNT/B at 1.8 Å.[11,12] The two structures taken together identified for the first time the correlation between the three stages of toxicity, which are binding, translocation, and catalytic action with the three well-defined structural domains.

The three-domain organization is similar to many soluble bacterial toxins, and the structure of BoNT/B is shown in Figure 2-1.[12]

The author of this chapter has not reported any conflicts of interest.

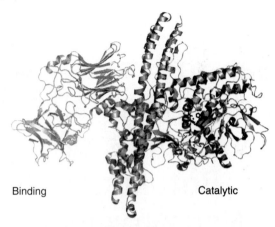

Binding   Catalytic

Translocation

FIGURE 2-1. Ribbons diagram of botulinum neurotoxin type B. The three functional domains are labeled as binding, translocation, and catalytic. The active site residues and the catalytic zinc ion are shown in the catalytic domain. The three-dimensional structure clearly demarcated the three functional domains. The lower half of the binding domain is involved in ganglioside and receptor binding. *See Color Plate*

The sequence homology and functional similarity suggest that the domain organization of all serotypes of BoNTs will be similar. Very recently, from single particle electron microscope analysis, it is suggested that the domain organization may be different in BoNT/E.[15] However, three populations of varying organization are identified. It is not clear whether this difference is due to the mode of sample preparation for EM studies. Only an x-ray structure could further verify this domain organization.

BoNT consists of three structural domains of similar molecular mass, the first one third (N-terminal) corresponding to the catalytic domain, the middle one third corresponding to the translocation domain, and the last (C-terminal) one third corresponding to the binding domain. The most intriguing aspect of the structure is a long stretch of amino acids (~50 residues) belonging to the translocation domain in sequence but associated with the catalytic domain, forming a 'belt' wrapped around the catalytic domain. The significance and the function of the belt region are poorly understood now and are under structural and biophysical investigation.

The crystal structures of BoNT/A and B helped in analyzing each domain and in mutagenic studies to identify amino acids important for each stage of toxicity. In the following sections, each domain will be discussed separately

to correlate the structure-function relationships. The discussion will be of general nature and will be applicable to all serotypes (except for some minor variations) because all serotypes share significant sequence homology and functional similarity. However, important differences exist in their pharmacologic effects.

STRUCTURE-FUNCTION RELATIONSHIPS

Binding Domain

BoNT is approximately 1250 residues long and residues from 870 (in the case of BoNT/A) to the C-terminal end form the receptor binding domain. It consists of two subdomains. The following discussion pertains to BoNT/B. The BoNT/B serotype is chosen here because the high-resolution structure of both the intact holotoxin and the recombinant C-fragment or binding domain are available.[12,16] The N terminal half of the binding domain consists of two 7-stranded antiparallel β sheets sandwiched together to form a 14-stranded β barrel in a jelly roll motif. This particular motif is very similar to that observed in legume lectins, which are also carbohydrate proteins.[17] The C-terminal half of the binding domain contains a β-trefoil motif.[18] The two subdomains are connected by an α-helix. The entire binding domain is tilted away from the translocation domain and makes minimal contact with it. The binding domain of BoNT/B is very similar to the binding domain in holotoxin BoNT/A and the C-fragment of tetanus toxin. The crystal structure of the recombinant C-fragment of BoNT/B is similar to that in holotoxin of B.[16] However, the N-terminal helix is differently oriented in the recombinant protein. This may be an artifact of recombinant protein because the interactions between the translocation domain and this helix is absent in the C-fragment alone. Such a direct comparison of the binding domain in the holotoxin and the individual domain is not possible for A or tetanus toxin because the structure of only one of them is available. Even though the overall sequence homology is weak for all clostridial neurotoxins in the C-terminal half of the binding domain, it is suggested that they would adopt the same fold, with the differences in sequences accounted for by the extended loop regions.[17] This is shown to be valid at least for BoNT/A, and B and the tetanus toxin.

The first stage in botulinum toxicity is the binding of neurotoxin to the presynaptic cell receptors. The clostridial neurotoxins bind first to the large negatively charged surface of the presynaptic membrane, which consists of polysialogangliosides and other acidic lipids.[5] Studies have revealed that neurotoxins bind to di- and trisialogangliosides such as GD1a, GT1b and GD1b.[19,20] But, in order to produce the level of intoxication by such minute concentrations of toxins (subpicomolar), the binding affinity to receptors must be very high. Therefore, a double-receptor model for binding has been proposed.[19] The toxin binds to the negatively charged surface of presynaptic membranes through low-affinity interactions with the polysialogangliosides that are present in high concentrations, and then moves laterally to bind to a protein receptor specific for each serotype. Because the final binding constant is the product of these two binding constants, a very high affinity can be achieved.[19] Different serotypes of BoNT are thought to have different specific protein receptors, and it has been shown that BoNT/B binds to a synaptotagmin protein.[21] The structural studies over the past decade combined with biochemical and mutational analysis of amino acids in the binding domain have given a reliable model for double-receptor binding, which might lead to therapeutics to prevent the toxin binding, thereby blocking the toxicity.

Ganglioside Binding Site

Binding studies have revealed that neurotoxins bind to disialogangliosides and trisialogangliosides. BoNT/B has been shown to bind to GT1b, although with weak affinity. The crystal structure of intact botulinum neurotoxin in complex with sialyllactose, a partial mimic of one branch of GT1b, has mapped the binding region. There are two cavities (site 1 and site 2, Fig. 2-2) at the C-terminal half of the binding domain of all clostridial toxins, based on known structures. In BoNT/B, Site 1 is formed by residues Glu1188, Glu1189, His 1240, and Tyr 1262 and sialyllactose binds to this side. Accordingly, it was identified as the ganglioside binding site for all clostridial neurotoxins (Fig. 2-3). Site 2 is formed by residues Gly 1118, Trp 1177, Try 1180, Try 1184, Phe 1193, Leu 1194, Ile 1197, Pro 1196, and Asp1199.[22] In the sialyllactose-BoNT/B complex structure, this site was unoccupied.[12]

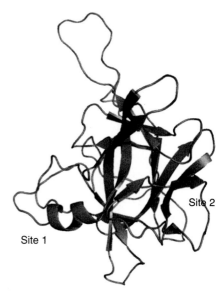

FIGURE 2-2. The C-terminal domain of the receptor binding domain of botulinum neurotoxin B forms a β-trefoil fold. The trefoil domain forms a subdomain of the binding domain, and both ganglioside and the protein receptor bind to this subdomain. The two binding sites are marked as site 1 and site 2, and will form the binding sites for ganglioside and protein receptor. *See Color Plate*

The location of site 2 with respect to 1 also ruled out the possibility that the second branch of GT1b sugar could occupy that site. Accordingly, it was concluded that the binding site for GT1b sugar is site 1 in BoNT/B and by extension in other serotypes.

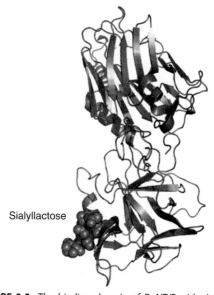

FIGURE 2-3. The binding domain of BoNT/B with sialyllactose at site 1. Sialyllactose is shown in sphere model. This binding site also validated most of the mutagenesis studies. *See Color Plate*

However, sugar complexes with TeNT binding domain suggested that they could bind to both the sites. Gt1b binds to TeNT also. Owing to technical difficulties in using GT1b sugar, the structure of TeNT binding domain in complex with a GT1b analog was determined.[23,24] Interestingly, the synthetic GT1b molecule binds to both sites and acts as a cross-linker between TeNT binding domains. This scenario is totally different from that observed for BoNT. Accordingly, although there is only one binding site for BoNT, there are two for TeNT. Later, this has been shown to be true with mass spectroscopy and mutational analysis of BoNT and TeNT.[25,26] It was also suggested from mass spectrum analysis that although both sites are required for TeNT binding, the ganglioside molecule bound to site 2 may be displaced by a receptor protein.[22]

Protein Receptor Binding Site

The crystal structure of TeNT binding domain with disialyllactose or a tripeptide (Tyr-Glu-Trp) later showed that both of them bind at site 2. Disialyllactose (the GD3 sugar moiety) forms one branch of GT1b oligosaccharide (Fig. 2-4). Also, we found that these two compete for binding, and the tripeptide binds with greater affinity. This prompted us to suggest that in TeNT, the ganglioside bound to this site may be replaced by the protein receptor, which has much higher affinity than ganglioside.[22] We further suggested that in BoNT, site 2, which is not occupied by ganglioside, will be the site for the receptor protein.

Double Receptor Mode

Interestingly, this was proved to be right by two exquisite structures of BoNT/B in complex with a short polypeptide corresponding to the luminal part of synaptotagmin, a receptor protein for BoNT/B.[27,28] It has been shown that the SYT-II peptide binds at site 2, as suggested previously[22] (Fig. 2-5). However, the residues in BoNT/B at this site are hydrophobic, whereas they are hydrophilic in TeNT.[27] Nevertheless, the structures taken together have identified the binding sites for gangliosides and the protein receptor, and support the double-receptor model proposed by Montecucco.[19] In addition to providing experimental evidence for the double-receptor model, these structures may also help in identifying small molecules to block either the ganglioside, the protein receptor, or both.

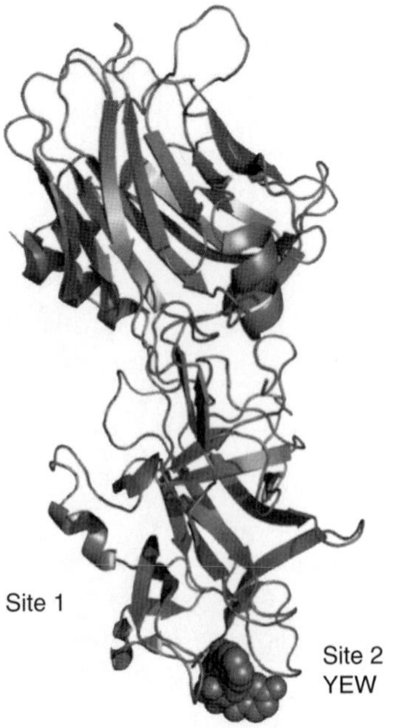

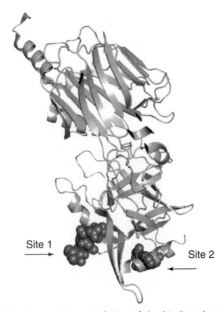

FIGURE 2-4. Binding domain of tetanus toxin with a tripeptide (Tyr-Glu-Trp) bound at site 2. The tripeptide is shown in sphere model. The orientation is similar to that shown in Figure 2-3. *See Color Plate*

FIGURE 2-5. A composite figure of the binding domain of BoNT/B with sialyllactose and the tripetide as it is bound in tetanus (both shown in sphere model). The helical fragment of Syt II from Chai et al. is superposed.[27] The helical fragment occupies the same place as the tripeptide in tetanus. This strongly supports our earlier prediction that site 2 may be the site where the receptor protein would bind. *See Color Plate*

Drug Design With the Receptor Binding Domain as a Therapeutic Target

Structural and computational docking work on BoNT/B has already shown that doxorubicin can be used to block gangliosides.[29,30] However, the BoNT/B-doxorubicin complex structure showed that the orientation of doxorubicin is different from that predicted by docking studies.[29,30] This underscores the importance of crystallographic study for understanding the interactions of drug molecules with toxins (Fig. 2-6). Even though the affinity of doxorubicin to neurotoxins may not be strong, it certainly presents itself as a strong lead compound because a number of analogs of doxorubicin have already been synthesized and may present a better candidate.[31] With the knowledge that doxorubicin competes with gangliosides to bind to the toxin and the mechanism is similar to ganglioside binding, it would be a potential lead compound for drug design to treat botulism caused by type B (and G). Although catalytic domain remains an attractive target for botulinum therapeutics, binding domain now can be used as an additional or alternative target because both the ganglioside and protein receptor binding sites have been identified.

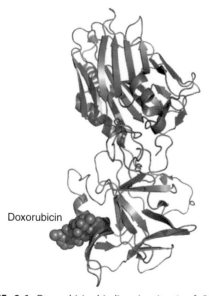

Doxorubicin

FIGURE 2-6. Doxorubicin binding in site 1 of BoNT/B. Sialyllactose, a mimic of GT1b, binds in the same site. Also, doxorubicin has been shown to compete with gangliosides for binding to this site. The fact that it competes with gangliosides or displaces sialyllactose (during crystallization) shows that this site can be blocked and used for drug design. *See Color Plate*

Translocation Domain

To attack the targets in the cytosol, the catalytic domain must cross the hydrophobic barrier of the vesicle membrane. The acidification of the vesicle lumen by a proton-pumping ATPase leads to pH-dependent conformational changes in the toxin. The acidic conformation then exposes a hydrophobic area of the toxin molecule, creates an ion channel in the membrane, and translocates the L chain into the cytosol.[1,6,32,33] It has been shown that the translocation domain forms channels in lipid vesicles, but its role on the neuroparalytic activity was unclear.[34] The heavy chain forms channels in planar phospholipid bilayers also, and the channel formation has been visualized.[35,36] It is still not clear how these channels are formed or whether oligomerization of the toxin is required. Even if such a channel is created, it is unclear whether it can translocate the 50-kDa light chain without unfolding it. The size of the pore formed by BoNT/B heavy chain has been estimated to be about 8-15 Å.[37,38] It has been suggested that the light chain might unfold and thread through the created channel and then refold in the cytosol.[39] It has been suggested that BoNT heavy chain acts as chaperone for the L chain, allowing it to enter through the membrane[38]; recent findings on this topic are detailed in Chapter 4.

In the holotoxin this domain consists of two long α-helices, each about 105 Å long, forming a coiled coil. Two kinks in the coiled coil split the helices into four, each ~50 Å long. The core of the translocation domain consists of four-helical bundle at one end and a three-helical bundle on the other. Attempts are under way to study the mechanism of translocation and pore formation via challenging structural work, but not much progress has been made.

Catalytic Domain

The N-terminal one third of botulinum neurotoxin corresponds to the catalytic domain. In the holotoxin, the catalytic domain and the rest of the molecule (heavy chain consisting of the binding and translocation domains) are held together by a disulfide bridge. This interchain disulfide bond is essential for translocation of catalytic domain into cytosol and for toxicity[38,40]; its eventual reduction precedes release of the L chain. The translocated catalytic domain cleaves a specific target of the soluble

N-ethylmaleimide-sensitive factor attachment protein receptor (SNARE) complex in the cytosol. The L chains of BoNTs and TeNT contain a HEXXH+E sequence identified as a zinc-binding motif in other zinc endopeptidases.

The inhibition of exocytosis in the cytosol involves the zinc-dependent proteolysis of specific components of the neuroexocytosis apparatus: BoNT/B, D, F, and G specifically cleave the vesicle-associated membrane protein (VAMP, also called synaptobrevin); BoNT/A and E cleave a synaptosomal associated protein of 25 kDa (SNAP-25) by specific hydrolysis, although at different places, and BoNT/C is unique and cleaves both syntaxin and SNAP-25.[41-48] Söllner et al[49] have shown that these proteins together form the SNARE complex responsible for mediating vesicle docking and fusion. The formation of this complex is inhibited by the BoNT-catalyzed proteolysis of any one of the components; although some BoNT-cleaved SNAREs can also form complexes, truncation by the toxins of their targets blocks vesicle fusion and thereby inhibits exocytosis (see Chapter 1).

Structurally, the catalytic domain is a compact globular domain consisting of a mixture of α-helices and β sheets and strands (Fig. 2-7). The active site zinc is bound deep inside a large open cavity that has a high negative electrostatic potential. The zinc ion is coordinated by two histidines in the same α-helix and a glutamate from a different α-helix. The fourth coordination is provided by a water molecule that acts as a nucleophile during the hydrolysis of the target protein. This arrangement is very similar to that in thermolysin and carboxypeptidase, which are also zinc endopeptidases.[41,50,51] The water molecule makes strong hydrogen bond contacts with the carboxylate side chain of Glu in the HEXXH motif. This Glu is conserved in all Clostridium neurotoxins and is suggested to act as a base for catalytic action.

The structures for the catalytic domain of all serotypes are now available.[52-59] The fold is similar and agrees within experimental errors (1.6 Å between C-α atoms). However, there are differences in the loop regions. These loop regions also differ from their conformation in the holotoxin. For example, there are three loop regions called 50 loop, 200 loop, and 250 loop.[59] They change their conformation dramatically in the catalytic domain structures because they lose interactions with the translocation domain. These changes also help in catalytic action. In addition to the similarity in fold, there are other remarkable similarities that suggest that the catalytic mechanism of all these serotypes is similar.

About 40 to 45 residues are present within a sphere of radius of 10 Å centered on the zinc atom. A few interactions are common to all of them, and they all involve conserved residues across serotypes (Fig. 2-8). The sequence numbers corresponding to BoNT/E are used in the

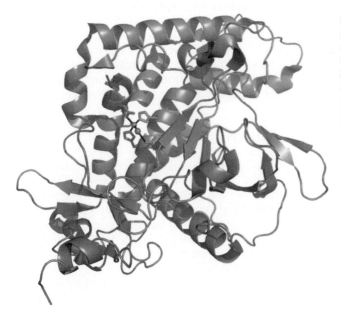

FIGURE 2-7. The catalytic domain of BoNT/E shown in ribbons representation. The active site residues, zinc, and the nucleophilic water are shown in ball and stick model. In BoNT/E, the zinc is coordinated by His211, His215, Glu250, and the nucleophilic water. Glu212, which acts as a base for catalytic action, is hydrogen bonded to the nucleophilic water. This arrangement is similar in all BoNTs. *See Color Plate*

```
BXC1_CLOBO    MPITINNFNYSDPVDNKNILYLDTHLNTLANEPEKAFRITGNIWVIPDRFSRNSNPNLNK 60
BXD_CLOBO     MTWPVKDFNYSDPVNDNDILYLRIPQNKLITTPVKAFMITQNIWVIPERFSSDTNPSLSK 60
BXB_CLOBO     MPVTINNFNYNDPIDNNNIIMMEPPFARGTGRYYKAFKITDRIWIIPERYTFGYKPEDFN 60
BXG_CLOBO     MPVNIKXFNYNDPINNDDIIMMEPFNDPGPGTYYKAFRIIDRIWIVPERFTYGFQPDQFN 60
BXE_CLOBO     MP-KINSFNYNDPVNDRTILYIKP---GGCQEFYKSFNIMKNIWIIPERNVIGTTPQDFH 56
BXF_CLOBO     MPVAINSFNYNDPVNDDTILYMQIPYEEKSKKYYKAFEIMRNVWIIPERNTIGTNPSDFD 60
BXA1_CLOBO    MPFVNKQFNYKDPVNGVDIAYIKIP-NVGQMQPVKAFKIHNKIWVIPERDTFTNPEEGDL 59
              *.   :  ***.**::.  *   :    *:* *  .:*::*:*          .

BXC1_CLOBO    PPRVTSPKSG--YYDPNYLSTDSDKDPFLKEIIKLFKRINSREIGEELIYRLSTDIPFPG 118
BXD_CLOBO     PPRPTSKYQS--YYDPSYLSTDEQKDTFLKGIIKLFKRINERDIGKKLINYLVVGSPFMG 118
BXB_CLOBO     KSSGIFNRDVCEYYDPDYLNTNDKKNIFLQTMIKLFNRIKSKPLGEKLLEMIINGIPYLG 120
BXG_CLOBO     ASTGVFSKDVYEYYDPTYLKTDAEKDKFLKTMIKLFNRINSKPSGQRLLDMIVDAIPYLG 120
BXE_CLOBO     PPTSLKNGDS-SYYDPNYLQSDEEKDRFLKIVTKIFNRINNNLSGGILLEELSKANPYLG 115
BXF_CLOBO     PPASLKNGSS-AYYDPNYLTTDAEKDRYLKTTIKLFKRINSNPAGKVLLQEISYAKPYLG 119
BXA1_CLOBO    NPPPEAKQVPVSYYDSTYLSTDNEKDNYLKGVTKLFERIYSTDLGRMLLTSIVRGIPFWG 119
                       ***. **  ::  .*: :*:    *:*:**   .   *:    *: *

BXC1_CLOBO    NNNTPINTFDFDVDFNSVDVKTRQGNNWVKTGSINPSVIITGPRENIIDPETSTFKLTNN 178
BXD_CLOBO     DSSTPEDTFDFTRHTTNIAVEKFENGSWKVTNIITPSVLIFGPLPNILDYTASLTLQGGQ 178
BXB_CLOBO     DRRVPLEEFNTNIASVTVNKLISNPGEVERKKGIFANLIIFGPGPVLNENETIDIGIQNH 180
BXG_CLOBO     NASTPPDKFAANVANVSINKKIIQPGAEDQIKGLMTNLIIFGPGPVLSDNFTDSMIMNGH 180
BXE_CLOBO     NDNTPDNQFH-IGDASAVEIKFSN----GSQDILLPNVIIMGAEPDLFETNSSNISLRNN 170
BXF_CLOBO     NDHTPIDEFSPVTRTTSVNIKLST----NVESSMLLNLLVLGAGPDIFESCCYPVRKLID 175
BXA1_CLOBO    G--STIDTELKVIDTNCINVIQPD----GSYRSEELNLVIIGPSADIIQFECKSFGHEVL 173
                .     .  :             :         .:::  *.    :  : 

BXC1_CLOBO    ----TFAAQEGFGALSIISISPRFMLTYSNATNDVGEGRFSKSEFCMDPILILMHELNHA 234
BXD_CLOBO     ----SNPSFEGFGTLSILKVAPEFLLTFSDVTSNQSSAVLGKSIFCMDPVIALMHELTHS 234
BXB_CLOBO     -----FASREGFGGIMQMKFCPEYVSVFNNVQENKGASIFNRRGYFSDPALILMHELIHV 235
BXG_CLOBO     -----SPISEGFGARMMIRFCPSCLNVFNNVQENKDTSIFSRRAYFADPALTLMHELIHV 235
BXE_CLOBO     ----YMPSNHRFGSIAIVTFSPEYSFRFNDN---------CMNEFIQDPALTLMHELIHS 217
BXF_CLOBO     PDVVYDPSNYGFGSINIVTFSPEYEYTFNDISGGHNS---STESFIADPAISLAHELIHA 232
BXA1_CLOBO    N-----LTRNGYGSTQYIRFSPDFTFGFEESLEVDTNPLLGAGKFATDPAVTLAHELIHA 228
                   :*    :  ..*     :.:         :   ** : * *** *

BXC1_CLOBO    MHNLYGIAIPNDQTISSVTSNIFYSQYNVKLEYAEIYAFGGPTIDLIPKSARKYFEEKAL 294
BXD_CLOBO     LHQLYGINIPSDKRIRPQVSEGFFSQDGPNVQFEELYTFGGLDVEIIPQIERSQLREKAL 294
BXB_CLOBO     LHGLYGIK-VDDLPIVPNEKKFFMQSTDA-IQAEELYTFGGQDPSIITPSTDKSIYDKVL 293
BXG_CLOBO     LHGLYGIK-ISNLPITPNTKEFFMQHSDP-VQAEELYTFGGHDPSVISPSTDMNIYNKAL 293
BXE_CLOBO     LHGLYGAKGITTKYTITQKQNPLITNIRG-TNIEEFLTFGGTDLNIITSAQSNDIYTNLL 276
BXF_CLOBO     LHGLYGARGVTYEETIEVKQAPLMIAEKP-IRLEEFLTFGGQDLNIITSAMKEKIYNNLL 291
BXA1_CLOBO    GHRLYGIAINPNR-VFKVNTNAYYEMSGLEVSFEELRTFGGHDAKFIDSLQENEFRLYYY 287
              *  ***    *:          :  : ::**   ..*

BXC1_CLOBO    DYYRSIAKRLNSITTANPSSFNKYIGEYKQKLIRKYRFVVESSGEVTVNRNKFVELYNEL 354
BXD_CLOBO     GHYKDIAKRLNNINKTIPSSWISNIDKYKKIFSEKYNFDKDNTGNFVVNIDKFNSLYSDL 354
BXB_CLOBO     QNFRGIVDRLNKV-LVCISDPNININIYKNKFKDKYKFVEDSEGKYSIDVESFDKLYKSL 352
BXG_CLOBO     QNFQDIANRLN-I-VSSAQGSGIDISLYKQIYKNKYDFVEDPNGKYSVDKDKFDKLYKAL 351
BXE_CLOBO     ADYKKIASKLS---KVQVSNPL--LNPYKDVFEAKYGLDKDASGIYSVNINKFNDIFKKL 331
BXF_CLOBO     ANYEKIATRLS---EVNSAPPEYDINEYKDYFQWKYGLDKNADGSYTVNENKFNEIYKKL 348
BXA1_CLOBO    NKFKDIASTLN--KAKSIVGTTASLQYMKNVFKEKYLLSEDTSGKFSVDKLKFDKLYKML 345
              :. *. *.          :    *.   ** :  **   :  ::  .* .::. *

BXC1_CLOBO    TQIFTEFNYAKIYNVQNRKIYLSNVYTPVTAN-ILDDNVYDIQNGFNIPKSNLNVLFMGQ 413
BXD_CLOBO     TNVMSEVVYSSQYNVKNRTHYFSRHYLPVFAN-ILDDNIYTIRDGFNLTNKGFNIENSGQ 413
BXB_CLOBO     MFGFTETNIAENYKIKTRASYFSDSLPPVKIKNLLDNEIYTIEEGFNISDKDMEKEYRGQ 412
BXG_CLOBO     MFGFTETNLAGEYGIKTRYSYFSEYLPPIKTEKLLDNTIYTQNEGFNIASKNLKTEFNGQ 411
BXE_CLOBO     YS-FTEFDLRTKFQVKCRQTYIGQYKY-FKLSNLLNDSIYNISEGYNIN--NLKVNFRGQ 387
BXF_CLOBO     YS-FTESDLANKFKVKCRNTYFIKYEF-LKVPNLLDDDIYTVSEGFNIG--NLAVNNRGQ 404
BXA1_CLOBO    TEIYTEDNFVKFFKVLNRKTYLNFDKAVFKIN-IVPKVNYTIYDGFNLRNTNLAANFNGQ 404
              :*.  :   : .       :: .  *  .  :*:*:.  .: ..  **

BXC1_CLOBO    NLSRNP-ALRKVN-PENMLYLFTKFCHKAIDGRSLYNK---------------------- 449
BXD_CLOBO     NIERNP-ALQKLS-SESVVDLFTKVCLRLTK----------------------------- 442
BXB_CLOBO     NKAINKQAYEEIS-KEHLAVYKIQMCKSVK----------------------------- 441
BXG_CLOBO     NKAVNKEAYEEIS-LEHLVIYRIAMCKPVMYK---------------------------- 442
BXE_CLOBO     NANLNPRIITPIT-GRGLVKKIIRFCKNIVSVKGIR------------------------ 422
BXF_CLOBO     SIKLNPKIIDSIP-DKGLVEKIVKFCKSVIPRK--------------------------- 436
BXA1_CLOBO    NTEINNMNFTKLKNFTGLFEFYKLLCVRGIITSKTKSLDKGYNK--------------- 448
              .        *       :    :   .   *
```

FIGURE 2-8. ClustalW[84] alignment of the seven serotypes of botulinum neurotoxins (only the catalytic domain is shown). The HEXXH+E motif and the conserved residues shown in Figure 2-9 are highlighted in gray. Identical residues are marked with '*', semiconserved residues with ':' and less conserved with '.'. Variable residues have no marking.

following discussion because high-resolution structures are available for both wild type and several mutants. However, the analysis is applicable to other serotypes.[53,60] BoNT/E-LC and its mutant structures all contain two monomers per asymmetric unit. In most cases, the conformation and architecture are similar except where noted. The side chain carboxylate of Glu 212 makes strong hydrogen bonds with the nucleophilic water coordinated to zinc. Glu 335 makes hydrogen bonding contacts with Arg 347 and His 211. Glu 249 interacts with His 215 and His 218, stabilizing the structure and electrostatic forces. These interactions stabilize the side chain conformations of His 211 and 215, allowing them to be properly oriented for zinc coordination. Because these residues are conserved in all serotypes, their role may be the same in all of them. Arg 347 and Tyr 350 are in the active-site region and are similarly placed in all of them with respect to zinc and the nucleophilic water (Fig. 2-9). Mutational analyses of these conserved residues have identified the extent to which they are involved in the catalytic mechanism.

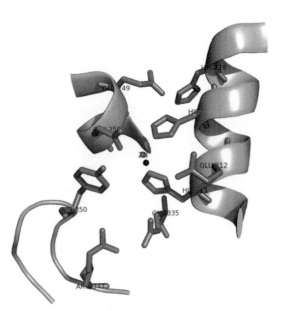

FIGURE 2-9. Active site residues and other conserved residues that play an important role in catalytic activity are shown. Here, BoNT/E is shown as a representative structure. The conserved residues shown are His211, Glu212, His215, His218, Glu249, Glu250, Glu335, Arg347, and Tyr350. The effects of mutation of most of them are discussed in the text.

Correlation of Mutational and Structural Analysis

Here we will correlate the structural analysis of various mutants of the residues discussed earlier in BoNT/E with their role in catalytic action. Results from similar mutational analysis on other serotypes and tetanus toxin show that these results are valid for all serotypes.[53,60-63] When Arg 347 was mutated to Ala, the general conformation of the active site remained the same. Because Arg 347 makes a salt bridge with Glu 335, which, in turn, is hydrogen bonded to His 211 and keeps it in proper orientation for zinc coordination, it was thought the disruption of the salt bridge might affect the architecture. But the only change was that the nucleophilic water moved away from zinc ion. The crystal structure of Tyr350Ala mutant showed some interesting features.[60] As in the case of Arg347Ala, the conformation of the active site remains the same. In one of the monomers, the nucleophilic water moves away from zinc, as in the case of Arg347Ala structure. Interestingly, in one monomer (molecule A), the nucleophilic water is replaced by a sulfate ion similar to what was observed in the holotoxin structure of BoNT/B.[12] Although this may be an artifact of crystallization, the results reiterated our

original suggestion that the sulfate ion represents the tetrahedral transition state of the carbonyl carbon of the scissile bond.[64] As discussed later, this helped in modeling the catalytic mechanism of botulinum neurotoxins. The activity for both Arg347Ala and Tyr350Ala is multifold less than for the wild type and almost not detectable. In Glu212Gln mutant structure, the hydrogen bonding interactions with the water coordinated to zinc are completely lost. Moreover, the electrostatic distribution near the active site has changed from highly negative to neutral. This results in the loss of activity of Glu212Gln. The Glu335Gln mutant structure showed another interesting feature. The active site zinc was not present in both the monomers causing ~7000 fold less activity than the wild type. Glu 335 forms a bridge between Arg 347 and His 211 in the wild type. These interactions are much weaker in Glu335Gln, and the orientation of His 211 has changed. This also results in the original nucleophilic water moving away. Although the conformation was not affected, the activity was lost. This study showed that Glu335Gln is an apo enzyme and underscored the role of zinc in catalytic activity.[60]

The Role of Zinc—Is It Structural or Catalytic?

The role of zinc has been extensively analyzed in BoTNs. Although it has been suggested to be structural, it has now been shown unequivocally that it is catalytic.[65,66] BoNT/B structure determined at pH 4.0 was devoid of zinc, but the architecture of the active site was not altered. A similar observation was also made when zinc was removed by treating BoNT/B with ethylenediaminetetraacetic acid (EDTA).[65] It has also been shown later with BoNT/E with one of its mutants that had lost zinc because of mutation.[60] Recently, the structure of BoNT/A catalytic domain treated with EDTA has been determined.[67] The active site was not perturbed by the removal of zinc. Simpson et al.[68] have shown that while Zn stripped neurotoxins are inactive in cell free assays, they are active against intact neuromuscular junction since internalized toxin presumably binds to cytosolic zinc.

Modeling the Transition State

BoNTs and thermolysin share a similar HEXXH+E motif, and both are zinc endopeptidase. The active site residues and the coordination geometry of zinc are also similar. Thermolysin has been studied extensively, and a large number of structures with transition state analogs are available for thermolysin. The superposition of Tyr350Ala (of BoNT/E-LC) with bound sulfate ion on the structure of thermolysin-inhibitor complex model shows an interesting similarity.[60] The sulfate ion superimposes on the phosphate ion of the inhibitor very well and has similar interactions. The sulfate ion mimics the transitional tetrahedral geometry of the scissile bond carbonyl carbon, as in the case of BoNT/B structure with sulfate ion.[12,64] The sulfur atom of sulfate ion imitates the carbonyl carbon of the scissile bond (Fig. 2-10). O1 and O3 of the sulfate ion at distances 2.40 and 2.61 Å from zinc, respectively, and mimic the positions of scissile peptide bond carbonyl oxygen and the displaced nucleophilic water. The O3 of sulfate makes hydrogen bonds with Glu212 OE1 and OE2 at 2.80 and 2.53 Å, respectively, and the O1 of sulfate with Glu250 OE1 at distance 2.84 Å. O4 of the sulfate represents the amide nitrogen of the scissile bond, which is in hydrogen bonding distance to Glu159 O as in thermolysin.

Based on the model of thermolysin with its inhibitors, it was proposed that Tyr350 and Arg347 interact with the carbonyl oxygens of P1 and P1′ of the substrate (here SNAP-25).[60] When these interactions are not available, the catalytic activity is affected. This model could not be directly compared with the BoNT/A-SNAP-25 complex. Although this complex structure helped in identifying the exosites, because the enzyme was a double mutant and an inactive form, some of the relevant interactions with the substrate near the active site are lost, specifically the interaction between Tyr and the substrate.[69] The P1 and P1′ of the substrate SNAP-25 peptide is bulging and not very close to the active site. The electron density in that region was also weak. For example, since Tyr has been mutated to Phe, the interaction between its OH group and the substrate is lost. In this structure, the scissile bond carbonyl oxygen is >6.5 Å away from zinc instead of 3.6 Å or so due to the absence of Tyr required for stabilization of the substrate.[69] It has recently been suggested that residues from Arg198 to Leu203 of the substrate complex structure may not represent the true conformation of the active complex.[70] Or it may be that the inactive mutant-substrate complex may not provide a realistic picture of the active site interaction. The overall comparison suggests that the substrate docking at the active site as well as the orientation of the peptide bond may be similar in all BoNTs and tetanus neurotoxin, even though the substrate and scissile bonds are different.

Our prediction that Tyr350 OH and Arg347 NH2 hydrogen bond with the carbonyl oxygens of P1 and P1′ has been recently shown to be valid.[67] In the crystal structure BoNT/A-LC in complex with arginine hydroxamate, the carbonyl oxygen and the hydroxamate oxygen coordinate with zinc. Also, the carbonyl oxygen makes a hydrogen bond (3.31 Å) with Tyr366 OH. However, there is no interaction with Arg363 because the inhibitor here is a single peptide and lacks the scissile bond. These interactions are absent in BaNT/A-LC:SNAP-25 peptide complex, probably because the enzyme is an inactive double mutant. Similar interactions are also observed in BoNT/A-LC structure in complex with a small molecule inhibitor.[71] In a recent structure from our laboratory with a tetrapeptide that binds tightly at the active site, we see hydrogen bonds from side chains of Tyr366 and Arg363 with P1 and P1′ carbonyl oxygens validating our previous models.[71a] This also supports the hypothesis that Tyr366 and Arg363 are required for the stabilization of substrate to position it for peptide bond cleavage and explains the lack of activity

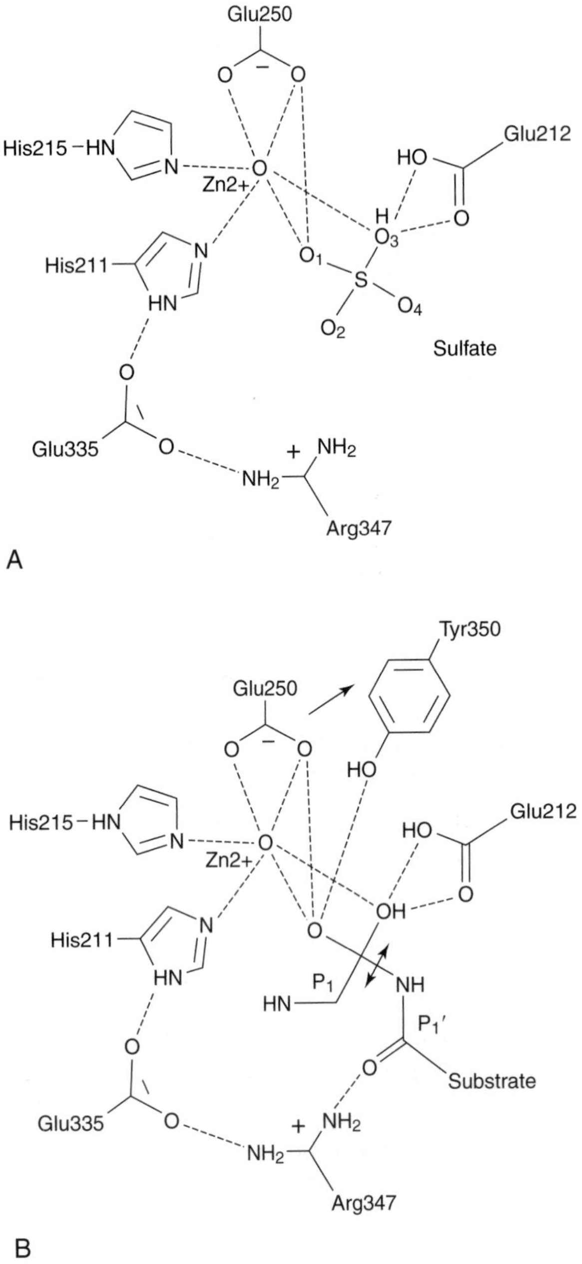

FIGURE 2-10. Proposed docking of substrate at the active site based on the interactions of the sulfate ion bound to the Tyr350 mutant molecule A (BoNT/E) and inhibitor bound thermolysin (2TMN). **A,** O1 of the sulfate ion at a distance of 2.4 Å from zinc corresponds to the carbonyl oxygen of the scissile bond (P1), whereas O3 corresponds to the nucleophilic water, which moves closer to Glu212 but still interacts with zinc. O2 and O4 will correspond to the Cα and scissile bond nitrogen. Thus, the sulfate ion mimics the tetrahedral transition state of the substrate. **B,** Proposed interactions of the carbonyl oxygens of P1 and P1' of the substrate during catalytic pathway. Tyr350 OH interacts with P1 carbonyl oxygen while Arg347 NH2 hydrogen bonds, with P1' stabilizing the substrate docking. An arrow mark between Glu250 and Tyr350 represents the anion-aromatic interaction. The scissile bond is marked with a double-headed arrow mark. (Reprinted from Agarwal R, Binz T, Swaminathan S. Analysis of active site residues of botulinum neurotoxin E by mutational, functional and structural studies: Glu335Gln is an apoenzyme. *Biochemistry.* 2005;44:8291-8302.)

when these two are mutated to alanine. Based on this information, we propose a common model for the catalytic mechanism of all serotypes and tetanus toxin.

Mechanism of Catalytic Activity of Botulinum Neurotoxins

These observations taken together with the movement of nucleophilic water gives a model for the catalytic activity and the importance of the nucleophilic water and Glu 212.

It is evident that Glu 212 helps the leaving group by transferring/shuttling two protons from the nucleophilic water. Our model here is consistent with what we had proposed for BoNT/B.[64] Carbonyl oxygen of the scissile bond is polarized by the nucleophilic water, which moves closer to Glu 212 but still maintains interaction with zinc. The transition tetrahedral state of the carbonyl carbon is stabilized by Arg 347 and Tyr 350. Protons are shuttled to the leaving group in two stages.

The crystal structure of BoNT/B-LC with substrate peptide has also provided a model for the catalytic mechanism in which Tyr372 (corresponding to Tyr350 in BoNT/E) is presumed to provide a proton to the leaving group.[59] The crystal structures of holo-BoNT/B with and without a sulfate ion at the active site have also provided a model for the catalytic mechanism and the presumed transition state.[64] In our model, the proton is shuttled by Glu230 to the leaving group and is similar to what is proposed for thermolysin. But it is clear from our published and unpublished structures that this Tyr is not in proper orientation with respect to the leaving nitrogen to donate a proton for the leaving group (Fig. 2-11). This scenario is slightly in variance with that proposed for TeNT, in which the corresponding tyrosine is suggested to be the proton donor.[63] It may be that the scheme is somewhat different for TeNT from BoNTs or that it needs further investigation. This is a classic example as how structural, mutational, and biochemical data can come together to arrive at the functional mechanism of an enzyme.

Catalytic Domain as a Target for Botulinum Therapeutics

Structural work on the catalytic domain in complex with substrate peptide and small molecules has given an impetus to use the catalytic domain as a target for drug discovery for BoNTs.[67,69,71-73] One important consideration in designing drugs using the catalytic domain as a target is their side effects. Because BoNTs are zinc endopeptidases, the effect of inhibiting them on other zinc peptidases that are essential for other biologic functions is a concern. The BoNT/A-SNAP-25 complex shows that in addition to the active site, the exosites can be used for blocking the toxicity. In this section, the structural and biochemical work leading to strategies for developing effective inhibitors will be discussed.

Traditional drug discovery begins with a lead molecule that is known to act as an inhibitor from biochemical studies. But high-speed computers and advanced computer algorithms have allowed millions of compounds to be screened in a high throughput manner before biochemical screening is even attempted.

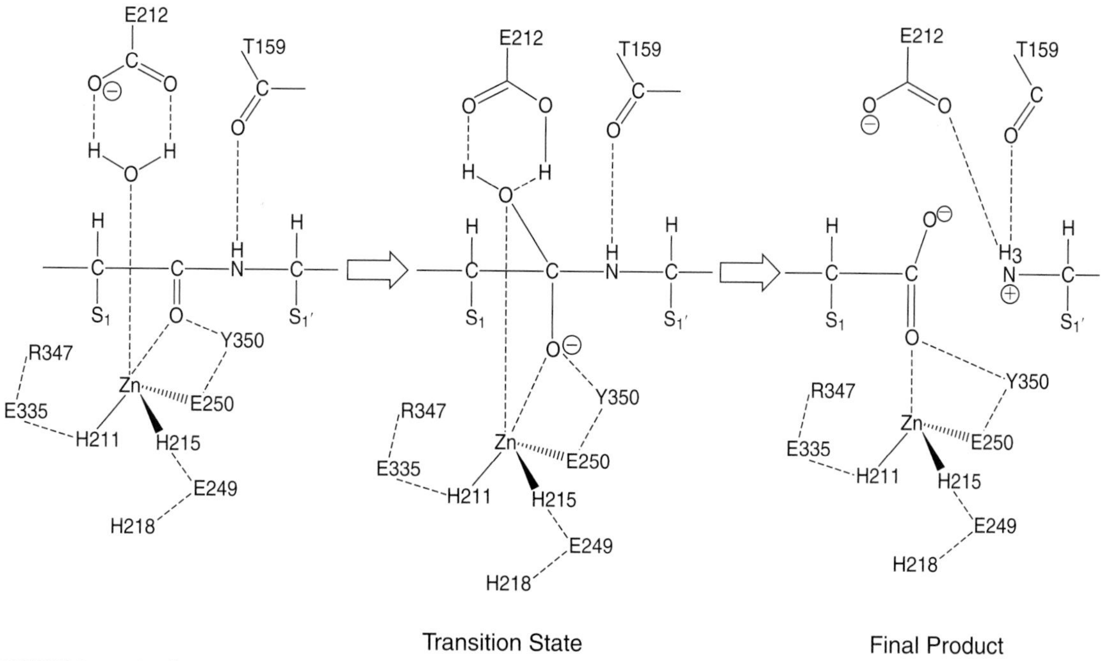

Transition State   Final Product

FIGURE 2-11. Catalytic pathway model for BoNT/E-LC based on our present and previous results. Glu212 serves as a general base for the catalytic activity and shuttles two protons to the leaving group. His218, Glu249, Glu335, Arg347, and Tyr350 stabilizing the orientation of the histidines or the transition state are also shown along with Thr159. Although experimental evidence for the role of Glu249 and His218 is not yet available, Thr159 is included here in analogy with our work on BoNT/B.[64] S1 and S1' are Arg180 and Ile181 of SNAP-25. Hydrogen bond interactions and anion-aromatic interaction (Tyr350–Glu250) are shown in dashed lines. (Reprinted from Agarwal R, Eswaramoorthy S, Kumaran D, Binz T, Swaminathan S. Structural analysis of botulinum neurotoxin type E catalytic domain and its mutant Glu212->Gln reveals the pivotal role of the Glu212 carboxylate in the catalytic pathway. *Biochemistry.* 2004;43:6637-6644.)

Potential molecules are first selected and then modified to produce first- and second-generation drug compounds. The success of this method is also due to high-resolution structures that are being determined. Several groups are now working with the available structures of BoNT catalytic domains to develop efficient drugs. Kim Janda has been working on BoNT/A and has come up with a number of lead molecules.[74-77] One such molecule is arginine hydroxamate, which inhibits the catalytic activity at the micromolar level. In this study, the inhibitor molecule was cocrystallized with a mutant of BoNT/A (Arg363Ala/Tyr366Phe). The carbonyl and N hydroxyl oxygens bound to the zinc, and the arginine submoiety was positioned at the S1' site. However, this work was done with a mutant, as in the case of BoNT/A-SNAP-25 peptide. Karen Allen's group have recently repeated this work with the wild type and have shown that the interactions are similar. Based on this complex structure and the knowledge derived from that study, two inhibitors have been designed and the structures of inhibitor—enzyme complexes have been determined by Allen's group. They have identified two compounds, 4-chlorocinnamic hydroxamate and 2,4-dichlorocinnamic hydroxamate, both very potent inhibitors. The second compound has IC50 in the nanomolar range.

Bavari et al. have taken a different approach to identifying potent inhibitors, They have started with short peptides (e.g., CRATKML) and combined the information from crystal structures of the wild-type and substrate complex using molecular dynamics. Combining molecular dynamics, docking, and visual inspection and manual adjustments, they have identified the pharmacaphore at the active site. Using this information with virtual screening of selected compounds, they have arrived at a few potent inhibitors.[70,72,78-80]

In our laboratory, we are combining our structural information with virtual screening of small molecules from different libraries. In addition, we are also using known peptidic inhibitors to identify pharmacaphores and to use this for the design of potent drugs. We have also shown in the case of bis(5-amidino-2-benzimidazolyl) methane (BABIM), how it could bind to the enzyme at the active site of BoNT/B.[73] In summary, the structural studies on BoNTs have helped in understanding the mechanism of action of this toxins and also in the drug discovery program.

Metal Ions as Inhibitors

Simpson et al.[81] have shown that the catalytic activity could be inhibited by mercury ions because they might attach to thiol groups of cysteine residues near the active site. In BoNT/A, there is one cysteine close to the active site zinc, whereas there are two consecutive cysteines in BoNT/F.[52] We have shown that the mercury ion binds to Cys 364, which is closer to Arg 365 in BoNT/F (Swaminathan, unpublished). Recently, the cocrystal structure of BoNT/A-LC with silver ion shows that it binds to one of the histidines in HEXXH motif thereby disrupting the zinc coordination (Pdb id: 2G7N). It has also been shown that mercury compounds in general inhibit the activity of BoNT/A.[82] Further work is needed to exploit this possibility.

Feasibility of Designing a Set of Common Inhibitors for a Majority of Serotypes of Botulinum Neurotoxins

As of now, the structures of catalytic domains of most of the serotypes of BoNTs and tetanus neurotoxin have been determined. The structures show remarkable similarity, especially near the active site. We have shown that residues within 10 Å radius from the active site zinc are conserved in all of them and the interactions between the active site residues are also maintained in all structures.[60] Comparison of the active sites of these shows that the active site geometry is similar and superimposable. Because the geometry and the sequence are conserved, it is possible to design or identify a common inhibitor that will have similar interaction with the protein residues of all serotypes leading to a common drug. Variations in and around the active site may be responsible for the specificity of substrates. As long as the active site zinc is blocked, it should be possible to block the catalytic activity. These small molecule inhibitors may be better than substrate-based peptide inhibitors because they are not serotype specific. However, it has also been pointed out that subtype variability within a serotype may affect the broad spectrum of small molecule ligands.[83]

CONCLUSIONS

In summary, the structural work on BoNT and its individual fragments has provided ample information on the molecular mechanism of this family of toxins. This information coupled with virtual screening and biochemical work will lead to the development of effective therapeutics against this deadly poison.

ACKNOWLEDGMENTS

This research was supported by the U.S Army Medical Research Acquisition Activity (Award No. DAMD17-02-2-011) and Defense Threat Reduction Agency BO742081 under DOE prime contract No. DE-AC02-98CH10886 with Brookhaven National Laboratory. The author is thankful to Drs. Eswaramoorthy, Kumaran, and Agarwal for their help in this research.

References

1. Schiavo G, Rossetto O, Montecucco C. Clostridial neurotoxins as tools to investigate the molecular events of neurotransmitter release. *Semin Cell Biol.* 1994;5:221-229.
2. Dasgupta BR, Rasmussen S. Purification and amino acid composition of type E botulinum neurotoxin. *Toxicon.* 1983;21:535-545.
3. Sathyamurthy V, Dasgupta BR. Separation, purification, partial characterization and comparison of the heavy and light chains of botulinum neurotoxin types A, B and E. *J Biol Chem.* 1985;260:10461-10466.
4. Montecucco C, Papini E, Schiavo G. Bacterial protein toxins penetrate cells via a four-step mechanism. *FEBS Lett.* 1994;346:92-98.
5. Montecucco C, Schiavo G. Mechanism of action of tetanus and botulinum neurotoxins. *Mol Microbiol.* 1994;13:1-9.
6. Menestrina G, Schiavo G, Montecucco C. Molecular mechanisms of action of bacterial protein toxins. *Mol Aspects Med.* 1994;15:79-193.
7. Oguma K, Fujinaga Y, Inoue K. Structure and function of Clostridium botulinum toxins. *Microbiol Immunol.* 1995;39:161-168.
8. Simpson LL: Identification of the characteristics that underlie botulinum toxin potency: Implications for designing novel drugs. *Biochemie.* 2000;82:943-953.
9. Simpson LL. Molecular pharmacology of botulinum toxin and tetanus toxin. *Annu Rev Pharmacol Toxicol.* 1986;26:427-453.
10. Simpson LL, ed. *Botulinum Neurotoxins and Tetanus Toxin.* New York: Academic Press; 1989.
11. Lacy DB, Tepp W, Cohen AC, DasGupta BR, Stevens RC. Crystal structure of botulinum neurotoxin type A and implications for toxicity. *Nat Struct Biol.* 1998;5:898-902.
12. Swaminathan S, Eswaramoorthy S. Structural analysis of the catalytic and binding sites of Clostridium botulinum neurotoxin B. *Nat Struct Biol.* 2000;7:693-699.
13. Jankovic J, Brin MF. Therapeutic uses of botulinum toxin. *N Engl J Med.* 1992;324:1186-1194.
14. Johnson EA, Goodnough MC. Preparation and properties of botulinum toxin type A for medical use. In Tsui JKC, Calne DB, eds. *Handbook of Dystonia.* New York: Marcel Decker, Inc.; 1995:347-365.
15. Fischer A, Garcia-Rodriguez C, Geren I, Lou J, Marks JD, Nakagawa T, et al. Molecular architecture of Botulinum neurotoxin E revealed by single particle electron microscopy. *J Biol Chem.* 2007;283:3997-4003.
16. Jayaraman S, Eswaramoorthy S, Ahmed SA, Smith LA, Swaminathan S. N-terminal helix reorients in recombinant C-fragment of Clostridium botulinum type B. *Biochem Biophys Res Commun.* 2005;330:97-103.
17. Umland TC, Wingert LM, Swaminathan S, Furey WF, Schmidt JJ, Sax M. Structure of the receptor binding fragment Hc of tetanus neurotoxin. *Nat Struct Biol.* 1997;4:788-792.
18. Murzin AG, Lesk AM, Chothia C. beta-Trefoil fold. Patterns of structure and sequence in the Kunitz inhibitors interleukins-1 beta and 1 alpha and fibroblast growth factors. *J Mol Biol.* 1992;223:531-543.
19. Montecucco C. How do tetanus and botulinum toxins bind to neuronal membranes? *Trends Biochem Sci.* 1986;11:314-317.
20. Pierce EJ, Davison MD, Parton RG, Habig WH, Critchley DR. Characterization of tetanus toxin binding to rat brain membranes: Evidence for a high-affinity proteinase-sensitive receptor. *Biochemical J.* 1986;236:845-852.
21. Nishiki T-I, Tokuyama Y, Kamata Y, Nemoto Y, Yoshida A, Sato K, et al. The high-affinity binding of Clostridium botulinum type B neurotoxin to synaptotagmin II associated gangliosides GT1b/GD1a. *FEBS Lett.* 1996;378:253-257.
22. Jayaraman S, Eswaramoorthy S, Kumaran D, Swaminathan S. Common binding site for disialyllactose and tri-peptide in C-fragment of tetanus neurotoxin. *Proteins.* 2005;61:288-295.
23. Emsley P, Fotinou C, Black I, Fairweather NF, Charles IG, Watts C, et al. The structures of the H(C) fragment of tetanus toxin with carbohydrate subunit complexes provide insight into ganglioside binding. *J Biol Chem.* 2000;275:8889-8894.
24. Fotinou C, Emsley P, Black I, Ando H, Ishida H, Kiso M, et al. The crystal structure of tetanus toxin Hc fragment complexed with a synthetic Gt1b analogue suggests cross-linking between ganglioside receptors and the toxin. *J Biol Chem.* 2001;276:32274-32281.
25. Rummel A, Bade S, Alves J, Bigalke H, Binz T. Two carbohydrate binding sites in the H(CC)-domain of tetanus neurotoxin are required for toxicity. *J Mol Biol.* 2003;326:835-847.
26. Rummel A, Mahrhold S, Bigalke H, Binz T. The HCC-domain of botulinum neurotoxins A and B exhibits a singular ganglioside binding site displaying serotype specific carbohydrate interaction. *Mol Microbiol.* 2004;51:631-644.
27. Chai Q, Arndt JW, Dong M, Tepp WH, Johnson EA, Chapmann ER, et al. Structural basis of cell surface receptor recognition by botulinum neurotoxin B. *Nature.* (London) 2006;444:1019-1020.
28. Jin R, Rummel A, Binz T, Brunger AT. Botulinum neurotoxin B recognizes its protein receptor with high affinity and specificity. *Nature.* (London) 2006;444:1092-1095.
29. Eswaramoorthy S, Kumaran D, Swaminathan S. Crystallographic evidence for doxorubicin binding to the receptor-binding site in Clostridium botulinum neurotoxin B. *Acta Cryst.* 2001;D57:1743-1746.
30. Lightstone FC, Prieto MC, Singh AK, Piqueras MC, Whittal RM, Knapp MS, et al. Identification of novel small molecule ligands that bind to tetanus toxin. *Chem Res Toxicol.* 2000;13:356-362.
31. Cirilli M, Bachechi F, Ughetto G. Interactions between Morpholinyl anthracyclines and DNA. *J Mol Biol.* 1992;230:878-889.

32. Oblatt-Montal M, Yamazaki M, Nelson R, Montal M. Formation of ion channels in lipid bilayers by a peptide with the predicted transmembrane sequence of botulinum neurotoxin A. *Protein Sci.* 1995;4: 1490-1497.

33. Montal MS, Blewitt R, Tomich JM, Montal M. Identification of an ion channel-forming motif in the primary structure of tetanus and botulinum neurotoxins. *FEBS Lett.* 1992;313:12-18.

34. Shone CC, Hambleton P, Melling J. A 50-kDa fragment from the NH2-terminus of the heavy subunit of Clostridium botulinum neurotoxin forms channels in lipid vesicles. *Eur J Biochem.* 1987;167:175-180.

35. Flicker PF, Robinson JP, DasGupta BR. Is formation of visible channels in a phospholipid bilayer by botulinum neurotoxin type B sensitive to its disulfide? *J Struct Biol.* 1999;128:297-304.

36. Schmid MF, Robinson JP, DasGupta BR. Direct visualization of botulinum neurotoxin induced channels in phospholipid vesicles. *Nature.* 1993;364:827-830.

37. Hoch DH, Romero-Mira M, Ehrlich BE, Finkelstein A, DasGupta BR, Simpson LL. Channels formed by botulinum, tetanus, and diphtheria toxins in planar lipid bilayers: relevance to translocation of proteins across membranes. *Proc Natl Acad Sci U S A.* 1985;82:1692-1696.

38. Koriazova L, Montal M. Translocation of botulinum neurotoxin light chain protease through the heavy chain channel. *Nat Struct Biol.* 2003;10:13-18.

39. Lebeda FJ, Olson MA. Structural predictions of the channel-forming region of botulinum neurotoxin heavy chain. *Toxicon.* 1995;33:559-567.

40. de-Paiva A, Poulain B, Lawrence GW, Shone CC, Tauc L, Dolly JO. A role for the interchain disulfide or its participating thiols in the internalization of botulinum neurotoxin A revealed by a toxin derivative that binds to ecto-acceptors and inhibits transmitter release intracellularly. *J Biol Chem.* 1993;268:20838-20844.

41. Schiavo G, Shone CC, Rossetto O, Alexander FCG, Montecucco C. Botulinum neurotoxin serotype F is a zinc endopeptidase specific for VAMP/synaptobrevin. *J Biol Chem.* 1993;268:11516-11519.

42. Schiavo G, Benfenati F, Poulain B, Rossetto O, de-Lauretto PP, Dasgupta BR, et al. Tetanus and botulinum-B neurotoxins block neurotransmitter release by a proteolytic cleavage of synaptobrevin. *Nature.* 1992;359:832-835.

43. Schiavo G, Rossetto O, Catsicas S, Polverino-de-Laureto P, Dasgupta BR, Benfenati F, et al. Identification of the nerve terminal targets of botulinum neurotoxin serotypes A, D and E. *J Biol Chem.* 1993;268:23784-23787.

44. Schiavo G, Santucci A, Dasgupta BR, Metha PP, Jontes J, Benfenati F, et al. Botulinum neurotoxins serotypes A and E cleave SNAP-25 at distinct COOH-terminal peptide bonds. *FEBS Lett.* 1993;335:99-103.

45. Schiavo G, Malizio C, Trimble WS, Polverino-de-Laureto P, Milan G, Sugiyama H, et al. Botulinum G neurotoxin cleaves VAMP/synaptobrevin at a single Ala-Ala peptide bond. *J Biol Chem.* 1994;269: 20213-20216.

46. Schiavo G, Matteoli M, Montecucco C. Neurotoxins affecting neuroexocytosis. *Physiol Rev.* 2000;80: 717-766.

47. Blasi J, Chapman ER, Yamasaki S, Binz T, Niemann H, Jahn R. Botulinum neurotoxin C blocks neurotransmitter release by means of cleaving HPC-1/syntaxin. *EMBO J.* 1993;12:4821-4828.

48. Foran P, Lawrence GW, Shone CC, Foster KA, Dolly JO. Botulinum neurotoxin C1 cleaves both syntaxin and SNAP-25 in intact and permeabilized chromaffin cells: correlation with its blockade of catecholamine release. *Biochemistry.* 1996;35:2630-2636.

49. Sollner T, Whiteheart SW, Brunner M, Erdjument-Bromage H, Geromanos S, Tempst P, et al. SNAP receptors implicated in vesicle targeting and fusion. *Nature.* 1993;362:318-324.

50. Schiavo G, Rossetto O, Santucci A, Dasgupta BR, Montecucco C. Botulinum neurotoxins are zinc proteins. *J Biol Chem.* 1992;267:23479-27483.

51. Schiavo G, Poulain B, Rossetto O, Benfenati F, Tauc L, Montecucco C. Tetanus toxin is a zinc protein and its inhibition of neurotransmitter release and protease activity depend on zinc. *EMBO J.* 1992;11:3577-3583.

52. Agarwal R, Binz T, Swaminathan S. Structural analysis of botulinum neurotoxin serotype F light chain: implications on substrate binding and inhibitor design. *Biochemistry.* 2005;44:11758-11765.

53. Agarwal R, Eswaramoorthy S, Kumaran D, Binz T, Swaminathan S. Structural analysis of botulinum neurotoxin type E catalytic domain and its mutant Glu212->Gln reveals the pivotal role of the Glu212 carboxylate in the catalytic pathway. *Biochemistry.* 2004;43:6637-6644.

54. Arndt JW, Chai Q, Christian T, Stevens RC. Structure of botulinum neurotoxin type D light chain at 1.65 A resolution: Repercussions for VAMP-2 substrate specificity. *Biochemistry.* 2006;45:3255-3262.

55. Arndt JW, Yu W, Bi F, Stevens RC. Crystal structure of botulinum neurotoxin type G light chain: serotype divergence in substrate recognition. *Biochemistry.* 2005;44:9574-9580.

56. Jin R, Sikorra S, Stegmann CM, Pich A, Binz T, Brunger AT. Structural and biochemical studies of botulinum neurotoxin serotype C1 light chain protease: implications for dual substrate specificity. *Biochemistry.* 2007;46:10685-10693.

57. Rao KN, Kumaran D, Binz T, Swaminathan S: Structural studies on the catalytic domain of clostridial tetanus toxin. *Toxicon.* 2005;45:929-939.

58. Segelke B, Knapp M, Kadkhodayan S, Balhorn R, Rupp B. Crystal structure of Clostridium botulinum neurotoxin protease in a product-bound state: Evidence for noncanonical zinc protease activity. *Proc Natl Acad Sci U S A.* 2004;101:6888-6893.

59. Hanson MA, Stevens RC. Cocrystal structure of synaptobrevin-II bound to botulinum neurotoxin type B at 2.0 A resolution. *Nat Struct Biol.* 2000;7:687-692.

60. Agarwal R, Binz T, Swaminathan S. Analysis of active site residues of botulinum neurotoxin E by mutational, functional and structural studies: Glu335Gln is an apo-enzyme. *Biochemistry.* 2005;44:8291-8302.

61. Binz T, Bade S, Rummel A, Kollewe A, Alves J. Arg362 and Tyr365 of the botulinum neurotoxin type A light chain are involved in transition state stabilization. *Biochemistry.* 2002;41:1717-1723.

62. Rigoni M, Caccin P, Johnson EA, Montecucco C, Rossetto O. Site-directed mutagenesis identifies active-site residues of the light chain of botulinum neurotoxin type A. *Biochem Biophys Res Commun.* 2001;288:1231-1237.

63. Rossetto O, Caccin P, Rigoni M, Tonello F, Bortoletto N, Stevens RC, et al. Active-site mutagenesis of tetanus neurotoxin implicates TYR-375 and GLU-271 in metalloproteolytic activity. *Toxicon.* 2001;39: 115-1159.

64. Swaminathan S, Eswaramoorthy S, Kumaran D. Structure and enzymatic activity of botulinum neurotoxins. *Move Dis.* 2004;19(suppl 8):S17-S22.

65. Eswaramoorthy S, Kumaran D, Keller J, Swaminathan S. Role of metals in the biological activity of Clostridium botulinum neurotoxins. *Biochemistry.* 2004;43:2209-2216.

66. Li L, Singh BR. Role of zinc binding in type A botulinum neurotoxin light chain's toxic structure. *Biochemistry.* 2000;39:10581-10586.

67. Fu Z, Chen S, Baldwin MR, Boldt GE, Crawford A, Janda KD, et al. Light chain of botulinum neurotoxin-serotype A: structural resolution of a catalytic intermediate. *Biochemistry.* 2006;45:8903-8911.

68. Simpson LL, Maksymowych AB, Hao S. The role of zinc binding in the biological activity of botulinum toxin. *J Biol Chem.* 2001;276:27034-27041.

69. Breidenbach MA, Brunger A. Substrate recognition strategy for botulinum neurotoxin serotype A. *Nature.* 2004;432:925-929.

70. Burnett JC, Ruthel G, Stegmann CM, et al. Inhibition of metalloprotease botulinum serotype A from a pseudo-peptide binding mode to a small molecule that is active in primary neurons. *J Biol Chem.* 2007;282:5004-5014.

71. Silvaggi NR, Boldt GE, Hixon MS, Kennedy JP, Tzipori S, Janda KD, et al. Structures of Clostridium botulinum Neurotoxin Serotype A Light Chain complexed with small-molecule inhibitors highlight active-site flexibility. *Chem Biol.* 2007;14:533-542.

71a. Kumaran D, Rawat R, Ludivico ML, Ahmed SA, Swaminathan S. Structure- and substrate-based inhibitor design for Clostridium botulinum neurotoxin A. *J Mol Biol.* 2008;283:18883-18891.

72. Burnett JC, Schmidt JJ, Stafford RG, Panchal RG, Nguyen TL, Hermone AR, et al. Novel small molecule inhibitors of botulinum neurotoxin A metalloprotease activity. *Biochem Biophys Res Commun.* 2003;310:84-93.

73. Eswaramoorthy S, Kumaran D, Swaminathan S. A novel mechanism for Clostridium botulinum neurotoxin inhibition. *Biochemistry.* 2002;41:9795-9802.

74. Boldt GE, Dickerson TJ, Janda KD. Emerging chemical and biological approaches for the preparation of discovery libraries. *Drug Discov Today.* 2006;11: 143-148.

75. Boldt GE, Eubanks LM, Janda KD. Identification of a botulinum neurotoxin A protease inhibitor displaying efficacy in a cellular model. *Chem Commun.* 2006;7:3063-3065.

76. Boldt GE, Kennedy JP, Hixon MS, McAllister LA, Barbieri JT, Tzipori S, et al. Synthesis, characterization and development of a high-throughput methodology for the discovery of botulinum neurotoxin a inhibitors. *J Comb Chem.* 2006;8:513-521.

77. Boldt GE, Kennedy JP, Janda KD. Identification of a potent botulinum neurotoxin a protease inhibitor using in situ lead identification chemistry. *Org Lett.* 2006;8:1729-1732.

78. Burnett JC, Henchal EA, Schmaljohn AL, Bavari S. The evolving field of biodefence: therapeutic developments and diagnostics. *Nat Rev Drug Discov.* 2005;4:281-297.

79. Burnett JC, Opsenica D, Sriraghavan K, Panchal RG, Ruthel G, Hermone AR, et al. A refined pharmacophore identifies potent 4-amino-7-chloroquinoline-based inhibitors of the botulinum neurotoxin serotype A metalloprotease. *J Med Chem.* 2007;50:2127-2136.

80. Burnett JC, Schmidt JJ, McGrath CF, Nguyen TL, Hermone AR, Panchal RG, et al. Conformational sampling of the botulinum neurotoxin serotype A light chain: implications for inhibitor binding. *Bioorg Med Chem.* 2005;13:333-341.

81. Simpson LL, Maksymowych AB, Park J-B, Bora RS. The role of the interchain disulfide bond in governing the pharmacological actions of botulinum toxin. *J Pharmacol Exp Ther.* 2004;308:857-864.

82. Ahmed SA, Smith LA. Light chain of botulinum A neurotoxin expressed as an inclusion body from a synthetic gene is catalytically and functionally active. *J Protein Chem.* 2000;19:475-487.

83. Arndt JW, Jacobson MJ, Abola EE, Forsyth CM, Tepp WH, Marks JD, et al. A structural perspective of the sequence variability within botulinum neurotoxin subtypes A1-A4. *J Mol Biol.* 2006;362:733-742.

84. Chenna R, Sugawara H, Koike T, Lopez R, Gibson TJ, Higgins DG, et al. Multiple sequence alignment with the Clustal series of programs. *Nucleic Acids Res.* 2003;31:3497-3500.

Botulinum Neurotoxin—a Modular Nanomachine

3

Audrey Fischer, Lilia Koriazova, Myrta Oblatt-Montal, and Mauricio Montal

INTRODUCTION

Botulinum neurotoxin (BoNT) proteases disable synaptic vesicle exocytosis by cleaving their cytosolic soluble N-ethylmaleimide-sensitive factor (NSF) attachment protein receptor (SNARE) substrates.[1-7] However, the mechanism underlying the translocation of the endocytosed protease from acidic endosomes into the cytosol is poorly understood. A major thrust of our endeavor is the in-depth analysis of protein translocation by BoNT, a modular nanomachine in which one of its modules—the heavy chain (HC) channel—operates as a specific protein-translocating transmembrane chaperone for another of its component modules—the light chain (LC) protease. The challenge is to understand the intimate relationship between the LC and the HC, two entities which in isolation are harmless yet when associated together by nature are transformed into the most potent toxin known.[8] Mechanistic insights into how this protein machine[9] evolved to this level of sophistication may be derived from the biophysical analysis of the interaction between these two modules in the context of the full-length toxin embedded in a membrane. This is precisely what we review in this chapter.

How do the BoNT proteases reach their cytosolic substrates? Structurally, BoNT consists of three modules[5,10-12]: the LC protease; and the HC, which encompasses the translocation domain (TD), and the receptor-binding domain (RBD). This structural modularity has a physiologic counterpart. The RBD determines the cellular specificity mediated by the high-affinity interaction with a surface protein receptor, SV2, for BoNT/A[13,14] and synaptotagmins I and II for BoNT/B and BoNT/G,[15] and a ganglioside (GT_{1B}) coreceptor.[13-16] Then, BoNTs enter sensitive cells via receptor-mediated endocytosis.[5,17-22] Exposure of the BoNT-receptor complex to the acidic milieu of endosomes[21-25] induces a major conformational change, leading to the insertion of the HC into the endosomal bilayer membrane, thereby forming transmembrane channels.[26-29] The HC of BoNT/A acts as both a channel and a transmembrane chaperone for the LC to ensure a translocation-competent conformation during its transit from the acidic endosome into the cytosol.[30] These findings provided compelling evidence of retrieval of a folded LC protease that is capable of proteolyzing its SNARE substrate only after productive translocation across bilayers and release from the channel.[30] Together, these results support the view that the TD module is the conduit for the passage of the LC module from the interior of the endosome into the cytosol, allowing contact between the protease and the SNARE substrates.[5,21,28] Cleavage of the SNAREs,[31,32] which are essential for synaptic vesicle fusion and neurotransmitter release, aborts synaptic transmission, thereby causing severe paralysis.[4,5]

The authors of this chapter do not report any conflicts of interest.

BoNT CHANNEL ACTIVITY UNDER CONDITIONS PREVALENT AT ENDOSOMES

Figure 3-1 depicts a model of the sequence of events underlying BoNT LC translocation through the HC channel, which is consistent with the findings collected thus far[30,33-36] and reviewed in this chapter. Step 1 shows the crystal structure BoNT/A before insertion into the membrane[10]: LC is purple, TD is orange, and RBD is red. Then is shown a schematic representation of the membrane inserted BoNT/A at the onset of translocation (step 2) with a partially unfolded LC (purple) trapped within the HC channel (orange), a series of transfer steps (steps 3 and 4), and an exit event at the completion of LC translocation (step 5), leaving the HC channel within the membrane. Translocation proceeds under conditions that recapitulate those across endosomes: the interchain disulfide bridge (green) is intact in the low pH, oxidizing environment of the *cis* compartment, corresponding to the endosome interior. The presence of reductant and neutral pH in the *trans* compartment, corresponding to the cytosol, promotes refolding of LC and release from HC after completion of translocation.

What is the evidence for the model? Figures 3-2 and 3-3 summarize the evidence for the beginning (see Fig. 3-1, steps 1 and 2) and the end (see Fig. 3-1, step 5) of translocation.[30,33-35] First, we probed the role of the disulfide bridge in the translocation process.[30] We exploited the differential accessibility of the disulfide cross-link between the HC and the LC to a membrane-impermeant reductant

(tris-[2-carboxyethyl] phosphine [TCEP]) to identify requirements for translocation across membranes. We showed that channel formation and LC translocation across membranes require both a pH gradient and a redox gradient, acidic and oxidizing on the *cis* compartment in which BoNT/A is present and neutral and reducing on the *trans* compartment in which the substrate synaptosomal-associated protein with Mr = 25 kDa (SNAP-25) is present. These conditions emulate the pH and redox gradients across endosomes[30,33-35] and allow the formation of transmembrane channels by BoNT/A and BoNT/E, as shown in Figure 3-2A and 3-2D. The initial results were obtained from planar lipid bilayer membranes devoid of any additional cellular components.[30] As shown in Figure 3-2, the equivalent pattern of activity is recorded from membrane patches isolated from neuroblastoma cells.[33,34] The channel activity of BoNT/A displays the prototypical discrete square events that are characteristic of unitary channel currents.[37] In contrast, unreduced BoNT/A does not form channels under otherwise equivalent conditions (see Fig. 3-2B). Given that prereduced BoNT/A (see Fig. 3-2C) forms channels with properties equivalent to those of the isolated HC,[30,33-35] and that the HC is a channel irrespective of the redox state,[30,33,34] the inescapable conclusion is that in unreduced holotoxin the anchored LC cargo occludes the HC channel (see Fig. 3-1, step 2; and Fig. 3-2B). Is this occlusion terminated at the end of translocation and release of cargo? How and when is cargo release triggered at the membrane interface after translocation? Is the protease activity of cargo detectable in the *trans* compartment after completion of translocation?

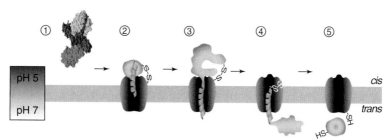

FIGURE 3-1. Sequence of events underlying BoNT LC translocation through the HC channel. (1) BoNT/A holotoxin prior to insertion in the membrane (*gray bar*); BoNT/A is represented by the crystal structure rendered on YASARA (www.YASARA.org) using the Protein Data Bank accession code 3BTA.[10] Then, schematic representation of the membrane inserted BoNT/A during an entry event (2), a series of transfer steps (3, 4), and an exit event (5) under conditions that recapitulate those across endosomes. (Reproduced with permission from Fischer A, Montal M. Single molecule detection of intermediates during botulinum neurotoxin translocation across membranes. *Proc Natl Acad Sci U S A.* 2007;104:10447-10452. Copyright [2007], National Academy of Sciences, U S A.) *See Color Plate*

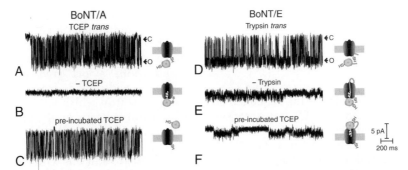

FIGURE 3-2. Release of cargo from chaperone is necessary for productive translocation. BoNT/A and BoNT/E holotoxin channels in excised patches of Neuro 2A cells. Diagrams on the right side of each record depict an interpretation. Top and bottom represent *cis* and *trans* compartments; LC cargo (*light gray*), HC (*dark gray and black*), disulfide linkage (-S-S-), and the membrane (*gray bar*). **A.** Single-channel currents for holotoxin BoNT/A; the *trans* compartment contained 0.25 mM TCEP. C and O denote the closed and open states. The characteristic fast transitions between the closed and open states are clearly discernible; γ is determined from the amplitude of the fluctuations between the closed and open states. **B.** Nonreduced holotoxin BoNT/A does not form channels; note the absence of current fluctuations. **C.** Single-channel currents of reduced holotoxin BoNT/A by preincubation with reductant TCEP (0.25 mM). **D.** Single-channel currents of holotoxin BoNT/E in the presence of both trypsin and TCEP in the *trans* compartment. **E.** Single-channel currents of holotoxin BoNT/E in the absence of trypsin in the TCEP-containing *trans* compartment. **F.** Single-channel currents of reduced holotoxin BoNT/E by pre-incubation with 10 mM TCEP and in the presence of 4 mM trypsin in the *trans* compartment. Single-channel currents were recorded at −100 mV in symmetric 0.2 M NaCl; all other conditions were identical to those previously described.[34,35] Other conventions as in Figure 3-1. *See Color Plate*

RETRIEVAL OF ENDOPEPTIDASE ACTIVITY OF BoNT LC IN THE *TRANS* COMPARTMENT AT THE COMPLETION OF TRANSLOCATION

To examine if the LC protease goes through the HC channel (see Fig. 3-1, step 5), we developed a high-sensitivity enzyme-linked immunosorbant assay (ELISA) and scaled up the single-channel measurements to detect numerous (≥ 1000) channels.[30] Cleavage of SNAP-25 required the presence of the reductant TCEP on the *trans* compartment and pH 5.0 on the *cis* compartment (see Fig. 3-3A), a condition that correlates tightly with the insertion of multiple channels in the bilayer membrane (see Fig. 3-3B). This correlation argues that only under conditions in which the channel activity of the holotoxin is detected (see Figs. 3-2A and 3-3B), proteolytic activity of the LC on the *trans* compartment is confirmed (see Fig. 3-3A). This result is consistent with

the concomitant absence of channel activity (see Fig. 3-3B) and LC protease activity (see Fig. 3-3A) when the pH on the *cis* compartment was 4.5. A tight correlation was uncovered between the decrease in α-helical content of the LC at pH 5.0 (see Fig. 3-3C) with the occurrence of channel (see Fig. 3-3B) and protease (see Fig. 3-3A) activities of holotoxin[30]; such correlation is highlighted by the blue box on Figure 3-3. At pH 4.5, there is a drastic increase in LC helicity (see Fig. 3-3C) coincident with the absence of channel (see Fig. 3-3B) and protease (see Fig. 3-3A) activities. Together, the data indicate that only the unfolded conformation of the LC correlates with both channel and protease activities of BoNT/A. The decrease in α-helical content of the LC necessarily constrains the LC cargo to be either extended or α-helical segments in order to fit into a channel of ~15 Å in diameter, as calculated from the single-channel conductance (γ) of BoNT/A.[30] Collectively, these findings provide convincing evidence of recovery of endopeptidase activity of BoNT LC in the *trans* compartment only after productive translocation across synthetic lipid bilayer

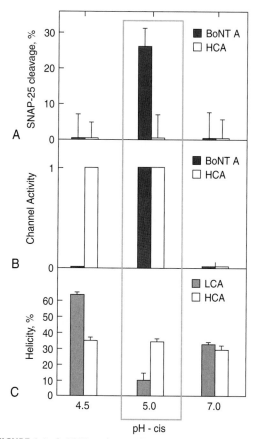

FIGURE 3-3. BoNT/A endopeptidase activity correlates with BoNT/A channel activity and the unfolding of LC/A. **A.** Endopeptidase activity in samples collected from the *trans* chamber of bilayer experiments as function of pH in the *cis* compartment; the *trans* compartment pH was 7.0. **B.** Channel activity of BoNT/A and HC/A as function of pH in the *cis* compartment; the *trans* compartment pH was 7.0. Absence or presence of channel activity is arbitrarily defined as 0 or 1; number of experiments (n) = 6 for HC/A and n = 10 for BoNT/A. **C.** α-Helical content of LC/A and HC/A as function of pH calculated from far UV-CD measurements carried out at 25°C; n = 3. (Modified and reproduced with permission from Koriazova LK, Montal M. Translocation of botulinum neurotoxin light chain protease through the heavy chain channel. *Nat Struct Biol.* 2003;10:13-18.) *See Color Plate*

membranes[30] (see Fig. 3-1, step 5). Evidence for the importance of unfolding and a propensity toward α-helical structure for efficient translocation has been subsequently obtained for BoNT/D using an entirely different experimental approach.[38] Similarly, a requirement for acid-induced unfolding has been reported for the translocation of the 263-residue N-terminal domain of anthrax lethal factor, the cargo, through the protective antigen heptameric pore.[39,40]

RELEASE OF CARGO FROM CHAPERONE IS NECESSARY FOR PRODUCTIVE TRANSLOCATION

For BoNT/A, the disulfide cross-link between LC and HC must be on the *trans* (cytosolic) compartment to achieve productive translocation of the LC cargo (see Fig. 3-1, step 5; Fig. 3-2A, 2B).[30,34,35] Disulfide reduction on the *cis* compartment dissociates the LC cargo from the HC before translocation and therefore generates a HC channel devoid of translocation activity (see Fig. 3-2C).[30,33] Disulfide disruption within the bilayer during translocation aborts it.[35] We infer that completion of LC translocation occurs as the disulfide bridge, C-terminus of the LC, enters the cytosolic compartment. This analysis supports a model of N- to C-terminal orientation of cargo during translocation with the C-terminus as the last portion to be translocated and exit the channel (see Fig. 3-1, step 5). We propose that an intact disulfide bridge is a necessary condition for translocation but not for channel insertion, as demonstrated by the fact that the isolated HC channel is unperturbed by chemical reductants.[30] The tight coupling of translocation completion with disulfide reduction strongly argues in favor of the view that LC refolding precludes retrotranslocation. From this viewpoint, refolding in cytosol may be interpreted as a trap that prevents retrotranslocation and dictates the unidirectional nature of the translocation process. The disulfide linkage is, therefore, a crucial aspect of the BoNT toxicity (see also Chapter 2 and references 41 and 42) and is required for chaperone function, acting as a principal determinant for cargo translocation and release.

Is the intact disulfide bridge specifically required for LC translocation? Whereas BoNT/A is cleaved to the mature di-chain within the *Clostridium* bacteria, BoNT/E is not cleaved before secretion.[43] Therefore, the single-chain BoNT/E holotoxin provides a path to explore the linkage requirements for LC translocation. For BoNT/E, completion of LC translocation occurs only after proteolytic cleavage by trypsin and disulfide reduction in the *trans* compartment, implying that release of cargo from chaperone is necessary for productive translocation[34] (see Fig. 3-1, step 5). Experimental evidence for this condition is illustrated in Figures 3-2D and 3-2E. In the absence of trypsin in the *trans* compartment (see Fig. 3-2E), channel insertion and onset of translocation proceed, as shown by the appearance of channels that remain in an occluded state for the lifetime of the experiment. This is consistent with the unrelieved occlusion of the HC channel by the LC. In contrast, the presence of trypsin in the *trans* compartment (see Fig. 3-2D) leads to the appearance of channels with single-channel properties equivalent to those of isolated HC, a hallmark of unoccluded channels. Furthermore, single-chain BoNT/E, reduced before the translocation assay, displays channel activity (see Fig. 3-2F). However, despite the fact that trypsin is present in the *trans* compartment, the channel remains occluded for the lifetime of the experiment. Therefore, proteolytic cleavage of LC from HC and disulfide reduction during the exit event are required for productive translocation (see Fig. 3-1, step 5). These findings also imply that the transformation of an occluded state characterized by low γ intermediates with prolonged pore occupancy into an unoccluded channel with $\gamma \sim 65$ pS only occurs after the LC completes translocation from the *cis* to the *trans* compartment and is physically separated from the HC channel by both reduction of the disulfide bridge and cleavage of the scissile bond. Thus, the chaperone-cargo anchor must be severed to complete productive translocation.[34]

DISCRETE INTERMEDIATES DURING BoNT TRANSLOCATION REVEAL THE CONFORMATIONAL DYNAMICS OF CARGO-CHANNEL INTERACTIONS

To decipher how the tight interplay between the HC and LC modules underlies the conspicuously potent neurotoxicity of BoNT we developed an assay that monitors the translocation of BoNT LC by the BoNT HC channel in real time and at the single-molecule level in excised membrane patches[37] from BoNT-sensitive Neuro 2A neuroblastoma cells.[34,35] The assay allows us to probe Steps 2, 3, 4 and 5 of Figure 3-1, namely, the conformational transitions of both HC and LC linked to translocation across membranes, and the requirements for LC refolding and release at

the endosome surface after translocation. The type of questions that we investigate are as follows: What is the nature of the interactions between the cargo and the channel during translocation and after completion of translocation? How is cargo conformation protected by the channel during translocation to ensure proper refolding after translocation is completed? What determines refolding of cargo after translocation? When is refolding initiated?

A key feature of the single-molecule translocation assay is sensitivity, which led us to discover a succession of discrete transient intermediate channel conductances, which reflect permissive stages during LC translocation for both BoNT/A and BoNT/E. This is illustrated in Figure 3-4 for BoNT/A; the top panel shows the absence of channel currents before BoNT/A insertion into the membrane. The time course of channel conductance change after exposure to BoNT/A (defined as zero time), is shown in the next four panels, which display representative consecutive segments recorded at the indicated times during a single, 1- hour long experiment. Intermediate conductances were discerned at $\gamma \cong 20$ pS (after 5 min), $\cong 37$ pS (after 9 min), and $\cong 55$ pS (after 5.5 min) before entering the stable γ of 65 pS. Note that the γ values for each of the intermediate conductances fluctuate, yet they clearly exhibit a trend toward higher γ values with time, as depicted by the dotted lines. This pattern of channel activity characteristic of holotoxin (see Fig. 3-4) allows us to operationally define three states of the BoNT channel. First, a closed state, and second, an "occluded state" with the partially unfolded LC trapped within the channel during the translocation process (see Fig. 3-1, steps 2, 3 and 4). This occluded state is identified as a set of intermediate conductances corresponding to transitions between the closed state and several blocked open states. Third, an "unoccluded state" is visible upon completion of translocation and release of the LC associated to transitions between the closed state and the fully open state (see Fig. 3-1, step 5). The terminal and stable γ for holotoxin channels ($\cong 67$ pS,) and the distinctive γ of HC channels ($\cong 66$ pS) (see Fig. 3-2C) exhibit similar characteristics, thereby supporting the view of the HC channel as an end point achieved after completion of LC translocation through the HC channel, as observed in holotoxin/A (see Fig. 3-2A) and holotoxin/E (see Fig. 3-2D) channels[30,33,34] (see Fig. 3-1, Step 5).

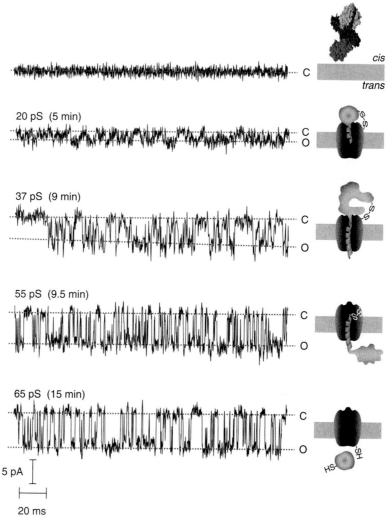

FIGURE 3-4. Single-molecule detection of discrete intermediates during BoNT translocation. High-gain and fast-time resolution of BoNT/A single-channel currents recorded at −100 mV in excised patches of Neuro 2A cells, with schematic representation (*right*). Top panel shows absence of channel currents prior to exposure to BoNT/A. Subsequent panels represent the time course of change of channel conductance. Each segment indicates the representative γ at the recorded time; the dotted lines are traced on the average current for the closed and open states. All other conditions were identical to those previously described[30,32] and other conventions as in Figure 3-1. *See Color Plate*

We interpret the progressive, stepwise increase in channel conductance with time as the progress of LC translocation during which the protein-conducting HC channel conducts Na^+ and partially unfolded LC (illustrated as a helix in Fig. 3-1, step 2; Fig. 3-4) detected as channel block. After translocation is complete, the channel is unoccluded (see Fig. 3-1, step 5). In other words, during translocation the HC channel conducts gradually more Na^+ around the unfolded LC polypeptide chain before entering an exclusively ion-conductive state.

What is the significance of the newly identified intermediate states? We conjecture that the residence time at each intermediate reflects the conformational changes of cargo within the chaperone pore and that these determine the efficiency and outcome of translocation. Within the occluded state, the low conductance intermediates (see Fig. 3-4, $\gamma \cong 20$ pS) exhibit the longest occupancy time, consistent with an energetic barrier associated with the initiation of LC unfolding, presumably into a molten globule state, at the onset of translocation—an entry event (see Fig. 3-1, step 2). By contrast, intermediates with γ values $\gamma \cong 40$ pS (see Fig. 3-4) have shorter lifetimes, presumably a result of overcoming the activation energy (see Fig. 3-1, step 3). This sequence of transfer steps leads to a transition into the final γ intermediate with $\gamma \cong 55$ pS (see Fig. 3-1, step 4). This last intermediate in the sequence (see Fig. 3-4) is relatively long lived, plausibly limited by the refolding of the LC at the channel exit interface in the *trans* compartment and reduction of the disulfide bridge before final release from the HC channel, an exit event (see Fig. 3-1, step 5; Fig. 3-4). Thus, the main consequence of this analysis is the resolution of LC translocation into an entry event, a series of transfer steps, and an exit event. The key unanswered questions are now centered on an understanding of the precise conformational state at each one of the identified intermediates; what we can say is that the trend is to preserve partially unfolded conformers, (evidenced by the occluded intermediates) (see Fig. 3-1, steps 2–4; Fig. 3-4)[34] and native-like conformers (evidenced by the recovery of LC protease activity at the end of translocation) (see Fig. 3-1, step 5; Fig. 3-2A; Fig. 3-3).[30]

THE BoNT HC CHANNEL AS A CHAPERONE FOR THE LC PROTEASE

At the root of the BoNT translocation process is the interaction between an unfolded LC cargo embedded within the HC protein-conducting channel (see Fig. 3-1, steps 2-4). An analogous scheme has been invoked for the translocation of the catalytic domain (A chain) by the transmembrane (T) domain of diphtheria toxin,[44-46] and for the translocation of the anthrax toxin lethal factor by the protective antigen pore.[39,40] That channel activity has been documented for BoNT/A,[27,29,30,33] BoNT/E,[29] BoNT/B,[28] BoNT/C,[26] and tetanus neurotoxin,[28,47,48] and protein translocation activity has been shown for BoNT/A,[30] BoNT/E,[34,35] and BoNT/D[38] points to the general validity of the idea. This notion is reminiscent of the maintenance of an unfolded or partially folded state of polypeptides by chaperones. Therefore, it is fitting to consider plausible similarities. The translocon, the universally conserved protein-conducting channel responsible for the translocation of nascent proteins across membranes or for the insertion of integral membrane proteins into targeted membranes, has been the subject of intense inquiry.[49,50] The translocon is a membrane protein complex composed of three different protein subunits: $\alpha\beta\gamma$ in the ER Sec61 complex of eukaryotes, SecYEG in eubacteria, and SecYEβ in archae. The structures of protein-conducting channels of the *Escherichia coli* SecYEG bound to a translating ribosome, ~15 Å resolution,[51] and the archaeon *Methanococcus jannaschii* SecYEβ, 3.2 Å resolution,[52] are instructive because they provide detailed information on protein-conducting channels pertaining to both cotranslational and post-translational translocation systems. They define blueprints for protein-conducting channels for which the underlying protein fold is a compact transmembrane α-helical bundle. Both of these complexes evoke a tantalizing resemblance to the occluded BoNT channel. The reconstruction of the SecYEG led to the view that the nascent polypeptide chain is tightly accommodated within the channel hindering conductance and, given a channel constriction of ~15 Å, it is permissive to accommodate α-helices.[51,53,54] The structure of the SecYEβ shows that the protein-conducting channel is occluded by a short helix. The channel lumen is lined by hydrophobic residues around the major constriction of only 3 Å; however, the channel must change conformation to an open state in order to accommodate translocation of α-helices (12–14 Å) through the center of the channel.[55,56] Indeed, reconstitution of the purified SecY complex into lipid bilayers shows that the channel is nonconductive[57]; however, deletion of the short helix or mutations in the pore ring render the SecY channel open.[57] The structures of these two translocons outline the intricacies of the initial stages of protein translocation and are consistent with the occurrence of discrete transient intermediates involving extensive interactions between the chaperone and the cargo in a dynamic succession that dictates the progress and directionality of translocation and, ultimately, determines the fate of cargo either as a folded secreted protein or as an integral membrane polypeptide.

Protein import in mitochondria and chloroplasts occurs posttranslationally and involves unfolded proteins.[58-60] A number of protein translocase complexes have been identified: the inner mitochondrial membrane TIM23 translocase,[61] and the outer (Toc75)[62] and inner (Tic110)[63] chloroplast membrane translocases display pore diameters of ~13 Å,

~14 Å, and 15 Å, respectively. The secondary structure of the precursor polypeptide cargos are therefore necessarily constrained to be either extended or α-helical segments in order to fit into a channel of ~15 Å in diameter. An analogous requirement for unfolded cargo is required by protein translocases for which the underlying protein fold is a transmembrane hollow β-barrel. A case in point is the protective antigen (PA) PA_{63} pore of anthrax toxin, a 14-stranded β-barrel formed at the center of the homoheptameric assembly that exhibits a central pore with a cross-section of ~15 Å.[40] Similar schemes have emerged from single-channel measurements on the interactions between helical cargo peptides and the transmembrane β-barrel of the α-hemolysin protein pore.[64]

Compared with the molecular complexity of the mitochondrial and chloroplast protein translocases, and the translocons in eukarya, bacteria, and archae, the BoNT protein highlights the simplicity of its modular design to achieve its exquisite activity. The analogy that emerges from the findings summarized here for BoNT is probably more than coincidental and points to a fundamental common principle of molecular design for BoNT and the translocases, all of which clearly catalyze the concerted and intertwined unfolding, translocation, and refolding of cargo proteins.

BoNT HC CHANNEL AS A TARGET FOR INTERVENTION

The body of evidence summarized suggests the notion that the BoNT channel may represent a potential target for intervention to attenuate BoNT neurotoxicity. A search for channel blockers and their eventual identification may provide proof-of-principle thereby paving the way toward the development of BoNT-selective antidotes. Open channel blockers are small molecules that enter the open channel and transiently occlude the passageway by interacting with the main chain or side chains of the channel protein exposed to the channel lumen. The seminal affinity labeling studies of Changeux and colleagues[65] using chlorpromazine as an open channel blocker of the nicotinic acetylcholine receptor established that this type of blocker indeed probes the accessibility of pore-lining residues.[65] Open channel blockers are notorious for their broad selectivity.[66] Despite such limitations, they are valuable tools for proof-of-principle validation.

Accordingly, our focus has been to screen the activity of known open channel blockers of cation-selective channels on the BoNT channel reconstituted in lipid bilayers.[30,36] The results collected thus far are exciting and promising. The initial survey uncovered three classes of drugs with HC channel blocker activity in the μM concentration range; these drugs conspicuously attenuate the single-channel conductance, shorten the open channel lifetime, and reduce the channel open probability.[66,67] Indeed, chlorpromazine exhibits μM potency in the HC channel blocking assay (Fig. 3-5) (unpublished results). QX-222, a trimethyl quaternary ammonium derivative of the ionizable amine local anesthetic lidocaine,[66] is a blocker of voltage-gated cation-selective channels and also of the nicotinic cholinergic receptor channel.[66,67] QX-222 blocks the BoNT HC channel in the micromolar concentration range. A sample recording illustrating the effect of QX-222 is shown in Figure 3-5. In the absence of drug (panel A), the occurrence of up to five independent unoccluded BoNT channels undergoing transitions from closed (C) to open (O) states is clearly discerned. In contrast, in the presence of 40-μM QX-222 (panel B), the pattern of channel activity is drastically altered: the frequency of openings is reduced and long quiescent periods dominate the records. Such a pattern is archetypical for the action of channel blockers.[66,67] Second, antimalarial agents such as chloroquine and quinacrine, known to affect intracellular processing of BoNTs by collapsing the pH gradient across endocytic vesicles, exert a direct blocking action on the HC channel in the high micromolar concentration range.[68] Third, antiviral agents such as amantadine, an anti-influenza drug that acts by blocking the channels formed by the M2 protein of influenza virus,[69,70] or its analog, memantine (1-amino-3,5-dimethyladamantane), a well known, clinically tolerated open channel blocker of the NMDA-subtype of glutamate receptor,[71] also block the HC channel. Memantine, approved by the the US Food and Drug Administration for the treatment of dementia, blocks the N-methyl-D-aspartate (NMDA) receptor channel with a Ki of 300 nM, whereas it blocks the HC channel at concentrations of 30 μM or more.

This analysis presents a new paradigm for the screen of small molecule blockers of the BoNT channel that may evolve into a platform for antidote discovery aimed at abrogating this crucial activity, which is essential for BoNT neurotoxicity.

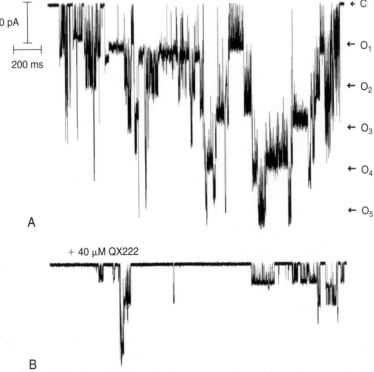

FIGURE 3-5. QX-222 blocks the BoNT HC channel. Single-channel recordings of BoNT/A holotoxin reconstituted in planar lipid bilayers in the absence (**A**) and presence (**B**) of 40-μM QX-222. Records obtained at −100 mV in symmetric 0.5 M KCl, 1 mM CaCl$_2$, 2.5 mM citrate pH 5.5. Final protein concentration was 0.5 μg/mL. In the absence of QX-222, the current histogram is fitted with the sum of five Gaussians (excluding the closed state) corresponding to the occurrence of five channels with a γ ≅ 110 pS. In the presence of QX-222, there is a marked reduction in both γ and in the number of openings; the open states are scarcely populated to allow a meaningful fit to the data points, and the histogram is best fitted with a single Gaussian corresponding to the closed state. Other conditions as for Figure 3-3B. (Unpublished data, experimental method from Koriazova and Montal.) *See Color Plate*

CONCLUDING REMARKS

This endeavor has demonstrated that the BoNT protein-conducting channel acts as a chaperone and requires acidification in *cis* and reduction in *trans*. Identification of translocation intermediates allowed us to define that LC translocation by the HC protein–conducting channel involves an entry event, a series of transfer steps, and an exit event. Under these conditions, the LC protease activity is retrieved in the *trans* compartment, consistent with the translocation of the cargo protease through the channel. The collective findings represent a significant advance in our understanding of BoNT translocation; yet they also raise a new set of questions needing further study, particularly regarding the precise conformers of the cargo within the channel/chaperone at each one of the identified intermediate states (see Fig. 3-1, steps 2-4).[30,34] Overall, the findings imply that within the cell, the LC protease unfolds inside acidic oxidizing endosomes, goes through the HC protein–conducting channel, refolds at the interface, and dissociates from the channel in the cytosolic reducing milieu, where it cleaves its substrate SNARE. Given that the translocation process is essential for BoNT neurotoxicity, the BoNT protein-conducting channel emerges as a potential target for antidote design and discovery.

ACKNOWLEDGMENTS

This work was supported by the U.S. Army Medical Research and Materiel Command (DAMD17-02-C-0106), National Institutes of Health Training Grant T32 GM08326, and a Pacific Southwest Regional Center of Excellence Grant AI-65359.

References

1. Schiavo G, Rossetto O, Catsicas S, Polverino de Laureto P, DasGupta BR, Benfenati F, et al. Identification of the nerve terminal targets of botulinum neurotoxin serotypes A, D, and E. *J Biol Chem.* 1993;268:23784-23787.

2. Weber T, Zemelman BV, McNew JA, Westermann B, Gmachl M, Parlati F, et al. SNAREpins: minimal machinery for membrane fusion. *Cell.* 1998;92:759-772.

3. Sutton RB, Fasshauer D, Jahn R, Brunger AT. Crystal structure of a SNARE complex involved in synaptic exocytosis at 2.4 A resolution. *Nature.* 1998;395:347-353.

4. Jahn R, Lang T, Sudhof TC: Membrane fusion. *Cell.* 2003;112:519-533.

5. Schiavo G, Matteoli M, Montecucco C. Neurotoxins affecting neuroexocytosis. *Physiol Rev.* 2000;80:717-766.

6. Schiavo G, Benfenati F, Poulain B, Rossetto O, Polverino de Laureto P, DasGupta BR, et al. Tetanus and botulinum-B neurotoxins block neurotransmitter release by proteolytic cleavage of synaptobrevin. *Nature.* 1992;359:832-835.

7. Blasi J, Chapman ER, Link E, Binz T, Yamasaki S, De Camilli P, et al. Botulinum neurotoxin A selectively cleaves the synaptic protein SNAP-25. *Nature.* 1993;365:160-163.

8. Arnon SS, Schechter R, Inglesby TV, Henderson DA, Bartlett JG, Ascher MS, et al. Botulinum toxin as a biological weapon: medical and public health management. *JAMA.* 2001;285:1059-1070.

9. Alberts B. The cell as a collection of protein machines: preparing the next generation of molecular biologists. *Cell.* 1998;92:291-294.

10. Lacy DB, Tepp W, Cohen AC, DasGupta BR, Stevens RC. Crystal structure of botulinum neurotoxin type A and implications for toxicity. *Nat Struct Biol.* 1998;5:898-902.

11. Lacy DB, Stevens RC: Sequence homology and structural analysis of the clostridial neurotoxins. *J Mol Biol.* 1999;291:1091-1104.

12. Swaminathan S, Eswaramoorthy S. Structural analysis of the catalytic and binding sites of Clostridium botulinum neurotoxin B. *Nat Struct Biol.* 2000;7:693-699.

13. Dong M, Yeh F, Tepp WH, Dean C, Johnson EA, Janz R, et al. SV2 is the protein receptor for botulinum neurotoxin A. *Science.* 2006;312:592-596.

14. Mahrhold S, Rummel A, Bigalke H, Davletov B, Binz T. The synaptic vesicle protein 2C mediates the uptake of botulinum neurotoxin A into phrenic nerves. *FEBS Lett.* 2006;580:2011-2014.

15. Rummel A, Karnath T, Henke T, Bigalke H, Binz T. Synaptotagmins I and II act as nerve cell receptors for botulinum neurotoxin G. *J Biol Chem.* 2004;279:30865-30870.

16. Nishiki T, Tokuyama Y, Kamata Y, Nemoto Y, Yoshida A, Sekiguchi M, et al. Binding of botulinum type B neurotoxin to Chinese hamster ovary cells transfected with rat synaptotagmin II cDNA. *Neurosci Lett.* 1996;208:105-108.

17. Dolly JO, Black J, Williams RS, Melling J. Acceptors for botulinum neurotoxin reside on motor nerve terminals and mediate its internalization. *Nature.* 1984;307:457-460.

18. Black JD, Dolly JO. Interaction of 125I-labeled botulinum neurotoxins with nerve terminals. I. Ultrastructural autoradiographic localization and quantitation of distinct membrane acceptors for types A and B on motor nerves. *J Cell Biol.* 1986;103:521-534.

19. Black JD, Dolly JO. Interaction of 125I-labeled botulinum neurotoxins with nerve terminals. *J Cell Biol.* 1986;103:535-544.

20. Dolly JO, De Paiva A, Foran P, Lawrence G, Daniels-Holgate PU, Ashton AC. Probing the process of transmitter release with botulinum and tetanus neurotoxins. *Semin Neurosci.* 1994;6:149-158.

21. Simpson LL. Identification of the major steps in botulinum toxin action. *Annu Rev Pharmacol Toxicol.* 2004;44:167-193.

22. Simpson LL. Ammonium chloride and methylamine hydrochloride antagonize clostridial neurotoxins. *J Pharmacol Exp Ther.* 1983;225:546-552.

23. Puhar A, Johnson EA, Rossetto O, Montecucco C. Comparison of the pH-induced conformational change of different clostridial neurotoxins. *Biochem Biophys Res Commun.* 2004;319:66-71.

24. Lawrence G, Wang J, Chion CK, Aoki KR, Dolly JO. Two protein trafficking processes at motor nerve endings unveiled by botulinum neurotoxin e. *J Pharmacol Exp Ther.* 2007;320:410-418.

25. Montecucco C, Schiavo G, Dasgupta BR: Effect of pH on the interaction of botulinum neurotoxins A, B and E with liposomes. *Biochem J.* 1989;259:47-53.

26. Donovan JJ, Middlebrook JL. Ion-conducting channels produced by botulinum toxin in planar lipid membranes. *Biochemistry.* 1986;25:2872-2876.

27. Blaustein RO, Germann WJ, Finkelstein A, DasGupta BR. The N-terminal half of the heavy chain of botulinum type A neurotoxin forms channels in planar phospholipid bilayers. *FEBS Lett.* 1987;226:115-120.

28. Hoch DH, Romero-Mira M, Ehrlich BE, Finkelstein A, DasGupta BR, Simpson LL. Channels formed by botulinum, tetanus, and diphtheria toxins in planar lipid bilayers: relevance to translocation of proteins across membranes. *Proc Natl Acad Sci U S A.* 1985;82:1692-1696.

29. Sheridan RE. Gating and permeability of ion channels produced by botulinum toxin types A and E in PC12 cell membranes. *Toxicon.* 1998;36:703-717.

30. Koriazova LK, Montal M. Translocation of botulinum neurotoxin light chain protease through the heavy chain channel. *Nat Struct Biol.* 2003;10:13-18.

31. Jahn R, Scheller RH. SNAREs—engines for membrane fusion. *Nat Rev Mol Cell Biol.* 2006;7:631-643.

32. Starai VJ, Jun Y, Wickner W. From the Cover: Feature Article: Excess vacuolar SNAREs drive lysis and Rab bypass fusion. *Proc Natl Acad Sci U S A.* 2007;104:13551-13558.

33. Fischer A, Montal M. Characterization of Clostridial botulinum neurotoxin channels in neuroblastoma cells. *Neurotox Res.* 2006;9:93-100.

34. Fischer A, Montal M. Single molecule detection of intermediates during botulinum neurotoxin translocation across membranes. *Proc Natl Acad Sci U S A.* 2007;104:10447-10520.

35. Fischer A, Montal M. Crucial role of the disulfide bridge between botulinum neurotoxin light and heavy chains in protease translocation across membranes. *J Biol Chem.* 2007;282:29604-29611.

36. Oblatt-Montal M, Yamazaki M, Nelson R, Montal M. Formation of ion channels in lipid bilayers by a peptide with the predicted transmembrane sequence of botulinum neurotoxin A. *Protein Sci.* 1995;4:1490-1497.

37. Hamill OP, Marty A, Neher E, Sakmann B, Sigworth FJ. Improved patch-clamp techniques for high-resolution current recording from cells and cell-free membrane patches. *Pflugers Arch.* 1981;391:85-100.

38. Bade S, Rummel A, Reisinger C, Karnath T, Ahnert-Hilger G, Bigalke H, et al. Botulinum neurotoxin type D enables cytosolic delivery of enzymatically active cargo proteins to neurones via unfolded translocation intermediates. *J Neurochem.* 2004;91:1461-1472.

39. Krantz BA, Finkelstein A, Collier RJ. Protein translocation through the anthrax toxin transmembrane pore is driven by a proton gradient. *J Mol Biol.* 2006;355:968-979.

40. Zhang S, Udho E, Wu Z, Collier RJ, Finkelstein A. Protein translocation through anthrax toxin channels formed in planar lipid bilayers. *Biophys J.* 2004;87:3842-3849.

41. de Paiva A, Poulain B, Lawrence GW, Shone CC, Tauc L, Dolly JO. A role for the interchain disulfide or its participating thiols in the internalization of botulinum neurotoxin A revealed by a toxin derivative that binds to ecto-acceptors and inhibits transmitter release intracellularly. *J Biol Chem.* 1993;268:20838-20844.

42. Antharavally B, Tepp W, DasGupta BR. Status of Cys residues in the covalent structure of botulinum neurotoxin types A, B, and E. *J Protein Chem.* 1998;17:187-196.

43. Sathyamoorthy V, DasGupta BR. Separation, purification, partial characterization and comparison of the heavy and light chains of botulinum neurotoxin types A, B, and E. *J Biol Chem.* 1985;260:10461-10466.

44. Collier RJ. Understanding the mode of action of diphtheria toxin: a perspective on progress during the 20th century. *Toxicon.* 2001;39:1793-1803.

45. Ren J, Kachel K, Kim H, Malenbaum SE, Collier RJ, London E. Interaction of diphtheria toxin T domain with molten globule-like proteins and its implications for translocation. *Science.* 1999;284:955-957.

46. Oh KJ, Senzel L, Collier RJ, Finkelstein A. Translocation of the catalytic domain of diphtheria toxin across planar phospholipid bilayers by its own T domain. *Proc Natl Acad Sci U S A.* 1999;96:8467-8470.

47. Gambale F, Montal M. Characterization of the channel properties of tetanus toxin in planar lipid bilayers. *Biophys J.* 1988;53:771-783.

48. Borochov-Neori H, Yavin E, Montal M: Tetanus toxin forms channels in planar lipid bilayers containing gangliosides. *Biophys J.* 1984;45:83-85.

49. Blobel G, Walter P, Chang CN, Goldman BM, Erickson AH, Lingappa VR. Translocation of proteins across membranes: the signal hypothesis and beyond. *Symp Soc Exp Biol.* 1979;33:9-36.

50. Blobel G. Intracellular protein topogenesis. *Proc Natl Acad Sci U S A.* 1980;77:1496-1500.

51. Mitra K, Schaffitzel C, Shaikh T, Tama F, Jenni S, Brooks CL 3rd, et al. Structure of the E. coli protein-conducting channel bound to a translating ribosome. *Nature.* 2005;438:318-324.

52. Van den Berg B, Clemons WM Jr, Collinson I, Modis Y, Hartmann E, Harrison SC, et al. X-ray structure of a protein-conducting channel. *Nature.* 2004;427:36-44.

53. Beckmann R, Spahn CM, Eswar N, Helmers J, Penczek PA, Sali A, et al. Architecture of the protein-conducting channel associated with the translating 80S ribosome. *Cell.* 2001;107:361-372.

54. Mitra K, Frank J. A model for co-translational translocation: ribosome-regulated nascent polypeptide translocation at the protein-conducting channel. *FEBS Lett.* 2006;580:3353-3360.

55. Cannon KS, Or E, Clemons WM Jr, Shibata Y, Rapoport TA. Disulfide bridge formation between SecY and a translocating polypeptide localizes the translocation pore to the center of SecY. *J Cell Biol.* 2005;169:219-225.

56. Gumbart J, Schulten K. Molecular dynamics studies of the archaeal translocon. *Biophys J.* 2006;90:2356-2367.

57. Saparov SM, Erlandson K, Cannon K, Schaletzky J, Schulman S, Rapoport TA, et al. Determining the conductance of the SecY protein translocation channel for small molecules. *Mol Cell.* 2007;26:501-509.

58. Mokranjac D, Neupert W. Protein import into mitochondria. *Biochem Soc Trans.* 2005;33(Pt 5):1019-1023.

59. Rehling P, Brandner K, Pfanner N. Mitochondrial import and the twin-pore translocase. *Nat Rev Mol Cell Biol.* 2004;5:519-530.

60. Schnell DJ, Hebert DN. Protein translocons: multifunctional mediators of protein translocation across membranes. *Cell.* 2003;112:491-505.

61. Truscott KN, Kovermann P, Geissler A, Merlin A, Meijer M, Driessen AJ, et al. A presequence- and voltage-sensitive channel of the mitochondrial preprotein translocase formed by Tim23. *Nat Struct Biol.* 2001;8:1074-1082.

62. Hinnah SC, Wagner R, Sveshnikova N, Harrer R, Soll J. The chloroplast protein import channel toc75: pore properties and interaction with transit peptides. *Biophys J.* 2002;83:899-911.

63. Heins L, Mehrle A, Hemmler R, Wagner R, Kuchler M, Hormann F, et al. The preprotein conducting channel at the inner envelope membrane of plastids. *EMBO J.* 2002;21:2616-2625.

64. Movileanu L, Schmittschmitt JP, Scholtz JM, Bayley H. Interactions of peptides with a protein pore. *Biophys J.* 2005;89:1030-1045.

65. Giraudat J, Dennis M, Heidmann T, Scholtz JM, Bayley H. Structure of the high-affinity binding site for non-competitive blockers of the acetylcholine receptor: serine-262 of the delta subunit is labeled by [3H]chlorpromazine. *Proc Nat Acad Sci U S A.* 1986;83:2719-2723.

66. Hille B: *Ion Channels of Excitable Cells,* 3rd ed. Sunderland, MA, Sinauer, 2001.

67. Lester HA. The permeation pathway of neurotransmitter-gated ion channels. *Annu Rev Biophys Biomol Struct.* 1992;21:267-292.

68. Schmid A, Benz R, Just I, Aktories K. Interaction of Clostridium botulinum C2 toxin with lipid bilayer membranes. Formation of cation-selective channels and inhibition of channel function by chloroquine. *J Biol Chem.* 1994;269:16706-16711.

69. Wang C, Takeuchi K, Pinto LH, Lamb RA. Ion channel activity of influenza A virus M2 protein: characterization of the amantadine block. *J Virol.* 1993;67:5585-5594.

70. Pinto LH, Holsinger LJ, Lamb RA. Influenza virus M2 protein has ion channel activity. *Cell.* 1992;69:517-528.

71. Chen HS, Lipton SA: Mechanism of memantine block of NMDA-activated channels in rat retinal ganglion cells: uncompetitive antagonism. *J Physiol.* 1997;499(Pt 1):27-46.

Interactions Between Botulinum Neurotoxins and Synaptic Vesicle Proteins

4

Axel T. Brunger, Rongsheng Jin, and Mark A. Breidenbach

INTRODUCTION

Clostridial neurotoxins (CNTs) are produced by species of anaerobic, gram-positive, spore-forming, rod-shaped, bacteria within the genus *Clostridium*. Botulinum neurotoxins (BoNTs), expressed by *Clostridium botulinum*, cause botulism, a severe neurologic disease associated with a life-threatening flaccid paralysis affecting both humans and animals.[1] Tetanus toxin (TeNT), expressed by *Clostridium tetani*, causes tetanus, a disease characterized by spastic paralysis that causes opposing skeletal muscles to contract spasmodically.[2] The first scientific observations of the paralytic syndrome botulism were made by Justinus Kerner in 1820,[3] who discovered that the disease can be caused by the intake of contaminated smoked sausages (Latin: *botulus*). Tetanus has been recognized since ancient times and was already described by Hippocrates; in 1867, it was hypothesized that an infectious agent is the cause.[1] CNTs interfere with the acetylcholine release process itself but not with acetylcholine storage or the entry of Ca^{2+}, implying that CNTs block neuronal exocytosis.[4] CNTs block neurotransmitter release by proteolytic cleavage of soluble N-ethylmaleimide-sensitive fusion protein attachment protein receptors (SNAREs), proteins that play a key role in Ca^{2+}-triggered neurotransmitter release.[5,6]

Botulism and tetanus are no longer considered major threats to public health, but occasionally small botulism outbreaks are still reported.[7] Rather, BoNTs (usually in complex with hemagglutinin) have become powerful therapeutic agents. For example, controlled application of very low doses of BoNT/A has proven to be an effective treatment for certain neurologic disorders associated with an abnormal increase in muscle tone or activity, such as spasticity and focal dystonias.[8] Recently, BoNT/A-containing treatments have also been shown to be beneficial for conditions such as achalasia,[9] chronic headache,[10] and hyperhidrosis.[11] These and other therapeutic applications of CNT are reviewed in detail in other chapters of this book. Moreover, CNTs have become powerful research tools to study the function of SNARE proteins in Ca^{2+}-triggered neurotransmitter release.[12] This chapter focuses on structural insights of the interactions between BoNTs and their proteolytic targets and cell surface receptors.

MODULAR ARCHITECTURE AND MECHANISM OF ACTION

CNTs are synthesized as single polypeptide chains of approximately 150 kDa. This single chain is post-translationally cleaved by certain bacterial and tissue proteases into a 50-kDa light chain (LC) and a 100-kDa heavy chain (HC).[13,14] On cleavage, the LC and HC of

The authors of this chapter do not report any conflicts of interest.

CNTs remain covalently and reversibly linked by a disulfide bond until being exposed to reducing conditions in the neuronal cytosol[15,16] (Fig. 4-1A). CNTs associate with non-neurotoxin components such as hemagglutinins, that may assist with the intoxication process and contribute to antigenic distinctness.[17]

There are seven serotypes of BoNTs (termed A to G) and one TeNT.[2,18] All BoNTs have a high degree of primary sequence conservation, although all are antigenically distinct.[19] Crystal structures of full-length BoNT/A holotoxin[20] and of BoNT/B holotoxin[21] are available (Fig. 4-2A). Both structures are very similar; they exhibit a modular architecture: the LC protease, translocation (the N-terminal subdomain of HC, HC_N) and the receptor binding domains (the C-terminal subdomain of HC, HC_C). It is important to note that in these crystal structures, the translocation domain is in its soluble conformation; the structure of its membrane-inserted conformation remains to be elucidated.

All BoNTs employ a similar mechanism of toxicity, suggesting that these toxins have a common evolutionary origin.[16] The HCs mediate the neuronal cell surface binding, internalization by receptor-mediated endocytosis, and transportation of the LC across the membrane into the cytosol and reduction of the disulfide bond (see Fig. 4-1A). Once the LC is released into the cytosol, SNARE targets are proteolysed by the LC.[22,23]

Primary sequence analyses of LC proteases revealed a Zn^{2+}-binding His-Glu-X-X-His motif. This motif is found in a variety of Zn^{2+}-dependent metalloproteases such as thermolysin, and it suggests that LCs may use a similar enzymatic mechanism.[24] The CNT-LCs cleave specific peptide bonds within the neuronal SNARE proteins (synaptobrevin, syntaxin, and SNAP-25) (see Fig. 4-1B). BoNT/A and E specifically cleave SNAP-25, whereas serotypes B, D, F, and G of BoNTs cleave synaptobrevin. BoNT/C1 is unique in that it is able to hydrolyze two substrates: syntaxin[25,26] and SNAP-25.[27-29]

SNARES AND CA2+-TRIGGERED NEUROTRANSMITTER RELEASE

Much of our understanding of the critical role SNAREs play in neurotransmission can be

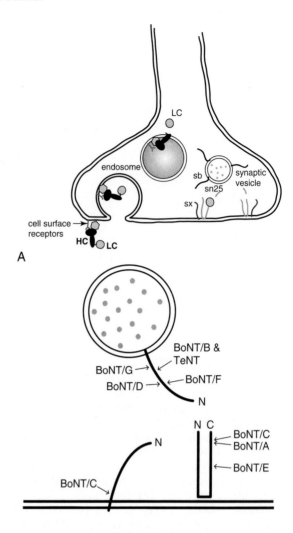

FIGURE 4-1. Synaptic SNAREs are targeted by CNT light chains. **A,** A four-step model for CNT intoxication includes (1) neurospecific cell-surface binding, (2) receptor-mediated endocytosis, (3) translocation of the light chain, and (4) SNARE-specific proteolysis.[16,111,112] The toxin heavy chain (HC, *black*) mediates cell-surface binding with ganglioside and glycoprotein receptors. Following endocytosis, the HC also mediates translocation of the light chain (LC, *gray*) if the endosome is acidified. LCs can target the synaptic SNAREs, including vesicle-bound synaptobrevin (sb), presynaptic membrane-bound syntaxin (sx), and SNAP-25 (sn25) before ternary SNARE complex formation. **B,** The relative locations of the peptide bonds hydrolyzed by LCs in the core domains of SNARE proteins are shown. The cut sites of the seven botulinum neurotoxin serotypes (BoNT/A-G) and that of tetanus toxin (TeNT) are indicated by arrows. *See Color Plate*

directly traced to the finding that botulism and tetanus toxins block Ca^{2+}-triggered neurotransmitter release. At neuromuscular junctions (NMJs), acetylcholine is predominantly secreted via full vesicle fusion events rather than by a transient "kiss-and-run" mechanism, which likely plays a more prominent role in the central nervous system.[30-32] A continuous cycle of synaptic vesicle formation, delivery, fusion, and local recycling occurs such that a steady supply of vesicles is available for neurotransmitter release when triggered by the arrival of an action potential.[33]

As the nerve terminal is depolarized during the arrival of an action potential, a rapid influx of Ca^{2+} enters the nerve cytosol through voltage-gated Ca^{2+}-channels, triggering fusion events.[30] Although tethering complexes hold docked vesicles in close proximity to their target membranes, an additional set of proteins interact to bring the two membranes close enough such that phospholipid bilayer reorganization into a fused state becomes energetically favorable.[34] Among the essential proteins for this task are the SNAREs.[35,36] Neuronal SNAREs are membrane bound, either via a single transmembrane region as in the cases of synaptobrevin and syntaxin,[37] or by post-translational palmitoylation as in the case of SNAP-25.[38] SNARE proteins contain at least one core domain that can adopt a parallel, coiled-coil conformation when given the opportunity to interact with other SNARE proteins[39] (Fig. 4-2B).

Intense biochemical and biophysical scrutiny of SNARE proteins has yielded the "zipper model" of membrane fusion.[40-43] The principle of this model is simple: SNAREs protruding from the synaptic vesicle membrane (mainly synaptobrevin) assemble into low-energy core complexes, with SNAREs anchored to the presynaptic membrane (mainly syntaxin and SNAP-25). The core domains of SNARE proteins are mostly unstructured in the absence of binding partners,[44-46] but they are entirely helical when the ternary complex is formed.[39] The helices formed by SNARE proteins are amphipathic, and the coiled-coil structure is largely stabilized by hydrophobic packing.[47] A notable exception is the conserved "ionic layer" formed at the center of the complex by a network of salt bridges and hydrogen bonds.[39] The resulting structure is remarkably stable, resisting extreme chemical and thermal denaturing conditions.[48-50] The stepwise assembly of these low-energy complexes is thought to counter the energetic penalty of bringing phospholipid headgroups from opposing membranes together at a distance where membrane reorganization into a fusogenic state becomes favorable.[51] SNARE-mediated docking and fusion appears to be a general strategy for combining independent

compartments in eukaryotic cells, but SNAREs are not the only factors imparting targeting specificity between intracellular membranes as originally believed. A number of additional proteins form tethering complexes to assist in this process.[52,53] In addition, SNARE assembly is not inherently Ca^{2+}-sensitive; additional factors are required for regulation of synaptic vesicle fusion. Synaptotagmin 1, a Ca^{2+}-binding protein, has been shown to be a sensor for Ca^{2+}-induced fusion events.[54,55] Other factors such as Munc18 (nSec1), Munc13, and complexin bind to SNAREs and may play a role in regulating SNARE complex assembly.[56-59] However, the precise sequence of events and role of the various components of Ca^{2+}-triggered neurotransmitter release remain to be elucidated.[60]

The crucial role of SNAREs in synaptic exocytosis was illuminated by the discovery that they are the physiologic targets of the CNTs; in 1992, Schiavo and colleagues[6] reported that the intracellular proteolytic target of TeNT and BoNT/B is synaptobrevin. The target sites of the other BoNT serotypes are summarized in (see Fig. 4-1B).[5,6,26,61,62] Remarkably, all CNT LCs target sites within the core domains of SNARE proteins.

CNT LC PROTEASES

BoNT and TeNT LCs are among the most selective proteases known.[63] As mentioned earlier, primary sequence and structural analysis of LCs suggest that their enzymatic mechanism is related to that of other Zn^{2+}-metalloproteases,[20,21,64-66] but the structural basis of SNARE target selectivity is unusual. Oddly, the LCs do not appear to recognize a consensus site, or even have rigorous requirements for particular side chains flanking the scissile bond.[67] Also, the LCs generally require long stretches of their target SNAREs for optimal efficiency.[28,67-71] Indeed, point mutations in SNARE regions remote from the scissile bond can dramatically reduce LC efficiency.[71-74] The cleavage-site selectivity of CNT-LCs is remarkable. For example, the scissile bond in SNAP-25 for BoNT/A (Gln197-Arg198) is shifted by exactly one residue compared with that for BoNT/C1 (Arg198-Ala199). BoNT/C1 cleaves only one of two identical neighboring peptide bonds (Lys253-Ala254 and Lys260-Ala261) in syntaxin-1A.[26]

The apo structures of all members of the family of CNT-LCs are now available: BoNT/A,[20,74,75] BoNT/B,[21] BoNT/C1,[76] BoNT/D,[77]

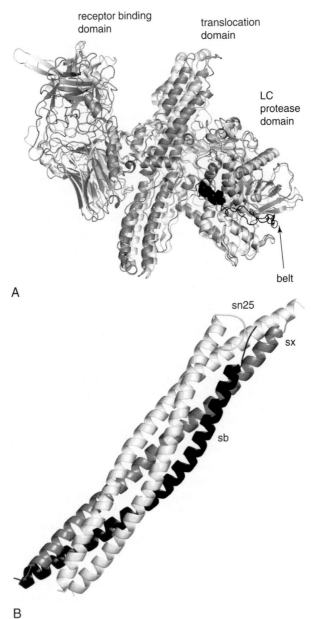

FIGURE 4-2. Structures of apo CNTs and a ternary SNARE complex. **A,** Apo holotoxin structures: BoNT/A (PDB code 3BTA)[20] (*dark gray*) and BoNT/B (PDB code 1EPW)[21] (*light gray*). The LC protease, translocation, and receptor binding domains are indicated. The structures were superimposed using the backbone atoms of the LC protease domain. The belt region is colored black. **B,** Crystal structure of the neuronal SNARE complex[39] consisting of synaptobrevin (sb, *dark gray*), syntaxin (sx, *medium gray*), and SNAP-25 (sn25, *light gray*) (PDB code 1SFC). This structure represents the post-fusion state of the SNARE complex. *See Color Plate*

BoNT/E,[64] BoNT/F,[78] BoNT/G,[79] and TeNT[65,66] (see Fig. 4-2C). The structural differences among the CNT-LCs are mostly limited to solvent-exposed loops and potential substrate interaction sites. The striking similarity of LC active sites naturally leads to the question of which LC features are determinants of substrate selectivity. Furthermore, none of the LCs efficiently cleave truncated substrate peptides less than 20–30 residues. Rather, unusually long stretches of residues of the substrates are required for optimal cleavage.[28,67,69-71]

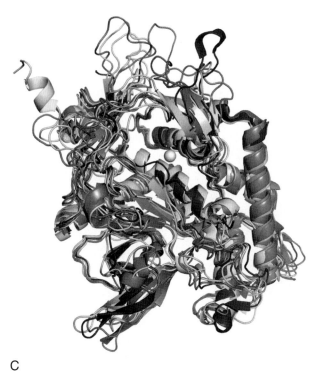

C

FIGURE 4-2 cont'd. C, An overall superposition of the LC protease structures from all seven serotypes of BoNTs and TeNT: BoNT/A (PDB code 1XTF),[20,74,75] BoNT/B (1EPW),[21] BoNT/C1 (2QN0), BoNT/D (2FPQ),[77] BoNT/E (1T3A),[64] BoNT/F (2A8A),[78] BoNT/G (1ZB7),[79] and TeNT (1Z7H).[65] Despite their different substrate specificities, CNT-LCs display high structural similarity. *See Color Plate*

In general, long sequences that are located near the N-termini of the scissile bonds appear to be important for cleavage, as revealed by mutagenesis studies on synaptobrevin and SNAP-25.[68,80] For example, the optimal portion of SNAP-25 required for maximally efficient cleavage by BoNT/A spans residues 146 to 202.[28,81] Other CNTs require 30 to 60 residue stretches of their substrate for efficient cleavage, regardless of scissile-bond location.[68-70] Moreover, point mutations in SNAREs far remote from the scissile bond can dramatically reduce the proteolysis efficiency.[72-74]

The structure of a BoNT/A·SNAP-25 complex[74] finally provided insights into the basis of LC substrate selectivity. To date, this is the only structure of a complex between a CNT-LC and its substrate; a previous report of the structure of a complex between BoNT/A-LC and synaptobrevin[82] is not supported by the experimental data.[74,83] Remarkably, SNAP-25 wraps around most of the LC's circumference; the extensive interface between the enzyme and its substrate is not restricted to the active site (Fig. 4-3A). Moreover, in contrast to the contiguous helical conformation observed in the ternary SNARE complex,[39] SNAP-25 adopts three distinct types of secondary structure upon binding to BoNT/A. The N-terminal residues of SNAP-25 (147–167) form an α-helix, the C-terminal residues (201–204) form a distorted β-strand, and residues in between are mostly extended.[74] Mutagenesis and kinetics experiments demonstrated that the N-terminal α-helix and the C-terminal β-sheet are critical for an efficient substrate binding and cleavage, and are termed α- and β-exosites, respectively. The structure confirmed the existence of such exosites, which had been postulated before based on biochemical experiments.[72,84]

The highly unusual extended enzyme-substrate interface used by BoNT/A serves to properly orient its conformationally variable SNARE target such that the scissile peptide bond is placed within close proximity of the catalytic motif of the enzyme. Notably, many

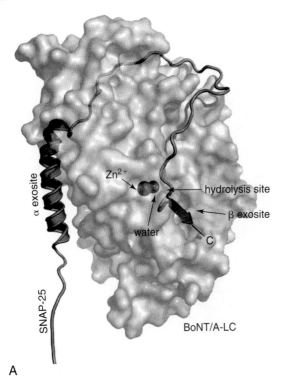

A

FIGURE 4-3. Interactions between BoNTs and synaptic vesicle proteins. **A,** Structure of the BoNT/A·SNAP-25 complex. The protease component of BoNT/A forms an extended interface with the C-terminal core domain of SNAP-25. Multiple sites of enzyme-substrate interaction remote from the catalytic Zn^{2+} and associated nucleophile extend around most of the toxin's circumference, imparting the protease with exquisite specificity. SNAP-25 is unstructured in the absence of a binding partner but adopts a mix of α-helix, β-sheet, and extended conformations when complexed with BoNT/A. *See Color Plate*

of the interactions that impart substrate specificity occur on the face of the protease that is opposite to its active site (α-exosite), and the C-terminus of the substrate (β-exosite) induces a conformational change in the active site pocket, probably rendering the protease competent for catalysis. The multisite binding strategy used by BoNT/A accounts for the extreme selectivity of this enzyme. The structure of the BoNT/A·SNAP-25 complex vividly illustrates the extent of substrate that must be available for efficient proteolysis to occur. SNAREs exhibit considerable conformational variability; they can exist as monomeric components with little secondary structure, as partially structured SNARE complexes or subcomplexes, or in complex

with regulatory factors.[85] Thus, BoNT/A probably cannot efficiently hydrolyze SNAP-25 if any portion of the C-terminal core domain is already incorporated into a ternary SNARE complex (see Fig. 4-2B) or bound to a regulatory factor.

The structural and enzyme kinetics studies of the BoNT/C1-LC have provided further information regarding the toxin-substrate interaction.[76] BoNT/C1-LC is unique among all BoNTs in that it exhibits dual specificity toward both syntaxin and SNAP-25. Interestingly, although both BoNT/A and BoNT/C1 cleave SNAP-25, the scissile bond is shifted by only a single residue (Gln197-Arg198 for BoNT/A and Arg198-Ala199 for BoNT/C1). Structural modeling revealed that the remote α-exosite that was previously identified in the complex of BoNT/A-LC and SNAP-25 is structurally conserved in BoNT/C1. Single site mutations in the predicted α-exosite of BoNT/C1 had a significant but less severe effect on SNAP-25 cleavage in comparison to that of BoNT/A, suggesting that this region plays a less stringent role on substrate discrimination. Such a "promiscuous" substrate-binding strategy by the α-exosite could account for its dual substrate specificity. As a crucial supplement to the function of the remote α-exosite, the scissile-bond proximal exosites probably ensure the correct register for hydrolysis. This includes the β-exosite as observed on BoNT/A and key residues surrounding the scissile peptide bond. A small, distinct pocket (S1′) near the active site of BoNT/C1 was found that potentially ensures the correct register for the cleavage site by only allowing alanine as the P1′ residue for both SNAP-25 and syntaxin. Mutations of this SNAP-25 residue dramatically reduced enzymatic activity of BoNT/C1.[76]

The crystal structure of the BoNT/A-LC·SNAP-25 complex revealed a small loop (residues 183–190) that detaches from the surface of BoNT/A-LC and separates the α-exosite from the active site. This loop may be able to accommodate the necessary "slack" for the cleavage-site register shift between BoNT/A and BoNT/C1 while maintaining the approximate position of the α-exosite. Consistent with this notion, there is little effect on substrate cleavage on insertion of up to three extra residues in this loop.[76] The divided roles for substrate discrimination among different exosites could provide some flexibility of the precise scissile bond position while ensuring high overall substrate specificity.

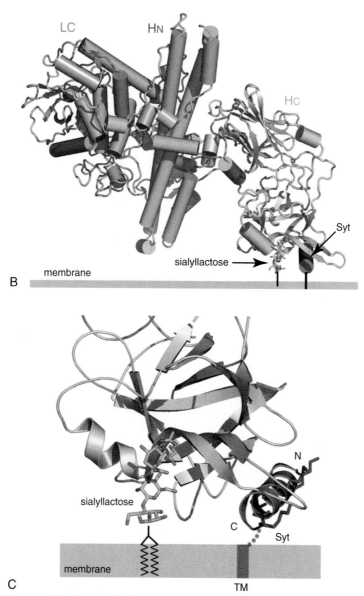

FIGURE 4-3 cont'd. B, Proposed binding mode of BoNT/B on the membrane surface. The structure of a sialyllactose-bound BoNT/B (PDB code 1F31) was superimposed on the complex of BoNT/B-HC$_C$ and synaptotagmin II by using the coordinates of the HC$_C$ fragment for the alignment. The LC, the amino-terminal part of the heavy chain (HC$_N$), and the carboxy-terminal domain of the heavy chain (HC$_C$) are shown. **C,** A close-up view of the proposed interface between BoNT/B and membrane. Four lysine residues that are conserved in synaptotagmins I and II are shown as sticks. *See Color Plate*

RECEPTOR INTERACTIONS

Complex gangliosides, a class of glycosphingo-lipids that are particularly abundant in the outer leaflet of nerve cell membranes, have long been recognized to function as receptors for CNT-HCs. Later, the existence of two classes of binding sites distinguished by different affinities and protease-sensitivities[86,87] led to a dual-receptor concept: complex ganglio-sides first accumulate CNTs on the plasma membrane surface before protein receptors subsequently mediate their endocytosis, with a different protein receptor being recognized by each BoNT.[22,88,89] Such a dual-receptor binding process could account for the extraordinary binding affinity and specificity of CNTs.

Ganglioside-binding sites have been identified for several CNTs.[21,90,91] The structure of a complex between BoNT/B and sialyllactose revealed a conserved binding pocket,[21] which was also shown to be essential for ganglioside recognition of BoNT/A, BoNT/B, and TeNT.[91,92] The amino acids that form this binding site are conserved among all CNTs except BoNT/D. The trisialoganglioside GT1b was found to interact with the receptor binding domains of BoNT/A, BoNT/B, and TeNT.[91,92] At present, the only protein receptors to have been identified are synaptotagmin I and synaptotagmin II for BoNT/B and BoNT/G, respectively, and synaptic vesicle protein SV2 (isoforms A, B and C) for BoNT/A.[93-97] Furthermore, BoNT/A and B were observed to bind synaptic vesicle protein complexes in synaptosome lysates.[98] The complexes comprised several proteins including synaptotagmin I, SV2, synaptophysin, VAMP2, and the vacuolar proton pump. However, it is unknown if any of these proteins play a role in the toxin binding and endocytosis processes in addition to synaptotagmins and SV2. In contrast to these CNTs, TeNT may have two ganglioside binding sites and no protein receptor has yet been found.[92]

The BoNT protein receptors SV2 and synaptotagmins I and II are localized to synaptic vesicles. The luminal domains of these protein receptors become exposed to the extracellular space when synaptic vesicles fuse with the presynaptic membrane on depolarization of the presynaptic terminal. This is likely the temporal window through which BoNTs interact with their specific receptors. Similarly, it is probably during this period that passive neutralizing antitoxins can act.[99]

Synaptotagmins are a family of transmembrane proteins that trigger Ca^{2+}-dependent neurotransmitter release. Synaptotagmins I and II are essential for synaptic transmission in neuromuscular junctions.[100] BoNT/B and BoNT/G bind to the luminal domains of synaptotagmins I and II when they are exposed on the neuronal cell surface. The carboxy-terminal domain of the heavy chain (HC_C) of BoNT/B is solely responsible for specific binding with the luminal domains of synaptotagmins I and II.[93,97] The luminal domain of synaptotagmin II is unstructured in solution.[101] Upon binding to BoNT/B, it folds

into an α-helix, which binds at the distal tip of the HC_C of BoNT/B in a saddle-shaped crevice on the surface (see Fig. 4-3B).[101,102] The extensive intermolecular interface has a buried surface area of about 1200 $Å^2$, involving mostly hydrophobic residues and complementary salt bridges.

The toxin-receptor interactions are highly specific. Mutations in the synaptotagmin binding cleft greatly reduce the toxicity of BoNT/B by up to 1000-fold and are more significant than mutations in the ganglioside-binding pocket.[101] The structure of the BoNT/B synaptotagmin II complex also sheds light on the interaction of BoNT/G with its receptor. BoNT/G is the closest homolog to BoNT/B and also binds to the membrane-proximal region of synaptotagmin I and II.[97] Primary sequence analysis revealed that the synaptotagmin binding site is conserved among BoNT/B and BoNT/G but not in other toxin family members. Mutations of some of the BoNT/G residues that are equivalent to the synaptotagmin-interacting residues on BoNT/B significantly decrease the binding affinities between synaptotagmins and BoNT/G.[103] Taken together, BoNT/B and G likely employ the same strategy for receptor binding.

The dual-receptor hypothesis for BoNTs was proposed more than 20 years ago,[88] but the spatial and functional relationship between these two receptors had been unclear. Crystal structures now offer clues about this relationship: the luminal domain of synaptotagmin II and a sialyllactose carbohydrate moiety occupy two adjacent but nonoverlapping binding sites (see Fig. 4-3C).[21,90,91,101] Ganglioside or synaptotagmin binding does not cause significant structural changes in the HC_C domain. However, they appear to act synergistically; the dissociation constant between the receptor-binding domain of BoNT/B and the luminal domain of synaptotagmin II in solution is more than 100-fold larger than that measured between BoNT/B and full-length synaptotagmin II (including the transmembrane region) in the presence of gangliosides and micelles.[96] Deletion of the transmembrane domain of synaptotagmin I abolishes ganglioside-dependent binding.[104] Clearly, further experiments are needed to characterize potential intramembrane interactions between the two receptors. Nevertheless, toxin-receptor interactions may be different for other members of the CNT family. As mentioned earlier, two carbohydrate-binding sites in the C-terminal part of the heavy chain fragment of TeNT are required for its function.[92] These different mechanisms of cell-surface recognition may explain the differences in CNT trafficking in peripheral neurons. Characterization of both the protein and lipid receptor sites could provide an approach to retarget BoNTs to different cell types by site-directed mutagenesis. Such modified BoNTs could possibly be used as drug delivery systems.[105]

For CNTs, proper orientation on the membrane surface is important for efficient endocytosis and subsequent translocation of the light chain to the cytosol.[106,107] In the case of BoNT/B, the simultaneous attachment of synaptotagmin and ganglioside ligands imposes geometric restrictions on the position of BoNT/B with respect to the membrane surface (see Fig. 4-3B–C). Two strongly negatively charged molecular surfaces, which remain charged even in an acidic endosomal lumen, further restrict the orientation of BoNT/B on the membrane surface. In addition, four solvent-exposed lysine residues are conserved in both synaptotagmins I and II (see Fig. 4-3C), which may interact with phospholipid headgroups. The interactions between the toxin's heavy chain and nearby negatively charged phospholipids appear to stabilize the toxin on membranes.[22] Interestingly, the receptor binding region, especially around the synaptotagmin II binding site, was recognized by mouse anti-BoNT/B antibodies.[108]

It is conceivable that CNTs first interact with the oligosaccharide portion of polysialogangliosides, which are highly enriched at nerve terminals, causing the CNT to adhere to the neuronal cell surface. Upon binding to exposed gangliosides, the toxins will be constrained to the plasma membrane surface, thereby significantly increasing localized toxin concentration.[109] The toxin-ganglioside complex could then diffuse laterally before binding to a second, less abundant, protein receptor. The abundance of polysialogangliosides ensures high trapping efficiency, whereas enhanced specificity is conferred by the protein receptor.

CONCLUSIONS

The remarkable specificity of the CNT-LC proteases is attributed to the existence of multiple substrate-binding sites including exosites that are remote from the scissile bond. In addition, CNTs also exhibit high specificity for neuronal cell-surface receptors. It is noteworthy that CNTs bind to one component of the synaptic vesicle fusion machinery (synaptotagmins or SV2s), and then cleave another on entry (SNAREs). Clearly, more structures of the CNTs in complex with their substrates or receptors are needed to investigate if the receptor and substrate recognition mechanisms are conserved among CNTs and to provide starting points for structure-based inhibitor development.

Very limited information is currently available regarding the function of the N-terminal part of the heavy chain (belt domain) and the translocation domain (see Fig. 4-2A). As discussed in a recent review, the CNT heavy chain belt might act as a surrogate pseudosubstrate inhibitor of the LC protease or as a chaperone during the translocation step.[110] A better molecular understanding of the mechanism of action of CNTs has the potential to yield new clinical applications.

ACKNOWLEDGMENTS

ATB acknowledges support by the Department of Defense and Defense Threat Reduction Agency proposal number 3.10024_06_RD_B.

References

1. Hatheway CL. Toxigenic clostridia. *Clin Microbiol Rev.* 1990;3:66-98.
2. Montecucco C, Schiavo G. Structure and function of tetanus and botulinum neurotoxins. *Q Rev Biophys.* 1995;28:423-472.
3. Erbguth FJ. Historical notes on botulism, Clostridium botulinum, botulinum toxin, and the idea of the therapeutic use of the toxin. *Mov Disord.* 2004;19(Suppl 8):S2-S6.
4. Kao I, Drachman DB, Price DL. Botulinum toxin: mechanism of presynaptic blockade. *Science.* 1976;193:1256-1258.
5. Blasi J, Chapman ER, Link E, Binz T, Yamasaki S, De Camilli P, et al. Botulinum neurotoxin A selectively cleaves the synaptic protein SNAP-25. *Nature.* 1993;365:160-163.
6. Schiavo G, Benfenati F, Poulain B, Rossetto O, Polverino de Laureto P, et al. Tetanus and botulinum-B neurotoxins block neurotransmitter release by proteolytic cleavage of synaptobrevin. *Nature.* 1992;359:832-835.
7. Sobel J, Tucker N, Sulka A, McLaughlin J, Maslanka S. Foodborne botulism in the United States, 1990-2000. *Emerg Infect Dis.* 2004;10:1606-1611.
8. Kessler KR, Benecke R. Botulinum toxin: from poison to remedy. *Neurotoxicology.* 1997;18:761-770.
9. Gui D, Rossi S, Runfola M, Magalini SC. Review article: botulinum toxin in the therapy of gastrointestinal motility disorders. *Aliment Pharmacol Ther.* 2003;18:1-16.
10. Charles PD. Botulinum neurotoxin serotype A: a clinical update on non-cosmetic uses. *Am J Health Syst Pharm.* 2004;61(Suppl 6):S11-S23.

11. Munchau A, Bhatia KP. Uses of botulinum toxin injection in medicine today. *BMJ.* 2000;320:161-165.

12. Niemann H, Blasi J, Jahn R. Clostridial neurotoxins: new tools for dissecting exocytosis. *Trends Cell Biol.* 1994;179-185.

13. Helting TB, Parschat S, Engelhardt H. Structure of tetanus toxin. Demonstration and separation of a specific enzyme converting intracellular tetanus toxin to the extracellular form. *J Biol Chem.* 1979;254:10728-10733.

14. Weller U, Dauzenroth ME, Meyer ZU, Heringdorf D, Habermann E. Chains and fragments of tetanus toxin. Separation, reassociation and pharmacological properties. *Eur J Biochem.* 1989;182:649-656.

15. Schiavo G, Papini E, Genna G, Montecucco C. An intact interchain disulfide bond is required for the neurotoxicity of tetanus toxin. *Infect Immun.* 1990;58:4136-4141.

16. Turton K, Chaddock JA, Acharya KR. Botulinum and tetanus neurotoxins: structure, function and therapeutic utility. *Trends Biochem Sci.* 2002;27:552-558.

17. Fujinaga Y, Inoue K, Watarai S, Sakaguchi Y, Arimitsu H, Lee JC, et al. Molecular characterization of binding subcomponents of Clostridium botulinum type C progenitor toxin for intestinal epithelial cells and erythrocytes. *Microbiology.* 2004;150(Pt 5):1529-1538.

18. Binz T, Kurazono H, Wille M, Frevert J, Wernars K, Niemann H. The complete sequence of botulinum neurotoxin type A and comparison with other clostridial neurotoxins. *J Biol Chem.* 1990;265:9153-9158.

19. Lacy DB, Stevens RC. Sequence homology and structural analysis of the clostridial neurotoxins. *J Mol Biol.* 1999;291:1091-1104.

20. Lacy DB, Tepp W, Cohen AC, DasGupta BR, Stevens RC. Crystal structure of botulinum neurotoxin type A and implications for toxicity. *Nat Struct Biol.* 1998;5:898-902.

21. Swaminathan S, Eswaramoorthy S. Structural analysis of the catalytic and binding sites of Clostridium botulinum neurotoxin B. *Nat Struct Biol.* 2000;7:693-699.

22. Schiavo G, Matteoli M, Montecucco C. Neurotoxins affecting neuroexocytosis. *Physiol Rev.* 2000;80:717-766.

23. Simpson LL. Identification of the major steps in botulinum toxin action. *Annu Rev Pharmacol Toxicol.* 2004;44:167-193.

24. Kurazono H, Mochida S, Binz T, Eisel U, Quanz M, Grebenstein O, et al. Minimal essential domains specifying toxicity of the light chains of tetanus toxin and botulinum neurotoxin type A. *J Biol Chem.* 1992;267:14721-14729.

25. Blasi J, Chapman ER, Yamasaki S, Binz T, Niemann H, Jahn R. Botulinum neurotoxin C1 blocks neurotransmitter release by means of cleaving HPC-1/syntaxin. *Embo J.* 1993;12:4821-4828.

26. Schiavo G, Shone CC, Bennett MK, Scheller RH, Montecucco C. Botulinum neurotoxin type C cleaves a single Lys-Ala bond within the carboxyl-terminal region of syntaxins. *J Biol Chem.* 1995;270:10566-10570.

27. Foran P, Lawrence GW, Shone CC, Foster KA, Dolly JO. Botulinum neurotoxin C1 cleaves both syntaxin and SNAP-25 in intact and permeabilized chromaffin cells: correlation with its blockade of catecholamine release. *Biochemistry.* 1996;35:2630-2636.

28. Vaidyanathan VV, Yoshino K, Jahnz M, Dorries C, Bade S, Nauenburg S, et al. Proteolysis of SNAP-25 isoforms by botulinum neurotoxin types A, C, and E: domains and amino acid residues controlling the formation of enzyme-substrate complexes and cleavage. *J Neurochem.* 1999;72:327-337.

29. Williamson LC, Halpern JL, Montecucco C, Brown JE, Neale EA. Clostridial neurotoxins and substrate proteolysis in intact neurons: botulinum neurotoxin C acts on synaptosomal-associated protein of 25 kDa. *J Biol Chem.* 1996;271:7694-7699.

30. Van der Kloot W. Loading and recycling of synaptic vesicles in the Torpedo electric organ and the vertebrate neuromuscular junction. *Prog Neurobiol.* 2003;71:269-303.

31. Aravanis AM, Pyle JL, Tsien RW. Single synaptic vesicles fusing transiently and successively without loss of identity. *Nature.* 2003;423:643-647.

32. Gandhi SP, Stevens CF. Three modes of synaptic vesicular recycling revealed by single-vesicle imaging. *Nature.* 2003;423:607-613.

33. Sudhof TC. The synaptic vesicle cycle. *Annu Rev Neurosci.* 2004;27:509-547.

34. Harbury PA. Springs and zippers: coiled coils in SNARE-mediated membrane fusion. *Structure.* 1998;6:1487-1491.

35. Schuette CG, Hatsuzawa K, Margittai M, Stein A, Riedel D, Kuster P, et al. Determinants of liposome fusion mediated by synaptic SNARE proteins. *Proc Natl Acad Sci U S A.* 2004;101:2858-2863.

36. Sollner TH. Intracellular and viral membrane fusion: a uniting mechanism. *Curr Opin Cell Biol.* 2004;16:429-435.

37. Sollner T. SNAREs and targeted membrane fusion. *FEBS Lett.* 1995;369:80-83.

38. Veit M, Sollner TH, Rothman JE. Multiple palmitoylation of synaptotagmin and the t-SNARE SNAP-25. *FEBS Lett.* 1996;385:119-123.

39. Sutton RB, Fasshauer D, Jahn R, Brunger AT. Crystal structure of a SNARE complex involved in synaptic exocytosis at 2.4 A resolution. *Nature.* 1998;395:347-353.

40. Otto H, Hanson PI, Jahn R. Assembly and disassembly of a ternary complex of synaptobrevin, syntaxin, and SNAP-25 in the membrane of synaptic vesicles. *Proc Natl Acad Sci U S A.* 1997;94:6197-6201.

41. Hanson PI, Roth R, Morisaki H, Jahn R, Heuser JE. Structure and conformational changes in NSF and its membrane receptor complexes visualized by quick-freeze/deep-etch electron microscopy. *Cell.* 1997;90:523-535.

42. Lin RC, Scheller RH. Structural organization of the synaptic exocytosis core complex. *Neuron.* 1997;19:1087-1094.

43. Matos MF, Mukherjee K, Chen X, Rizo J, Sudhof TC. Evidence for SNARE zippering during Ca2+-triggered exocytosis in PC12 cells. *Neuropharmacology.* 2003;45:777-786.

44. Fasshauer D, Bruns D, Shen B, Jahn R, Brunger AT. A structural change occurs upon binding of syntaxin to SNAP-25. *J Biol Chem.* 1997;272:4582-4590.

45. Hazzard J, Sudhof TC, Rizo J. NMR analysis of the structure of synaptobrevin and of its interaction with syntaxin. *J Biomol NMR.* 1999;14:203-207.

46. Fiebig KM, Rice LM, Pollock E, Brunger AT. Folding intermediates of SNARE complex assembly. *Nat Struct Biol.* 1999;6:117-123.

47. Ossig R, Schmitt HD, de Groot B, Riedel D, Keranen S, Ronne H, et al. Exocytosis requires asymmetry in the central layer of the SNARE complex. *EMBO J.* 2000;19:6000-6010.

48. Fasshauer D, Eliason WK, Brunger AT, Jahn R. Identification of a minimal core of the synaptic

SNARE complex sufficient for reversible assembly and disassembly. *Biochemistry*. 1998;37:10354-10362.

49. Ernst JA, Brunger AT. High resolution structure, stability, and synaptotagmin binding of a truncated neuronal SNARE complex. *J Biol Chem*. 2003;278:8630-8636.

50. Kubista H, Edelbauer H, Boehm S. Evidence for structural and functional diversity among SDS-resistant SNARE complexes in neuroendocrine cells. *J Cell Sci*. 2004;117(Pt 6):955-966.

51. Fasshauer D. Structural insights into the SNARE mechanism. *Biochim Biophys Acta*. 2003;1641:87-97.

52. Chen YA, Scheller RH. SNARE-mediated membrane fusion. *Nat Rev Mol Cell Biol*. 2001;2:98-106.

53. Sollner T, Whiteheart SW, Brunner M, Erdjument-Bromage H, Geromanos S, Tempst P, et al. SNAP receptors implicated in vesicle targeting and fusion. *Nature*. 1993;362:318-324.

54. Fernandez-Chacon R, Shin OH, Konigstorfer A, Matos MF, Meyer AC, Garcia J, et al. Structure/function analysis of Ca2+ binding to the C2A domain of synaptotagmin 1. *J Neurosci*. 2002;22:8438-8446.

55. Fernandez-Chacon R, Konigstorfer A, Gerber SH, Garcia J, Matos MF, Stevens CF, et al. Synaptotagmin I functions as a calcium regulator of release probability. *Nature*. 2001;410:41-49.

56. Misura KM, Scheller RH, Weis WI. Three-dimensional structure of the neuronal-Sec1-syntaxin 1a complex. *Nature*. 2000;404:355-362.

57. Dulubova I, Khvotchev M, Liu S, Huryeva I, Sudhof TC, Rizo J. Munc18-1 binds directly to the neuronal SNARE complex. *Proc Natl Acad Sci U S A*. 2007;104:2697-2702.

58. Tang J, Maximov A, Shin OH, Dai H, Rizo J, Sudhof TC. A complexin/synaptotagmin 1 switch controls fast synaptic vesicle exocytosis. *Cell*. 2006;126:1175-1187.

59. Basu J, Shen N, Dulubova I, Lu J, Guan R, Guryev O, et al. A minimal domain responsible for Munc13 activity. *Nat Struct Mol Biol*. 2005;12:1017-1018.

60. Rizo J, Chen X, Arac D. Unraveling the mechanisms of synaptotagmin and SNARE function in neurotransmitter release. *Trends Cell Biol*. 2006;16:339-350.

61. Schiavo G, Santucci A, Dasgupta BR, Mehta PP, Jontes J, Benfenati F, et al. Botulinum neurotoxins serotypes A and E cleave SNAP-25 at distinct COOH-terminal peptide bonds. *FEBS Lett*. 1993;335:99-103.

62. Yamasaki S, Binz T, Hayashi T, Szabo E, Yamasaki N, Eklund M, et al. Botulinum neurotoxin type G proteolyses the Ala81-Ala82 bond of rat synaptobrevin 2. *Biochem Biophys Res Commun*. 1994;200:829-835.

63. Oost T, Sukonpan C, Brewer M, Goodnough M, Tepp W, Johnson EA, et al. Design and synthesis of substrate-based inhibitors of botulinum neurotoxin type B metalloprotease. *Biopolymers*. 2003;71:602-619.

64. Agarwal R, Eswaramoorthy S, Kumaran D, Binz T, Swaminathan S. Structural analysis of botulinum neurotoxin type E catalytic domain and its mutant Glu212–>Gln reveals the pivotal role of the Glu212 carboxylate in the catalytic pathway. *Biochemistry*. 2004;43:6637-6644.

65. Breidenbach MA, Brunger AT. 2.3 A crystal structure of tetanus neurotoxin light chain. *Biochemistry*. 2005;44:7450-7477.

66. Rao KN, Kumaran D, Binz T, Swaminathan S. Structural analysis of the catalytic domain of tetanus neurotoxin. *Toxicon*. 2005;45:929-939.

67. Schmidt JJ, Bostian KA. Endoproteinase activity of type A botulinum neurotoxin: substrate requirements and activation by serum albumin. *J Protein Chem*. 1997;16:19-26.

68. Yamasaki S, Baumeister A, Binz T, Blasi J, Link E, Cornille F, et al. Cleavage of members of the synaptobrevin/VAMP family by types D and F botulinal neurotoxins and tetanus toxin. *J Biol Chem*. 1994;269:12764-12772.

69. Foran P, Shone CC, Dolly JO. Differences in the protease activities of tetanus and botulinum B toxins revealed by the cleavage of vesicle-associated membrane protein and various sized fragments. *Biochemistry*. 1994;33:15365-15374.

70. Cornille F, Martin L, Lenoir C, Cussac D, Roques BP, Fournie-Zaluski MC. Cooperative exosite-dependent cleavage of synaptobrevin by tetanus toxin light chain. *J Biol Chem*. 1997;272:3459-3464.

71. Schmidt JJ, Bostian KA. Proteolysis of synthetic peptides by type A botulinum neurotoxin. *J Protein Chem*. 1995;14:703-708.

72. Rossetto O, Schiavo G, Montecucco C, Poulain B, Deloye F, Lozzi L, et al. SNARE motif and neurotoxins. *Nature*. 1994;372:415-416.

73. Pellizzari R, Rossetto O, Lozzi L, Giovedi S, Johnson E, Shone CC, et al. Structural determinants of the specificity for synaptic vesicle-associated membrane protein/synaptobrevin of tetanus and botulinum type B and G neurotoxins. *J Biol Chem*. 1996;271:20353-20358.

74. Breidenbach MA, Brunger AT. Substrate recognition strategy for botulinum neurotoxin serotype A. *Nature*. 2004;432:925-929.

75. Segelke B, Knapp M, Kadkhodayan S, Balhorn R, Rupp B. Crystal structure of Clostridium botulinum neurotoxin protease in a product-bound state: Evidence for noncanonical zinc protease activity. *Proc Nat Acad Sci U S A*. 2004;101:6888-6893.

76. Jin R, Sikorra S, Stegmann CM, Pich A, Binz T, Brunger AT. Structural and biochemical studies of botulinum neurotoxin serotype c1 light chain protease: implications for dual substrate specificity. *Biochemistry*. 2007;46:10685-10693.

77. Arndt JW, Chai Q, Christian T, Stevens RC. Structure of botulinum neurotoxin type D light chain at 1.65 A resolution: repercussions for VAMP-2 substrate specificity. *Biochemistry*. 2006;45:3255-3262.

78. Agarwal R, Binz T, Swaminathan S. Structural analysis of botulinum neurotoxin serotype F light chain: implications on substrate binding and inhibitor design. *Biochemistry*. 2005;44:11758-11765.

79. Arndt JW, Yu W, Bi F, Stevens RC. Crystal structure of botulinum neurotoxin type G light chain: serotype divergence in substrate recognition. *Biochemistry*. 2005;44:9574-9580.

80. Binz T, Blasi J, Yamasaki S, Baumeister A, Link E, Sudhof TC, et al. Proteolysis of SNAP-25 by types E and A botulinal neurotoxins. *J Biol Chem*. 1994;269:1617-1620.

81. Chen S, Barbieri JT. Unique substrate recognition by botulinum neurotoxins serotypes A and E. *J Biol Chem*. 2006;281:10906-10911.

82. Hanson MA, Stevens RC. Cocrystal structure of synaptobrevin-II bound to botulinum neurotoxin type B at 2.0 A resolution. *Nat Struct Biol*. 2000;7:687-692.

83. Rupp B, Segelke B. Questions about the structure of the botulinum neurotoxin B light chain in complex with a target peptide. *Nat Struct Biol*. 2001;8:663-664.

84. Washbourne P, Pellizzari R, Baldini G, Wilson MC, Montecucco C. Botulinum neurotoxin types A and E require the SNARE motif in SNAP-25 for proteolysis. *FEBS Lett*. 1997;418:1-5.

85. Brunger AT. Structure and function of SNARE and SNARE-interacting proteins. *Q Rev Biophys.* 2006;38: 1-47.

86. Lazarovici P, Yavin E. Affinity-purified tetanus neurotoxin interaction with synaptic membranes: properties of a protease-sensitive receptor component. *Biochemistry.* 1986;25:7047-7054.

87. Pierce EJ, Davison MD, Parton RG, Habig WH, Critchley DR. Characterization of tetanus toxin binding to rat brain membranes. Evidence for a high-affinity proteinase-sensitive receptor. *Biochem J.* 1986;236:845-852.

88. Montecucco C. How do tetanus and botulinum neurotoxins bind to neuronal membranes? *Trends Biochem Sci.* 1986;11:314-317.

89. Dolly JO. Probing the process of transmitter release with botulinum and tetanus neurotoxin. *Semin Neurosci.* 1994;6:149-158.

90. Eswaramoorthy S, Kumaran D, Swaminathan S. Crystallographic evidence for doxorubicin binding to the receptor-binding site in Clostridium botulinum neurotoxin B. *Acta Crystallogr D Biol Crystallogr.* 2001;57(Pt 11):1743-1746.

91. Rummel A, Mahrhold S, Bigalke H, Binz T. The HCC-domain of botulinum neurotoxins A and B exhibits a singular ganglioside binding site displaying serotype specific carbohydrate interaction. *Mol Microbiol.* 2004;51:631-643.

92. Rummel A, Bade S, Alves J, Bigalke H, Binz T. Two carbohydrate binding sites in the H(CC)-domain of tetanus neurotoxin are required for toxicity. *J Mol Biol.* 2003;326:835-847.

93. Dong M, Richards DA, Goodnough MC, Tepp WH, Johnson EA, Chapman ER. Synaptotagmins I and II mediate entry of botulinum neurotoxin B into cells. *J Cell Biol.* 2003;162:1293-1303.

94. Dong M, Yeh F, Tepp WH, Dean C, Johnson EA, Janz R, et al. SV2 is the protein receptor for botulinum neurotoxin A. *Science.* 2006;312:592-596.

95. Mahrhold S, Rummel A, Bigalke H, Davletov B, Binz T. The synaptic vesicle protein 2C mediates the uptake of botulinum neurotoxin A into phrenic nerves. *FEBS Lett.* 2006;580:2011-2014.

96. Nishiki T, Tokuyama Y, Kamata Y, Nemoto Y, Yoshida A, Sato K, et al. The high-affinity binding of Clostridium botulinum type B neurotoxin to synaptotagmin II associated with gangliosides GT1b/GD1a. *FEBS Lett.* 1996;378:253-257.

97. Rummel A, Karnath T, Henke T, Bigalke H, Binz T. Synaptotagmins I and II act as nerve cell receptors for botulinum neurotoxin G. *J Biol Chem.* 2004;279: 30865-30870.

98. Baldwin MR, Barbieri JT. Association of botulinum neurotoxin serotypes A and B with synaptic vesicle protein complexes. *Biochemistry.* 2007;46:3200-3210.

99. Tacket CO, Shandera WX, Mann JM, Hargrett NT, Blake PA. Equine antitoxin use and other factors that predict outcome in type A foodborne botulism. *Am J Med.* 1984;76:794-798.

100. Pang ZP, Sun J, Rizo J, Maximov A, Sudhof TC. Genetic analysis of synaptotagmin 2 in spontaneous and Ca2+-triggered neurotransmitter release. *EMBO J.* 2006;25:2039-2050.

101. Jin R, Rummel A, Binz T, Brunger AT. Botulinum neurotoxin B recognizes its protein receptor with high affinity and specificity. *Nature.* 2006;444: 1092-1095.

102. Chai Q, Arndt JW, Dong M, Tepp WH, Johnson EA, Chapman ER, et al. Structural basis of cell surface receptor recognition by botulinum neurotoxin B. *Nature.* 2006;444:1096-1100.

103. Rummel A, Eichner T, Weil T, Karnath T, Gutcaits A, Mahrhold S, et al. Identification of the protein receptor binding site of botulinum neurotoxins B and G proves the double-receptor concept. *Proc Natl Acad Sci U S A.* 2007;104:359-364.

104. Kozaki S, Kamata Y, Watarai S, Nishiki T, Mochida S. Ganglioside GT1b as a complementary receptor component for Clostridium botulinum neurotoxins. *Microb Pathog.* 1998;25:91-99.

105. Bade S, Rummel A, Reisinger C, Karnath T, Ahnert-Hilger G, Bigalke H, et al. Botulinum neurotoxin type D enables cytosolic delivery of enzymatically active cargo proteins to neurones via unfolded translocation intermediates. *J Neurochem.* 2004;91: 1461-1472.

106. Hoch DH, Romero-Mira M, Ehrlich BE, Finkelstein A, DasGupta BR, Simpson LL. Channels formed by botulinum, tetanus, and diphtheria toxins in planar lipid bilayers: relevance to translocation of proteins across membranes. *Proc Natl Acad Sci U S A.* 1985;82:1692-1696.

107. Koriazova LK, Montal M. Translocation of botulinum neurotoxin light chain protease through the heavy chain channel. *Nat Struct Biol.* 2003;10:13-18.

108. Dolimbek BZ, Steward LE, Aoki KR, Atassi MZ. Immune recognition of botulinum neurotoxin B: Antibody-binding regions on the heavy chain of the toxin. *Mol Immunol.* 2007;45:910-924.

109. Montecucco C, Rossetto O, Schiavo G. Presynaptic receptor arrays for clostridial neurotoxins. *Trends Microbiol.* 2004;12:442-446.

110. Brunger AT, Breidenbach MA, Jin R, Fischer A, Santos JS, Montal M. Botulinum neurotoxin heavy chain belt as an intramolecular chaperone for the light chain. *PLoS Pathog.* 2007;3:e113.

111. Humeau Y, Doussau F, Grant NJ, Poulain B. How botulinum and tetanus neurotoxins block neurotransmitter release. *Biochimie.* 2000;82:427-446.

112. Lalli G, Bohnert S, Deinhardt K, Verastegui C, Schiavo G. The journey of tetanus and botulinum neurotoxins in neurons. *Trends Microbiol.* 2003; 11:431-437.

Immune Recognition of Botulinum Neurotoxins A and B: Molecular Elucidation of Immune Protection Against the Toxins

5

M. Zouhair Atassi and K. Roger Aoki

INTRODUCTION

We had previously localized the regions on the H chain of botulinum neurotoxin A (BoNT/A) that are recognized by mouse, horse, chicken and human anti-BoNT/A antibodies (Abs) and block the activity of the toxin *in vivo*. The human Abs were from cervical dystonia (CD) patients who had been treated with BoNT/A and had become unresponsive to the treatment. We also localized the regions involved in BoNT/A binding to mouse brain synaptosomes (snps). In the 3-D structure, the Ab-binding regions, except for one, and the snps-binding regions either coincide or overlap. Thus occupancy of these sites by the Abs prevents the toxin from binding to nerve synapse and block toxin entry into the neuron. The ability of the Abs to inhibit toxin binding to snps permitted us to develop an in vitro assay for neutralizing Abs based on the ability of the Abs to inhibit BoNT/A-snps binding. We also determined the regions on BoNT/B that bind neutralizing anti-BoNT/B Abs from horse, mouse and human (BoNT/B-treated CD patients) and found that some of the

Ab-binding sites are also involved in the binding of BoNT/B to mouse and rat synaptotagmin II. Thus analysis of the locations of the Ab-binding on BoNT/A and /B, the snps-binding regions on BoNT/A and the synaptotagmin II binding regions on BoNT/B provides a molecular rationalization for the ability of protecting Abs to block BoNT/A and BoNT/B actions in vivo.

Botulinum neurotoxins (BoNTs) are produced by *Clostridium botulinum* in seven serotypes (A through G, with many subtypes for each serotype). BoNTs are the most potent toxins known. They act on the nervous system by blocking the release of acetylcholine from nerve terminals at the neuromuscular junction, thereby causing paralysis. The action is initiated by binding of BoNT to a receptor on the cell surface at the presynaptic neuromuscular junction. Then endocytosis of the toxin-receptor complex ensues and the internalized toxin blocks neurotransmitter release (see Chapter 1). The binding of BoNTs A and B to cell surface receptor is a function of the H chain,[1-13] whereas the L chain, a zinc endopeptidase,[14] is required for intracellular activity. It is now well

Dr. Atassi is a NAC member of the NTI, and he also receives research support from Allergan, Inc. Dr. Aoki is an employee of Allergan, Inc., the manufacturer and marketer of Botox(r), a botulinum toxin based product described in this chapter.

established that the H chain binds to the receptor,[15,16] thereby allowing the L chain, or a combination of H and L chains, to be internalized and cause paralysis.

In recent studies, we mapped the regions on BoNTs A and B that bind neutralizing Abs against the correlate toxin from human, mouse, and other species.[17-21] These localizations were achieved by employing a panel of 60 uniform-size synthetic overlapping peptides that encompassed the entire H chain of each toxin serotype and determining their abilities to bind Abs against the correlate toxin. We also used the BoNT/A H-chain peptides to localize the regions on the H chain that are involved in BoNT/A binding to snps.[11] Synaptotagmin (Syt-II) has been identified as a cell-surface receptor for BoNT/B. The binding surfaces between BoNT/B and rat synaptotagmin II (Syt-II)[12] or mouse Syt-II[13] were recently determined by x-ray crystallography. A region that bound mouse Abs overlapped[21] with a recently defined site on BoNT/B that binds to mouse and rat synaptotagmin II, thus providing a molecular explanation for the neutralizing (protecting) activity of these Abs.

Because intramuscular injection of BoNTs produces a reversible local reduction of motor neuron activity at the affected neuromuscular junctions, the toxins (mostly BoNT/A and /B) are used to treat a variety of clinical conditions associated with involuntary muscle spasm and contractions, as well as in cosmetic and other therapeutic applications.[22-31] However, the therapeutic benefits are not permanent, and therefore, the injections have to be repeated every 3 to 6 months. After a few treatments, some patients (less in the case of BoNT/A than BoNT/B), the injections elicit neutralizing Abs against the correlate toxin, which reduce the benefit or render the patient completely unresponsive to further treatment.[22,32-42]

We have studied the molecular immune responses to BoNT/A and /B in cervical dystonia (CD) patients. CD is associated with neck-muscle spasms that produce pain and involuntary contractions, resulting in abnormal neck movements and posture.[37] Symptoms of CD can be relieved by injecting the affected muscle with a BoNT (usually type A or type B). We will describe in the present article the molecular specificity of neutralizing anti-BoNT/A and anti-BoNT/B Abs from human (CD patients who have become non-responsive

to BoNT treatment), mouse, and other species and explain how these Abs thwart toxin action by blocking the binding of each toxin to its receptor.

METHOD FOR LOCALIZING THE REGIONS OF IMMUNE RECOGNITION ON THE H CHAINS OF BoNT/A AND /B, AND REGIONS THAT BIND TO CELL RECEPTOR

This laboratory had previously introduced[43] a comprehensive synthetic method that was designed to localize the entire profile of the continuous regions on a protein that are involved in immune (Ab and T-cell) recognition,[17,22,43-52] as well as regions involved in other binding activities.[53] For example, it has been used to localize the binding regions on hemoglobin for haptoglobin[54,55] on acetylcholine receptor for a-neurotoxins,[56,57] the subunit interacting surfaces in oligomeric proteins[58-60] and the extracellular topography of membrane-bound receptors.[61,62] The approach employs consecutive synthetic overlapping peptides that encompass the entire protein chain and have a uniform size and fixed overlaps.

To localize the regions of immune recognition and receptor binding on the H chain of BoNT/A and BoNT/B, we synthesized two panels of 60 peptides each (29 H_N and 31 H_C) that encompassed entire H chain of the respective toxin.[17,19-22] The peptides were 19 residues each in size (except for peptide C31, which was 22 and 24 residues in BoNT/A and BoNT/B, respectively) and overlapped consecutively by five residues (Table 5-1). We determined the regions of T-cell recognition in selected mouse strains[63-65] and those recognized by Abs from various species against the correlate toxin.[18,19,21] We also used these two 60-peptide panels to localize the regions recognized by blocking Abs of mouse protection assay (MPA)–positive sera from CD patients[20,21] who were treated with BoNT/A or BoNT/B and had become resistant to further treatment with the correlate toxin. To localize the BoNT/A regions on the H chain that are involved in the toxin's binding to snps, we employed the same panel of BoNT/A peptides and determined their ability in

TABLE 5-1 Synthetic Overlapping Peptides of the Heavy Chains of BoNT/A and /B

Peptide Toxin	Residue Number	Numbers	Amino Acid Sequence
BoNT/A	N1	449–467	a l n d l c i k v n n w d l **f f s p s**
BoNT/B	N1	442–460	a P G I C I D V D n E D L F **f I A D K**
BoNT/A	N2	463–481	**f f s p s** e d n f t n d l n **k g e e i**
BoNT/B	N2	456–474	**f I A D K** N S F S D D L S K **N E R I E**
BoNT/A	N3	477–495	**k g e e i** t s d t n i e a a **e e n I s**
BoNT/B	N3	470–488	**N E R I E** Y N T Q S N Y I E **N D F P I**
BoNT/A	N4	491–509	**e e n I s** l d l i q q y y L **t f n f d**
BoNT/B	N4	484–502	**N D F P I** N E l i L D T D L **I S K I E**
BoNT/A	N5	505–523	**t f n f d** n e p e n i s I e **n l s s d**
BoNT/B	N5	498–516	**I S K I E** L P S e n T E S L **T D F N V**
BoNT/A	N6	519–537	**n l s s d** i i g q l e l m p **n I e r f**
BoNT/B	N6	512–530	**T D F N V** D V P V Y e K Q p **A I K K I**
BoNT/A	N7	533–551	**n I e r f** p n g k k y e l d **k y t m f**
BoNT/B	N7	526–544	**A I K K I** F T D E N T I F Q **Y L Y S Q**
BoNT/A	N8	547–565	**k y t m f** h y l r a q e f e **h g k s r**
BoNT/B	N8	540–558	**Y L Y S Q** T F P L D I R D I **S L T s S**
BoNT/A	N9	561–579	**h g k s r** i a l t n s v n e **a l l n p**
BoNT/B	N9	554–572	**S L T s S** F D D A L L F S N **K V Y S F**
BoNT/A	N10	575–593	**a l l n p** s r v y t f f s s **d y v k k**
BoNT/B	N10	568–586	**K V Y S F** F S M D Y I K T A **N K v V E**
BoNT/A	N11	589–607	**d y v k k** v n k a t e a a m **f l g w v**
BoNT/B	N11	582–600	**N K v V E** A G L F A G W V K **Q I V N D**
BoNT/A	N12	603–621	**f l g w v** e q l v y d f t d **e t s e v**
BoNT/B	N12	596–614	**Q I V N D** F V I E A N K S N **T M D K I**
BoNT/A	N13	617–635	**e t s e v** s t t d k i a d i **t i i i p**
BoNT/B	N13	610–628	**T M D K I** A D I S L i V P Y **I G L A L**
BoNT/A	N14	631–649	**t i i i p** y i g p a l n i g n **m l y k**
BoNT/B	N14	624–642	**I G L A L** N V g N E T A K g **n F E N A**
BoNT/A	N15	645–663	**n m l y k** d d f v g a l I f **s g a v i**
BoNT/B	N15	638–656	**n F E N A** F E I A g a S I L **L E F I P**
BoNT/A	N16	659–677	**s g a v i** l l e f i p e i a **i p v l g**
BoNT/B	N16	652–670	**L E F I P** E l L I P V V G a **F L L E S**
BoNT/A	N17	673–691	**i p v l g** t f a l v S Y i a **n k v l t**
BoNT/B	N17	666–684	**F L L E S** Y I D N K N K i i **K T I D N**
BoNT/A	N18	687–705	**n k v l t** v q t i d n a l s **k r n e k**
BoNT/B	N18	680–698	**K T I D N** A L t K R n E K W **S D M Y G**
BoNT/A	N19	701–719	**k r n e k** w d e v y k y i v **t n w l a**
BoNT/B	N19	694–712	**S D M Y G** L I V A Q W L S T **V n T Q F**
BoNT/A	N20	715–733	**t n w l a** k v n t q I d l i **r k k m k**
BoNT/B	N20	708–726	**V n T Q F** Y T I K E G M Y K **A L N Y Q**
BoNT/A	N21	729–747	**r k k m k** e a l e n q a e a **t k a i i**
BoNT/B	N21	722–740	**A L N Y Q** A Q A L E E I I K **Y R Y N i**
BoNT/A	N22	743–761	**t k a i i** n y q y n q y t e **e e k n n**
BoNT/B	N22	736–754	**Y R Y N i** Y S E K E K S N I **N I D F n**
BoNT/A	N23	757–775	**e e k n n** i n f n i d d l s **s k l n e**
BoNT/B	N23	750–768	**N I D F n** D I N S K L N E G **I N Q A I**

Continued

TABLE 5-1 Synthetic Overlapping Peptides of the Heavy Chains of BoNT/A and /B—Cont'd

Peptide Toxin	Residue Number	Numbers	Amino Acid Sequence
BoNT/A	N24	771–789	**sklne**sinkamIni**nkfln**
BoNT/B	N24	764–782	**INQAI**DNINNFInG**CSVSY**
BoNT/A	N25	785–803	**nkfln**qcsvsylmn**smipy**
BoNT/B	N25	778–796	**CSVSY**LMKKMIPLA**VEKLL**
BoNT/A	N26	799–817	**smipy**gvkrledfd**aslkd**
BoNT/B	N26	792–810	**VEKLL**DFDNTLKKN**LLNYI**
BoNT/A	N27	813–831	**aslkd**allkyiydn**rgtli**
BoNT/B	N27	806–824	**LLNYI**DENkLYLIG**SAEYE**
BoNT/A	N28	827–845	**rgtli**gqvdrlkdk**vnntl**
BoNT/B	N28	820–838	**SAEYE**KSKVNKYLk**TIMPF**
BoNT/A	N29	841–859	**vnntl**stdipfqls**kyvdn**
BoNT/B	N29	834–852	**TIMPF**DLSiYTNDT**ILIEM**

H_C peptides

Peptide Toxin	Residue Number	Numbers	Amino Acid Sequence
BoNT/A	C1	855-873	**KYVDN**QRLLSTFTEY**IKNI**
BoNT/B	C1	848-866	**ILIEM**FNKYNSEIL**NNIIL**
BoNT/A	C2	869-887	**YIKNI**INTSILNLR**YESNH**
BoNT/B	C2	862-880	**NNIIL**NLRYKDNNL**IDLSG**
BoNT/A	C3	883-901	**YESNH**LIDLSRYAS**KINIG**
BoNT/B	C3	876-894	**IDLSG**YGAKVEVYD**GVELN**
BoNT/A	C4	897-915	**KINIG**SKVNFDPID**KNQIQ**
BoNT/B	C4	890-908	**GVELN**DKNQFKLTS**SANSK**
BoNT/A	C5	911-929	**KNQIQ**LFNLESSKI**EVILK**
BoNT/B	C5	904-922	**SANSK**IRVTQNQNI**IFNSV**
BoNT/A	C6	925-943	**EVILK**NAIVYNSMY**ENFST**
BoNT/B	C6	918-936	**IFNSV**FLDFSVSFW**IRIPK**
BoNT/A	C7	939-957	**ENFST**SFWIRIPKY**FNSIS**
BoNT/B	C7	932-950	**IRIPK**YKNDGIQNY**IHNEY**
BoNT/A	C8	953-971	**FNSIS**LNNEYTIINC**MENN**
BoNT/B	C8	946-964	**IHNEY**TIINCMKNN**SGWKI**
BoNT/A	C9	967-985	**CMENN**SGWKVSLNY**GEIIW**
BoNT/B	C9	960-978	**SGWKI**SIRGNRIIW**TLIDI**
BoNT/A	C10	981-999	**GEIIW**TLQDTQEIK**QRVVF**
BoNT/B	C10	974-992	**TLIDI**NGKTKSVFF**EYNIR**
BoNT/A	C11	995-1013	**QRVVF**KYSQMINIS**DYINR**
BoNT/B	C11	988-1006	**EYNIR**EDISEYINR**WFFVT**
BoNT/A	C12	1009-1027	**DYINR**WIFVTITNN**RLNNS**
BoNT/B	C12	1002-1020	**WFFVT**ITNNLNNAK**IYING**
BoNT/A	C13	1023-1041	**RLNNS**KIYINGRLI**DQKPI**
BoNT/B	C13	1016-1034	**IYING**KLESNTDIK**DIREV**
BoNT/A	C14	1037-1055	**DQKPI**SNLGNIHAS**NNIMF**
BoNT/B	C14	1030-1048	**DIREV**IANGEIIFK**LDGDI**
BoNT/A	C15	1051-1069	**NNIMF**KLDGCRDTH**RYIWI**
BoNT/B	C15	1044-1062	**LDGDI**DRTQFIWMK**YFSIF**
BoNT/A	C16	1065-1083	**RYIWI**KYFNLFDKE**LNEKE**
BoNT/B	C16	1058-1076	**YFSIF**NTELSQSNI**EERYK**
BoNT/A	C17	1079-1097	**LNEKE**IKDLYDNQS**NSGIL**

TABLE 5-1 Synthetic Overlapping Peptides of the Heavy Chains of BoNT/A and /B—Cont'd

Peptide Toxin	Residue Number	Numbers	Amino Acid Sequence
BoNT/B	C17	1072-1090	**E E R Y K** I Q S Y S E Y L K **D F W G N**
BoNT/A	C18	1093-1111	**N S G I L** K D F W G D Y L Q **Y D K P Y**
BoNT/B	C18	1086-1104	**D F W G N** P L M Y N K E Y Y **M F N A G**
BoNT/A	C19	1107-1125	**Y D K P Y** Y M L N L Y D P N **K Y V D V**
BoNT/B	C19	1100-1118	**M F N A G** N K N S Y I K L K **K D S P V**
BoNT/A	C20	1121-1139	**K Y V D V** N N V G I R G Y M **Y L K G P**
BoNT/B	C20	1114-1132	**K D S P V** G E I L T R S K Y **N Q N S K**
BoNT/A	C21	1135-1153	**Y L K G P** R G S V M T T N I **Y L N S S**
BoNT/B	C21	1128-1146	**N Q N S K** Y I N Y R D L Y I **G E K F I**
BoNT/A	C22	1149-1167	**Y L N S S** L Y R G T K F I I **K K Y A S**
BoNT/B	C22	1142-1160	**G E K F I** I R R K S N S Q S **I N D D I**
BoNT/A	C23	1163-1181	**K K Y A S** G N K D N I V R N **N D R V Y**
BoNT/B	C23	1156-1174	**I N D D I** V R K E D Y I Y L **D F F N L**
BoNT/A	C24	1177-1195	**N D R V Y** I N V V V K N K E **Y R L A T**
BoNT/B	C24	1170-1188	**D F F N L** N Q E W R V Y T Y **K Y F K K**
BoNT/A	C25	1191-1209	**Y R L A T** N A S Q A G V E K **I L S A L**
BoNT/B	C25	1184-1202	**K Y F K K** E E E K L F L A P **I S D S D**
BoNT/A	C26	1205-1223	**I L S A L** E I P D V G N L S **Q V V V M**
BoNT/B	C26	1198-1216	**I S D S D** E F Y N T I Q I K **E Y D E Q**
BoNT/A	C27	1219-1237	**Q V V V M** K S K N D Q G I T **N K C K M**
BoNT/B	C27	1212-1230	**E Y D E Q** P T Y S C Q L L F **K K D E E**
BoNT/A	C28	1233-1251	**N K C K M** N L Q D N N G N D **I G F I G**
BoNT/B	C28	1226-1244	**K K D E E** S T D E I G L I G **I H R F Y**
BoNT/A	C29	1247-1265	**I G F I G** F H Q F N N I A K **L V A S N**
BoNT/B	C29	1240-1258	**I H R F Y** E S G I V F E E Y **K D Y F C**
BoNT/A	C30	1261-1279	**L V A S N** W Y N R Q I E R S **S R T L G**
BoNT/B	C30	1254-1272	**K D Y F C** I S K W Y L K E V **K R K P Y**
BoNT/A	C31	1275-1296	**S R T L G** C S W E F I P V D D G W G E **R P L**
BoNT/B	C31	1268-1291	**K R K P Y** N L K L G C N W Q F I P K D **E G W T E**

BoNT/A, botulinum neurotoxin A; BoNT/B, botulinum neurotoxin B.
Synthetic overlapping peptides of the heavy (H) Chains of BoNT/A and /B, which we have prepared.[17,19-22] The 60 peptides for each toxin covered the entire sequence of the respective BoNT H Chain (residues 449-1296 of BoNT/A and 442–1291 of BoNT/B). For a given toxin, each peptide overlapped by 5 residues with its consecutive neighbor. The peptides although displayed one under the other are not intended to be aligned here for sequence homology. For sequence homology of toxin serotypes, see Atassi and Oshima.[22]

solution to inhibit the binding of BoNT/A to mouse brain snps.[11]

This strategy is intended to localize the regions within which binding sites reside[43-47] but not to define the boundaries of the sites. The approach has enabled mapping of the *continuous* regions of molecular recognition on the H chains of BoNT/A and /B but does not ordinarily localize *discontinuous* recognition sites, which might also play an important role in the recognition of the two BoNTs by T cells, Abs, and presynaptic cell surface receptor (for definition of *continuous* and *discontinuous* binding regions, see Atassi and Smith[66]).

IMMUNE RECOGNITION AND RECEPTOR BINDING OF BoNT/A

REGIONS ON THE H CHAIN OF BoNT/A THAT BIND ANTITOXIN ANTIBODIES FROM DIFFERENT HOST SPECIES

We mapped the Ab and T-cell recognition regions on the 848-residue H chain (residues 449–1296) of BoNT/A.[17-19,22,63-65] Human, horse, mouse, and chicken anti-BoNT/A Abs recognized similar regions that exhibited in some cases a frame shift of two to three residues to the left or to the right.[18] The shift and the variability observed with different antisera in the amounts of Abs bound to a given peptide are consistent with what is known about the immune recognition of proteins.[44,47,49,67]

The Ab-recognition regions on the H chain occupy surface areas in the BoNT/A three-dimensional (3-D) structure, but the great part of the surface is not immunogenic. Regions recognized by the protective antisera of the four different species are prime candidates for inclusion in synthetic vaccine designs.

Although the work was designed to localize the immunodominant regions, this is not to imply in any way that the regions binding lower amounts of Abs are of lesser immunologic significance. Protection by Abs is not only a function of their levels in the antisera and the regions to which they bind but also of their affinity and often their immunoglobulin class (see next section). The studies were designed to localize the Ab-binding regions and the amounts of Abs against each region but not their affinity.[17,18,63-65]

MOLECULAR SPECIFICITY OF NEUTRALIZING AND NON-NEUTRALIZING ANTI-BoNT/A ANTIBODIES

We have investigated in two high responder (to BoNT/A) mouse strains (BALB/c, H2^d, and SJL, H2^S), the H-chain regions recognized by Abs in the last bleed of non-neutralizing anti-BoNT/A antisera and of neutralizing antisera in the bleed immediately following it in the bleeding schedule.[68] Although the neutralizing antisera bound slightly higher amounts of total (IgG + IgM) Abs, non-neutralizing and neutralizing BALB/c Abs showed similar peptide-binding profiles involving peptides N6/N7, N25, C2/C3, C9/C10/C11, C15, C18, C24, C30, and C31 and, at lower amounts of bound Abs, peptides N19, C6/C7, and C28. The total (IgG + IgM) Abs of the neutralizing SJL antisera recognized peptides N5, N22, and C21, and these peptides were only slightly recognized (N22, C21) or unrecognized (N5) by the non-neutralizing antisera. Additionally, peptides N7/N8, N25, C11, C15, and less so N27/N28 bound two-fold or more Abs from the SJL neutralizing antisera than the non-neutralizing antisera. The Abs bound to peptides C4 and C29 were of relatively lower affinity. Peptides C2/C3, C7, C18/C19, C24, C30, and C31 bound higher amounts of Abs in the SJL neutralizing versus the non-neutralizing antisera, but the differences were less than double. We also mapped the binding profiles of the IgG Abs in these sera. BALB/c and SJL had 13- to 36-fold higher levels of IgG Abs that bound to BoNT/A in the neutralizing antisera relative to non-neutralizing antisera. The IgG Abs in the neutralizing antisera of each mouse haplotype bound to the same peptides that bound total Abs in the correlate antiserum. But in both mouse strains, the non-neutralizing Abs showed little or no IgG Abs that bound to these peptides. In the SJL haplotype, the IgG response to peptide N5 was transient, appearing strongly in early neutralizing Abs and disappearing by day 70. It is not clear why the response to region N5 plays a role in initiating and contributing to the neutralizing activity of the toxin in the SJL strain in the early stages but does not appear to be needed in later hyperimmune stages of the Ab response.

It was concluded[68] that the switch in the BALB/c and SJL mouse strains from non-neutralizing to neutralizing Abs is not accompanied, in a given strain, with major changes in the epitope-recognition profile. Although there were some slight differences between non-neutralizing and neutralizing antisera in the levels of Abs bound by some peptides, these differences were not sufficient to explain the disparity in protection properties.[68] Protection was mostly linked to the immunoglobulin class of the Abs. IgM Abs were non-neutralizing, whereas IgG Abs, which were produced after the switch, were neutralizing.[68]

THE SYNAPTOSOME-BINDING REGIONS ON THE H CHAIN OF BoNT/A

In order for BoNTs to exert their toxic activity, they need to bind to the neuron's presynaptic cell surface in the first step. The binding is a function of the H subunit. We have determined the regions on the H chain that bind to snps.[11] Inhibition of the binding of ^{125}I-labeled BoNT/A (50,000 cpm) to synaptosome (4 µL) was done with unlabeled toxin or with the individual peptides. The snps, in the absence or in the presence of different amounts of unlabeled toxin, were incubated with ^{125}I-labeled toxin, (5 minutes, 37°C) in 0.1 mL of Ringer's solution. The experiments were done in triplicates as described.[11] The levels of binding of ^{125}I-labeled toxin in the presence of different amounts of unlabeled toxin or peptide relative to the uninhibited controls were used to determine the percent of inhibition. The binding was completely inhibited by unlabeled BoNT/A but not by unrelated proteins, indicating that the binding of ^{125}I-labeled BoNT/A to snps was entirely specific. The 50% inhibition value (IC50) was obtained at an inhibitor concentration of 1.198 $\times 10^{-8}$ M. Inhibition studies with the individual peptides showed that, on the H_N domain, inhibitory activities greater than 10% were displayed, in decreasing order, by peptides 799–817, 659–677, 729–747, 533–551, 701–719, and 757–775. Lower inhibitory activities (between 5.6% and 8.7%) were exhibited by five other peptides, 463–481, 505–523, 519–537, 603–621, and 645–663. The remaining 18 H_N peptides had little or no inhibitory activity. In the H_C domain, peptides 1065–1083, 1163–1181, and 1275–1296 had the highest inhibitory activities (between 25% and 29%), followed (10%–12% inhibitory activity) by peptides 1107–1125, 1191–1209, and 1233–1251. Two other peptides, 1079–1097 and 1177–1195, had very low (5.8% and 4.9%) inhibitory activities. The remaining 23 H_C peptides had no inhibitory activity. Inhibition with mixtures of equimolar quantities of the six most active peptides of H_N, 5 of H_C or all 11 of H_N and H_C revealed that the peptides contain independent non-competing binding regions.[11]

The H_C domain of BoNT/A has at least five major snps-binding regions (Table 5-2 and Fig. 5-1).[11] Except for CS1, the snps-binding regions within the H_C domain mapped to the C-terminal portion or H_{CC} subdomain. The finding that the H_N carries significant snps-binding regions was unexpected because the domain itself does not bind to snps. It is possible that the conformations of the binding regions in the isolated H_N domain are disrupted by the proteolytic scission of the H chain that is necessary to separate the H_N and H_C domains. Furthermore, the free peptide in solution displays conformational flexibility due to equilibrium among conformational states whose time average is random. When a conformational state approaches the shape needed for binding, it will do so and is removed thus

TABLE 5-2 Regions on the H Chain of BoNT/A Corresponding to Synaptosome-Inhibiting Peptides

Regions Inhibiting BONT/A-snp Binding	Sequence Position
H_N Domain	
NS1	510–546
NS2	659–670
NS3	703–717
NS4	731–745
NS5	759–773
NS6	794–812
H_C Domain	
CS1	1070–1083
CS2	1109–1123
CS3	1165–1204
CS4	1235–1249
CS5	1281–1295

BoNT/A, botulinum neurotoxin A; snp, mouse brain synaptosomes.
The table provides the approximate regions corresponding to peptides inhibiting synaptosome binding by 10% or more. When peptides immediately adjacent to strong inhibitors (i.e., greater then 10%) demonstrated inhibition, the peptides were merged in order to define a region. For example NS1 contains the majority of peptides N5 and N7, bounding the entirety of peptide N6.
From Maruta T, Dolimbek BZ, Aoki KR, Steward LE, Atassi MZ. Mapping of the synaptosome-binding regions on the heavy chain of botulinum neurotoxin A by synthetic overlapping peptides encompassing the entire chain. *Protein J.* 2004;23:539-552.

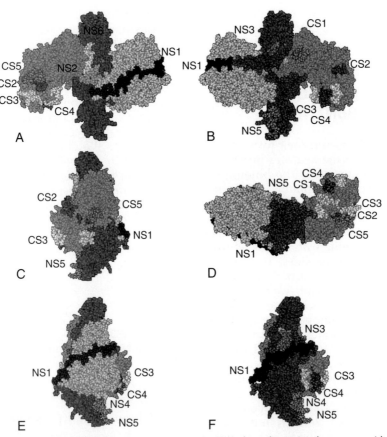

FIGURE 5-1. Space-filling images of botulinum neurotoxin A (BoNT/A) three-dimensional structure with the mouse brain synaptosome (snps)–binding regions (**A**) front view, (**B**) back view (rotated 180 degrees on the Y-axis, relative to [**A**]), (**C**) side view looking through the H_C domain (rotated −90 degrees on the Y-axis, relative to [**A**]), (**D**) bottom view (rotated 90 degrees on the X-axis, relative to [**B**]), (**E**) side view looking through the L chain (rotated 90 degrees on the Y-axis, relative to [**A**]), (**F**) same view as (**E**) but with the L chain removed. The snps-binding regions in the H_N domain are labeled NS1–NS6, and those in the H_C domain are labeled CS1–CS5, corresponding to the designations in Table 5-2. The H_N domain is shown in *red*, the H_C domain is shown in *green*, and the L chain is shown in *yellow*. The images were generated with the x-ray structure coordinates of BoNT/A.[76] (From Maruta T, Dolimbek BZ, Aoki KR, Steward LE, Atassi MZ. Mapping of the synaptosome-binding regions on the heavy chain of botulinum neurotoxin A by synthetic overlapping peptides encompassing the entire chain. *Protein J.* 2004;23:539-552.) *See Color Plate*

shifting the equilibrium in its favor. No one peptide completely inhibited BoNT/A binding to snps, which suggested that the receptor has a large binding area with multi-subsite attachments. Of particular interest is snps-binding region NS1 that is entirely contained within the unique structural element that has been termed the belt and surrounds the catalytic L chain. The role that the belt plays in receptor binding, translocation, and L chain delivery through the membrane is currently unknown.

Five of the six snps-binding regions mapped onto H_N domain surfaces that display negative electrostatic charges[11] (Fig. 5-2). Two of these regions, NS3 and NS4, occupy surfaces with very strong electrostatic negative charges and also correspond to regions that are largely

located at the interface of the L and H chains. Unlike the snps-binding regions on the H_N domain, those on the H_C domain exhibit no particular pattern or surface potential charge uniqueness but are a mix of electrostatic positive, negative, and neutral surface charges.

The peptides that bind protecting mouse anti-BoNT/A Abs[17,18,68] and those that bind to mouse snps[11] are compared in Figure 5-3. In the H_N domain, the major snps-binding regions within peptides N16, N19, N21 and N23, as well as the minor regions within peptides N2, N12, and N15, did not correspond to binding regions of mouse Abs. But the major snps-binding region within the overlap N6/N7 coincided with an Ab-binding region, and the one within peptide N26

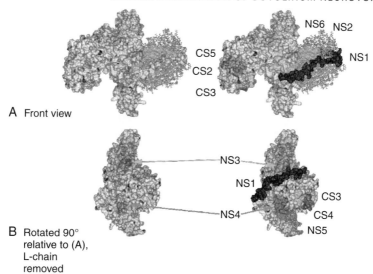

FIGURE 5-2. Electrostatic potential surfaces of botulinum neurotoxin A (BoNT/A), with *(right panel)* and without *(left panel)* mouse brain synaptosome (snps)–binding regions mapped on the surface (**A**) front view with and without snps-binding regions mapped on the structure *(right and left panels, respectively)*, (**B**) side view (rotated 90 degrees relative to [**A**] and with the L chain removed), with and without snps-binding regions mapped on the surface *(right and left panels, respectively)*. The significant overlap of snps-binding regions NS3 and NS4 with negative electrostatic potential is highlighted with arrows. Positive, negative, and neutral electrostatic potential surfaces are shown in *blue, red,* and *white,* respectively. The L chain is shown in *yellow* stick form. The images were generated with the x-ray structure coordinates of BoNT/A from Lacy et al[76] and the electrostatic potential surfaces were calculated with DelPhi[96-97] and mapped onto a solvent-accessible surface as computed by INSIGHTII. (From Maruta T, Dolimbek BZ, Aoki KR, Steward LE, Atassi MZ. Mapping of the synaptosome-binding regions on the heavy chain of botulinum neurotoxin A by synthetic overlapping peptides encompassing the entire chain. *Protein J.* 2004;23:539-552.) *See Color Plate*

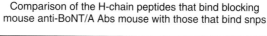

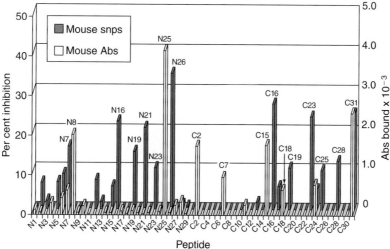

FIGURE 5-3. Comparison of the H-chain peptides that bind mouse brain synaptosomes (snps) with those that bind blocking (i.e., protecting) mouse anti–botulinum neurotoxin A (BoNT/A) antibodies. (From Maruta T, Dolimbek BZ, Aoki KR, Steward LE, Atassi MZ. Mapping of the synaptosome-binding regions on the heavy chain of botulinum neurotoxin A by synthetic overlapping peptides encompassing the entire chain. *Protein J.* 2004;23:539-552.) *See Color Plate*

shared an overlap with the Ab-binding region within peptide N25. Therefore, Abs that bind to the overlap N6/N7/N8 and to peptide N25 will be expected to block the ability of regions N5/N6/N7 and N26, respectively, to bind to snps. In the H_C domain, the major snps-binding regions C16/C17, C19, C23/C24/C25, and C31 either correspond to or overlap with Ab-binding regions. Only the region within peptide C28 was uniquely a snps-binding region and did not bind mouse anti-BoNT/A Abs. The limited set of snps-binding regions that correspond to Ab-binding regions are mapped onto the 3-D structure of BoNT/A in Figure 5-4. The extensive correspondence between the snps-binding and the Ab-binding regions on the H_C domain could explain the high neutralizing capacity of anti-H_C Abs.[69-71]

The initial step of receptor-mediated endocytosis of BoNT involves binding to the cell surface. In the endosomes, exposure of the toxin to low pH causes it to undergo conformational changes that induce the H chain to form a membrane channel that allows the light chain to pass into the cytosol.[72-75] The formation of the channel was proposed to involve, in addition to initial the binding regions, other contact regions on both the H_C and H_N domains.[11] Because Abs against a protein antigen bind to surface locations on the 3-D structure of the correlate protein,[18,47,53] neutralizing Abs would for the most part block the initial

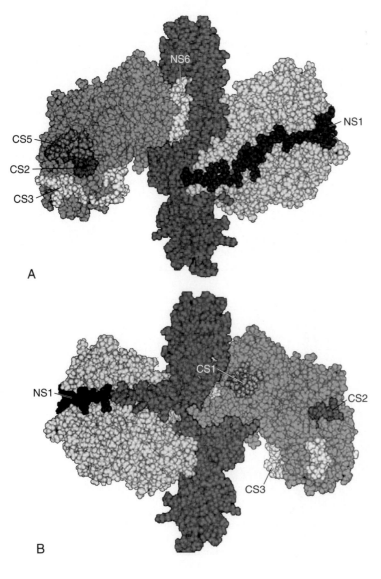

FIGURE 5-4. Space-filling images ([**A**] front view, [**B**] back view rotated 180 degrees on the Y-axis, relative to [**A**]) showing the locations in the three-dimensional structure of botulinum neurotoxin A (BoNT/A) of the limited set of major regions on the H chain that bind to mouse brain synaptosomes and which either coincide or overlap with the regions that bind protective (i.e., blocking) mouse anti-BoNT/A antibodies. The H_N domain is shown in *red* and the HC domain is in *green*, whereas the L chain is shown in *yellow*. The antigenic regions were obtained from Atassi and Dolimbek,[18] and the images were generated with the x-ray structure coordinates of BoNT/A.[76] (From Maruta T, Dolimbek BZ, Aoki KR, Steward LE, Atassi MZ. Mapping of the synaptosome-binding regions on the heavy chain of botulinum neurotoxin A by synthetic overlapping peptides encompassing the entire chain. *Protein J.* 2004;23:539-552.) *See Color Plate*

binding regions. We deduced[11] that the initial binding areas on the 3-D structure of BoNT/A[76] form the correspondence or overlap between regions to which Abs bind and those that bind to snps (see Fig. 5-4). The highest clustering of snps-binding regions resides on the second half of the H_C domain, a region of BoNT/A that plays a critical role in receptor binding. But there are also some binding areas on the H_N domain.

THE REGIONS ON THE H-CHAIN OF BoNT/A RECOGNIZED BY ANTIBODIES OF CERVICAL DYSTONIA PATIENTS WHO BECAME UNRESPONSIVE TO BoNT/A TREATMENT

CD is due to neck-muscle spasms that cause pain and involuntary contractions, resulting in abnormal neck movements and posture. Symptoms can be relieved by injecting the affected muscle with a BoNT (usually type A or B). The therapeutic benefits are impermanent, and toxin injections need to be repeated every 3 to 6 months. In a very small percentage of patients (less with BoNT/A than with BoNT/B), the treatment elicits neutralizing antitoxin antibodies, which reduce or terminate the patient's responsiveness to further treatment. We have recently reported[20] the localization of the regions on the H chain of BoNT/A that bind Abs in sera that have neutralizing anti-BoNT/A Abs by the MPA from CD patients who had been treated with BoNT/A (Botox, Allergan, Irvine, CA). In previous studies,[77] we found that human antitetanus neurotoxin (TeNT) Abs cross-react with BoNT/A and BoNT/B. So we devised an assay procedure for measuring specific anti-BoNT/A Abs in human sera by absorbing out or inhibiting the anti-TeNT Abs with TeNT before analyzing the sera for the anti-BoNT/A Abs. The sera were obtained from 28 CD patients who had become unresponsive to treatment with BoNT/A and in an in vivo assay protected mice against a lethal dose of BoNT/A. It should be noted that the Ab-binding profiles of the patients' sera were more restricted than the profile of the hyperimmune sera.[20] The pattern of Ab recognition varied from patient to patient (Fig. 5-5), but a very limited set of peptides were recognized by most of the patients. These were, in decreasing amounts of Ab binding, peptide N25 (H chain residues 785–803), C9/C10 (967–985/981–999), C31 (1275–1296), C15 (1051–1069), C20 (1121–1139), N16 (659–677), N22 (743–761), and N4 (491–509). However, not every serum recognized all of these peptides. The finding that the binding profile was not the same for all the patients is consistent with previous observations that immune responses to protein antigens are under genetic control and that the response to each epitope within a protein is under separate genetic control.[47,78-81] Except for the region within C9/C10 (967–985/981–999), the other regions either coincided (N16 [659–677] and C31 [1275–1296]), or overlapped (N22, N25, C15, and C20), with the snps-binding regions on the H chain described in the preceding section (Table 5-3 and Fig. 5-6).

We compared[11] the spatial proximities in the 3-D structure[76] of the Ab-binding regions to the snps-binding regions. The results (Figs. 5-7 and 5-8) showed that, except for one, the Ab-binding regions either coincide or overlap with the snps regions. Thus, N16 on the translocation domain is involved in both Ab binding as well as snps binding. The Ab-binding region N22 overlaps significantly with the snps-binding regions on N21 and N23. The Ab-binding region N25 is sandwiched between the snps-binding regions N16 (which also binds Abs) and N26. The Ab-binding region on C15 is immediately adjacent to region C31 that binds both snps as well as Abs. Region C31 is also adjacent to region C19 that also binds snps. Furthermore, region C19 is located between the Ab-binding regions N4 and C20. Therefore, it appears that only the Ab-binding regions located on C9–C10 do not coincide or overlap with, or are adjacent to, any snps-binding region. Of course, it is expected that snps-binding regions that coincide or overlap with Ab-binding regions would be prevented, in the presence of neutralizing Abs, from binding to nerve synapse, and therefore, toxin entry into the neuron would be blocked. Thus, analysis of the locations of the Ab-binding and the snps-binding regions in the 3-D structure provides a molecular rationalization for the ability of protecting Abs to block BoNT/A action in vivo.

Determination of the submolecular regions on the BoNT/A H chain that bind anti-BoNT/A Abs and the regions that bind snps has had immediate applications. It has enabled us to

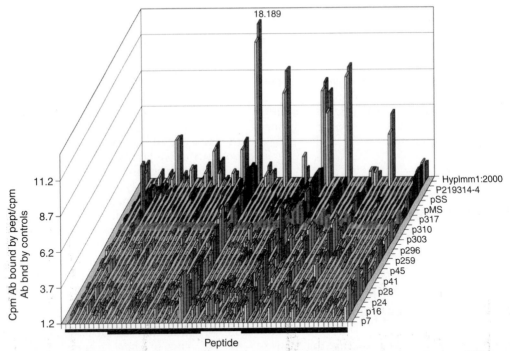

FIGURE 5-5. Mapping of the antibody (Ab)-recognition profiles for the individual 28 mouse protection assy (MPA)–positive cervical dystonia (CD) sera. The results, which represent the average of four experiments that varied ± 5% or less, are expressed in ratio of Abs bound to peptides in the CD serum/Abs bound by the four peptides N2, N12, C17, and C23, which as a rule showed no Ab binding with any of the 28 sera studied and were therefore used as negative control. (From Dolimbek BZ, Aoki KR, Steward LE, Jankovic J, Atassi MZ. Mapping of the regions on the heavy chain of botulinum neurotoxin A (BoNT/A) recognized by antibodies of cervical dystonia patients with immunoresistance to BoNT/A. *Mol Immunol.* 2007;44:1029-1041.) *See Color Plate*

develop a useful assay for neutralizing anti-BoNT/A Abs based on their ability to interfere with the toxin binding to snps[82] and also a peptide-based immunoassay for antibodies against BoNt/A.[83] These assays are outlined in the next two sections.

A NEW ASSAY FOR NEUTRALIZING AND NON-NEUTRALIZING ANTI-BoNT/A ABS BASED ON INHIBITION OF BoNT/A BINDING TO SYNAPTOSOMES

The MPA, which is an in vivo assay, is currently the most widely used method for monitoring neutralizing Abs in BoNT-treated patients. In the previous section, we showed[20] that a number of the BoNT/A regions on the H sub-unit that bind blocking mouse Abs coincided,

or overlapped, with regions that bind to snps. This indicated that blocking anti-BoNT/A Abs would be predicted to inhibit BoNT/A binding to snps.[82] We analyzed sera from 58 CD patients who had been treated with BoNT/A (Botox) for neutralizing Abs by MPA and determined their abilities to inhibit in vitro the binding of active BoNT/A or inactive toxin (toxoid) to mouse brain snps.[82] With active ^{125}I-labeled BoNT/A-snps binding, the MPA-positive sera (n = 30) showed distinctly higher inhibition levels (mean = 21.1 ± 5.8) than those obtained with MPA-negative sera (n = 28) (mean = -1.3 ± 3.9; $P < 0.0001$) or with control sera (n = 19) (mean = -3.4 ± 2.8; $P < 0.0001$). Similarly, inhibition levels by MPA-positive sera of ^{125}I-labeled inactive toxin (toxoid) binding to snps (mean = 48.6 ± 8.7) were distinctly higher than inhibition by MPA-negative sera (mean = 10.0 ± 7.6; $P < 0.0001$) or control sera (mean = 1.8 ± 6.9; $P < 0.0001$). In Figure 5-9, we show a comparison of the results of inhibition by MPA-positive sera (n = 30), MPA-negative sera (n = 28) and control sera (n = 19) of the

TABLE 5-3 Comparison of the Regions that Bind Abs in MPA-Positive Sera of BoNT/A-Treated CD Patients and Regions that Bind to Mouse snps*

Peptide	Residue	MPA +ve CD Sera	snps
H$_N$ Domain			
N4	491–509	+	-
N7	533-551	-	+
N8	547-565	±	-
N16	**659–677**	+	++
N19	701–719	-	+
N21	**729–747**	-	++
N22	**743–761**	+	-
N23	**757–775**	-	+
N25	**785–803**	+++	-
N26	**799–817**	-	+++
H$_C$ Domain			
C2	869–887	±	-
C3	883–901	±	-
C6	925–943	±	-
C7	939–957	+	-
C9	967–985	+	-
C10	981–999	++	-
C15	**1051–1069**	++	-
C16	**1065–1083**	-	+++
C19	**1107–1125**	-	+
C20	**1121–1139**	++	-
C23	**1163–1181**	-	++
C24	**1177–1195**	+	±
C25	**1191–1209**	-	+
C28	1233–1251	-	+
C31	**1275–1296**	++	++

abs, antibodies; MPA, mouse protective assay; snps, mouse brain synaptosomes.
*The table shows only the peptides that bind either Abs in MPA-positive sera from CD patients and/or mouse snps. Peptides and/or their overlap that possess both bindings are shaded. Please see the below listed reference for explanation on the number of + signs for the binding peptides.
From Dolimbek BZ, Aoki KR, Steward LE, Jankovic J, Atassi MZ. Mapping of the regions on the heavy chain of botulinum neurotoxin A (BoNT/A) recognized by antibodies of cervical dystonia patients with immunoresistance to BoNT/A. *Mol Immunol.* 2007;44:1029-1041.

binding of ^{125}I-labeled active BoNT/A and ^{125}I-labeled toxoid binding to snps. It is evident that active toxin and the toxoid gave comparable results that clearly distinguished the MPA-positive sera from MPA-negative sera and controls. Inhibitions by the sera of the latter two groups were virtually undistinguishable. Thus, using labeled active toxin or toxoid, the inhibition assay correlated very well with the MPA. The inhibitory activity of the non-neutralizing sera generally correlated with the length of survival after toxin challenge (correlation coefficients of inhibition: active toxin = 0.445; P = 0.0167; inactive toxoid = 0.774; P < 0.0001).[82]

It was concluded[82] that the snps-inhibition assay is reliable and reproducible, and correlates very well with the MPA. It requires much less serum (0.75% of the amount needed for the MPA) and is considerably less costly than the MPA. With either ^{125}I-labeled active toxin or toxoid, it is possible to distinguish CD sera that have neutralizing Abs from those that lack such Abs. Because the results with the toxoid

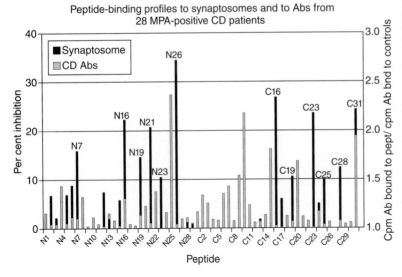

FIGURE 5-6. Comparison of profiles of peptide-binding to mouse brain synaptosomes (snps)[11] and to antibodies (Abs) in an antiserum pool of equal volumes from the 28 mouse protective assay (MPA)–positive patients with cervical dystonia (CD)[20] analyzed in Figure 5-5. *See Color Plate*

were as discriminating as those of the active toxin, it would not even be necessary to use active toxin in these assays.

A PEPTIDE-BASED IMMUNOASSAY FOR ANTI-BoNT/A ANTIBODIES

The aforementioned determination[20] of the Ab-binding profile of the CD sera showed that Abs in CD sera bound to one or more of the peptides N25 (785–803), C10 (981–999), C15 (1051–1069), and C31 (1275–1296). This suggested to us the possibility that binding to these peptides could be used for assay of Abs in CD sera. We recently found[83] that Ab binding to these regions showed very significant deviations from the control responses. Of these four peptides, C10 showed the most significant level of separation between patient and control groups ($P = 5 \times 10^{-7}$) and the theoretical resolution (i.e., ability to distinguish CD patients from control), 84%, was about 4% higher than the least resolved response, C31 ($P = 6 \times 10^{-6}$, resolution 80%). Because the amounts of Abs bound to a given peptide varied with the patient and not all the patients necessarily recognized all four peptides, there was the possibility that binding to combinations of two or more peptides might give a better discriminatory capability. Using two peptides, C10 plus C31, the resolution improved to 87% ($P = 4 \times 10^{-8}$). These two peptides appeared to compliment each other and negate the lower resolution of C31. A combination of three peptides

(Fig. 5-10) gave resolutions that ranged from 85 (N25 + C15 + C31; $P = 2 \times 10^{-7}$) to 88% (C10 + C15 + C31; $P = 1 \times 10^{-8}$). Finally, using the data of all four peptides, N25 + C10 + C15 + C31, gave (see Fig. 5-10) a resolution of 86% ($P = 1 \times 10^{-7}$). Although these levels of resolution are somewhat lower than that obtained with whole BoNT/A (resolution 97%; $P = 6 \times 10^{-12}$), it was concluded[83] that the two-peptide combination C10 + C31, or the three-peptide combination C10 + C15 + C31 (affording resolutions of 87% and 88%, respectively) provide a good diagnostic, toxin-free procedure for assay of total specific anti-toxin Abs in BoNT/A-treated CD patients.

IMMUNE RECOGNITION AND RECEPTOR BINDING OF BoNT/B

ANTIBODY BINDING REGIONS ON THE BoNT/B H CHAIN AND THEIR RELATIONSHIP TO RECEPTOR BINDING

We have commenced studies aimed at elucidating the molecular and cellular immune responses to BoNT/B and have recently

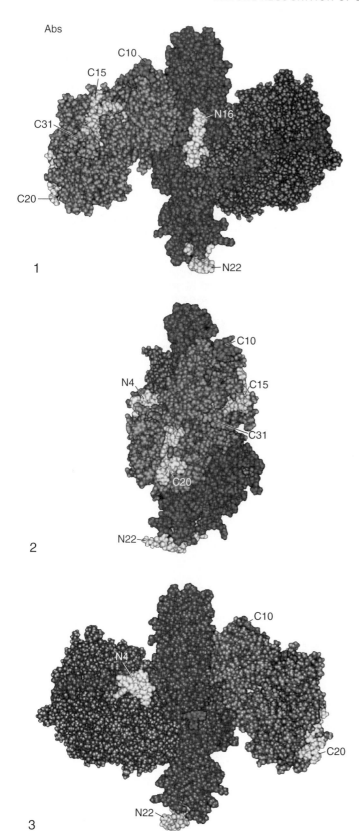

FIGURE 5-7. Images of the three-dimensional structure of botulinum neurotoxin (BoNT/A) showing the locations of the regions that bind anti-BoNT/A antibodies (Abs) in mouse protective assay (MPA)–positive sera from BoNT/A-treated patients with cervical dystonia (CD). The regions are colored *white* (low amounts of Ab binding), *pink* (medium levels of binding), *rose* (high binding) and *red* (very high binding). Image 2 is obtained by rotating the molecule in image 1 90 degrees counterclockwise around the vertical axis, and image 3 is obtained by rotating image 2 again 90 degrees counterclockwise around the vertical axis. (From Dolimbek BZ, Aoki KR, Steward LE, Jankovic J, Atassi MZ. Mapping of the regions on the heavy chain of botulinum neurotoxin A [BoNT/A] recognized by antibodies of cervical dystonia patients with immunoresistance to BoNT/A. *Mol Immunol.* 2007;44:1029-1041.) *See Color Plate*

Abs & Snps

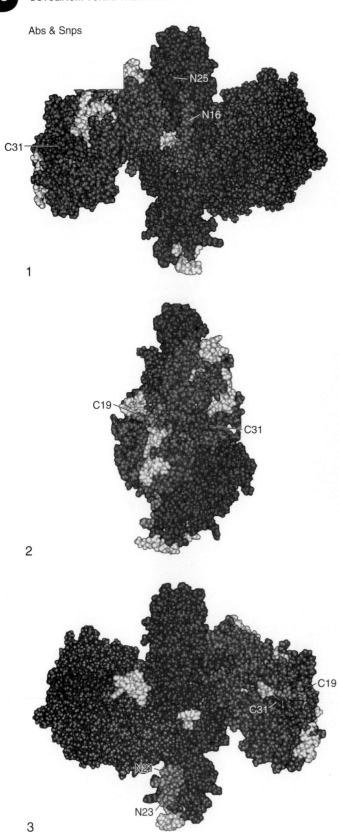

FIGURE 5-8. Images of the three-dimensional representations of botulinum neurotoxin A (BoNT/A) showing the antibody (Ab)–binding regions localized with mouse protective assay (MPA)–positive sera[20] from BoNT/A-treated patients with cervical dystonia (CD) and the mouse brain synaptosome (snps)–binding regions on BoNT/A. The Ab-binding regions that do not coincide but might overlap with snps binding regions are colored *white*. The snps-binding regions, two of which (N16 and C31) coincide completely with Ab-binding regions, are colored *rose* or *red*. Images in panels 2 and 3 are obtained by rotating the image in panel 1 90 and 180 degrees, respectively, counterclockwise around the vertical axis. (From Dolimbek BZ, Aoki KR, Steward LE, Jankovic J, Atassi MZ. Mapping of the regions on the heavy chain of botulinum neurotoxin A (BoNT/A) recognized by antibodies of cervical dystonia patients with immunoresistance to BoNT/A. *Mol Immunol.* 2007;44:1029-1041.) *See Color Plate*

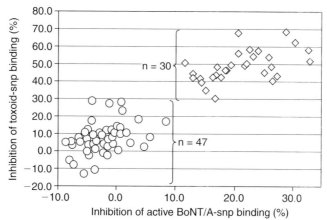

FIGURE 5-9. Comparison of the inhibition levels by human sera of the binding of active botulinum neurotoxin A (BoNT/A) and inactive toxin (toxoid) to mouse brain synaptosomes (snps). The figure compares the results of inhibition by ($\diamond$) mouse protective assay (MPA)–positive sera (n = 30), ($\bigcirc$) MPA-negative sera (n = 28) and control sera (n = 19) of the binding of ^{125}I-labeled active BoNT/A and ^{125}I-labeled toxoid binding to snps. The figure shows that active toxin and toxoid gave comparable results that clearly differentiated the MPA-positive sera from MPA-negative sera and controls. The inhibitions by sera of latter two groups were not distinguishable. (From Maruta T, Dolimbek BZ, Aoki KR, Atassi MZ. Inhibition by human sera of botulinum neurotoxin-A binding to synaptosomes: A new assay for blocking and non-blocking antibodies *J Neurosci Methods.* 2006;151:90-96.) *See Color Plate*

localized the regions on the BoNT/B H chain that are recognized by neutralizing (neutralizing) human, horse, and outbred mouse anti-BoNT/B Abs.[21] Human antisera were a pool of equal volumes from 10 CD patients who had been treated with Myobloc (a BoNT/B product from Solstice Neurosciences, Inc., South San Francisco, CA)

and had become unresponsive to treatment. We are currently determining the recognition profiles of neutralizing Abs in individual MPA-positive sera from a large number of BoNT/B-treated CD patients.

Abs from the three host species recognized similar, but not identical, peptides. There were also peptides recognized by two or only by one

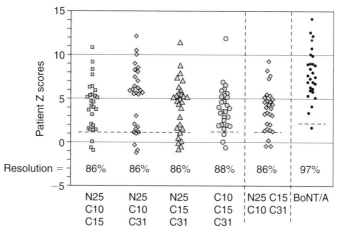

FIGURE 5-10. Binding of antibodies (Abs) in mouse protective assay (MPA)–positive sera from patients with cervical dystonia (CD) (n=28), normalized to 10 normal controls, to peptide combinations shown on the x-axis and to botulinum neurotoxin (BoNT/A). Patient and control response (gray zone) distribution are taken after accumulation. The percent values represent optimal resolution between the two groups (equal proportion of false-positive and false-negative findings at a particular Z value [-]).Control mean and deviation were determined and patient values were normalized by (sample value-control mean)/ control standard deviation. (From Atassi MZ, Dolimbek BZ, Deitiker P, Jankovic J, Aoki KR. A peptide-based immunoassay for antibodies against botulinum neurotoxin A. *J Mol Recognition.* 2007;20:15-21.)

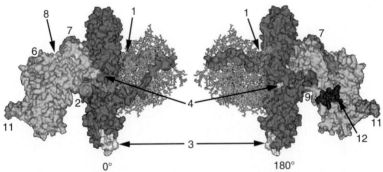

FIGURE 5-11. Three-dimensional images of botulinum neurotoxin B (BoNT/B) showing the locations of antigenic regions that are recognized by human and mouse anti-BoNT/B antibodies (Abs) with overlaps of seven or more residues.[21] The H_C domain of the heavy chain is in *green* and the translocation (H_N) domain is in *red*. The L chain, displayed in wire style, is *yellow*. The right image is obtained by 180 degrees rotation of the left image. The numbers labeling the regions refer to the numbers and sequences.[21] Regions that describe a distinct patch on the surface and may form in each case a single unique antigenic site that binds the polyclonal Abs directed against that site. The three-dimensional coordinates used for these images were from the RCSB Protein Data Bank (PDB), accession code 1EPW.[84] (From Dolimbek BZ, Steward LE, Aoki KR, Atassi MZ. Immune recognition of botulinum neurotoxin B: Antibody-binding regions on the heavy chain of the toxin. *Mol Immunol.* 2007, doi:10.1016/j.molimm.2007.08.007) *See Color Plate*

host species. Where a peptide was recognized by Abs of more than one host species, these Abs were present at different levels in their antisera. Human, horse, and mouse Abs bound, although in different amounts, to regions within peptides 736–754, 778–796, 848–866, 932–950, 974–992, 1058–1076, and 1128–1146. Human and horse Abs bound to peptides 890-908 and 1170-1188. Human, and mouse Abs recognized peptides 470–488/484–502 overlap, 638–656, 722–740, 862–880, 1030–1048, 1072–1090, 1240–1258 and 1268–1291. We concluded that the antigenic regions localized with the three antisera are similar, in some cases exhibiting a small shift to the left or to the right.[21]

Of the regions that are recognized by human, mouse and horse anti-BoNT/B Abs (see Table 5-3), regions 3 and 5 show 1–2 residue shift in the relative positions by human and mouse Abs, whereas regions 8 and 9 exhibit left and right shifts of 5 and 6–7 residues, respectively. The locations in the 3-D structure[84-87] of the antigenic regions that bind human and mouse Abs are shown in Figures 5-11 and 5-12. The regions recognized by human and mouse Abs occupy predominantly equivalent or comparable surface locations on the toxin molecule (see Fig. 5-11) that either coincide completely or display only minor shifts.

The aforementioned shift and variability with different antisera are consistent with what is known about the immune recognition of proteins. Whereas locations of the immune recognition regions on a protein are inherent in

their 3-D locations and depend on the covalent structure of the protein,[43,44,47,88] recognition is under control of the major histocompatibility complex (MHC), and the response to each site is under separate genetic control.[78-81] Therefore, immunodominance of Abs directed against a given site varies with the host species and even with individuals within a given species. A given site can show a frame shift with Abs of different host species and among individuals within the same species.[43,44,47,67,88] The MHC of the host is in all likelihood a major cause of the frame shift and the level of the Ab response.

Region 4, at the interface between the H_C and H_N domains, seems to be partially inaccessible. However, the flexibility of the H_C-H_N interface of the molecule would quite likely allow region 4 to become accessible during binding to the cell receptor and/or translocation. Examination of the 3-D locations of the antigenic regions revealed that regions 1, 3, and 10 occupy discrete locations and most probably form independent antigenic sites.[21] However, certain regions occupy immediately contiguous locations and appear to constitute a single patch on the surface (see Fig. 5-12). Region combinations that seem to fall in this category and were concluded to form quite likely in each case a single antigenic site are: regions 2–4; 5-8 and two residues of 4; 6–7; 9 and part of 11.[21] The polyclonal Ab population directed against a given site comprises Ab molecules that may not necessarily perceive the site in a uniformly identical manner.

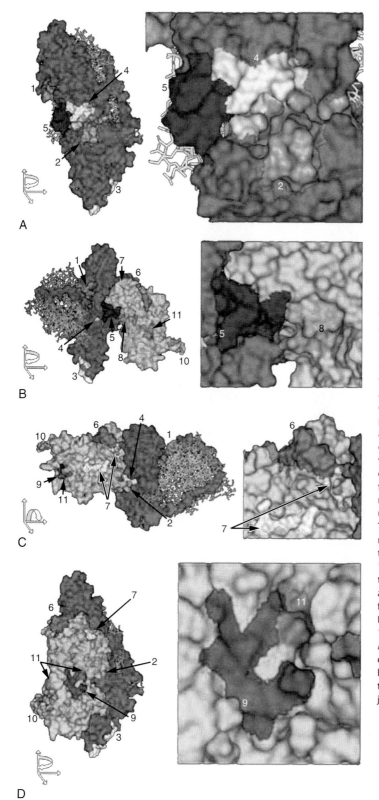

FIGURE 5-12. Contiguous regions that describe distinct patches on the surface. These combinations may each form a single site. Three-dimensional surface-mapped images of botulinum neurotoxin B (BoNT/B) illustrating antigenic regions on the surface that are recognized by human and mouse anti-BoNT/B antibodies (Abs) (see Table 5-3).[21] The numbers correspond with the peptide numbers and sequences listed in Table 5-3.[21] The orientations and close-ups in this figure highlight contiguous surface regions that are formed by discontinuous peptides. **A,** The left panel is a view of the BoNT/B structure with the H_C domain removed. The image is rotated 80 degrees around the y-axis compared with the 0 degree image in Figure 5-11 (see panel D for a similar display with the H_C domain present). The right panel is a close-up view and clearly illustrates that regions 2, 4, and 5 form a contiguous surface patch. Although regions 2 and 5 are accessible when the H_C domain is present (see Fig. 5-11), the solution accessibility of region 4 to antibodies is unknown (see the discussion). **B,** The left panel is a view of the structure rotated 40 degrees around the y-axis compared with the 180-degree structure in Figure 5-11. The right panel shows a close-up view of regions 5 and 8, illustrating that these regions form a contiguous surface. **C,** The left panel is a view of the BoNT/B structure rotated 70 degrees around the x-axis compared with the 0-degree structure in Figure 5-11. The right panel is a close-up view of the contiguous surface between regions 6 and 7. **D,** The left panel is a view of the structure rotated 90 degrees around the y-axis relative to the 0-degree structure in Figure 5-11. The right panel is a close-up of the contiguous surface formed between regions 9 and 11. The three-dimensional coordinates for these images were from the RCSB Protein Data Bank (PDB), accession code 1EPW.[84] (From Dolimbek BZ, Steward LE, Aoki KR, Atassi MZ. Immune recognition of botulinum neurotoxin B: Antibody-binding regions on the heavy chain of the toxin. *Mol Immunol.* 2007, doi:10.1016/j.molimm.2007.08.007) *See Color Plate*

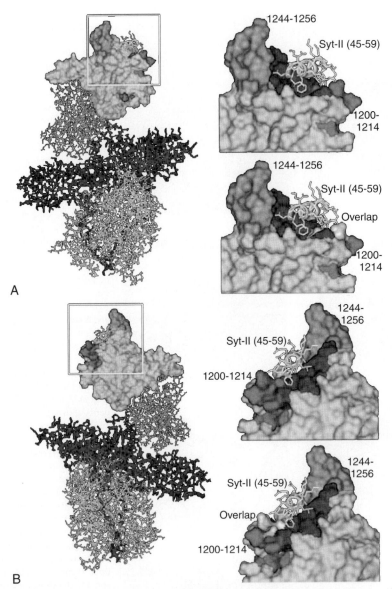

FIGURE 5-13. Proximity of the mouse synaptotagmin II (Syt-II) binding site to mouse Ab-binding epitopes on botulinum neurotoxin B (BoNT/B). **A,** The left panel is a view of the three-dimensional structure of BoNT/B showing the locations on the molecule of the mouse anti-BoNT/B antibody (Ab)-binding epitopes within residues 1200–1214 and 1244–1256 relative to the area to which mouse Syt-II binds. The boxed area is detailed in the right panels. **Upper Panel,** The antigenic sites and Syt-II binding site are independently colored as follows: *Magenta,* Ab-binding region 1200–1214; *blue,* 1244–1256; *dark red,* Syt-II binding pocket. **Lower Panel,** Colors signify the same but in addition the overlap of Syt-II binding site and 1200–1214 is shown in *silver-gray.* **B,** Back view obtained by rotating the BoNT/B structure in A by 180 degrees. The labels and colors connote the same information as described in **A**. Note that there are residues that actually overlap between region 1200-1214 and the Syt-II binding site, whereas region 1244–1256 is immediately adjacent to the Syt-II binding site (see text for details). These images make it clear why binding of Abs to either region 1200–1214 or 1244–1256 would be expected to block the binding of Syt-II to BoNT/B. The three-dimensional coordinates used for these images were from the RCSB Protein Data Bank (PDB), accession code 2NPO.[13] Note that rat Syt-II binds to the same BoNT/B area.[12] (From Dolimbek BZ, Steward LE, Aoki KR, Atassi MZ. Immune recognition of botulinum neurotoxin B: Antibody-binding regions on the heavy chain of the toxin. *Mol Immunol.* 2007, doi:10.1016/j.molimm.2007.08.007) *See Color Plate*

The Ab response, in all likelihood, describes a bell-shaped specificity curve whose apex is directed against the middle of the site, but each Ab molecule within that population perceives the site somewhat differently, emphasizing different regions of the surface of the site. This phenomenon was described for antigenic sites of other proteins.[47,67] Thus although the overlapping peptide strategy was designed to localize *continuous* binding regions of a protein, it would appear that the method is also capable of identifying some *discontinuous* antigenic sites.[21]

The binding surfaces between BoNT/B and rat synaptotagmin II (Syt-II)[12] or mouse Syt-II,[13] a cell surface receptor for BoNT/B,[3,4,89-91] have been determined. Figure 5-13 shows the location of the Syt-II binding crevice relative to regions involved in the binding of mouse anti-BoNT/B Abs. Residues S1116, P1117, and V1118 are located within the horse anti-BoNT/B Abs binding region 1115–1129, whereas residue D1115 on one ridge of the binding crevice is within 6.5 Å from the Syt-II binding surface in the complex. On the same ridge of the crevice and within 6.5 Å are residues Y1244, E1245, S1246, and K1254 within region 1244–1256 of BoNT/B that binds mouse anti-BoNT/B Abs. On the other side of the crevice, the ridge has the Syt-II contact residues S1201, E1203, and F1204, which reside in the mouse Ab-binding region 1200–1214. These overlaps (see Fig. 5-13) would explain the blocking activity of horse and mouse Abs, which by competing for, and blocking, the Syt-II binding region on BoNT/B prevent toxin binding to Syt-II. However, the results indicated that human neutralizing Abs may also be directed against other BoNT/B regions that are not involved in the toxin-Syt-II binding. These may interact with other cell surface molecules involved in BoNT/B binding.[92-95] We have recently analyzed the BoNT/B residues that bind neutralizing human anti-BoNT/B Abs and found that at least one epitope (unpublished work) is very close to the trisaccharide binding site.[84] This work will be published in detail soon.

CONCLUSIONS

BoNTs act at the presynaptic neuromuscular junction by blocking acetylcholine release at nerve terminals, thereby causing temporary paralysis. The action is initiated by the binding of BoNT, through its H chain, to a presynaptic cell surface receptor, thereby allowing the L chain, or a combination of H and L chains, to be internalized and cause paralysis. Because of these properties, BoNTs (particularly types A and B) have been exploited in therapeutic conditions associated with involuntary muscle spasm and contractions, as well as in cosmetic and other applications. However, periodic injections are needed, and the immune system responds (less to BoNT/A than to BoNT/B) by mounting T-cell responses and Abs that may block the initial binding of the toxin to its receptor (i.e., neutralizing Abs). We have determined on the H chains of BoNT/A and /B the covalent and 3-D locations of the regions recognized by blocking Abs. Not all anti-BoNT Abs will block its action. Blocking (and hence protection) by Abs is a function of Ab affinity, class, and isotype. The Ab-binding regions reside on the surface of the respective toxin, and neutralizing Abs against a given toxin bind to regions that the toxin uses to bind to its correlate receptor. So when these regions are occupied by Abs of sufficient affinity, they are unable to bind to receptor. These findings provide a molecular basis for how neutralizing Abs obstruct toxin action and are important for designing effective synthetic peptide vaccines and devising, for certain clinical needs, tolerization strategies against preselected epitopes.

ACKNOWLEDGMENTS

This work was supported by a grant from Allergan and by the Welch Foundation due to the award to M. Z. Atassi of the Robert A. Welch Chair of Chemistry.

References

1. Williams RS, Tse CK, Dolly JO, Hambleton P, Melling J. Radioiodination of botulinum neurotoxin type A with retention of biological activity and its binding to brain synaptosomes. *Eur J Biochem.* 1983;131:437-445.
2. Evans DM, Williams RS, Shone CC, Hambleton P, Melling J, Dolly JO. Botulinum neurotoxin type B. Its purification, radioiodination and interaction with rat-brain synaptosomal membranes. *Eur J Biochem.* 1986;154:409-416.
3. Nishiki T, Kamata Y, Nemoto Y, Omori A, Ito T, Takahashi M, et al. Identification of protein receptor for Clostridium botulinum type B neurotoxin in rat brain synaptosomes. *J Biol Chem.* 1994;269:10498-10503.
4. Nishiki T, Tokuyama Y, Kamata Y, Nemoto Y, Yoshida A, Sekiguchi M, et al. Binding of botulinum type B neurotoxin to Chinese hamster ovary cells transfected with rat synaptotagmin II cDNA. *Neurosci Lett.* 1996;208:105-108.

5. Nishiki T, Tokuyama Y, Kamata Y, Nemoto Y, Yoshida A, Sato K, et al. The high-affinity binding of Clostridium botulinum type B neurotoxin to synapto-tagmin II associated with gangliosides GT1b/GD1a. *FEBS Lett*. 1996;378:253-257.

6. Kozaki S, Akira M, Yoichi K, Jun O, Genji S. Immunological characterization of papain-induced fragments of Clostridium botulinum type A neurotox-in and interaction of the fragments with brain synap-tosomes. *Infect Immun*. 1989;57:2634-2639.

7. Simpson LL. Molecular pharmacology of botulinum toxin and tetanous toxin. *Ann. Rev. Pharmacol Toxicol*. 1986;26:427-453.

8. Simpson LL. Peripheral actions of the botulinum toxins. *Botulinum Neurotoxin and Tetanus Toxin*. New York: Academic Press; 1989:153-178.

9. Bandyopadhyay S, Clark AW, Das Gupta B, Sathyamoorthy V. Role of the heavy and light chains of botulinum neurotoxin in neuromuscular paralysis. *J Biol Chem*. 1987;262:2660-2663.

10. Li L, Singh BR. In vitro translation of type A Clostridium botulinum neurotoxin heavy chain and analysis of its binding to rat synaptosomes. *J Prot Chem*. 1999;18:89-95.

11. Maruta T, Dolimbek BZ, Aoki KR, Steward LE, Atassi MZ. Mapping of the synaptosome-binding regions on the heavy chain of botulinum neurotoxin A by synthetic overlapping peptides encompassing the entire chain. *Protein J*. 2004;23:539-552.

12. Jin R, Rummel A, Binz T, Brunger AT. Botulinum neurotoxin B recognizes its protein receptor with high affinity and specificity. *Nature*. 2006;444: 1092-1095.

13. Chai Q, Arndt JW, Dong M, Tepp WH, Johnson EA, Chapman ER, et al. Structural basis of cell surface receptor recognition by botulinum neurotoxin B. *Nature*. 2006;444:1096-1100.

14. Role of zinc in the structure and toxic activity of botu-linum neurotoxin. *Biochemistry*. 1998;37:5267-5278.

15. Dong M, Yeh F, Tepp WH, Dean C, Johnson EA, Janz R, et al. SV2 is the protein receptor for botulinum neu-rotoxin A. *Science*. 2006;312:592-596.

16. Mahrhold S, Rummel A, Bigalke H, Davletov B, Binz T. The synaptic vesicle protein 2C mediates the uptake of botulinum neurotoxin A into phrenic nerves. *FEBS Lett*. 2006;580:2011-2014.

17. Atassi MZ, Dolimbek BZ, Hayakari M, Middlebrook JL, Whitney B, Oshima M. Mapping of the antibody-bind-ing regions on botulinum neurotoxin H-chain domain 855-1296 with anti-toxin antibodies from three host species. *J Prot Chem*. 1996;15:691-700.

18. Atassi MZ, Dolimbek BZ. Mapping of the antibody-binding regions on the HN-domain (residues 449-859) of botulinum neurotoxin A with antitoxin antibodies from four host species. Full profile of the continuous antigenic regions of the H-chain of botulinum neurotoxin A. *Protein J*. 2004;23:39-52.

19. Dolimbek GS, Dolimbek BZ, Aoki KR, Atassi MZ. Mapping of the antibody and T cell recognition pro-files of the HN domain (residues 449-859) of the heavy chain of botulinum neurotoxin A in two high-responder mouse strains. *Immunol Investig*. 2005;34:119-142.

20. Dolimbek BZ, Aoki KR, Steward LE, Jankovic J, Atassi MZ. Mapping of the regions on the heavy chain of botulinum neurotoxin A (BoNT/A) recognized by anti-bodies of cervical dystonia patients with immunoresis-tance to BoNT/A. *Mol Immunol*. 2007;44:1029-1041. Epub 2006 May 2.

21. Dolimbek BZ, Steward LE, Aoki KR, Atassi MZ. Immune recognition of botulinum neurotoxin B: Antibody-binding regions on the heavy chain of the toxin. *Mol Immunol*. 2007, doi:10.1016/j.molimm.2007.08.007

22. Atassi MZ, Oshima M. Structure, activity and immune (T and B cell) recognition of botulinum neurotoxin. *Crit Revs Immunol*. 1999;19:219-260.

23. Silberstein SD. Review of botulinum toxin type A and its clinical applications in migraine headache. *Expert Opin Pharmacother*. 2001;10:1649-1654.

24. Silberstein SD. Preventive treatment of migraine. *Trends Pharmacol Sci*. 2006;27:410-415.

25. Borodic GE, Acquadro M, Johnson EA. Botulinum toxin therapy for pain and inflammatory disorders: mechanisms and therapeutic effects. *Expert Opin Investig Drugs*. 2001;10:1531-1544.

26. Becker-Wegerich PM, Rauch L, Ruzicka T. Botulinum toxin A: Successful decollete rejuvenation. *Dermatol Surg*. 2002;28:168-171.

27. Binder WJ, Brin MF, Blitzer A, Pogoda JM. Botulinum toxin type A (BOTOX) for treatment of migraine. *Dis Mon*. 2002;48:323-335.

28. Turton K, Chaddock JA, Acharya KR. Botulinum and tetanus neurotoxins: structure, function and therapeu-tic utility. *Trends Biochem Sci*. 2002;27:552-558.

29. Gui D, Rossi S, Runfola M, Magalini SC. Review article: botulinum toxin in the therapy of gastrointestinal motility disorders. *Aliment Pharmacol Ther*. 2003;18: 1-16.

30. Brashear A, McAfee AL, Kuhn ER, Fyffe J. Botulinum toxin type B in upper-limb poststroke spasticity: a double-blind, placebo-controlled trial. *Arch Phys Med Rehabil*. 2004;85:705-709.

31. Diamond A, Jankovic J. Botulinum toxin in dermatol-ogy - beyond wrinkles and sweat. *J Cosmet Dermatol*. 2006;5:169.

32. Göschel H, Wohlfarth K, Frevert J, Dengler R, Bigalke H. Botulinum A toxin therapy: neutralizing and nonneutralizing antibodies—therapeutic conse-quences. *Exp Neurol*. 1997;147:96-102.

33. Dressler D, Bigalke H. Antibody-induced failure of botulinum toxin type B therapy in de novo patients. *Eur Neurol*. 2004;52:132-135.

34. Dressler D, Bigalke H. Botulinum toxin type B de novo therapy of cervical dystonia. Frequency of antibody in-duced therapy failure. *J Neurol*. 2005;252:904-907.

35. Jankovic J. Botulinum toxin: Clinical implications of antigenicity and immunoresistance. In: Brin MF, Hallett M, Jankovic J, eds. *Scientific and Therapeutic Aspects of Botulinum Toxin*. Philadelphia, PA: Lippincott Williams & Wilkins. 2002;409-415.

36. Jankovic J. Botulinum toxin in clinical practice. *J Neurol Neurosurg Psychiatry*. 2004;75:951-957.

37. Jankovic J. Treatment of cervical dystonia with botulinum toxin. *Mov Disord*. 2004;19(suppl 8): S109-S115.

38. Jankovic J, Vuong KD, Ahsan J. Comparison of efficacy and immunogenicity of original versus current botuli-num toxin in cervical dystonia. *Neurology*. 2003;60:1186-1188.

39. Jankovic J, Hunter C, Atassi MZ, Dolimbek BZ, Dolimbek GS, BOS Research Group. Botulinum toxin type B observational study (BOS). *Mov Disord*. 2005;20(suppl 10):S31.

40. Jankovic J, Hunter C, Dolimbek BZ, Dolimbek GS, Adler CH, Brashear A, et al. Clinico-immunologic aspects of botulinum toxin type B treatment of cervical dystonia. *Neurology*. 2006;67:2233-2235.

41. Atassi MZ. Basic immunological aspects of botulinum toxin therapy. *Move Dis.* 2004;19(suppl 8):S68-84.

42. Atassi MZ. On the enhancement of anti-neurotoxin antibody production by subcomponents, HA1 and HA3b, of Clostridium botulinum type B 16S toxin-hemagglutinin. *Microbiology.* 2006;152:1891-1895.

43. Kazim AL, Atassi MZ. A novel and comprehensive synthetic approach for the elucidation of protein antigenic structures. Determination of the full antigenic profile of the alpha-chain of human haemoglobin. *Biochem J.* 1980;191:261-264.

44. Kazim AL, Atassi MZ. Structurally inherent antigenic sites. Localization of the antigenic sites of the alpha-chain of human haemoglobin in three host species by a comprehensive synthetic approach. *Biochem J.* 1982;203:201-208.

45. Bixler GS Jr, Atassi MZ. Molecular localization of the full profile of the continuous regions recognized by myoglobin primed T-cells using synthetic overlapping peptides encompassing the entire molecule. *Immunol Commun.* 1983;12:593-603.

46. Bixler GS, Atassi MZ. T cell recognition of myoglobin. Localization of the sites stimulating T cell proliferative responses by synthetic overlapping peptides encompassing the entire molecule. *J Immunogen.* 1984;11:339-353.

47. Atassi MZ. Antigenic structures of proteins. Their determination has revealed important aspects of immune recognition and generated strategies for synthetic mimicking or protein binding sites. *Eur J Biochem.* 1984;145:1-20.

48. Kurisaki JI, Atassi H, Atassi MZ. T-cell recognition of ragweed Allergen Ra3: Localization of the full T-cell recognition profile by synthetic overlapping peptides representing the entire protein chain. *Eur J Immuol.* 1986;16:236-240.

49. Yoshioka N, Atassi MZ. Antigenic structure of human haemoglobin: Localization of the antigenic sites of the ß-chain in three host species by synthetic overlapping peptides representing the entire chain. *Biochem J.* 1986;234:441-447.

50. Mulac-Jericevic B, Kurisaki JI, Atassi MZ. Profile of the continuous antigenic regions on the extracellular part of the α-chain of an acetylcholine receptor. *Proc Natl Acad Sci U S A.* 1987;84:3633-3637.

51. Ulrich RG, Atassi H, Lutz P, Cresswell P, Atassi MZ. Immune recognition of human major histocompatibility antigens: Localization by a comprehensive synthetic strategy of the continuous antigenic sites in the first domain of HLA-DR2 β Chain. *Eur J Immuol.* 1987;17:497-502.

52. Ulrich RG, Atassi MZ. Mapping of the full profile of T-cell allorecognition regions on HLA-DR2β subunit. *Eur J Immunol.* 1990;20:713-721.

53. Atassi MZ. Strategies for the localization and synthesis of protein binding sites. In: Tschesche H. *Modern Methods in Protein Chemistry.* Berlin, Germany: de Gruyter; 1988;1-40.

54. Yoshioka N, Atassi MZ. Haemoglobin binding with haptoglobin: Localization of the haptoglobin binding sites on the β-chain of human haemoglobin by synthetic overlapping peptides encompassing the entire chain. *Biochem J.* 1986;234:453-456.

55. McCormick DJ, Atassi MZ. Hemoglobin binding with haptoglobin: Delineation of the haptoglobin binding site on the α-chain of human hemoglobin. *J Prot Chem.* 1990;9:735-742.

56. Mulac-Jericevic B, Atassi MZ. Profile of the α-bungarotoxin-binding regions on the extracellular part of the α-chain of Torpedo californica acetylcholine receptor. *Biochem J.* 1987;248:847-852.

57. Mulac-Jericevic B, Manshouri T, Yokoi T, Atassi MZ. The regions of α-neurotoxin binding on the extracellular part of the α-subunit of human acetylcholine receptor. *J Prot Chem.* 1988;7:173-177.

58. Yoshioka N, Atassi MZ. Subunit interacting surfaces of human haemoglobin: Localization of the α-β subunit interacting surfaces on the β-chain by a comprehensive synthetic strategy. *Biochem J.* 1986;234:457-461.

59. Yoshioka N, Atassi MZ. Subunit interacting surfaces of human hemoglobin in solution. Localization of the α-β subunit interacting surfaces on the α-chain by a comprehensive synthetic strategy. *J Prot Chem.* 1999;18:179-185.

60. Atassi MZ, Yoshioka N. Mapping of the subunit interacting surfaces of oligomeric proteins in solution by a comprehensive synthetic strategy. *J Prot Chem.* 1998;17:553-555.

61. Atassi MZ, Mulac-Jericevic B. Mapping the extracellular topography of the α-chain in free and in membrane-bound acetylcholine receptor by antibodies against overlapping peptides spanning the entire extracellular parts of the chain. *J Prot Chem.* 1994;13:37-47.

62. Atassi MZ, Mulac-Jericevic B, Ashizawa T. Mapping of the polypeptide chain organization of the main extracelluar domain of the α-subunit in membrane-bound acetylcholine receptor by anti-peptide antibodies spanning the entire domain. *Adv Exp Med Biol.* 1994;347:221-229.

63. Rosenberg JS, Middlebrook JL, Atassi MZ. Localization of the regions on the C-terminal domain of the heavy chain of botulinum toxin A recognized by T-lymphocytes and by antibodies after immunization of mice with pentavalent toxoid. *Immunol Investig.* 1997;26:491-504.

64. Oshima M, Hayakari M, Middlebrook JL, Atassi MZ. Immune recognition of botulinum neurotoxin type A: Regions recognized by T cells and antibodies against the protective HC fragment (Residues 855–1296) of the toxin. *Mol Immunol.* 1997;34:1031-1040.

65. Oshima M, Middlebrook JL, Atassi MZ. Antibodies and T cells against synthetic peptides of the C-terminal domain (HC) of botulinum neurotoxin type A and their cross-reaction with HC. *Immunol Lett.* 1998;60:7-12.

66. Atassi MZ, Smith JA. A proposal for the nomenclature of antigen sites in peptides and proteins. *Immunochemistry.* 1978;15:609-610.

67. Atassi MZ. Antigenic structure of myoglobin. The complete immunochemical anatomy of a protein and conclusions relating to antigenic structures of proteins. *Immunochemistry.* 1975;12:423-438.

68. Atassi MZ, Dolimbek GS, Deitiker PR, Aoki KR, Dolimbek BZ. Submolecular recognition profiles in two mouse strains of non-protective and protective antibodies against botulinum neurotoxin A. *Mol Immunol.* 2005;42:1509-1520.

69. Byrne MP, Smith LA. Development of vaccines for prevention of botulism. *Biochimie.* 2000;82:955-966.

70. Middlebrook JL. Protection strategies against botulinum toxin. *Adv Exp Med Biol.* 1995;383:93-98.

71. Woodward LA, Arimitsu HR, Hirst R, Oguma K. Expression of HC subunits from clostridium types C and D and their evaluation as candidate vaccine antigens in mice. *Infect Immun.* 2003;71:2941-2944.

72. Koriazova LK, Montal M. Translocation of botulinum neurotoxin light chain protease through the heavy chain channel. *Nat Struct Biol.* 2003;10:13-18.

73. Li L, Singh BR. Role of zinc binding in type A botulinum neurotoxin light chain's toxic structure. *Biochemistry*. 2000;39:10581-10586.

74. Simpson LL. Identification of the major steps in botulinum toxin action. *Annu Rev Pharmacol Toxicol*. 2004;44:167-193.

75. Montal MS, Blewitt R, Tomich JM, Montal M. Identification of an ion channel-forming motif in the primary structure of tetanus and botulinum neurotoxins. *Febs Lett*. 1992;313:12-18.

76. Lacy DB, Tepp W, Cohen AC, DasGupta BR, Stevens RC. Crystal structure of botulinum neurotoxin type A and implications for toxicity. *Nat Struct Biol*. 1998;5:898-902.

77. Dolimbek BZ, Jankovic J, Atassi MZ. Cross reaction of tetanus and botulinum neurotoxins A and B and the boosting effect of botulinum neurotoxins A and B on a primary anti-tetanus antibody response. *Immunol Investig*. 2002;31:247-262.

78. Okuda K, Christadoss PR, Twining SS, Atassi MZ, David CS. Genetic control of immune response to sperm whale myoglobin in mice. I. T lymphocyte proliferative response under H-2-linked Ir gene control. *J Immunol*. 1978;121:866-868.

79. Okuda K, Twining SS, David CS, Atassi MZ. Genetic control of immune response to sperm whale myoglobin in mice. II. T lymphocyte proliferative response to the synthetic antigenic sites. *J Immunol*. 1979;123:182-188.

80. Twining SS, David CS, Atassi MZ. Genetic control of the immune response to myoglobin. IV. Mouse antibodies in outbred and congenic strains against sperm whale myoglobin recognize the same antigenic sites that are recognized by antibodies raised in other species. *Mol Immunol*. 1981;18:447-450.

81. David CS, Atassi MZ. Genetic control and intersite influences on the immune response to sperm whale myoglobin. *Adv Exp Med Biol*. 1982;150:97-126.

82. Maruta T, Dolimbek BZ, Aoki KR, Atassi MZ. Inhibition by human sera of botulinum neurotoxin-A binding to synaptosomes: A new assay for blocking and non-blocking antibodies. *J Neurosci Methods*. 2006;151:90-96. Epub 2006 Feb 8.

83. Atassi MZ, Dolimbek BZ, Deitiker P, Jankovic J, Aoki KR. A peptide-based immunoassay for antibodies against botulinum neurotoxin A. *J Mol Recognition*. 2007;20:15-21.

84. Swaminathan S, Eswaramoorthy S. Structural analysis of the catalytic and binding sites of Clostridium botulinum neurotoxin B. *Nat Struct Biol*. 2000;7:693-699.

85. Swaminathan S, Eswaramoorthy S. Crystallization and preliminary X-ray analysis of Clostridium botulinum neurotoxin type B. *Acta Crystallogr D Biol Crystallogr*. 2000;56:1024-1026.

86. Eswaramoorthy S, Kumaran D, Swaminathan S. A novel mechanism for Clostridium botulinum neurotoxin inhibition. *Biochemistry*. 2002;41:9795-9802.

87. Eswaramoorthy S, Kumaran D, Keller J, Swaminathan S. Role of metals in the biological activity of Clostridium botulinum neurotoxins. *Biochemistry*. 2004;43:2209-2216.

88. Kazim AL, Atassi MZ. Prediction and confirmation by synthesis of two antigenic sites in human haemoglobin by extrapolation from the known antigenic structure of sperm whale wyoglobin. *Biochem J*. 1977;167:275-278.

89. Kozaki S, Kamata Y, Watarai S, Nishiki T, Mochida S. Ganglioside GT1b as a complementary receptor component for Clostridium botulinum neurotoxins. *Microb Pathog*. 1998;25:91-99.

90. Ihara H, Kohda T, Morimoto F, Tsukamoto K, Karasawa T, Nakamura S, et al. Sequence of the gene for Clostridium botulinum type B neurotoxin associated with infant botulism, expression of the C-terminal half of heavy chain and its binding activity. *Biochim Biophys Acta*. 2003;1625:19-26.

91. Dong M, Richards DA, Goodnough MC, Tepp WH, Johnson EA, Chapman ER. Synaptotagmins I and II mediate entry of botulinum neurotoxin B into cells. *J Cell Biol*. 2003;162:1293-1303.

92. Rummel A, Mahrhold S, Bigalke H, Binz T. The HCC-domain of botulinum neurotoxins A and B exhibits a singular ganglioside binding site displaying serotype specific carbohydrate interaction. *Mol Microbiol*. 2004;51:631-643.

93. Kohda T, Ihara H, Seto Y, Tsutsuki H, Mukamoto M, Kozaki S. Differential contribution of the residues in C-terminal half of the heavy chain of botulinum neurotoxin type B to its binding to the ganglioside GT1b and the synaptotagmin 2/GT1b complex. *Microb Pathog*. 2007;42:72-79.

94. Fischer A, Montal M. Crucial role of the disulfide bridge between botulinum neurotoxin light and heavy chains in protease translocation across membranes. *J Biol Chem*. 2007;40:29604-29611.

95. Fischer A, Montal M. Single molecule detection of intermediates during botulinum neurotoxin translocation across membranes. *Proc Natl Acad Sci U S A*. 2007;104:10447-10452.

96. Rocchia W, Alexov E, Honig B. Extending the applicability of the nonlinear Poisson-Boltzmann equation: multiple dielectric constants and multivalent ions. *J Phys Chem B*. 2001;105:6507-6514. Addition/Correction. 2001;105:6754-6754.

97. Rocchia W, Sridharan S, Nicholls A, Alexov E, Chiabrera A, Honig B. Rapid grid-based construction of the molecular surface and the use of induced surface charge to calculate reaction field energies: applications to the molecular systems and geometric objects. *J Comp Chem*. 2002;23:128-137.

Biology and Clinical Pharmacology of Botulinum Neurotoxin Type C and Other Non-A/Non-B Botulinum Neurotoxins

6

Roberto Eleopra, Valeria Tugnoli, and Cesare Montecucco

INTRODUCTION

The botulinum neurotoxin (BoNT) is one of the most potent neurotoxins in human and animals, and it exists in seven different serotypes designated as type A, B, C, D, E, F, and G.

The large majority of outbreaks of human botulism are caused by intoxication with BoNT serotype A, serotype B, or serotype E.[1] All seven serotypes are large proteins that act on cholinergic neuromuscular junctions to block transmission of synaptic vesicles. The molecular basis of the inhibition of neurotransmitter release caused by these BoNT serotypes have been recently unraveled.[2-6] Research on laboratory and animal preparations has shown that the toxins produce this effect by proceeding through a sequence of four steps: (1) binding to receptors on the plasma membrane, (2) penetration of the plasma membrane by receptor-mediated endocytosis, (3) penetration of the endosome membrane, and (4) intracellular expression of an enzymatic action that culminates in blockade of exocytosis.[7-11]

BoNTs are able to enter the neuronal cytosol, where they display a zinc-dependent proteinase activity specific for three proteins of the neuroexocytosis apparatus. BoNT serotype B (BoNT/B), D (BoNT/D), F (BoNT/F) and G (BoNT-G) cleave at single points. Synaptobrevin (VAMP), BoNT serotype A (BoNT/A), and BoNT serotype E (BoNT/E) act specifically on synaptosome-associated protein with Mr = 25 k (SNAP-25), whereas BoNT serotype C (BoNT/C) cleaves both SNAP-25 and syntaxin, two proteins located on the cytosolic face of the nerve plasmalemma.[3]

In the past decade, a great deal of attention has been focused on BoNTs, in part due to the discovery that the various serotypes are zinc-dependent endoproteases that cleave specific synaptic proteins implicated in docking and fusion of vesicles but also because the BoNT serotype A and B are now drugs that have been approved for medical use. They have various clinical applications and their use is now extended to different human diseases characterized by cholinergic hyperactivity of the somatic or autonomic nervous system. The therapeutic use of BoNT/A in humans is well established is rapidly expanding.[12]

The use of BoNT/A in humans has been done in consequence of the epidemiologic

The authors of this chapter have not reported any conflicts of interest.

77

findings on the occurrence of botulism, that have been used as the basis for deciding which serotypes should be tested as therapeutic agents. Epidemiologic data suggest that serotypes A, B, E, F, and G cause adult botulism, whereas serotypes C only sporadic cases (infant botulism) and D do not affect humans.[13,14]

In clinical practice, the use of non-BoNT/A serotypes could be useful when a specific immune response to BoNT/A is proved. There are reports of some nonresponders to BoNT/A,[15-18] particularly when repetitive injections are performed. These drawbacks can be overcome by using a different BoNT serotypes when a specific immune resistance to BoNT/A is proved, even if its actions have never been systematically studied in human tissues, such as in the neuromuscular junction.

Actually, no extensive data exist in humans on the comparative dose-response characteristics of the seven toxin serotypes. Indeed, there are no convincing data that demonstrate whether the human neuromuscular junction is actually sensitive to all seven serotypes.[3,5] The biochemical and cellular events at the basis of the different durations of action of the various toxins are unknown, but several factors may contribute to them: (a) the lifetime of the L chain in the cytosol; (b) the turnover of the truncated soluble SNARE protein; (c) secondary biochemical events triggered by the production of truncated SNARE proteins or the released peptides.[5]

Recent studies have advanced two schools of thought as to why various species of botulinum toxins differ in their time course. With respect to BoNT/A, one theory is that the toxin becomes compartmentalized and persists in the nerve terminal, allowing it to remain proteolytically active over a long period of time and able to cleave any newly synthesized SNAP-25.[19-21] A second line of thought is that truncated fragments (e.g., SNAP-25 when cleaved by BoNT/A or BoNT/E), once cleaved by the toxin, are unable to be degraded from the nerve terminal, preventing insertion of new SNAP-25 molecules.[21-23] At present, there is no consensus implicating a single, universal mechanism responsible for the disparity in time course among the different toxins.[24]

Therefore, the neurotoxin gene sequence comparisons of all of the toxin serotypes (serotypes A to G) suggest that the *BoNT* gene has evolved separately in different genomic backgrounds.[25] The presence of these toxins in different genetic backgrounds suggests their

movement both within species and among other species. Most of these bacteria are distributed throughout the world, yet there is no known geographic relationship to the genetic diversity. Actually, no extensive data exist in humans on the comparative dose-response characteristics of the seven toxin serotypes. Our experience in humans is related to the electrophysiologic comparison of BoNT/A, BoNT/E, BoNT/F, BoNT/B and BoNT/C injections in compound muscle action potential (CMAP) percentage amplitude variation of the abductor digitorum minimi (ADM) muscle of the hand,[26] and as shown in Figure 6-1, the temporal profile of the neuromuscular blockade induced is summarized for each BoNT serotype as percentage variation over the.

In this chapter, we will summarize the action and the effect of non-A/non-B BoNT serotypes, particularly in relation to their applications for human diseases.

BOTULINUM NEUROTOXIN SEROTYPE F

The BoNT/F is the first non-A serotype used in humans as an alternative to BoNT/A, and its choice has been related to the knowledge of human botulism and the detection that the seven BoNTs show different antigens with distinct immunogenic reactivity. BoNT/F demonstrates specificity for the vesicle-associated membrane protein (VAMP) synaptobrevin, a protein in the membrane of synaptic vesicles themselves. If the nerve terminal were to replenish the number of synaptic vesicles at a rate fast enough to compensate for those affected by type F toxin, then the normal neuromuscular transmission could resume within days.[3,27] Moreover, antibodies to BoNT/A toxoid (inactivated type A toxin) do not have significant neutralizing effect against BoNT/F,[28] suggesting that BoNT/F might be an alternative therapy for subjects patients who have developed antibodies to BoNT/A. BoNT/F was less lethal in animals than BoNT/A per unit protein,[29] and in rats, BoNT/F causes less muscle weakness and had a shorter duration of action than an equivalent LD_{50} of BoNT/A.[30]

The first use of BoNT/F in patients with antibodies to BoNT/A was reported in 1992; the toxin was used in two patients with torticollis, one patient with oromandibular dystonia, and one patient with stuttering in which the toxin has provided significant

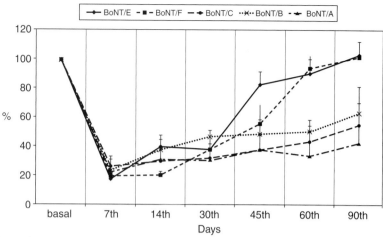

FIGURE 6-1. The figure shows the mean and standard deviation of the compound muscle action potential amplitude (CMAP) variations over time, elicited at the abductor digiti minimi of the hand after ulnar nerve stimulation in humans. Different BoNT serotypes are injected. After baseline value, 10 IU of BoNT/A, 10 IU of BoNT/F, 10 IU of BoNT/E, 10 IU of BoNT/C, and 1000 IU of BoNT/B were injected in 40 different muscles of 20 voluntary subjects. For each serotype, the mean and standard deviation of the CMAP was calculated and the values are shown in percentages by comparing to the initial value.

clinical improvement.[31] However, BoNT/F injection in nonresponders or in dystonic patients treated for the first time relieved symptoms for a shorter time period[24,32-37] and it appears to be beneficial only if injected at high doses when compared with BoNT/A.

Greene and Fahn[32] proposed that BoNT/F may be adequate for some clinical situations in which its effect not needed over long periods. Patients with severe torticollis and radiculopathy could need BoNT injections to relax muscle spasm in the postlaminectomy period, and in these cases, BoNT/F may be preferable to BoNT/A. Moreover, a high BoNT/F dosage can be used because excess neck weakness will short lived and development of immunity to BoNT/F does not preclude future treatment of torticollis with BoNT/A. BoNT/F could be also injected preoperatively to verify that weakness of the target muscles will result in functional improvement.

Recently, the injection of a mixture of different BoNT serotypes has been proposed because several sites of action could be targeted simultaneously. In fact, the mixture of different types of toxin might have a different and unique action, as compared with that of a single serotype. Also, the mixture may also help reduce the risk of eliciting antibodies.[33] In 1999, Mezaki and colleagues[33] treated patients with blepharospasm by injecting BoNT/A or BoNT/F into the orbicularis oculi muscle on one side and 1:1 mixture of both

serotypes into the other side, and thereby compared the peak effect and duration of action in a double-blind controlled study. They concluded that the peak effect of BoNTs was comparable between the single use of type A or F toxin and the combined use of both, and that the duration of action by the mixture was longer than that of BoNT/F but shorter than by BoNT/A alone. Because the effect of the toxin is dose dependent, the similarity of the peak effect supports for the implication that no clinically detectable augmentation or inhibition occurred by the simultaneous action of type A and F toxins on the nerve endings.

In conclusion, different clinical data suggest that BoNT/F is a valid alternative to BoNT/A when a shorter effect is desirable in clinical practice. A higher BoNT/F dosage may produce a seemingly better and longer duration of benefit, even if it is still substantially shorter than the average duration of benefit obtained from BoNT/A. The optimal dose of BoNT/F for an individual patient should be determined by the practitioner, but this study suggests that adverse effects could be a potential problem with doses of BNT-F exceeding 780 MU.[37] The possibility of developing immunity to BoNT/F after long-term treatment is still unknown. Larger series using higher doses of BoNT/F and studies evaluating higher and more frequent dosing with regard to antibody development are needed.

BOTULINUM NEUROTOXIN SEROTYPE C

BoNT/C cleaves both SNAP-25 and syntaxin, two proteins located on the cytosolic face of the nerve plasmalemma. BoNT/C is unique among botulinum neurotoxins because it cleaves two rather than one protein. This double-target specificity of BoNT/C suggested that it could be a valuable alternative to the use of BoNT/A and prompted us to evaluate its therapeutic potential.

In 1997, Coffield and associates[38] demonstrated the action of BoNT/C in human muscles by conducting the following experiment: (1) isolation and testing of BoNT/C from two different strains of clostridia, (2) neutralization of toxicity with specific antibodies, (3) demonstration that the human nervous system has high-affinity binding sites for BoNT/C, (4) demonstration that the human nervous system has a gene encoding syntaxin 1A, the major substrate for BoNT/C, and (5) demonstration that serotype C cleaves the translation product of the human syntaxin 1A gene. Taken together, these results offer compelling evidence that isolated human tissues are susceptible to the toxin.

The fact that BoNT/C does paralyze human neuromuscular transmission raises the question of why the toxin does not typically cause human botulism. In fact, only one isolated case of infant human botulism has been described until now.[39] Although there could be many possible explanations, two are particularly obvious: an apparent resistance may be due to "ecologic factors" (i.e., lack of human exposure) or to "physiologic factors" (i.e., poor human absorption).[5,19-23]

Before the BoNT/C injection was used as a therapeutic drug for dystonia, we compared the BoNT/C activity with that of BoNT/A by using the experiment performed with the isolated mouse hemidiaphragm preparations. This assay allowed us to define the range of doses of BoNTs to be used in humans.[2] Moreover, in a preclinical study in human, we describe the electrophysiologic results obtained with low-dosage injection in the extensor digitorum brevis (EDB) muscles of BoNT/C in comparison with BoNT/A[40,41] and, later, in the ADM of the hand of voluntary subjects,[26] illustrating that BoNT/C has an effect in human similar to BoNT/A. In this latter study, we injected in five ADMs 15 MU of BoNT/A, in five ADMs 15 MU of BoNT/C (prepared in 0.1 mL of phosphate buffer solution [PBS], containing 2% human serum albumin), in five ADMs BoNT/F (prepared in 0.1 mL of PBS, containing 2% human serum albumin), in five ADMs 1500 MU of BoNT/B (Neurobloc, Solstice Neurosciences, Inc., Malvern, PA) and in five ADMs 0.3 mL of saline solution (placebo) alone. Each subjects was blinded for the BoNT types or placebo injected. The neuromuscular blockade induced in the ADM injected with the drugs was quantified by the electrophysiologic evaluation of the CMAP amplitude, elicited by supramaximal electrical stimulation of the ulnar nerve at the wrist, before and after the treatment (at the 2, 4, 6, and 8 weeks). The electrical stimulation was done by using a single shock of 0.5 ms of duration, delivered in a random pattern at low frequency. The recording electrodes placements were the same for each patient, using similar environmental conditions, at the same time of the day and after checking the skin temperature. Before the study, we checked the long-term stability of the CMAP in 20 normal ADMs, by testing in various subjects this technique in different days and obtaining a CMAP percentage trend variation (test-retest amplitude variability) within 20% (our unpublished data).

Moreover, we also recorded the peak-to-peak amplitude of the CMAP evoked by supramaximal electrical stimulation of the ulnar and median nerves at the wrist and recorded with surface electrodes at the 4 DI, at the FDI and at the APB, before and after injection of BoNT at the same time intervals described earlier, in order to quantify the local diffusion of the drug. The neuromuscular block induced 2 weeks after BoNT application was similar among the different BoNTs. So, the following BoNT's temporal profile in recovery of function is not related to different amounts of the drug injected. In this study, the temporal profiles of BoNT/C and BoNT/A have been similar. In another study, BoNT/C injections have proved to be safe in humans because they did not affect the motor neuron counting after poisoning according to our previous study done by the motor unit number estimation (MUNE) technique.[42]

Following these preliminary data, few subjects with focal dystonia who had never been treated before with any BoNT were treated with BoNT/C with subsequent good clinical response.[40] More recently, four patients affected by facial dystonia (blepharospasm) and 10 subjects with torticollis resistant to BoNT/A underwent to BoNT/C therapy.[43]

These preliminary studies (open-label) revealed a good clinical improvement in all the subjects treated with BoNT/C in the dystonic muscles. The clinical benefit was maximal after 30 days for blepharospasm and torticollis, with a slow recovery afterward that extended for as long as 8 weeks, similar to that of BoNT/A. None of the individuals treated reported any collateral effect or adverse reaction in the muscles injected with the BoNT/C. So, BoNT/C injections appeared to be a valid therapy for dystonia and an alternative to BoNT/A.

OTHER BOTULINUM NEUROTOXIN SEROTYPES

BoNT/D was also studied on the human pyramidalis preparation in comparison to BoNT/C.[38,44] In contrast to BoNT/C, which appeared to block transmission in a similar to that of serotype A, BoNT/D produced no observable effect. Even when used at concentrations 10-fold higher than those of the other two serotypes, BoNT/D still produced no measurable effect over a period of 4 to 5 hours. The BoNT/D does not poison human preparations is in keeping with epidemiologic data. There has never been a confirmed case of type D human botulism. So, BoNT/D is not considered an alternative drug for treatment of dystonia in subjects resistant to BoNT/A.

Another serotype, BoNT/E, acts specifically on a protein called SNAP-25, in a manner similar to the way BoNT/A. BoNT/A and BoNT/E share their intracellular substrate. Both of them cleave SNAP-25 and remove nine amino acid residues (BoNT/A) or 26 amino acid residues (BoNT/E) from the carboxyl-terminus of the molecule, this leading to a substantial blockade of neurotransmitter release.[2,3] Hence, BoNT/E is expected to cause an inhibition of acetylcholine release, followed by recovery of function with a time course closely similar to that caused by BoNT/A. Hence, BoNT/E is expected to cause an inhibition of acetylcholine release, followed by recovery of function with a time course closely following that caused by BoNT/A. Hence, BoNT/E is expected to cause inhibition of acetylcholine release, followed by recovery of function with a time course closely similar to that caused by BoNT/A. Hence, BoNT/E is expected to cause an inhibition of acetylcholine release, followed by recovery of function with a time course closely

similar to that caused by BoNT/A. Hence, BoNT/E is expected to cause an inhibition of acetylcholine release, followed by recovery of function over a time course closely similar to that caused by BoNT/A. Hence, BoNT/E is expected to cause an inhibition of acetylcholine release, followed by recovery of function with a time course closely similar to that of BoNT/A. So, BoNT/E is expected to cause an inhibition of acetylcholine release, followed by recovery of function with a time course closely similar to that caused by BoNT/A.[22,44]

In our preclinical study,[22] we evaluated the effects of a double poisoning of the neuromuscular junction with simultaneous injection of both the serotypes (BoNT/A + BoNT/E) in two different dose proportions. In this study, 11 volunteers affected by cranial dystonia (idiopathic blepharospasm) with no previous history of botulism and never treated before with any kind of BoNT were examined. In each subject, 3 IU of Botox Allergan, Irvine, CA) (in 0.1 mL of saline solution) were injected in the EDB muscle of one foot and 3 IU of BoNT/E (prepared in 0.1 mL of PBS, containing 2% human serum albumin) in the EDB muscle of the contralateral side. BoNT/E was obtained from WAKO (Japan), trypsin activated, purified, and tested as previously described by Montecucco et al.[2]

In the second part of the same study, seven additional volunteers affected by idiopathic facial hemispasm (IFH) with no history of botulism and never treated before with any kind of BoNT were examined. Each subject was injected with 4 IU of Botox plus 2 IU of BoNT/E (in 0.1 mL of saline solution) in the EDB muscle of one foot and with 4 IU of BoNT/E pluse 2 IU of Botox (in 0.1 mL of saline solution) in the EDB muscle of the contralateral side.[22] In both groups, the neuromuscular blockade induced in the EDB muscles was calculated quantitatively by the electrophysiologic evaluation of the CMAP peak-to-peak amplitude, elicited by the supramaximal electrical stimulation of the peroneal nerve at the ankle before and after 7, 15, 30, 45, 60 and 90 days from injection. None of the individuals treated reported any adverse reaction in the muscles injected with the BoNTs. Muscles injected with BoNT/E recovered their function much faster than those injected with BoNT/A, and a significant statistical difference ($P < 0.001$) has been observed among all the EDB muscles treated with the two neurotoxins from 30th day onward. Another group of volunteers has been injected in the two EDB foot muscles with a mixture of the two toxins. The subjects received 4 IU of BONT/A plus 2 IU of BoNT/E in one foot and 2 IU of BoNT/A and 4 IU of BoNT/E in the other one. In both cases, after the injections, the EDB muscles recover with within a period similar to that of BoNT/E-treated muscles, clearly faster than that observed with BoNT/A.

The shorter duration of the BoNT/E-induced effects are not due to a shorter period inside the neuronal cytosol because neuromuscular junction paralyzed with a mixture of the two neurotoxins recover with the same, shorter time course found with BoNT/E. If the differential effect was due to BoNT/A remaining active longer in the cytosol and removing newly synthesized SNAP-25 molecules, the neuromuscular junction with the combination of neurotoxins should have recovered in time similarly to BoNT/A alone. Moreover, the time to recovery from BoNT/E or BoNT/A cannot be related to a different potency in the biologic activity of the units used, because they cause a similar maximal neuromuscular block at the seventh day. Although the difference in the time to recovery between the two neurotoxins is clearly established and highly reproducible, the present lack of knowledge of the turnover of SNAP-25 at the terminals of motoneurons does not allow one to explain at the molecular level the phenomenon uncovered here.

It is conceivable that the BoNT/A-cleaved SNAP-25, which preserves more than 95% of its sequence, is nonfunctional in neuroexocytosis but is not altered to such an extent as to be removed from the terminal as much as the BoNT/E-cleaved SNAP-25, which has lost more than 13% of its sequence. These data suggest that the strongly damaged BoNT/E-cleaved SNAP-25 is altered to such an extent as to be rapidly detected, removed, and replaced by newly synthesized molecules, resulting in a more rapid recovery of function. The present data do not permit to dismiss the alternative possibility that these toxins act on other intracellular as yet unknown targets, although there is no evidence that BoNTs act on other cytosolic substrates. Also the finding that the concurrent poisoning with the two BoNTs together does not provide an additive effect is in keeping with the proposal that all of their effects are mediated by SNAP-25 cleavage. Unlike the other two toxins, the shortest duration of action of BoNT/E dosage did not influence recovery time.[22,44]

Recently, other papers reported cases of wound or infantile botulism caused by C. botulinum type E[45,46] confirming as BoNT/E has an effect on humans. Tests of combinations of BoNT/A and /B and BoNT/A and /E were reported in the literature and shown to exacerbate paralysis compared with individually administered serotypes.[6,22,38]

Recovery from BoNT/A appeared to be biphasic, with recovery from the initial phase to be about two-fold faster than that of the final phase. Over 4 weeks, muscle activity had gradually improved following the highest dose of BoNT/A. Lower BoNT/A doses led to incrementally faster and more complete recovery. Persistence of maximum paralysis was exponentially related to the dosage of BoNT/A, with a doubling of the duration of the paralysis occurring with every 25% increase in the concentration of the toxin. In contrast, the rate of recovery from BoNT/B was monophasic relative to toxin dosage and the duration of maximum paralysis was linear relative to dosage.

DISCUSSION

There currently exist a number of experimental vaccines against botulinum toxin, including a pentavalent vaccine (A, B, C, D, and E) distributed by the Centers for Disease Control and Prevention. These vaccines were developed and had been administered long before it was realized that botulinum toxin has value as a therapeutic agent. As a result, there are vaccinated persons who, should they develop dystonia, would be unresponsive to botulinum toxin therapy. This is a relevant matter because botulinum toxin is the only therapeutic intervention that gives satisfactory results for most patients with dystonia, and vaccination can produce long-term resistance to toxin. These facts argue strongly that one must be cautious and thoughtful about administering vaccine.

In the past, the epidemiologic literature on naturally occurring botulism was used as a guide in selecting toxin serotypes for testing as medicinal agents. BoNT/A has long been implicated in human illness; it was the first serotype to be evaluated and used as a medicinal agent, and it has been approved for clinical use.[12] Other serotypes implicated in human illness (B, E, and F) are approved. BoNT/B is now commercially available, whereas BoNT/F and BoNT/E were tested in humans obtaining different clinical profiles, shorter in time when compared with BoNT/A.

So, BoNT/A is now considered the best BoNT serotype that could be used in humans for the treatment of focal movement disorders, even if some patients develop clinical resistance.[15-18] Subjects who are not sensitive to BoNT/A from the first injection or that become decreasingly sensitive to this therapy after prolonged treatment as a result of a specific immune response could be treated with a different BoNT serotype.

In these cases, the use of different BoNT serotypes could help in obtaining clinical improvement. The alternative use of BoNT/F has been proposed because experimental study showed that autoantibodies to BoNT/A do not affect BoNT/F, and because BoNT/F is often detected in human botulism. Moreover, BoNT/F is less lethal than BoNT/A in animal models. Different clinical data suggest that BoNT/F is a valid alternative to BoNT/A when a shorter duration of drug activity is required. Higher BoNT/F dosage may produce a subjectively better and longer duration of benefit, even if it is still substantially shorter than the average duration of benefit obtained from BoNT/A.

Similarly, in humans, muscles injected with BoNT/E injections showed a much faster recovery time than those injected with BoNT/A. This difference in recovery time is due to the strong intracytosol damage caused by BoNT/E-cleaved SNAP-25, which is altered to such an extent as to be rapidly detected, removed, and replaced by newly synthesized molecules, resulting in a rapid recovery of function. Even if it is not possible to exclude other alternative hypothesis about this mechanism.

The finding that BoNT/C blocks human neuromuscular transmission means that the practice of relying solely on epidemiology as a guide for choosing therapeutic agents is flawed. Clearly, BoNT/C warrants investigation for the treatment of neurologic disorders. Some preclinical studies have been reported in the literature regarding the therapeutic use of BoNT/C in humans,[26,40-42] revealing that BoNT/C could be considered a novel effective botulinum neurotoxin serotype for human use. BoNT/C showed a general profile of action similar to that of BoNT/A and is clearly longer acting than BoNT/F. Also, in a few subjects with focal dystonia treated with BoNT/C, a clinical benefit was present.[40] In addition, BoNT/C injections are safe in humans because they do not affect the motor neuron counting after poisoning.[42]

Until now only one case of human infantile botulism related to BoNT/C has been described in the literature[39] and the rare association of human botulism secondary to exposure to BoNT/C is probably related to the distribution of the spores of BoNT/C-producing *Clostridia* or the particular growth requirements of these bacteria.

The possibility that BoNT/C is efficacious carries a hidden benefit. If a situation were to arise in which it was necessary to provide immunization against naturally occurring botulism, there would be no need to include BoNT/C in the vaccine. This means that it would be possible to protect patients against food-borne botulism (e.g., BoNT/A, BoNT/E, BoNT/F) while not depriving them of the ability to respond to antidystonia medication (e.g., BoNT/C).

References

1. Cherington M. Clinical spectrum of botulism. *Muscle Nerve*. 1998;21:701-710.
2. Montecucco C, Schiavo G. Mechanism of action of tetanus and botulinum neurotoxins. *Mol Microbiol*. 1994;13:1-8.
3. Schiavo G, Matteoli M, Montecucco C. Neurotoxins affecting neuroexocytosis. *Physiol Rev*. 2000;80:717-766.
4. Humeau Y, Doussau F, Grant NJ, Poulain B. How botulinum and tetanus neurotoxins block neurotransmitter release. *Biochimie*. 2000;82:427-446.
5. Rossetto O, Seveso M, Caccina P., Schiavo G, Montecucco C. Tetanus and botulinum neurotoxins: turning bad guys into good by research. *Toxicon*. 2001;39:27-41.
6. Aoki KR. Physiology and pharmacology of therapeutic botulinum neurotoxins. *Curr Probl Dermatol*. 2002;30:107-116.
7. Simpson LL. Kinetic studies on the interaction between botulinum toxin type A and the cholinergic neuromuscular junction. *J Pharmacol Exp Ther*. 1980;212:16-21.
8. Simpson LL. The origin, structure, and pharmacological activity of botulinum toxin. *Pharmacol Rev*. 1981;33:155-188.
9. Simpson LL. *Botulinum Neurotoxin and Tetanus Toxin*. San Diego: Academic Press, 1989.
10. Habermann E, Dreyer F. Clostridial neurotoxins: Handling and action at the cellular level. *Curr Top Microbiol Immunol*. 1986;129:93-179.
11. Schiavo G, Rossetto O, Montecucco C. Clostridial neurotoxins as tools to investigate the molecular events of neurotransmitter release. *Semin Cell Biol*. 1994;5:221-229.
12. Jankovic J, Hallett M. *Therapy with Botulinum Toxin*. New York: Marcel Dekker, 1994.
13. Gangarosa EJ, Donadio JA, Armstrong RW, Meyer KF, Brachman PS, Dowell VR. Botulism in the United States, 1899-1969. *Am J Epidemiol*. 1971;93:93-101.
14. Dowell VR Jr. Botulism and tetanus: Selected epidemiologic and microbiologic aspects. *Rev Infect Dis*. 1984;6(suppl 1):202-207.
15. Borodic G, Johnson E, Goodnough M, Schantz E. Botulinum toxin therapy, immunologic resistance,

and problem with available materials. *Neurology.* 1996;46:26-29.

16. Brin M. Botulinum toxin: chemistry, pharmacology, toxicity, and immunology. *Muscle Nerve.* 1997;6 (suppl 6):S146-S165.

17. Hanna PA, Jankovic J. Mouse bioassay versus Western blot assay for botulinum toxin antibodies: correlation with clinical response. *Neurology.* 1998;50: 1624-1629.

18. Sankhla C, Jankovic J, Duane D. Variability of the immunologic and clinical response in dystonic patients immunoresistant to botulinum toxin injections. *Mov Disord.* 1998;13:150-154.

19. Adler M, Keller JE, Sheridan RE, Deshpande DD. Persistence of botulinum neurotoxin A demonstrated by sequential administration of serotypes A and E in the rat EDL muscle. *Toxicon.* 2001;39:233-243.

20. Bartels F, Heidrun B, Bigalke H, Frevert J, Halpern J, Middlebrook J. Specific antibodies against the Zn2+-binding domain of clostridial neurotoxins restore exocytosis in chromaffin cells treated with tetanus or botulinum neurotoxin. *J Biol Chem.* 1994;269:8122-8127.

21. de Paiva A, Meunier FA, Molgo J, Aoki KR, Dolly JO. Functional repair of motor endplates after botulinum neurotoxin type A poisoning: biphasic switch of synaptic activity between nerve sprouts and their parent terminals. *Proc Natl Acad Sci U S A.* 1999;96:3200-3205.

22. Eleopra R, Tugnoli V, Rossetto O, De Grandis D, Montecucco C. Different time courses of recovery after poisoning with botulinum neurotoxin serotypes A and E in humans. *Neurosci Lett.* 1998;256:135-138.

23. Raciborska DA, Charlton MP. Retention of cleaved synaptosome-associated protein of 25kDA (SNAP-25) in neuromuscular junctions: a new hypothesis to explain persistence of botulinum A poisoning. *Can J Physiol Pharmacol.* 1999;77:679-688.

24. Billante CR, Zealear DL, Billante M, Reyes JH, Sant'Anna G, Rodriguez R, et al. Comparison of neuromuscular blockade and recovery with botulinum toxins A and F. *Muscle Nerve.* 2002;26:395-403.

25. Hill KK, Smith TJ, Helma CH, Ticknor LO, Foley BT, Svensson RT, et al. Genetic diversity among botulinum neurotoxin-producing clostridial strains. *J Bacteriol.* 2007;189:818-832.

26. Eleopra R, Tugnoli V, Quatrale R, Rossetto O, Montecucco C. Different types of botulinum toxin in humans. *Mov Disord.* 2004;19(suppl 8):S53-S59.

27. Schiavo G, Shone CC, Rossetto O, Alexander FCG, Montecucco C. Botulinum neurotoxin serotype F is a zinc endopeptidase specific for VAMP/synaptobrevin. *J Biol Chem.* 1993;268:11516-11519.

28. Siegel LS. Evaluation of neutralizing antibodies to type A, B, E, and F botulinum toxins in sera from human rodients of botulinum pentavalent (ABCDE) toxoid. *J Clin Microbiol.* 1989;27:1906-1908.

29. Yang KH, Sugiyama H. Purification and properties of Clostridium botulinum type F toxin. *Appl Microbiol.* 1975;29:598-603.

30. Kaufman JA, Way JF, Siegel LS, Sellin LC. Comparison of the action of types A and F botulinum toxin at the rat neuromuscular junction. *Toxicol Appl Pharmacol.* 1985;79:211-217.

31. Ludlow CL, Hallett M, Rhew K, Cola R, Shinìizu T, Sakaguchi G, et al. Therapeutic use of type F botulinum toxin. *N Engl J Med.* 1992;326:349-350.

32. Greene PE, Fahn S. Use of botulinum toxin type F injections to treat torticollis in patients with immunity to botulinum toxin type A. *Mov Dis.* 1993;8:479-483.

33. Mezaki T, Kaji R, Kohara N, Fujii H, Katayama M, Shimizu T, et al. Comparison of therapeutic efficacies of type A and F botulinum toxins for blepharospasm: a double-blind, controlled study. *Neurology.* 1995;45:506-508.

34. Sheean GL, Lees AJ. Botulinum toxin F in the treatment of torticollis clinically resistant to botulinum toxin A. *J Neurol Neurosurg Psychiatry.* 1995;59:601-607.

35. Greene PE, Fahn S. Response to botulinum toxin F in seronegative botulinum toxin A-resistant patients. *Mov Dis.* 1996;11:181-184.

36. Chen R, Karp BI, Hallett M. Botulinum toxin type F for treatment of dystonia: long-term experience. *Neurology.* 1998;51:1494-1496.

37. Houser MK, Sheean GL, Lees AJ. Further studies using higher doses of botulinum toxin type F for torticollis resistant to botulinum toxin type A. *J Neurol Neurosurg Psychiatry.* 1998;64:577-580.

38. Coffield JA, Barkry N, Zhang R, Carlson J, Gomella LG, Simpson LL. In vitro characterization of botulinum toxin types A, C and D action on human tissues: combined electrophysiologic, pharmacologic and molecular biologic approaches. *J Pharmacol Exp Ther.* 1997; 280:1489-1498.

39. Oguma K, Yokota K, Hayashi S, Takeshi M, Kumagai M, Itoh N, et al. Infant botulism due to Clostridium botulinum type C toxin. *Lancet.* 1990;336:1449-1450.

40. Eleopra R, Tugnoli V, Rossetto O, Montecucco C, De Grandis D. Botulinum neurotoxin serotype C: a novel effective botulinum toxin therapy in human. *Neurosci Lett.* 1997;224:91-94.

41. Eleopra R, Tugnoli V, De Grandis D, Montecucco C. Botulinum toxin serotype C treatment in subjects affected by focal dystonia and resistant to botulinum toxin serotype A. *Neurology.* 1998;50(suppl 4):72.

42. Eleopra R, Tugnoli V, Quatrale R, Gastaldo E, Rossetto O, De Grandis D, et al. Botulinum neurotoxin serotypes A and C do not affect motor units survival in humans: an electrophysiological study by motor units counting. *Clin Neurophysiol.* 2002;113: 1258-1264.

43. Eleopra R, Tugnoli V, Quatrale R, Rossetto O, Montecucco C, Dressler D. Clinical use of non-A botulinum toxins: botulinum toxin type C and botulinum toxin type F. *Neurotox Res.* 2006;9:27-131.

44. Schiavo G, Rossetto O, Catsicas S, De Laureto PP, Dasgupta BR, Benfenati F, et al. Identification of the nerve terminal targets of botulinum neurotoxin serotypes A, D and E. *J Biol Chem.* 1993;268: 23784-23787.

45. Artin I, Björkman P, Cronqvist J, Radström P, Holst E. First case of type E wound botulism diagnosed using real-time PCR. *J Clin Microbiol.* 2007;45: 3589-3594.

46. Abe Y, Negasawa T, Monma C, Oka A. Infantile botulism caused by Clostridium butyricum type e toxin. *Pediatr Neurol.* 2008;38:55-57.

Effects of Botulinum Toxin on Central Nervous System Function   **7**

Carlo Trompetto, Giovanni Abbruzzese, Antonio Suppa, and Alfredo Berardelli

INTRODUCTION

Botulinum toxin type A (BoNT/A) is a metallo-proteinase that inhibits acetylcholine release from the presynaptic terminals by cleaving synaptosome-associated protein (SNAP-25), a presynaptic membrane protein required for fusion of neurotransmitter-containing vesicles. The toxin produces its therapeutic effect by inhibiting acetylcholine release from the presynaptic terminals of the spinal motoneurons, thus blocking neuromuscular transmission and weakening the hyperactive muscle fibers that are involved in involuntary movements.[1,2]

Studies in animals show that besides its peripheral action, BoNT/A also acts on central nervous system (CNS) structures. Evidence shows that intramuscular injected BoNT/A reaches the spinal cord through retrograde axonal transport. Approximately 2 days after radiolabeled BoNT/A was injected into gastrocnemius muscle of a cat, distal-proximal gradient of radioactivity developed first in the sciatic nerve, then in the ipsilateral spinal ventral roots, and ultimately in the spinal cord segments innervating the injected muscle.[3,4] A recent study performed in rats demonstrated that BONT/A is retrogradely transported by central neurons and motorneurones.[5] The toxin can also reach the CNS through the bloodstream and the blood-brain barrier. Using autoradiography of toxin marked with ^{125}I and indirect fluorescent labeling, Boroff and

Chen[6] detected the toxin in the brain parenchyma and blood vessels. Whether the toxin can be diffused through the bloodstream and the blood-brain barrier at low doses remains unclear. Within the CNS, the toxin may inhibit the release of acetylcholine and other neurotransmitters,[7,8] but with systemic injection, there is not likely to be sufficient CNS toxin to have any effect.

Animal studies have demonstrated that BoNT/A can also act on fusimotor synapses. The toxin blocks the gamma motor endings of jaw muscles in a rat, reducing the spindle afferent discharge without altering muscle tension.[9] In a morphologic study comparing the effects of BoNT/A on extrafusal and intrafusal fibers in a rat,[10] the toxin caused fiber atrophy and spread of Ach staining in the endplate, indicating parallel denervation of extrafusal and intrafusal fibers. Evidence of fusimotor denervation suggests that the toxin alters activity in muscle spindle afferents. The altered spindle afferent input may be indirectly responsible for functional changes in central neural networks at both segmental and suprasegmental levels.

Therefore, animal studies suggest that BoNT/A most likely exerts its effects within the CNS indirectly through perturbation of peripheral inputs bound to the CNS. Over the past 15 years, several studies have attempted to demonstrate the CNS effects of botulinum toxin in humans. In this chapter, we review those studies providing the most convincing evidence.

Drs. Trompetto, Suppa, and Berardelli do not report any conflicts of interest. Dr. Abbruzzese has received honoraria from Novartis and Orion Pharma, lecture fees from Boehringer Ingelheim and Wyeth Lederle, and a research grant to his Department from Allergan.

STUDIES OF SPINAL CORD FUNCTION

Two studies investigating reciprocal inhibition before and after BoNT/A injection in patients with dystonia[11] and essential tremor[12] showed that the toxin alters the excitability of the spinal interneurons. Both studies tested reciprocal inhibition with a simple technique by evoking test H-reflexes in the flexor muscles of the wrist, while low-intensity conditioning electric stimuli, designed to stimulate the Ia afferents, are applied to the radial nerve in the spiral groove.[13] If the radial nerve stimulation is given at the appropriate time, it suppresses the test H-reflex in the flexor muscles. In healthy subjects, reciprocal inhibition consists of two phases. The first phase, which peaks at an interval of 0 ms between the conditioning (radial nerve) shock and the test (median nerve) shock, is attributed to activation of a disynaptic pathway inhibiting the flexor spinal motoneurons (postsynaptic inhibition, mediated by Ia inhibitory interneurons).

The second phase, which peaks at an interval of 10 to 20 ms, is mediated by two interneurons organized in a trisynaptic linkage acting at the level of the flexor Ia afferents (presynaptic inhibition) (Fig. 7-1A and B).[14] Experiments performed in cats have shown that the interneurons responsible for presynaptic inhibition are separate from the Ia interneurons involved in disynaptic inhibition. Both groups of interneurons receive diverse supraspinal projections from the cortex and the brain stem.[15]

Before botulinum toxin injection, patients with dystonia and essential tremor had a decreased second phase of reciprocal inhibition, due to an impaired descending control of the spinal interneurons responsible for presynaptic inhibition.[15] One month after botulinum injections, the second presynaptic phase of inhibition increased (see Fig. 7-1C). Furthermore, through its action at the extrafusal motor endplate, the toxin reduced the size of the H reflex and the M wave to a similar extent. The unchanged H/M ratio suggests that the toxin had no effect on the excitability of spinal motoneurons and, therefore, makes it

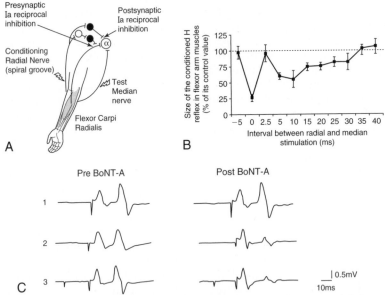

FIGURE 7-1. Radial-induced reciprocal inhibition of the H-reflex elicited in the flexor carpi radialis muscle. **A,** Schematic diagram showing presumed neuronal connections mediating reciprocal inhibition referred to in the text (black neurons are inhibitory). **B,** Time course of the first (postsynaptic) and second (presynaptic) phases of flexor H-reflex inhibition produced by radial nerve stimulation in a group of healthy subjects. Each point represents the mean, and the vertical bars show the standard error. Negative timing indicates that the median nerve test shock (used to evoke the test H-reflex in the flexor carpi radialis muscle) was given before the conditioning (radial nerve) shock. **C,** The recordings from one representative subject affected by idiopathic segmental forearm dystonia are shown: (A) before toxin injection; (B) 1 month after toxin injection; 1, test H reflex alone; 2, test H reflex conditioned by a shock delivered over the radial nerve (conditioning-test interval = 0 ms; postsynaptic inhibition); 3, test H reflex conditioned by a shock delivered over the radial nerve (conditioning-test interval = 20 ms; presynaptic inhibition). The toxin restored the presynaptic phase of reciprocal inhibition (B-3), which was absent before the injection (A-3).

unlikely that the toxin restored presynaptic inhibition by acting directly on the spinal cord. A more likely interpretation is that the toxin altered the tonic sensory inflow coming from the injected muscles, thus improving the function of the spinal circuitry mediating reciprocal inhibition. A BoNT/A-induced change in the spinal circuitry receives support first from the known reorganization of the corticospinal motor pathways induced by sensory inputs (for a recent review, see reference 16) and second from the observation that all the descending motor pathways project to the spinal interneurons mediating presynaptic inhibition.[17]

STUDIES OF CORTICAL MOTOR FUNCTION

Transcranial magnetic stimulation (TMS) of the motor cortex activates, both directly and trans-synaptically, the corticospinal cells, eliciting electromygrapic (EMG) responses in contralateral muscles, namely motor evoked potentials (MEPs).[18,19] TMS delivered by focal coils can be used for noninvasive mapping of the somatotopic representation of muscles within the motor strip. Cortical maps are constructed by stimulating different points on the scalp at a constant intensity and analyzing the number of sites from which MEPs can be elicited in the target muscle. These sites outline the extension of the cortical motor area.

Studies using TMS to construct cortical maps before and after BoNT/A injection in patients with writer's cramp,[20] cervical dystonia,[21] primary writing tremor[22] gave consistent results. In the patients with writer's cramp, the cortical maps of the muscles selected for the injection were displaced medially with respect to the nondominant (unaffected) side. One month after the injection, the maps had moved laterally, reaching a more normal position compared with the nondominant side. Three months after the injection, when the clinical effect of the toxin had worn off, the maps had moved medially, returning toward their original positions.[22] In the patients with cervical dystonia, before the toxin was injected into neck muscles, the cortical hand map on the side contralateral to the direction of the head rotation was laterally and posteriorly displaced. One month after the injection, the map moved closer to the vertex, returning to a more normal position.[21] In the single subject studied by the

authors with writing tremor, hand motor maps were displaced posteriorly on both sides compared with those obtained in 40 healthy volunteers. One month after BoNT/A injection in the forearm muscles, the maps became normal, moving closer to the vertex and to the interaural line on both sides.[22] In conclusion, in patients affected by dystonia, before treatment cortical maps were displayed from their normal position, and after injection became normal and when the toxin effects wore off, the maps returned abnormal.

These studies suggest that BoNT/A injection can cause changes in synaptic organization within the motor cortex that extend beyond the representation of the injected muscles. Because a large body of evidence states that sensory inputs can result in reorganization of corticomotor output (see reference 23), the investigators linked the transient reorganization of the motor cortex after the toxin injection to the modulation of the afferent inputs caused by the toxin's action in the periphery.

A sensitive way to measure changes in cortical excitability is to use paired TMS with stimuli in a conditioning-test paradigm. In healthy subjects, a conditioning stimulus delivered over the motor cortex and set to a low intensity that elicits no MEP on its own inhibits the MEP elicited by a subsequent suprathreshold test stimulus given 1 to 5 ms later.[24] This inhibitory response is thought to originate from the cortex and is termed short interval cortical inhibition (SICI). Drawing analogies from the results observed in animal experiments,[25-27] some investigators proposed that SICI reflects activation of the intracortical GABAergic neurons, which might be involved in maintaining the boundaries of the cortical motor maps and in brain plasticity (for a review, see reference 19). In this framework, the finding that afferent inputs can modulate SICI[23] assumes importance because motor cortical plasticity depends on changes in feedback from the periphery. Most importantly, reduced SICI in patients with dystonia[28] could explain the excessive and inappropriate muscle contraction typically seen in patients with dystonia.[28] To investigate the effects of BoNT/A at the level of the motor cortex, SICI was studied in 11 normal subjects and in 12 patients with dystonia involving the upper limb.[29] In the patients, SICI was assessed before the toxin was injected into the affected muscles, and 1 month and 3 months after. Before the injection, SICI was reduced in the affected muscles. One month after the injection, the level of SICI increased reaching normal values. When the patients were tested 3 months after the injection, their SICI levels had returned almost to the abnormally low levels seen before BoNT/A treatment. This study shows that BoNT/A can transiently modify the excitability of intracortical circuits. Given the physiology of SICI and in accordance with the current view of dystonia, these changes in cortical excitability have been attributed to the toxin's peripheral action on the muscle afferent input. The finding of changes of cortical excitability after BoNT/A has been confirmed by some authors[30] but not by others.[31,32] The contrasting results are possibly related to differences in the methodology used by the authors and in the clinical features of the patients studied.

STUDIES OF MUSCLE AFFERENTS

The studies we have reviewed support that BoNT/A in humans can alter the excitability of central neural circuits both at spinal and at cortical levels. Current evidence suggests that BoNT/A might induce changes in the excitability of CNS circuits by modulating peripheral sensory inputs. In all of the studies, the chemodenervation of intrafusal fibers is suggested to be the mechanism by which the toxin can modify sensory inputs. However, it must be stressed that also the toxin's action at the extrafusal endplates is likely to have a potent influence on sensory afferents.

The reduction of involuntary muscle contractions, caused by chemodenervation of extrafusal fibers, could induce several changes in muscle afferents. First, given the known linear relation between extrafusal fiber firing and the force produced by the homonymous muscle,[33] it should tone down the discharge rate of Ib fibers. Second, it could lengthen the muscle, in turn, increasing the firing rate in muscle spindles. Third, it could alter the firing of joint receptors, which are thought to respond to joint angle.[34] Finally, botulinum toxin might relieve pain also by altering sensory input.[35]

Whether the possible sensory changes induced by chemodenervation of intrafusal fibers can be distinguished from those induced at the extrafusal end plates is unclear. The role of intrafusal chemodenervation can be assessed by using vibration of limb and neck muscles.[36,37] Muscle or tendon vibration activates both primary and secondary spindle endings,[39] thus evoking a tonic vibration reflex (TVR) in the vibrated muscles, which is mediated by monosynaptic and polysynaptic circuits.[40] Besides this reflex activation of spinal motoneurons, the spindle inflow induced by muscle vibration facilitates the MEPs elicited by TMS,[41,42] acting at both spinal and cortical levels.[43] As spindle sensitivity to muscle vibration is increased by the fusimotor system,[44] both the TVR and the vibration induced MEP facilitation can be used to assess the chemodenervation after BoNT/A injection.

Urban and coworkers[36] investigated the vibration-induced facilitation of the MEPs recorded in the sternocleidomastoid muscle (SCM) in 20 healthy subjects and in 10 patients affected by idiopathic rotational torticollis. The patients were tested before (baseline measurements), and 6 and 12 weeks after BoNT-A injection in the affected SCM. The main result was that the vibration-induced facilitation in the treated SCM was lower 6 and 12 weeks after BoNT/A injection. This finding suggests that the toxin not only acts on extrafusal fibers, as shown by the reduction of the MEP elicited without vibration, but also on intrafusal fibers, as reflected by the extra and long-standing reduction of the vibrated-MEP.[36]

We investigated the TVR in the affected muscles of 10 patients with writer's cramp before and 3 weeks after BoNT/A injection.[45] In this study, we also measured the maximal M-wave (M_{max}) and the maximal voluntary contraction (MVC), parameters, which are known to be independent of muscle spindle afferents. In all subjects, BoNT/A injection reduced the TVR more than the M_{max} and MVC. Long-term evaluation of two patients disclosed that 7 months after the injection, M_{max} and MVC had fully recovered, whereas the TVR was still depressed. Hence, the TVR was significantly more depressed and remained depressed longer than the M_{max} and MVC. These findings cannot be explained by the concomitant denervation of extrafusal fibers, an event that should increase muscle spindle afferent discharge (because of reduced spindle unloading during vibration) and decrease Ib discharge (because of reduced muscle tension) mitigating the TVR reduction owing to extrafusal fiber denervation. This special sensitivity of the TVR to suppression by BoNT/A injection strongly suggests that the toxin can denervate the intrafusal muscle fibers, thereby reducing spindle

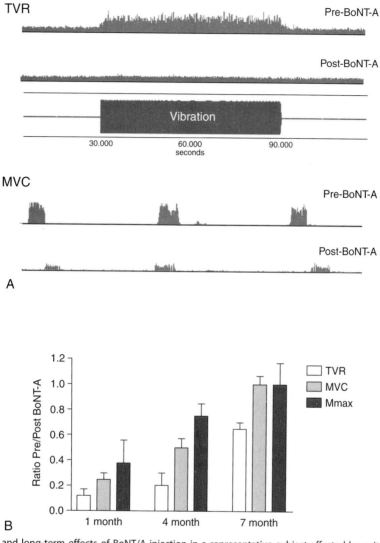

FIGURE 7-2. Short- and long-term effects of BoNT/A injection in a representative subject affected by writer's cramp. **A,** One month after injection, the tonic vibration reflex (TVR) was almost completely suppressed, whereas the maximal voluntary contraction (MVC) was only reduced. **B,** The histograms indicate the post-pre BoNT/A ratios at 1, 4, and 7 months after the injection. Seven months after BoNT/A injection, the TVR was still depressed, whereas MVC and maximal M wave (M_{max}) had fully regained their preinjection values.

inflow to the CNS during vibration (Fig. 7-2A and B).

Both studies investigating the intrafusal chemodenervation after BoNT/A injection gave consistent results about the action of the toxin on γ-efferents. It is undoubtedly easier to test vibration-induced MEP facilitation than the TVR, a parameter with a large inter- and intraindividual variability, which is influenced by many different factors.[46] However, Urban's method cannot be used in subjects affected by upper motor neuron syndrome (UMNS), in whom it is not possible to have an appropriate MEP test. This problem is not present using the TVR, which can be elicited also in the affected muscles of hemiplegic patients.[47] Recently, we were able to confirm the special sensitivity of the TVR to suppression by BoNT/A injection also in UMNS patients with spasticity, provided they retained the capability of moving the affected limb.[37] On the contrary, in plegic patients the extrareduction of the TVR was not found, suggesting the role of movement for the toxin action on γ-efferents.

CONCLUSIONS

Studies in humans provide evidence that BoNT/A alters sensory inputs to the CNS through reversible chemodenervation of extrafusal and intrafusal fibers. This peripheral action induces excitability changes in central neural circuits.

References

1. Simpson LL. The binary toxin produced by Clostridium botulinum enters cells by receptor-mediated endocytosis to exert its pharmacologic effects. *J Pharmacol Exp Ther.* 1989;251:1223-1228.
2. Simpson LL. Botulinum toxin: a deadly poison sheds its negative image. *Ann Intern Med.* 1996;125:616-617.
3. Habermann E. 125I-labeled neurotoxin from Clostridium botulinum A: preparation, binding to synaptosomes and ascent to the spinal cord. *Naunyn Schmiedebergs Arch Pharmacol.* 1974;281:47-56.
4. Wiegand H, Erdmann G, Wellhoner HH. 125I-labelled botulinum A neurotoxin: pharmacokinetics in cats after intramuscular injection. *Naunyn Schmiedebergs Arch Pharmacol.* 1976;292:161-165.
5. Antonucci F, Rossi C, Gianfranceschi L, Rossetto O, Caleo M. Long-distance retrograde effects of botulinum neurotoxin A. *J Neurosci.* 2008;28:3689-3696.
6. Boroff DA, Chen GS. On the question of permeability of the blood-barrier to BoNT. *Int Arch Allergy Applied Immunol.* 1975;48:495-504.
7. Bigalke H, Heller I, Bizzini B, Habermann E. Tetanus toxin and botulinum A toxin inhibit release and uptake of various transmitters, as studied with particulate preparations from rat brain and spinal cord. *Naunyn Schmiedebergs Arch Pharmacol.* 1981;316:244-251.
8. Janicki PK, Habermann E. Tetanus and botulinum toxins inhibit, and black widow spider venom stimulates the release of methionine-enkephalin-like material in vitro. *J Neurochem.* 1983;41:395-402.
9. Filippi GM, Errico P, Santarelli R, Bagolini B, Manni E. Botulinum A toxin effects on rat jaw muscle spindles. *Acta Otolaryngol.* 1993;113:400-404.
10. Rosales RL, Arimura K, Takenaga S, Osame M. Extrafusal and intrafusal muscle effects in experimental botulinum toxin-A injection. *Muscle Nerve.* 1996;19:488-496.
11. Priori A, Berardelli A, Mercuri B, Manfredi M. Physiological effects produced by botulinum toxin treatment of upper limb dystonia. Changes in reciprocal inhibition between forearm muscles. *Brain.* 1995;118:801-807.
12. Modugno N, Priori A, Berardelli A, Vacca L, Mercuri B, Manfredi M. Botulinum toxin restores presynaptic inhibition of group Ia afferents in patients with essential tremor. *Muscle Nerve.* 1998;21:1701-1705.
13. Day BL, Marsden CD, Obeso JA, Rothwell JC. Reciprocal inhibition between the muscles of the human forearm. *J Physiol.* 1984;349:519-534.
14. Berardelli A, Day BL, Marsden CD, Rothwell JC. Evidence favouring presynaptic inhibition between antagonist muscle afferents in the human forearm. *J Physiol.* 1987;391:71-83.
15. Nakashima K, Rothwell JC, Day BL, Thompson PD, Shannon K, Marsden CD. Reciprocal inhibition between forearm muscles in patients with writer's cramp and other occupational cramps, symptomatic

hemidystonia and hemiparesis due to stroke. *Brain.* 1989;112:681-697.
16. Miles TS. Reorganization of the human motor cortex by sensory signals: a selective review. *Clin Exp Pharmacol Physiol.* 2005;32:128-131.
17. Rudomin P, Jimenez I, Solodkin M, Duenas S. Sites of action of segmental and descending control of transmission on pathways mediating PAD of Ia- and Ib-afferent fibers in cat spinal cord. *J Neurophysiol.* 1983;50:743-769.
18. Currà A, Modugno N, Inghilleri M, Manfredi M, Hallett M, Berardelli A. Transcranial magnetic stimulation techniques in clinical investigation. *Neurology.* 2002;59:1851-1859.
19. Abbruzzese G, Trompetto C. Clinical and research methods for evaluating cortical excitability. *J Clin Neurophysiol.* 2002;19:307-321.
20. Byrnes ML, Thickbroom GW, Wilson SA, Sacco P, Shipman JM, Stell R, et al. The corticomotor representation of upper limb muscles in writer's cramp and changes following botulinum toxin injection. *Brain.* 1998;121:977-988.
21. Thickbroom GW, Byrnes ML, Stell R, Mastaglia FL. Reversible reorganisation of the motor cortical representation of the hand in cervical dystonia. *Mov Disord.* 2003;18:395-402.
22. Byrnes ML, Mastaglia FL, Walters SE, Archer SA, Thickbroom GW. Primary writing tremor: motor cortex reorganisation and disinhibition. *J Clin Neurosci.* 2005;12:102-104.
23. Ridding MC, Rothwell JC. Afferent input and cortical organisation: a study with magnetic stimulation. *Exp Brain Res.* 1999;126:536-544.
24. Kujirai T, Caramia MD, Rothwell JC, Day BL, Thompson PD, Ferbert A, et al. Corticocortical inhibition in human motor cortex. *J Physiol.* 1993;471:501-519.
25. Krnjevic K, Randic M, Straughan DW. Nature of a cortical inhibitory process. *J Physiol.* 1966;184:49-77.
26. Rosenthal J, Waller HJ, Amassian VE. An analysis of the activation of motor cortical neurons by surface stimulation. *J Neurophysiol.* 1967;30:844-858.
27. Matsumura M, Sawaguchi T, Kubota K. GABAergic inhibition of neuronal activity in the primate motor and premotor cortex during voluntary movement. *J Neurophysiol.* 1992;68:692-702.
28. Ridding MC, Sheean G, Rothwell JC, Inzelberg R, Kujirai T. Changes in the balance between motor cortical excitation and inhibition in focal, task specific dystonia. *Neurol Neurosurg Psychiatry.* 1995;59:493-498.
29. Gilio F, Curra A, Lorenzano C, Modugno N, Manfredi M, Berardelli A. Effects of botulinum toxin type A on intracortical inhibition in patients with dystonia. *Ann Neurol.* 2000;48:20-26.
30. Kanovsky P, Bares M, Streitova H, Klajblova D, Pavel D, Rektor I. The disorder of cortical excitability and cortical inhibition in focal dystonia is normalised following successful botulinum toxin treatment: an evidence from somatosensory evoked potentials and transcranial magnetic stimulation recordings. *Neurology.* 2005;64(suppl 1):A381.
31. Boroojerdi B, Cohen LG, Hallett M. Effects of botulinum toxin on motor system excitability in patients with writer's cramp. *Neurology.* 2003;61:1546-1550.
32. Allam N, Fonte-Boa PM, Tomaz CA, Brasil-Neto JP. Lack of effect of botulinum toxin on cortical excitability in patients with cranial dystonia. *Clin Neuropharmacol.* 2005;28:1-5.

33. Crago PE, Houk JC, Rymer WZ. Sampling of total muscle force by tendon organs. *J Neurophysiol.* 1982;47:1069-1083.

34. Gardner EP, Martin JH, Jessell TM. The bodily senses. In: Kandel ER, Schwartz JH, Jessell TM, eds. *Principles of Neural Science.* New York; McGraw-Hill, 2000: 430-450.

35. Guyer BM. Mechanism of botulinum toxin in the relief of chronic pain. *Curr Rev Pain.* 1999;3:427-431.

36. Urban PP, Rolke R. Effects of botulinum toxin type A on vibration induced facilitation of motor evoked potentials in spasmodic torticollis. *J Neurol Neurosurg Psychiatry.* 2004;75:1541-1546.

37. Trompetto C, Francavilla G, Ogliastro C, Avanzino L, Bove M, Berardelli A, et al. Intrafusal effects of botulinum toxin injection in patients with upper motor neurone syndrome. *Mov Disord.* 2007;22(Suppl 16):S3.

38. Burke D, Hagbarth KE, Lofstedt L, Wallin BG. The responses of human muscle spindle endings to vibration of non-contracting muscles. *J Physiol.* 1976;261: 673-693.

39. Burke D, Hagbarth KE, Lofstedt L, Wallin BG. The responses of human muscle spindle endings to vibration during isometric contraction. *J Physiol.* 1976;261:695-711.

40. Matthews PB. The reflex excitation of the soleus muscle of the decerebrate cat caused by vibration applied to its tendon. *J Physiol.* 1966;184:450-472.

41. Claus D, Mills KR, Murray NM. The influence of vibration on the excitability of alpha motoneurones. *Electroencephalogr Clin Neurophysiol.* 1988;69:431-436.

42. Siggelkow S, Kossev A, Schubert M, Kappels HH, Wolf W, Dengler R. Modulation of motor evoked potentials by muscle vibration: the role of vibration frequency. *Muscle Nerve.* 1999;22:1544-1548.

43. Kossev A, Siggelkow S, Schubert M, Wohlfarth K, Dengler R. Muscle vibration: different effects on transcranial magnetic and electrical stimulation. *Muscle Nerve.* 1999;22:946-948.

44. Morgan DL, Proske U, Gregory JE. Responses of primary endings of cat muscle spindles to locally applied vibration. *Exp Brain Res.* 1991;87:530-536.

45. Trompetto C, Curra A, Buccolieri A, Suppa A, Abbruzzese G, Berardelli A. Botulinum toxin changes intrafusal feedback in dystonia: a study with the tonic vibration reflex. *Mov Disord.* 2006;21:777-782.

46. Eklund G, Hagbarth KE. Normal variability of tonic vibration reflexes in man. *Exp Neurol.* 1966;16:80-92.

47. Hagbarth KE, Eklund G. Tonic vibration reflexes (TVR) in spasticity. *Brain Res.* 1966;2:201-203.

Botulinum Neurotoxin 8 Treatment of Cranial-Cervical Dystonia

Christopher Kenney and Joseph Jankovic

INTRODUCTION

Dystonia is a neurologic syndrome characterized by involuntary, sustained or spasmodic, patterned, repetitive muscle contractions, which causes twisting, flexing or extending, and squeezing movements or abnormal postures.[1] Dystonia can involve skeletal muscles in any part of the body; distribution of symptoms may be focal, multifocal, segmental, or generalized. Characteristic features include co-contraction of agonist/antagonist muscles and involuntary overflow contraction into adjacent muscle groups or in the opposite limb, the so-called mirror dystonia.[2,3] Dystonic movements are typically action-induced, although they may also occur at rest, particularly when severe or after peripheral injury.

Blepharospasm, an involuntary closure of the eye produced by spasmodic contractions of the eyelids and eyebrows is an example of focal dystonia. An increased frequency of blinking, associated with a feeling of irritation or dryness in the eyes, usually precedes sustained closure of the eyes. Only about 20% of patients with blepharospasm continue to have isolated blepharospasm, sometimes still called benign essential blepharospasm.[4,5] Blepharospasm is an increasingly recognized cause of disability affecting about 32 per 100,000 people.[6] Typically beginning in the 5th or 6th decade of life, women are effected more frequently than men in a ratio of 3:1.[7,8] Blepharospasm arises from excessive contractions of orbicularis oculi (pretarsal, preseptal, and periorbital portions), often involving adjacent muscles including procerus and corrugator. Overactivity of these muscles leads to excessive eye blinking and potentially persistent eye closure related to prolonged muscle spasms of the eyelids. In severe cases, patients may be functionally blind because of persistent eye closure. Quality of life may be markedly impaired with difficulty noted in reading, writing, and driving.[9] Bright light usually exacerbates blepharospasm, so many patients wear sunglasses both outside and inside. The spasms may be transiently alleviated by pulling on an upper eyelid, pinching the neck, talking, humming, yawning, singing, reading, looking down, and other maneuvers called sensory tricks ("geste antagonistique").[10] Blepharospasm may be confused with tic disorders manifested by frequent blinking or ptosis, and may be initially misdiagnosed as myasthenia gravis.[11] The majority of patients with blepharospasm display other involuntary movements in the face such as paranasal contractions, grimacing, or jaw opening/closing.[4] Some patients with blepharospasm may have associated inability to open eyes, the so-called apraxia of eyelid opening. This disorder may occur in isolation or in the setting of parkinsonism.[12,13] Often wrongly diagnosed as blepharospasm, apraxia of eyelid opening has been attributed to absence of contraction or inhibition of the levator palpebrae.[14]

Oromandibular dystonia consists of involuntary spasms of jaw, mouth, and tongue muscles that produce bruxism (tooth grinding); involuntary tongue movements; and opening, closure, or deviation of the jaw.[15] These symptoms may interfere with chewing, speaking, or swallowing. Secondary complications of

Dr. Jankovic has received relevant research grants from Allergan, Inc., Ipsen Limited, and Merz Pharmaceuticals, and has served as a consultant to Allergan, Inc., Benign Essential Blepharospasm Research Foundation, Dystonia Medical Research Foundation, Merz Pharmaceuticals, Michael J. Fox Foundation for Parkinson's Research, and the Neurotoxin Institute.

oromandibular dystonia include dental wear and the temporomandibular joint (TMJ) syndrome. Involuntary contractions of the mouth and jaw muscles can cause disabling dysarthria and chewing difficulties, as well as severe discomfort and social embarrassment. Some patients with oromandibular dystonia display involvement of the pharyngeal and laryngeal musculature, resulting in dysphagia, strained voice (spasmodic dysphonia), respiratory difficulties, and involuntary vocalizations. As in other forms of dystonia, alleviation of oromandibular dystonia may be attained by various sensory tricks, including touching the lips or chin, chewing gum, talking, or applying pressure in the submental area.[15]

Cervical dystonia is characterized by sustained, involuntary contractions of neck muscles that result in abnormal movements and postures of the head.[16] Onset occurs typically between the 3rd and 5th decades of life.[17] The term spasmodic torticollis is commonly used to describe this form of dystonia. However, because the movement is not always spasmodic and may consist of abnormal postures other than torticollis (e.g., turning of the head), such as laterocollis (head tilt), antercollis (neck flexion), and retrocollis (neck extension), the term cervical dystonia is preferred as a generic descriptor of dystonic movements or postures involving the neck.[18] Dystonic tremor, a component of the dystonia, is most obvious when the patient attempts to maintain primary position of the head by resisting the dystonic "pulling." About 25% of patients with cervical dystonia have postural tremor in their hands that is phenomenologically identical to essential tremor.[19] A majority of patients (2/3) note neck pain as a symptom of cervical dystonia.[20]

The combination of blepharospasm, oromandibular dystonia, and cervical dystonia is sometimes referred to as Meige syndrome, but the term cranial-cervical dystonia is more appropriate to describe this form of segmental dystonia. In most series of patients with cranial-cervical dystonia, women outnumber men at a ratio of 2:1, and the onset is usually in the sixth decade of life.[21] The disorder is a lifelong condition, and spontaneous remissions are rare.

ETIOLOGY

Because the muscle spasms of cranial-cervical dystonia are typically exacerbated by stress and relieved by relaxation, as well as by various sensory "tricks," the disorder is often incorrectly presumed to be psychological in nature. This misconception is fostered by the lack of diagnostic imaging or other laboratory tests for abnormalities, because the vast majority of these patients have "idiopathic" dystonia. The second most common cause of cranial-cervical dystonia is tardive dystonia, which is similar to tardive dyskinesia because it is caused by drugs that block dopamine receptors, such as the major tranquilizers and certain antiemetic drugs.[22] In contrast to orofacial and other stereotypic movements that are typically present in tardive dyskinesia, the movements in tardive dystonia are more sustained. Patients treated for Parkinson disease with levodopa may also experience cranial-cervical dystonia.[23] Structural lesions in the upper brain stem, diencephalon, and basal ganglia, resulting from stroke, multiple sclerosis, thalamotomy, hydrocephalus, and other causes, have been reported to cause cranial-cervical dystonia. In addition, cranial-cervical dystonia can be seen in patients with Wilson disease, and other metabolic and neurodegenerative disorders. Facial and jaw spasms, called oculomasticatory myorhythmia, can be a complication of central nervous system involvement in Whipple disease.[24] The rhythmic contractions of the eyelids, face, and mouth may be synchronous with convergent eye oscillations. Finally, trauma to the eyelids, jaw, or neck can trigger dystonic movements in the injured area, peripherally induced dystonia.[25]

PATHOPHYSIOLOGY

Dystonia is characterized by impaired inhibition at multiple levels of the central nervous system.[2] Overflow movements in adjacent muscles are thought to derive from a failure to suppress neuronal excitability in surrounding neural circuits (surround inhibition).[26] No specific abnormality or lesion has been identified on brain imaging studies or at autopsy of the brain of patients with cranial-cervical dystonia. Electrophysiologic studies of patients with cranial-cervical dystonia have demonstrated abnormalities in the R2 component of the blink reflex indicating increased excitation of the brainstem interneuronal pathway.[2] Other neurophysiologic and functional magnetic resonance imaging (fMRI) studies suggest evidence of disinhibition of the primary motor and premotor cortex, along with overactivity in the somatosensory cortex and caudal supplementary motor area.[27] Interestingly, botulinum toxin (BoNT) partially reverses the overactivity of the somatosensory cortex and caudal supplementary motor area after treatment.[28] Although generally regarded as a motor disorder, overactivity of the somatosensory cortex implicates the sensory system as well.[29] Existing clinical and experimental data lend support to the notion that sensorimotor integration is impaired in dystonia.

Clinical, pharmacologic, and biochemical studies have suggested dopaminergic and noradrenergic preponderance in some cases. This biochemical abnormality may be genetically determined, because family history of a movement disorder is present in at least one third of patients with cranial dystonia. A familial form of young-onset cervical dystonia with a dramatic response to levodopa has been reported, but the genetic mutation remains undiscovered.[30] Adult-onset cervical dystonia may occur in families with the DYT7 locus localized to the short arm of chromosome 18p by linkage analysis; however, the molecular basis is poorly understood.[31]

TREATMENT

While the cause of cranial-cervical dystonia is still poorly understood, the treatment has markedly improved in the last decade.[32,33] About one third of patients benefit from pharmacologic therapy with agents such as anticholinergics, benzodiazepines, or muscle relaxants (baclofen).[34] Dystonic patients usually require high doses of anticholinergic treatment (trihexyphenidyl 6–80 mg/day) for noticeable improvement. The pediatric population tolerates these doses more readily than adults.[35] Side effects, such as dry mouth, blurred vision, and confusion, may limit aggressive titration. Baclofen reduces spinal cord interneuron firing by activation of presynaptic GABA receptors.[35] As with trihexyphenidyl, slowly titrated doses may be required for amelioration of dystonia. Side effects include sedation, dizziness, and dry mouth. Tizanidine, a centrally acting muscle relaxant, improves dystonia and spasticity by stimulating noradrenergic α-2 receptors.[36] Longer acting benzodiazepines such as clonazepam provide symptomatic relief with less concern of addiction. In some patients, tardive dystonia responds well to tetrabenazine,

a dopamine-depleting drug.[37] Dose-limiting side effects include sedation, akathisia, depression, and parkinsonism.[38]

Clostridium botulinum produces toxin in seven structurally and immunologically distinct forms (A–G). These neurotoxins block the release of acetylcholine at the neuromuscular junction by cleaving peptides required for vesicular membrane fusion. Scott began using isolated botulinum type A (BoNT/A) to treat blepharospasm more than 20 years ago.[39] At present, two of seven serotypes are available commercially: type A (Botox [Allergan, Irvine, CA], Dysport [Ipsen, Milford, MA], Xeomin [Merz Pharma, Greensboro, NC], Prosigne [Lanzhou Institute of Biologic Products, Shanghai, China) and type B (Myobloc/NeuroBloc [Solstice Neurosciences, Malvern, PA]). Botulinum toxin has revolutionized the treatment of dystonia and a variety of other neurologic (spasticity, tics, migraine), ophthalmologic (strabismus, lacrimation, protective ptosis), urologic (overactive bladder, benign prostatic hyperplasia, pelvic floor dyssynergia), gastrointestinal (achalasia, sphincter of Oddi dysfunction, anal fissures), and dermatologic (hyperhidrosis, wrinkles, pruritus) conditions.[40]

Treatment of cranial-cervical dystonia with botulinum toxin requires a detailed knowledge of the local anatomy and the individual's condition. The potential side effects are related to the site of injection: an injection in the eyelids may cause ptosis, blurred vision, diplopia, tearing, or eyelid hematoma; an injection into the oromandibular muscles may cause chewing, speaking, and swallowing difficulties; and an injection into the cervical muscles can produce neck weakness and swallowing problems.[41,42] Complications usually improve spontaneously within 3 weeks.

For patients unresponsive to conventional pharmacologic intervention, options include intrathecal baclofen, selective peripheral denervation, and deep brain stimulation (DBS).[33] DBS is most appropriate for patients with disabling generalized dystonia rather than focal dystonia. To date, most investigators advocate targeting the globus pallidus interna (GPi) for the treatment of medically refractory dystonia.[43] Patients with DYT1 dystonia appear to have the most robust response. Case reports and case series of cervical dystonia and cranial-cervical dystonia look promising.[44-46] In contrast to essential tremor, the postoperative improvement of GPi-DBS may be delayed several months.[47] Phasic dystonic movements tend to improve more rapidly than tonic movements. DBS-related complications when targeting the GPi are infrequent but include intracerebral hemorrhage, infection, dysarthria, weakness, and numbness.[48]

BOTULINUM TOXIN FOR BLEPHAROSPASM

Although most physicians consider BoNT to be the most effective treatment for blepharospasm, few double-blind, placebo-controlled studies exist.[49] A Cochrane review on BoNT/A did not find any "suitable" studies that met their criteria for inclusion.[50] Nevertheless, many studies report that patients with blepharospasm improve dramatically using proper dosages and technique.

In 1985, Fahn reported results of eight blepharospasm patients injected with 10 units of BoNT/A in one eye and saline in the other.[51] Patients improved to a greater degree with active treatment based on electrophysiologic measurements, but a scale-to-measure clinical benefit was not used. Jankovic confirmed these findings 2 years later in a more conventional double-blind study in 12 blepharospasm patients, the majority of whom had dystonia of adjacent musculature (cranial-cervical dystonia).[52] Placebo-treated patients did not improve. Treatment with BoNT-A (25 units/eye) improved the severity rating score by 72% and the self-assessment score by 61%. The treatment effect started a mean of 3.7 days after injection and lasted 12.5 weeks. Adverse events included blurred vision, lacrimation, ecchymosis, ptosis, and diplopia.

The Jankovic Rating Scale (JRS), used in the aforementioned study, has been used to determine therapeutic efficacy by assessing the typical symptoms of blepharospasm, such as increased blinking, eyelid fluttering, and eyelid spasm.[53,54] The JRS total score ranges from 0 to 8 points and is calculated from the two items "Severity" and "Frequency," with five rating categories (0 to 4 points) each. The Blepharospasm Disability Index (BSDI) is a self-rating scale (0 to 4 points) for assessment of impairment of specific activities of daily living caused by blepharospasm, ranging from "no impairment", "slight/moderate/severe impairment" to "no longer possible due to my illness." The BSDI rates 6 domains that affect quality of life, such as "driving a vehicle," "reading," "watching TV," "shopping," "walking" and "doing everyday activities."

Following the initial placebo-controlled trial, several other studies provided evidence for the efficacy and safety of BoNT in the treatment of blepharospasm. Based on the findings of a randomized, double-blind study of 26 blepharospasm patients, Frueh and colleagues[55] recommended to avoid toxin injection in the "medial two thirds of the lower eyelid" to prevent diplopia from inferior oblique weakness. In a combined population of blepharospasm and hemifacial spasm (N = 112), Park and associates treated 11 blepharospasm patients in an open-label fashion, finding that 98.6% experienced "excellent" results lasting a mean of 16.5 weeks.[56] Side effects included dry eyes, ptosis, lid edema, and diplopia. Several studies have concluded that reduction in eyelid spasms from BoNT/A translates into improved quality of life.[9,57,58]

Several studies have compared different formulations of BoNT in the treatment of blepharospasm. Sampaio and coworkers[59] found no difference between Botox® and Dysport® with regard to duration of effect (primary end point) or adverse events in a single-blind, randomized comparison. A ratio of 4:1 was used to compare the two BoNT/A formulations. The duration of effect was 13.3 ± 5.9 for Dysport and 11.2 ± 5.8 weeks for Botox, but this difference was not statistically significant. Adverse events were noted in 50% of the Dysport group and 47% of the Botox group. Based on this study, the authors recommend a 4:1 conversion ratio in clinical practice. Using a double-blind crossover design, Nussgens studied 212 consecutive blepharospasm patients comparing Dysport and Botox. Duration of effect was identical in the two groups. Unfortunately, no attempt was made to measure the extent of spasm relief. Botox caused a significantly lower rate of side effects, particularly ptosis. The German formulation of BoNT/A (NT201/Xeomin), promoted as "free of complexing proteins," was compared with Botox in a 1:1 dose ratio in a randomized, double-blind parallel study of 300 patients with blepharospasm, 256 of whom completed the study; no difference in efficacy or adverse effects was found between the two products 3 weeks after injection.[53] The adjusted mean change in the JRS was −2.90 for the NT201 and −2.67 for the Botox group; the frequency of ptosis, the most common adverse effect, was 6.08% and 4.52% respectively. CBTX-A (Prosigne®) has not been widely investigated. In a small crossover study with eight blepharospasm and 18 hemifacial spasm patients Chinese BoNT/A appeared to provide equivalent global improvement, onset to response, and duration of efficacy with a similar side effect profile to Botox.[60]

Common reasons for lack of BoNT efficacy in patients with blepharospasm include underdosing, improper injection technique, presence of eyelid opening apraxia, and resistance from the development of antibody formation, especially in patients exposed to large doses and frequent injections. Levy and associates[61] investigated "supramaximal" doses of BoNT/A (>100 units) in patients with refractory blepharospasm in a prospective, open-label series of eight patients. Half of the cohort opted to continue high-dose BoNT/A. The authors concluded that in select cases, supramaximal doses of BoNT/A (maximum = 82.5 units/eye) may be well tolerated and effective in refractory blepharospasm. Based on a retrospective study, Pang and O'Day[62] also confirmed that higher doses than the recommended 50 units/eye may be needed for some patients. This is especially true for patients who have involvement of facial muscles other than orbicularis oculi.

Various injection techniques have been advocated to optimize the response to BoNT. In our experience and that of others, targeting the pretarsal rather than preseptal portion of orbicularis oculi yields the best results.[12] In 2002, Cakmur and coworkers[63] reported a retrospective comparison study of 25 blepharospasm patients using both techniques. Pretarsal BoNT/A produced a better response rate (97% vs. 90%) for a longer duration (11.4 weeks vs. 8.2 weeks). The most common side effect, ptosis, was less common in the pretarsal group (13% vs. 16%). The authors stated "that pretarsal injections of BoNT/A alone are sufficient to obtain optimum results and there is no reason or need to additionally inject the preseptal or orbital portion of the orbicularis oculi in patients with blepharospasm."[63] Several other investigators confirmed these findings.[12,64-66] As many as 50% of blepharospasm patients who are unresponsive to BoNT may fail because of the presence of apraxia of eyelid opening.[4] Surgical intervention may be required in these patients with suspension of frontalis or removal of the pretarsal orbicularis oculi. Maureillo and colleagues[67] suggest that upper eyelid surgery may increase the average duration of BoNT. After surgery, 14 patients experience a prolongation of effect from

122 days to 210 days. Finally, antibody production may render BoNT ineffective, but this is extremely unlikely because of relatively low dosages used and because the risk of blocking antibodies with new formation of Botox is rare.[68] In a retrospective chart review of 16 patients resistant to BoNT/A and then treated with BoNT/B, the mean effect duration equaled 7.3 weeks and rated as fair to excellent in the majority.[69] Side effects were, however, very common including pain at the site of injection (100%), ptosis (32.3%), and dry mouth (17.2%). Switching to an alternative botulinum toxin formulation may benefit refractory patients.

BOTULINUM TOXIN FOR OROMANDIBULAR DYSTONIA (See Chapter 16)

BOTULINUM TOXIN FOR CERVICAL DYSTONIA

Cervical dystonia consists of jerky or sustained, but nearly always patterned (same muscles involved) movements of the head and neck. The goal of treatment of cervical dystonia is not only to treat the abnormal postures and associated neck pain but also to prevent secondary complications such as contractures, cervical radiculopathy and myelopathy.[70]

Several muscles are involved in neck movement, particularly the sternocleidomastoid, splenius capitus, scalenus complex, and semispinalis capitis.[71] One of the challenges in BoNT treatment of cervical dystonia is to determine which muscles to inject.[18] This difficulty is compounded by the fact that multiple muscle combinations can produce the same movements, the particular pattern of abnormal muscle activity is highly individualized, and antagonist muscles may contract more intensely and may be more hypertrophic than agonist muscles. Only the latter group of muscles should be targeted for BoNT injection. Although some investigators have suggested that after injection of BoNT, the pattern of muscle activity may change,[72] this is rare in our experience. Some investigators have also shown that although there are no further changes in the electromyographic activity of the injected sternocleidomastoid subsequent to the first dose of BoNT, there may be a progressive change in the contralateral (i.e., antagonist) muscle.[73]

Selection methods (clinical inspection versus electromyographic analysis) to target and inject muscles remains controversial. Electromyography (EMG) can be used to confirm localization of the needle to a muscle or confirm and possibly quantify the occurrence of specific muscular activity during ongoing dystonic movements.[74-77] In comparison to an EMG mapping study, the clinical predictions of individual muscle involvement by four movement disorder specialists were only 59% sensitive and 75% specific.[78] One study showed that patients did better with EMG guidance compared with clinically guided injections.[79] The difference in the overall magnitude of this effect was, however, small and there was no difference between groups in the number of patients returning for booster injections. Although patients with retrocollis, head tilt, and shoulder elevation in particular demonstrated additional benefit with EMG-guided injections, the patients that did not have EMG-assistance received higher doses of BoNT, suggesting more severe disease.

The efficacy of BoNT in cervical dystonia has been demonstrated in both controlled and open-label trials[80-83] and in an evidence-based medicine criteria analysis.[84,85] In one double-blind, placebo-controlled trial, 61% of patients injected with BoNT/A improved; 74% of patients subsequently improved during a later open phase at a higher dose.[86] In general, improvement rates run from as low as 65%, to as high as 92%, and near-complete improvement in 83%, with further improvement after repeated treatments has been seen up to 5 years. A retrospective analysis of 616 patients treated with BoNT/A showed sustained significant benefit as measured by a disease severity score, independent of the type of cervical dystonia.[87] Pronounced individual differences were found in response to this treatment, even in patients with similar initial clinical scores and doses of BoNT/A. Although secondary nonresponse was seen in about 5% of patients, antibody tests revealed neutralizing serum antibodies in only 2%. Lew and associates reviewed studies[88] with BoNT/B, which taken together, showed about a 25% reduction in the Toronto Western Spasmodic Torticollis Scale (TWSTRS) and duration of action of 12 to 16 weeks.[89-91] The two pivotal studies, one using BoNT/A (Botox) and the other BoNT/B (Myobloc), that led to the approval of BoNT by the Food and Drug Administration (FDA) for cervical dystonia have not been published but have been previously reviewed.[81]

The most common complication of BoNT for cervical dystonia is pharyngeal weakness manifested by dysphagia. Although usually mild and rarely disabling, it may require a change to a soft diet to prevent aspiration.[92] In one study, 33% of patients receiving their first dose of BoNT experienced dysphagia and a greater number displayed radiographic swallowing abnormalities.[79] Dysphagia has been reported to occur on average 9.7 days after injection and last on average 3.5 weeks.[87] Dysphagia most commonly occurs with bilateral injections of the sternocleidomastoid or scalenus muscles, presumably because of local spread of the toxin from these muscles to posterior pharyngeal muscles. This complication may occur less frequently if the biologic activity of the toxin is contained within the target muscle by using multiple small injections rather than a single large bolus.[93] Neck weakness is the second most common local complication following BoNT treatment of cervical dystonia. In addition, BoNT/B has a relatively high incidence of injection site pain and dry mouth.[88-91]

Although BoNT has been considered the treatment of choice for cervical dystonia, it has been formally compared with medical therapy in only one study. Brans and coworkers[94] compared the effectiveness of BoNT/A with that of trihexyphenidyl in a prospective, randomized, double-blind design. Sixty-six consecutive patients with idiopathic cervical dystonia were randomized to treatment with trihexyphenidyl tablets plus placebo injection or placebo tablets plus BoNT/A injections. BoNT/A (Dysport) or saline was injected under electromyographic guidance at study entry and again after 8 weeks. Patients were assessed for efficacy at baseline and after 12 weeks by different clinical rating scales. Sixty-four patients completed the study, 32 in each group. The mean dose of BoNT/A was 292 U (first session) and 262 U (second session). The mean dose of trihexyphenidyl was 16.2 mg/day. The changes on the Disability section of the TWSTRS (primary outcome), Tsui Scale, and the General Health Perception Subscale were significantly improved in favor of BoNT/A. Furthermore, adverse effects were significantly less frequent in the BoNT/A group.

Several studies have attempted to determine optimum dosing in patients with cervical dystonia. Poewe and associates[95] performed a prospective, multicenter, placebo-controlled, double-blind, dose-ranging study in a group of previously untreated patients with rotational torticollis to obtain objective data on dose-response relations. Seventy-five patients were randomly assigned to receive treatment with placebo or total doses of 250, 500, and 1000 BoNT/A (Dysport) units divided between one splenius capitis and the contralateral sternocleidomastoid; 79% reported subjective improvement at one or more follow-up visits. Decreases in the modified Tsui score were significant at week 4 for the 500 and 1000 unit groups versus placebo. There was a positive relation between dose injected and the duration of clinical benefit. Ninety-four percent of patients treated with placebo and about 50% of patients receiving 200 and 500 units requested reinjection by 8 weeks. whereas only 39% of those having received 1000 units asked for a second treatment by this time. A dose relationship was also established for the number of adverse events overall and for the incidence of neck muscle weakness and voice changes. They concluded that although magnitude and duration of improvement was greatest after injections of 1000 units, it was at the cost of significantly more adverse events. They suggested a starting dose of 500 units, with upward titration if clinically necessary.

Another double-blind, randomized study, involving 31 patients with cervical dystonia who had previously received at least two previous injections, examined low-dose therapy.[96] The patients received either a mean total target dose of 547 ± 113 mouse units (MU) at a concentration of 500 MU Dysport/mL or a 4-times-diluted preparation of 130 ± 32 MU at a concentration of 125 MU Dysport/mL. TWSTRS and a self-rating rating before and after injection revealed comparable clinical improvement in both groups; however, three patients in the low-dose group received reinjections due to insufficient effects from the previous injection. These findings again suggest that low-dose treatment of cervical dystonia with Dysport may be clinically effective during maintenance therapy, at least for a limited period of time. The authors suggest that the low-dose Dysport effects may have been potentiated by the long-lasting effects of previous Dysport treatments at conventional doses.

Several factors can influence failure to respond to BoNT. Primary nonresponse is very rare and may be explained by the presence of blocking antibodies produced by prior vaccination, as required in some military personnel, contractures, insufficient dosage of BoNT, or injection of the incorrect muscles. In cervical dystonia, about half of these patients who initial fail to respond will subsequently benefit from BoNT. More recently, in a long-term study (median 5.5 years, range 1.5-10) in 78 patients with idiopathic cervical dystonia, treatment with BoNT-A was assessed using patient and treating neurologist scores, as well as global burden of disease, as expressed on Visual Analog Scales (VAS, 0–10).[97] By combining these outcome measures, 67% of the patients were characterized as having a good effect, and 33% an unsatisfactory effect. This outcome (good or unsatisfactory effect) was independent of the severity of head deviation or complexity pattern of cervical dystonia before treatment, the delay from onset to start of botulinum toxin treatment, or the number of treatments.

Cervical dystonia is due to a number of different etiologies including genetic predisposition, local trauma, and certain drugs, which may affect the responsiveness to BoNT. In one study, the response of patients with tardive cervical dystonia was similar to that of patients with idiopathic cervical dystonia, although the patients with tardive cervical dystonia required higher BoNT/A doses by about 30%, partly because of greater pain, larger muscles, and more complicated movements.[98] Acute-onset cervical dystonia (occurring within 4 weeks of trauma) is characterized by markedly reduced cervical mobility, prominent shoulder elevation with trapezius hypertrophy, isometric contraction of the affected muscles without involuntary movements, lack of effect of sensory tricks, or activation maneuvers. Although patients with post-traumatic cervical dystonia do not generally respond to BoNT injections as well as patients with idiopathic dystonia, this is usually the most effective treatment, particularly for pain relief. By contrast, delayed-onset cervical dystonia (between 3 months and 1 year after trauma) is clinically indistinguishable from nontraumatic idiopathic cervical dystonia with respect to BoNT.[99]

In a multicenter study of 100 patients with cervical dystonia, we examined the immunogenicity of BoNT/B and correlated the clinical response with the presence of blocking antibodies using a novel mouse protection assay.[100] A third of the patients who were negative for BoNT/B antibodies at baseline became positive for BoNT/B antibodies at last visit. Thus, the high antigenicity of BoNT/B limits its long-term efficacy.

In patients who appear to lose their response to BoNT treatment, detection of blocking antibodies should be sought by the mouse protection assay (MPA), which is considered the "gold standard" for detecting blocking antibodies.[68] If MPA is not readily available and the unilateral brow injection test is equivocal, then extensor digitorum brevis test may need to be performed, and if negative, it should be followed by carefully placed injections under electromygraphic guidance before switching to an immunologically alternative preparation of BoNT to improve results.[101,102]

CONCLUSION

A large body of data supports the conclusion that focal and segmental dystonias respond favorably to BoNT, particularly blepharospasm, oromandibular dystonia, cervical dystonia, and the combination of all three, cranial-cervical dystonia. Although earlier formulations of BoNT caused antibody production and loss of effect, this phenomenon has become exceedingly rare as long as the interval in between injections remains at 3 months or more.

References

1. Shahed J, Jankovic J. In: Stacy M, ed. *Handbook of Dystonia*. New York: Taylor & Francis Group, 2007. In press.
2. Hallett M. Pathophysiology of dystonia. *J Neural Transm Suppl*. 2006;70:485-488.
3. Sitburana O, Jankovic J. Focal hand dystonia, mirror dystonia and motor overflow. *J Neurol Sci*. 2007. In press.
4. Ben Simon GJ, McCann JD. Benign essential blepharospasm. *Int Ophthalmol Clin*. 2005;45:49-75.
5. Whitney CM. Benign essential blepharospasm. *Neurologist*. 2005;11:193-194.
6. Cossu G, Mereu A, Deriu M, Melis M, Molari A, Melis G, et al. Prevalence of primary blepharospasm in Sardinia, Italy: A service-based survey. *Mov Disord*. 2006;21:2005-2008.
7. Nutt JG, Muenter MD, Aronson A, Kurland LT, Melton LJ 3rd. Epidemiology of focal and generalized dystonia in Rochester, Minnesota. *Mov Disord*. 1988;3: 188-194.
8. Grandas F, Elston J, Quinn N, Marsden CD. Blepharospasm: a review of 264 patients. *J Neurol Neurosurg Psychiatry*. 1988;51:767-772.
9. Reimer J, Gilg K, Karow A, Esser J, Franke GH. Health-related quality of life in blepharospasm or hemifacial spasm. *Acta Neurol Scand*. 2005;111:64-70.
10. Jankovic J, Orman J. Blepharospasm: demographic and clinical survey of 250 patients. *Ann Ophthalmol*. 1984;16:371-376.
11. Mejia NI, Jankovic J. Secondary tics and tourettism. *Rev Bras Psiquiatr*. 2005;27:11-17.
12. Jankovic J. Apraxia of lid opening. *Mov Disord*. 1995;10:686-687.
13. Cardoso F, de Oliveira JT, Puccioni-Sohler M, Fernandes AR, de Mattos JP, Lopes-Cendes I. Eyelid dystonia in Machado-Joseph disease. *Mov Disord*. 2000;15:1028-1030.
14. Kerty E, Eidal K. Apraxia of eyelid opening: clinical features and therapy. *Eur J Ophthalmol*. 2006;16: 204-208.
15. Wessberg G. Management of oromandibular dystonia. *Hawaii Dent J*. 2003;34:15-16.
16. Brin MF, Benabou R. Cervical dystonia (torticollis). *Curr Treat Options Neurol*. 1999;1:33-43.
17. Claypool DW, Duane DD, Ilstrup DM, Melton LJ 3rd. Epidemiology and outcome of cervical dystonia (spasmodic torticollis) in Rochester, Minnesota. *Mov Disord*. 1995;10:608-614.
18. Jankovic J. Botulinum toxin therapy for cervical dystonia. *Neurotox Res*. 2006;9:145-148.
19. Pal PK, Samii A, Schulzer M, Mak E, Tsui JK. Head tremor in cervical dystonia. *Can J Neurol Sci*. 2000;27:137-142.
20. Kutvonen O, Dastidar P, Nurmikko T. Pain in spasmodic torticollis. *Pain*. 1997;69:279-286.
21. Soland VL, Bhatia KP, Marsden CD. Sex prevalence of focal dystonias. *J Neurol Neurosurg Psychiatry*. 1996;60:204-205.
22. van Harten PN, Kahn RS. Tardive dystonia. *Schizophr Bull*. 1999;25:741-748.
23. Jankovic J. Motor fluctuations and dyskinesias in Parkinson's disease: clinical manifestations. *Mov Disord*. 2005;20(Suppl 11):S11-S16.
24. Lynch T, Fahn S, Louis ED, Odel JG. Oculofacial-skeletal myorhythmia in Whipple's disease. *Mov Disord*. 1997;12:625-626.
25. Jankovic J. Can peripheral trauma induce dystonia and other movement disorders? Yes! *Mov Disord*. 2001;16:7-12.
26. Ljubisavljevic M, Kacar A, Milanovic S, Svetel M, Kostic VS. Changes in cortical inhibition during task-specific contractions in primary writing tremor patients. *Mov Disord*. 2006;21:855-859.
27. van Eimeren T, Siebner HR. An update on functional neuroimaging of parkinsonism and dystonia. *Curr Opin Neurol*. 2006;19:412-419.
28. Naumann M, Reiners K. Long-latency reflexes of hand muscles in idiopathic focal dystonia and their modification by botulinum toxin. *Brain*. 1997;120(Pt 3):409-416.
29. Dresel C, Haslinger B, Castrop F, Wohlschlaeger AM, Ceballos-Baumann AO. Silent event-related fMRI reveals deficient motor and enhanced somatosensory activation in orofacial dystonia. *Brain*. 2006;129: 36-46.
30. Schneider SA, Mohire MD, Trender-Gerhard I, Asmus F, Sweeney M, Davis M, et al. Familial doparesponsive cervical dystonia. *Neurology*. 2006;66: 599-601.
31. Nasir J, Frima N, Pickard B, Malloy MP, Zhan L, Grunewald R. Unbalanced whole arm translocation resulting in loss of 18p in dystonia. *Mov Disord*. 2006;21:859-863.
32. Jankovic J. Botulinum toxin in clinical practice. *J Neurol Neurosurg Psychiatry*. 2004;75:951-957.
33. Jankovic J. Treatment of dystonia. *Lancet Neurol*. 2006;5:864-872.
34. Berardelli A, Curra A. Pathophysiology and treatment of cranial dystonia. *Mov Disord*. 2002;17(suppl 2): S70-S74.
35. Greene P. Baclofen in the treatment of dystonia. *Clin Neuropharmacol*. 1992;15:276-288.

36. Lang AE, Riley DE. Tizanidine in cranial dystonia. *Clin Neuropharmacol.* 1992;15:142-147.

37. Kenney C, Jankovic J. Tetrabenazine in the treatment of hyperkinetic movement disorders. *Expert Rev Neurother.* 2006;6:7-17.

38. Kenney C, Hunter C, Jankovic J. Long-term tolerability of tetrabenazine in the treatment of hyperkinetic movement disorders. *Mov Disord.* 2007;22:193-197.

39. Scott AB, Kennedy RA, Stubbs HA. Botulinum A toxin injection as a treatment for blepharospasm. *Arch Ophthalmol.* 1985;103:347-350.

40. Truong DD, Jost WH. Botulinum toxin: clinical use. *Parkinsonism Relat Disord.* 2006;12:331-355.

41. Naumann M, Albanese A, Heinen F, Molenaers G, Relja M. Safety and efficacy of botulinum toxin type A following long-term use. *Eur J Neurol.* 2006;13(suppl 4):35-40.

42. Mejia NI, Vuong KD, Jankovic J. Long-term botulinum toxin efficacy, safety, and immunogenicity. *Mov Disord.* 2005;20:592-597.

43. Vidailhet M, Vercueil L, Houeto JL, Krystkowiak P, Lagrange C, Yelnik J, et al. Bilateral, pallidal, deep-brain stimulation in primary generalised dystonia: a prospective 3 year follow-up study. *Lancet Neurol.* 2007;6:223-229.

44. Hung SW, Hamani C, Lozano AM, Poon YY, Piboolnurak P, Miyasaki JM, et al. Long-term outcome of bilateral pallidal deep brain stimulation for primary cervical dystonia. *Neurology.* 2007;68:457-459.

45. Houser M, Waltz T. Meige syndrome and pallidal deep brain stimulation. *Mov Disord.* 2005;20:1203-1235.

46. Ostrem JL, Marks WJ Jr, Volz MM, Heath SL, Starr PA. Pallidal deep brain stimulation in patients with cranial-cervical dystonia (Meige syndrome). *Mov Disord.* 2007;22:1885-1891.

47. Kupsch A, Benecke R, Muller J, Trottenberg T, Schneider GH, Poewe W, et al. Pallidal deep-brain stimulation in primary generalized or segmental dystonia. *N Engl J Med.* 2006;355:1978-1990.

48. Kenney C, Simpson R, Hunter C, Ondo W, Almaguer M, Davidson A, et al. Short-term and long-term safety of deep brain stimulation in the treatment of movement disorders. *J Neurosurg.* 2007;106:621-625.

49. Kenney C, Jankovic J. Botulinum toxin in the treatment of blepharospasm and hemifacial spasm. *J Neural Transm.* 2007;115:585-591.

50. Costa J, Espirito-Santo C, Borges A, Ferreira JJ, Coelho M, Moore P, et al. Botulinum toxin type A therapy for blepharospasm. *Cochrane Database Syst Rev.* 2005;CD004900.

51. Fahn S, List T, Moslowitz C, Brin M, Bressman SB, Burke RE, et al. Double-blind controlled study of botulinum toxin for blepharospasm. *Neurology.* 1985;35(suppl 1):271-272.

52. Jankovic J, Orman J. Botulinum A toxin for cranial-cervical dystonia: a double-blind, placebo-controlled study. *Neurology.* 1987;37:616-623.

53. Roggenkamper P, Jost WH, Bihari K, Comes G, Grafe S. Efficacy and safety of a new Botulinum Toxin Type A free of complexing proteins in the treatment of blepharospasm. *J Neural Transm.* 2006;113:303-312.

54. Iwashige H, Nemeto Y, Takahashi H, Maruo T. Botulinum toxin type A purified neurotoxin complex for the treatment of blepharospasm: a dose-response study measuring eyelid force. *Jpn J Ophthalmol.* 1995;39:424-431.

55. Frueh BR, Nelson CC, Kapustiak JF, Musch DC. The effect of omitting botulinum toxin from the lower eyelid in blepharospasm treatment. *Am J Ophthalmol.* 1988;106:45-47.

56. Park YC, Lim JK, Lee DK, Yi SD. Botulinum a toxin treatment of hemifacial spasm and blepharospasm. *J Korean Med Sci.* 1993;8:334-340.

57. MacAndie K, Kemp E. Impact on quality of life of botulinum toxin treatments for essential blepharospasm. *Orbit.* 2004;23:207-210.

58. Tucha O, Naumann M, Berg D, Alders GL, Lange KW. Quality of life in patients with blepharospasm. *Acta Neurol Scand.* 2001;103:49-52.

59. Sampaio C, Ferreira JJ, Simoes F, Rosas MJ, Magalhaes M, Correia AP, et al. DYSBOT: a single-blind, randomized parallel study to determine whether any differences can be detected in the efficacy and tolerability of two formulations of botulinum toxin type A—Dysport and Botox—assuming a ratio of 4:1. *Mov Disord.* 1997;12:1013-1018.

60. Rieder CR, Schestatsky P, Socal MP, Monte TL, Fricke D, Costa J, et al. A double-blind, randomized, crossover study of prosigne versus botox in patients with blepharospasm and hemifacial spasm. *Clin Neuropharmacol.* 2007;30:39-42.

61. Levy RL, Berman D, Parikh M, Miller NR. Supramaximal doses of botulinum toxin for refractory blepharospasm. *Ophthalmology.* 2006;113:1665-1668.

62. Pang AL, O'Day J. Use of high-dose botulinum A toxin in benign essential blepharospasm: is too high too much? *Clin Experiment Ophthalmol.* 2006;34:441-444.

63. Cakmur R, Ozturk V, Uzunel F, Donmez B, Idiman F. Comparison of preseptal and pretarsal injections of botulinum toxin in the treatment of blepharospasm and hemifacial spasm. *J Neurol.* 2002;249:64-68.

64. Albanese A, Bentivoglio AR, Colosimo C, Galardi G, Maderna L, Tonali P. Pretarsal injections of botulinum toxin improve blepharospasm in previously unresponsive patients. *J Neurol Neurosurg Psychiatry.* 1996;60:693-694.

65. Jankovic J. Pretarsal injection of botulinum toxin for blepharospasm and apraxia of eyelid opening. *J Neurol Neurosurg Psychiatry.* 1996;60:704.

66. Kowal L. Pretarsal injections of botulinum toxin improve blepharospasm in previously unresponsive patients. *J Neurol Neurosurg Psychiatry.* 1997;63:556.

67. Mauriello JA Jr, Keswani R, Franklin M. Long-term enhancement of botulinum toxin injections by upper-eyelid surgery in 14 patients with facial dyskinesias. *Arch Otolaryngol Head Neck Surg.* 1999;125:627-631.

68. Jankovic J, Vuong KD, Ahsan J. Comparison of efficacy and immunogenicity of original versus current botulinum toxin in cervical dystonia. *Neurology.* 2003;60:1186-1188.

69. Dutton JJ, White JJ, Richard MJ. Myobloc for the treatment of benign essential blepharospasm in patients refractory to Botox. *Ophthal Plast Reconstr Surg.* 2006;22:173-177.

70. Chawda SJ, Munchau A, Johnson D, Bhatia K, Quinn NP, Stevens J, et al. Pattern of premature degenerative changes of the cervical spine in patients with spasmodic torticollis and the impact on the outcome of selective peripheral denervation. *J Neurol Neurosurg Psychiatry.* 2000;68:465-471.

71. Zesiewicz TA, Stamey W, Sullivan KL, Hauser RA. Botulinum toxin A for the treatment of cervical dystonia. *Expert Opin Pharmacother.* 2004;5:2017-2024.

72. Gelb DJ, Yoshimura DM, Olney RK, Lowenstein DH, Aminoff MJ. Change in pattern of muscle activity

following botulinum toxin injections for torticollis. *Ann Neurol.* 1991;29:370-376.

73. Erdal J, Ostergaard L, Fuglsang-Frederiksen A, Werdelin L, Dalager T, Sjo O, et al. Long-term botulinum toxin treatment of cervical dystonia—EMG changes in injected and noninjected muscles. *Clin Neurophysiol.* 1999;110:1650-1654.

74. Buchman AS, Comella CL, Stebbins GT, Tanner CM, Goetz CG. Quantitative electromyographic analysis of changes in muscle activity following botulinum toxin therapy for cervical dystonia. *Clin Neuropharmacol.* 1993;16:205-210.

75. Dressler D, Rothwell JC. Electromyographic quantification of the paralysing effect of botulinum toxin in the sternocleidomastoid muscle. *Eur Neurol.* 2000;43: 13-16.

76. Ostergaard L, Fuglsang-Frederiksen A, Sjo O, Werdelin L, Winkel H. Quantitative EMG in cervical dystonia. *Electromyogr Clin Neurophysiol.* 1996;36: 179-185.

77. Brans JW, Aramideh M, Koelman JH, Lindeboom R, Speelman JD, Ongerboer de Visser BW. Electromyography in cervical dystonia: changes after botulinum and trihexyphenidyl. *Neurology.* 1998;51:815-819.

78. Van Gerpen JA, Matsumoto JY, Ahlskog JE, Maraganore DM, McManis PG. Utility of an EMG mapping study in treating cervical dystonia. *Muscle Nerve.* 2000;23: 1752-1756.

79. Comella CL, Buchman AS, Tanner CM, Brown-Toms NC, Goetz CG. Botulinum toxin injection for spasmodic torticollis: increased magnitude of benefit with electromyographic assistance. *Neurology.* 1992;42:878-882.

80. Comella CL, Jankovic J, Brin MF. Use of botulinum toxin type A in the treatment of cervical dystonia. *Neurology.* 2000;55:S15-S21.

81. Jankovic J. Treatment of cervical dystonia with botulinum toxin. *Mov Disord.* 2004;19(Suppl 8):S109-S115.

82. Factor SA, Molho ES, Evans S, Feustel PJ. Efficacy and safety of repeated doses of botulinum toxin type B in type A resistant and responsive cervical dystonia. *Mov Disord.* 2005;20:1152-1160.

83. Truong D, Duane DD, Jankovic J, Singer C, Seeberger LC, Comella CL, et al. Efficacy and safety of botulinum type A toxin (Dysport) in cervical dystonia: results of the first US randomized, double-blind, placebo-controlled study. *Mov Disord.* 2005;20:783-791.

84. Ceballos-Baumann AO. Evidence-based medicine in botulinum toxin therapy for cervical dystonia. *J Neurol.* 2001;248(suppl 1):14-20.

85. Jankovic J, Esquenazi A, Fehlings D, Freitag F, Lang AM, Naumann M. Evidence-based review of patient-reported outcomes with botulinum toxin type A. *Clin Neuropharmacol.* 2004;27:234-244.

86. Greene P, Kang U, Fahn S, Brin M, Moskowitz C, Flaster E. Double-blind, placebo-controlled trial of botulinum toxin injections for the treatment of spasmodic torticollis. *Neurology.* 1990;40:1213-1218.

87. Kessler KR, Skutta M, Benecke R. Long-term treatment of cervical dystonia with botulinum toxin A: efficacy, safety, and antibody frequency. *German Dystonia Study Group.* 1999;246:265-274.

88. Lew MF, Brashear A, Factor S. The safety and efficacy of botulinum toxin type B in the treatment of patients with cervical dystonia: summary of three controlled clinical trials. *Neurology.* 2000;55:S29-S35.

89. Brashear A, Lew MF, Dykstra DD, Comella CL, Factor SA, Rodnitzky RL, et al. Safety and efficacy of NeuroBloc (botulinum toxin type B) in type A–responsive cervical dystonia. *Neurology.* 1999;53:1439-1446.

90. Brin MF, Lew MF, Adler CH, Comella CL, Factor SA, Jankovic J, et al. Safety and efficacy of NeuroBloc (botulinum toxin type B) in type A–resistant cervical dystonia. *Neurology.* 1999;53:1431-1438.

91. Lew MF, Adornato BT, Duane DD, Dykstra DD, Factor SA, Massey JM, et al. Botulinum toxin type B: a double-blind, placebo-controlled, safety and efficacy study in cervical dystonia. *Neurology.* 1997;49:701-707.

92. Anderson TJ, Rivest J, Stell R, Steiger MJ, Cohen H, Thompson PD, et al. Botulinum toxin treatment of spasmodic torticollis. *J R Soc Med.* 1992;85:524-529.

93. Borodic GE, Pearce LB, Smith K, Joseph M. Botulinum a toxin for spasmodic torticollis: multiple vs single injection points per muscle. *Head Neck.* 1992;14:33-37.

94. Brans JW, Lindeboom R, Snoek JW, Zwarts MJ, van Weerden TW, Brunt ER, et al. Botulinum toxin versus trihexyphenidyl in cervical dystonia: a prospective, randomized, double-blind controlled trial. *Neurology.* 1996;46:1066-1072.

95. Poewe W, Deuschl G, Nebe A, Feifel E, Wissel J, Benecke R, et al. What is the optimal dose of botulinum toxin A in the treatment of cervical dystonia? Results of a double blind, placebo controlled, dose ranging study using Dysport. *German Dystonia Study Group.* 1998;64:13-17.

96. Laubis-Herrmann U, Fries K, Topka H. Low-dose botulinum toxin-a treatment of cervical dystonia—a double-blind, randomized pilot study. *Eur Neurol.* 2002;47:214-221.

97. Skogseid IM, Kerty E. The course of cervical dystonia and patient satisfaction with long-term botulinum toxin A treatment. *Eur J Neurol.* 2005;12:163-170.

98. Tarsy D. Comparison of acute- and delayed-onset posttraumatic cervical dystonia. *Mov Disord.* 1998;13:481-485.

99. Jankovic J, Schwartz KS. Use of botulinum toxin in the treatment of hand dystonia. *J Hand Surg [Am].* 1993;18:883-1887.

100. Jankovic J, Hunter C, Dolimbek BZ, Dolimbek GS, Adler CH, Brashear A, et al. Clinico-immunologic aspects of botulinum toxin type B treatment of cervical dystonia. *Neurology.* 2006;67:2233-2235.

101. Jankovic J. Botulinum toxin: Clinical implications of antigenicity and immunoresistance. In: Brin MF, Hallett M, Jankovic J, eds. *Scientific and Therapeutic Aspects of Botulinum Toxin.* Philadelphia: Lippincott Williams & Wilkins; 2002:409-416.

102. Cordivari C, Misra VP, Vincent A, Catania S, Bhatia KP, Lees AJ. Secondary nonresponsiveness to botulinum toxin A in cervical dystonia: the role of electromyogram-guided injections, botulinum toxin A antibody assay, and the extensor digitorum brevis test. *Mov Disord.* 2006;21:1737-1741.

Botulinum Neurotoxin 9 Treatment of Limb and Occupational Dystonias

Barbara Illowsky Karp

INTRODUCTION

Dystonia can affect either the upper or lower extremities, both as an isolated focal dystonia and as part of generalized or segmental dystonia. In primary dystonias, the leg is more likely to be involved in childhood-onset generalized dystonia and dopa-responsive dystonia, whereas the hand and arm are more commonly affected in adult-onset focal dystonia. Both upper and lower extremity dystonia are amenable to treatment with botulinum neurotoxin (BoNT).

FOCAL HAND DYSTONIA

The most common primary limb dystonia is focal hand dystonia. Reported as early as the 18th century, Ramazzini[1] described "the morbid affections" of scribes and notaries, who developed "intense fatigue of the hand and whole arm because of the continuous almost tonic strain on the muscles and tendons, which in the course of time results in failure of power ..." Similar hand dysfunction afflicted those engaged in a variety of occupations, especially workers who performed tasks requiring repetitive, finely coordinated movements of the hands. As described by Aitken in 1882[2]:

"The disease is not entirely limited to the operation of writing. Shoemakers, milkmaids (or milkers of cows, goats, and ewes), nailsmiths, musicians, compositors, saddlers, sempstresses, and men who handle small hard articles with considerable muscular grasp, are subject to similar cramps. Hence the disease is known under a variety of names—as cobbler's spasm, milker's spasm, nailer's spasm, writer's cramp."

It is still true that focal hand dystonia tends to arise in those whose occupations or pastimes involve frequent repetitive movement of the hand and fingers. Writer's cramp, musician's cramp, and typist/keyboarder's cramp are among the more common types currently seen. Hand dystonia may be more functionally disabling than dystonia affecting other body areas, interfering with writing and skilled hand use.

SIGNS AND SYMPTOMS

"Every attempt to write calls forth uncontrollable movements in the thumb, the index finger, and middle finger so that the pen starts up and down on the paper. The handwriting ceases to be legible—a mere scrawl results, or grotesque interrupted scribbling. The more the patient persists in the attempt to write, the more does the difficulty of steadying the hand and using the pen increase. The visible and sensible contractions of the muscles of the thumb and fingers are soon followed by similar contractions of the forearms, even extending in some cases to the upper arm."[3]

The symptoms of focal hand dystonia begin insidiously, often heralded by vague, poorly localized feelings of discomfort or tension. Difficulty using the hand arises, along with muscle tightness, usually

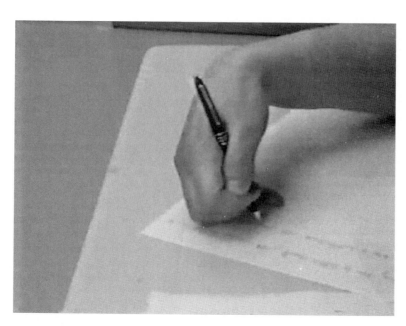

FIGURE 9-1. Wrist flexion in writer's cramp.

accompanied by abnormal hand posture (Fig. 9-1). Motor control is impaired, leading to difficulty writing or performing desired tasks. Although forearm aching and fatigue are common, overt pain is not.

Dystonia improves when the provoking activity ceases but returns quickly with resumption of the eliciting task, and worsens during attempts to continue with the activity. Focal hand dystonia can be remarkably task specific, leaving other tasks unaffected even if the same muscles are used or similar movements required. For example, musicians may have dystonic hand movements when playing one instrument but not another related instrument.[4] Some patients go through a progression, with initial symptoms being entirely task specific ("simple" cramp), followed by a later loss of specificity ("dystonic" cramp) so that dystonia is present during almost any hand use. When severe, dystonic posturing is

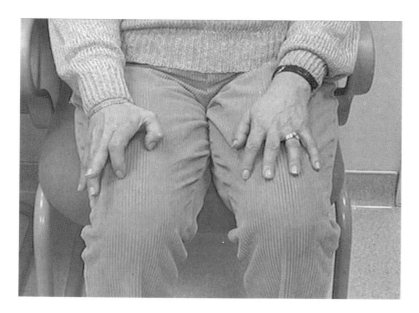

FIGURE 9-2. Dystonia at rest in a patient with writer's cramp.

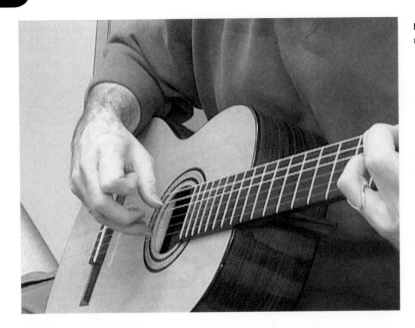

FIGURE 9-3. Finger flexion in musician's cramp.

elicited by thinking about a provoking task or even at rest (Fig. 9-2).

The motor symptoms of focal hand dystonia often progress over several months and then stabilize. Further progression, either to more proximal muscles of the arm or to the other hand, sometimes occurs.[5-7]

Strength and deep tendon reflexes are normal in primary focal hand dystonia. Mild rigidity or diminished arm swing may be present on the affected side.[5,6] Postural tremor, similar to essential tremor, is present in about 45% of patients with writer's cramp.[6,8] Routine sensory examination is normal in those with focal hand dystonia, although there may be subtle impairment of sensory discrimination.[9-11]

The combination of muscles involved in focal hand dystonia varies with the individual, and involvement of any combination of hand and arm flexors and extensors is possible. Certain patterns are, however, more common than others and may be characteristic of the provoking activity. In writer's cramp, the dominant hand is more commonly affected than the nondominant hand. In musicians, the pattern varies with the particular instrument being played.[12,13] Pianists tend to have dystonic flexion of the 4th and 5th fingers of the right hand, which often has more intricate passages to play than the left hand. In violinists, hyperflexion of the 4th and 5th fingers tends to affect the left, fingering hand rather than the right, bowing hand. Dystonic flexion of the 3rd finger of the right hand is a common pattern in guitar and banjo players, whereas extension of the 3rd finger of the right hand is more common in clarinetists (Fig. 9-3).

EPIDEMIOLOGY AND GENETICS

The prevalence of focal hand dystonia has been reported at 7 to 69 per million population.[14,15] Musician's dystonia is estimated to affect 0.2% to 0.5% of the general population.[16] Usually developing in middle age,[6] writer's cramp and musician's cramp are both more common in men, as opposed to other focal dystonias such as cervical dystonia or blepharospasm, which are more common in women.

A genetic component to focal hand dystonia is likely, with 5% to 20% of those with writer's cramp or musician's cramp reporting a family member with dystonia.[4,5,17] The DYT1 mutation is not common in either writer's cramp or musician's cramp,[18-21] however, focal hand dystonia has been reported in some members of families with DYT6, DYT7, DYT13, and DYT15 dystonias.[22-25]

DIFFERENTIAL DIAGNOSIS

Repetitive stress injury (RSI), also known as occupational overuse syndrome, is an important cause of hand disability that can be mistaken for focal hand dystonia. Similar to focal hand dystonia, RSI arises in those with repetitive movement or overuse of joints or muscles. Unlike focal hand dystonia, the predominant symptom of RSI is pain in the affected body part that worsens with continued use. There is no significant functional disability in RSI except as limited by pain. Repetitive stress injury is due to microtears and inflammation in the overused muscles and connective tissue, and is thus amenable to treatment with better ergonomic design, heat, massage, rest, and anti-inflammatory agents.[26,27] Even so, prognosis for this disorder has not been good.

Dystonic hand symptoms can arise in complex regional pain syndrome (CRPS), formerly known as reflex sympathetic dystrophy. In CRPS, dystonia may be accompanied by pain, allodynia, autonomic dysfunction, and skin changes.[28,29]

Mononeuropathies such as ulnar neuropathy or carpal tunnel syndrome may occasionally be mistaken for focal hand dystonia. Carpal tunnel syndrome causes pain as well as median nerve-distribution sensory loss and weakness, which are not present in focal hand dystonia. Focal hand dystonia and carpal tunnel syndrome can rarely coexist. When they do, the carpal tunnel symptoms may respond to carpal tunnel–specific treatment or surgery, whereas the focal hand dystonia symptoms do not.

Ulnar neuropathy can be similarly differentiated from focal hand dystonia by the presence of sensory loss and weakness in ulnar-innervated muscles. However, there have been reports of symptoms similar to focal hand dystonia in some patients with ulnar neuropathy, especially when the 4th and 5th fingers are involved, as is common in pianists. In such cases, near nerve recording may be able to detect a subtle ulnar neuropathy, and the dystonic as well as neuropathic symptoms may respond to ulnar nerve transposition.[30,31] The frequency of ulnar neuropathy leading to focal hand dystonia is uncertain.

Dystonia is common in psychogenic movement disorders.[32] Psychogenic dystonia should be suspected if the symptom onset is abrupt and if there are other somatizations or psychogenic neurologic symptoms.[33]

TREATMENT

With the onset of dystonic symptoms, most people first try resting the hand or performing their usual activities in a way that does not evoke dystonic symptoms. Those with writer's cramp try different grips or new pens. Switching to the nondominant hand for writing may be successful initially, but approximately 25% of those who switch develop dystonia in the second hand.[5,6] Musicians often try to change their technique and pattern of practice or to modify their instruments.

Nonpharmacologic approaches to focal hand dystonia, including massage therapy, chiropractic manipulation, splinting, limb immobilization, physical therapy, occupational therapy, biofeedback, hypnosis, and acupuncture, lead to little, if any, sustained improvement in focal hand dystonia. They may help, however, with some of the forearm discomfort and can be combined with medications.

Recent physiologic studies of focal hand dystonia have demonstrated distorted cortical sensory representation for individual fingers. Therapeutic strategies focused on trying to reverse these changes, including prolonged practice with sensory discrimination tasks,[34] limb immobilization,[35] and "sensory retuning"[36,37] have had some limited success. The initial success of limb immobilization has not been reproduced and cannot be recommended. Furthermore, limb immobilization has been reported to trigger the onset of "peripherally induced dystonia."[38] The use of repetitive transcranial magnetic stimulation to decrease cortical excitability in those with focal hand dystonia is also being explored.[39] A role for neurosurgical procedures, such as lesioning surgery (thalamotomy or pallidotomy) and deep brain stimulation, has not been established for focal hand dystonia. Few patients with idiopathic focal hand dystonia have undergone such procedures[40-42] and no controlled trials have been conducted.

Oral medications for focal hand dystonia include anticholinergics, dopaminergic agents, antidopaminergic drugs, benzodiazepines, and baclofen and other muscle relaxants. Anticholinergic drugs, such as trihexyphenidyl, which are the most successful oral medications for dystonia, usually bring little benefit in focal hand dystonia and often produce intolerable side effects.

Botulinum Toxin Treatment of Focal Hand Dystonia

The application of BoNT therapy to focal hand dystonia followed its use in blepharospasm, hemifacial spasm, and cervical dystonia in the late 1980s. Its efficacy and safety have been established over the past 25 years of use. In treating focal hand dystonia, the goals need to be clearly identified and realistic. Restoration of normal, full-time functional use of the hand is rarely achieved; better use of the hand for several weeks or months following injection is more likely. Muscle tightness and abnormal posture are more likely to respond than the loss of fine motor control.

Muscles are selected for injection on the basis of observation, clinical evaluation, patient report, or electromyographic evidence of excessive muscle activation. Because the pattern of dystonia varies widely among individuals, the selection of muscles must be tailored to the individual subject. Selection of muscles for injection may not be easy. Some patients have subjective muscles tightness without observable distortion of hand posture. Different muscles may contribute to similar patterns of movement in different individuals. In addition, the observed movement or posture is often a combination of dystonic and compensatory elements.

Separating dystonic from compensatory movements is often difficult, because compensatory actions may not be made consciously. It is crucially important to do so, however, in order to identify the correct muscles for injection. Several strategies may help. The person should be examined initially at rest and again while performing whatever actions elicit the dystonia, such as writing, typing, or playing an instrument, with an instruction to avoid making compensatory movements if possible. The patient should be further observed performing a variety of other motor tasks to see if dystonia can be brought out by actions that do not evoke compensatory movements. In one study, 45% of subjects with writer's cramp developed dystonic posturing in the affected hand when stressed by writing with the unaffected, usually nondominant hand.[43] Such "mirror dystonia" may be seen after a brief latency and may worsen with continued writing. If present, mirror dystonia may allow the examiner to appreciate dystonic elements or movements that are obscured during the performance of a task with the affected hand. Mirror dystonia may be helpful as a guide to determining which muscles to inject.[43,44]

Electromyography (EMG) of focal hand dystonia demonstrates muscle overcontraction and overflow into muscles not normally involved in the provoking activity.[45] In some cases, EMG recording through wire electrodes left in place during performance of the eliciting task can help clarify the involvement of small or deep muscles that are not obvious on simple observation.

As with the selection of muscles for injection, the dose of toxin must be individualized. The initial dose should be based on the size of the muscle to be injected, the number of muscles involved, and their proximity to each other. Because the degree of weakness from injection cannot be predicted, the initial dose should be one likely to produce benefit but low enough to make severe weakness unlikely.

The dilution of BoNT type A for limb injection can be adjusted by varying the volume of normal saline added to the vial. Dilution to low concentrations may allow accurate injection of very small doses, such as those required for intrinsic hand muscles. Preparation of the toxin in a higher concentration allows for a smaller injection volume, which may help limit the spread of toxin to contiguous muscles and thus decrease the likelihood of weakness in other than the desired muscles. Type B toxin can be similarly diluted to a lower concentration than the commercially available preparation, but cannot be concentrated.

After selection of the muscles for injection and determination of the dose and dilution, the toxin is injected intramuscularly into the belly of the chosen muscle, in the area of the innervation zone. EMG or ultrasound may be used to guide injections into specific muscles or muscle fascicles. For patients who cannot voluntarily activate or isolate the desired muscle, the location of the needle tip can be ascertained by eliciting muscle contraction via stimulation through the injection needle. Injection based on surface anatomy alone is inaccurate. In limb injections, the desired muscle or fascicle is entered in only 37% of attempts.[46] However, it has not been proven that careful localization enhances benefit or minimizes weakness in focal hand dystonia.

The effects of toxin injection are usually first apparent about 1 week after injection. Benefit peaks about 4 weeks after injection, then slowly abates over approximately 3 months, after which reinjection is needed. At each return visit, the patient should be questioned about the extent of maximal weakness and benefit experienced with the last injection and examined for residual effects. Toxin dose and selection of muscles may need to be adjusted in response to the previous injection. Over the course of several injection sessions, an optimal pattern of muscles and of doses for the individual subject can usually be determined. The benefit of injections can be maintained over years with repeated injection, often with - relatively stable choice of muscles and doses.[47,48]

The most common adverse effect of upper extremity injection of BoNT is weakness in injected muscles and those nearby. Weakness was seen in 53-100% of those participating in controlled clinical trials of boNT injection for limb dystonia.[49-52] Thus, some degree of weakness accompanies most limb injections but is rarely impairing.[49,50,53,54]

Overt weakness typically lasts 1 to 2 months, briefer than the period of benefit. Other reported adverse effects include the pain and discomfort of injection, bruising, and mild malaise for a few days after injection. Treated muscles may atrophy over time.

There are no widely accepted, validated rating scales for the assessment of writer's cramp or musician's dystonia. For writer's cramp, measures used include subjective estimate of the quality of handwriting, the time required to write a standard passage, physician rating of the extent of abnormal posture, and computerized writing analysis, as in the Writer's Cramp Rating Scale proposed by Wissel.[55] Validated rating tools are similarly

lacking for musician's dystonia, although a Musical Instrument Digital Interface (MIDI)–based scale may be useful in pianists.[56] Assessment of musician's cramp is especially difficult because of the variation in instruments and individual technique among those affected, as well as the difficulty physicians have in judging professional musician performance. In most types of focal hand dystonia, a simple visual analog scale or 5-point scale rating benefit as none, minimal, mild, moderate, or excellent may suffice for clinical evaluation. It is important to have patients similarly report their subjective sense of weakness from injection, because physical examination does not reflect the degree to which weakness interferes with function. Ultimately, it is an individual decision as to whether injections continue over time, usually based on consideration of whether the extent of benefit attained outweighs any weakness incurred and the cost and inconvenience of repeated injections.

Controlled clinical trials and open-label studies have established the efficacy of BoNT treatment for focal hand dystonia.[49-54,57-60] In randomized, placebo-controlled trials, muscles were selected for injection based on clinical examination, as were doses that ranged from 10 to 120 U Botox (Allergan,

TABLE 9-1 Controlled Trials of BoNT for Limb Dystonia

Reference	Study Population	BoNT Type and Trade Name	Outcome	Percentage of BoNT-Treated Subjects with Weakness
Kruisdijk et al[50]	39 with writer's cramp	A-Dysport	Significant subjective and objective improvement in writing	90
Yoshimura[49]	14 with upper extremity dystonia 3 with lower extremity dystonia	A (brand not specified)	Significant subjective improvement in writing; no objective improvement	53
Tsui[59]	20 with writer's cramp	A-Botox	Significant objective improvement in writing; no subjective improvement	100
Cole[51]	10 with focal hand dystonia	A-Botox	Significant subjective and objective improvement in writing	80

BoNT, botulinum neurotoxin.

Irvine, CA) per muscles and 10 to 300 U per treatment sessions (Table 9-1). Reinjection intervals ranged from 2 weeks to 9 months. In these studies, 67% to 93% of patients with focal hand dystonia benefited from injection. Benefit was first noted 5 to 28 days after injection and lasted 60 to 77 days. About 15% of patients did not improve with injection. Almost all patients with benefit had at least some noticeable weakness, which was severe in about 5% of injection sessions.

Despite the benefits of Botox injection, only about 1/3 of patients with focal hand dystonia continue injections longer than 2 to 3 years.[47,61] Musicians, especially professional musicians, are often dissatisfied with the extent of benefit. Performance can rarely be restored to the previous consistently high-level function.

Patients with Parkinson's disease and other parkinsonian disorders occasionally develop secondary fixed dystonia of the hand ("dystonic clenched fist"), which may benefit in terms of pain and hygiene from local BoNT injections.[64,65]

BOTULINUM TOXIN TREATMENT OF UPPER EXTREMITY SEGMENTAL DYSTONIA

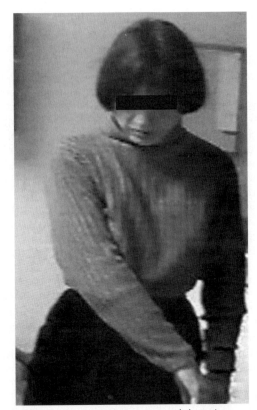

FIGURE 9-4. Upper extremity segmental dystonia.

Dystonia is termed segmental when it involves an extremity and proximal limb girdle musculature. Segmental dystonia is often unilateral and is more likely than focal hand dystonia to be symptomatic of a contralateral cerebral lesion. The BoNT treatment of arm segmental dystonia requires the injection of proximal shoulder muscles, often combined with distal injections of the arm or forearm. Therefore, higher doses are needed for segmental dystonia than for focal hand dystonia. In the upper extremity, arm adduction and internal rotation are common patterns, which may require the injection of muscles such as pectoralis major, latissimus dorsi, and teres major (Fig. 9-4).

Botulinum Toxin Treatment of Lower Extremity Dystonia

Although a common presentation of primary, generalized dystonia in children and of Parkinson's disease in adults, isolated idiopathic focal dystonia of the lower extremity is rare.

Singer and Papapetropoulos reported on four adults with primary focal foot dystonia and summarized three other cases from the literature, noting a mean age of onset of 53 years, mild to moderate impairment of gait, and pain in 50% of subjects.[62] The most common pattern of dystonia was foot inversion and toe flexion (Fig. 9-5). Foot position varied; both dorsiflexion and plantar flexion were seen. Similarly, toe extension rather than flexion was present in some subjects.

Physical therapy, surgery (including tendon transfer or lengthening), and oral medications have been tried for leg dystonia, but these therapeutic interventions are rarely effective.[63] Most patients with leg dystonia are given a trial of L-dopa, which can successfully treat dopa-responsive dystonia or leg dystonia associated with Parkinson's disease.

Leg dystonia can be treated by BoNT. Four of the patients reported by Singer received BoNT injection, with a marked response in three patients. Patients with leg dystonia have been included in larger trials on the efficacy of BoNT with reported benefit.[57] The large muscles of the leg require high doses of toxin. Despite

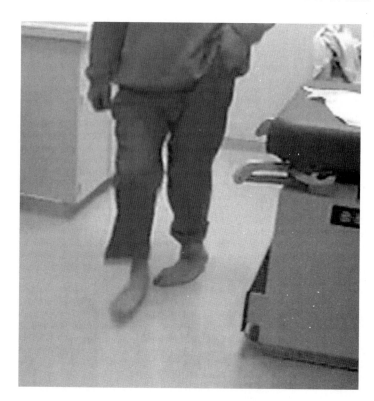

FIGURE 9-5. Foot dystonia.

the use of high doses, overt weakness is rare with leg injections of BoNT for dystonia. Similar to its use for dystonic clenched fists, BoNT injections have also been reported to improve "spastic toe clawing."[66]

SUMMARY

The most common limb dystonia, focal hand dystonia, commonly presents as a task-specific disorder such as writer's cramp or musician's cramp. Leg dystonia is much less common but can similarly be functionally disabling. BoNT injection is currently the most effective treatment available for both upper and lower extremity dystonia. Its use requires careful selection of muscles for injection and titration of dose. For patients responsive to the toxin, the benefit can be maintained for years with regular, repeated injection.

References

1. Ramazzini B. Diseases of scribes and notaries. In: *Diseases of Workers*. New York: Hafner Publishing Company; 1713:421-425.
2. Aitken W. *Outlines of the Science and Practice of Medicine*. 2nd ed. London: Charles Griffin and Company, Publisher; 1882:265.
3. Solly S. Scrivener's palsy, or the paralysis of writers. *Lancet*. 1864;2:709-711.
4. Altenmuller E. Focal dystonia: advances in brain imaging and understanding of fine motor control in musicians. *Hand Clin*. 2003;19(3):523-538,xi.
5. Sheehy MP, Marsden CD. Writer's cramp—a focal dystonia. *Brain*. 1982;105:461-480.
6. Marsden CD, Sheehy MP. Writer's cramp. *Trends Neurosci*. 1990;13:148-153.
7. Greene P, Kang UJ, Fahn S. Spread of symptoms in idiopathic torsion dystonia. *Mov Disord*. 1995;10:143-152.
8. Rosenbaum F, Jankovic J. Focal task-specific tremor and dystonia: categorization of occupational movement disorders. *Neurology*. 1988;38:522-527.
9. Bara-Jimenez W, Shelton P, Sanger TD, Hallett M. Sensory discrimination capabilities in patients with focal hand dystonia. *Ann Neurol*. 2000;47:377-380.
10. Sanger TD, Tarsy D, Pascual-Leone A. Abnormalities of spatial and temporal sensory discrimination in writer's cramp. *Mov Disord*. 2001;16:94-99.
11. Molloy FM, Carr TD, Zeuner KE, Dambrosia JM, Hallett M. Abnormalities of spatial discrimination in focal and generalized dystonia. *Brain*. 2003;23:23.
12. Brandfonbrener AG, Robson C. Review of 113 musicians with focal dystonia seen between 1985 and 2002 at a clinic for performing artists. *Adv Neurol*. 2004;94:255-256.
13. Altenmuller E. Causes and cures of focal limb dystonia in musicians. *Int Soc Study Tension Performance Journal*. 1998;9:13-17.
14. Nutt JG, Muenter MD, Aronson A, Kurland LT, Melton LJ. Epidemiology of focal and generalized dystonia in Rochester, Minn. *Mov Disord*. 1988;3:188-194.
15. The Epidemiological Study of Dystonia in Europe (ESDE) Collaborative Group. A prevalence study of

primary dystonia in eight European countries. *J Neurol.* 2000;247:787-792.

16. Frucht SJ. Focal task-specific dystonia in musicians. *Adv Neurol.* 2004;94:225-230.

17. Waddy HM, Fletcher NA, Harding AE, Marsden CD. A genetic study of idiopathic focal dystonias. *Ann Neurol.* 1991;29:320-324.

18. Kamm C, Castelon-Konkiewitz E, Naumann M, Heinen F, Brack M, Nebe A, et al. GAG deletion in the DYT1 gene in early limb-onset idiopathic torsion dystonia in Germany. *Mov Disord.* 1999;14: 681-683.

19. Kamm C, Naumann M, Mueller J, Mai N, Riedel L, Wissel J, et al. The DYT1 GAG deletion is infrequent in sporadic and familial writer's cramp. *Mov Disord.* 2000;15:1238-1241.

20. Friedman JR, Klein C, Leung J, Woodward H, Ozelius LJ, Breakefield XO, et al. The GAG deletion of the DYT1 gene is infrequent in musicians with focal dystonia. *Neurology.* 2000;55:1417-1418.

21. Schmidt A, Jabusch HC, Altenmuller E, Hagenah J, Bruggemann N, Hedrich K, et al. Dominantly transmitted focal dystonia in families of patients with musician's cramp. *Neurology.* 2006;67:691-693.

22. Almasy L, Bressman SB, Raymond D, Kramer PL, Greene PE, Heiman GA, et al. Idiopathic torsion dystonia linked to chromosome 8 in two Mennonite families. *Ann Neurol.* 1997;42:670-673.

23. Leube B, Hendgen T, Kessler KR, Knapp M, Benecke R, Auburger G. Evidence for DYT7 being a common cause of cervical dystonia (torticollis) in central Europe. *Am J Med Genet.* 1997;74:529-532.

24. Valente EM, Bentivoglio AR, Cassetta E, Dixon PH, Davis MB, Ferraris A, et al. DYT13, a novel primary torsion dystonia locus, maps to chromosome 1p36.13–36.32 in an Italian family with cranial-cervical or upper limb onset. *Ann Neurol.* 2001; 49:362-366.

25. Bhidayasiri R, Jen JC, Baloh RW. Three brothers with a very-late-onset writer's cramp. *Mov Disord.* 2005; 20:1375-1377.

26. Pitner MA. Pathophysiology of overuse injuries in the hand and wrist. *Hand Clin.* 1990;6:355-364.

27. Ranney D. Work-related chronic injuries of the forearm and hand: their specific diagnosis and management. *Ergonomics.* 1993;36:871-880.

28. van Hilten JJ, van de Beek WJ, Vein AA, van Dijk JG, Middelkoop HA. Clinical aspects of multifocal or generalized tonic dystonia in reflex sympathetic dystrophy. *Neurology.* 2001;56:1762-1765.

29. Birklein F, Riedl B, Sieweke N, Weber M, Neundorfer B. Neurological findings in complex regional pain syndromes-analysis of 145 cases. *Acta Neurol Scand.* 2000;101:262-269.

30. Ross MH, Charness ME, Lee D, Logigian EL. Does ulnar neuropathy predispose to focal dystonia? *Muscle Nerve.* 1995;18:606-611.

31. Charness ME, Ross MH, Shefner JM. Ulnar neuropathy and dystonic flexion of the fourth and fifth digits: clinical correlation in musicians. *Muscle Nerve.* 1996; 19:431-437.

32. Hinson VK, Cubo E, Comella CL, Goetz CG, Leurgans S. Rating scale for psychogenic movement disorders: scale development and clinimetric testing. *Mov Disord.* 2005;20:1592-1597.

33. Lang AE. Psychogenic dystonia: a review of 18 cases. *Can J Neurol Sci.* 1995;22:136-143.

34. Zeuner KE, Hallett M. Sensory training as treatment for focal hand dystonia: a 1-year follow-up. *Mov Disord.* 2003;18:1044-1047.

35. Priori A, Pesenti A, Cappellari A, Scarlato G, Barbieri S. Limb immobilization for the treatment of focal occupational dystonia. *Neurology.* 2001;57:405-409.

36. Candia V, Schafer T, Taub E, Rau H, Altenmuller E, Rockstroh B, et al. Sensory motor retuning: a behavioral treatment for focal hand dystonia of pianists and guitarists. *Arch Phys Med Rehabil.* 2002;83:1342-1348.

37. Candia V, Wienbruch C, Elbert T, Rockstroh B, Ray W. Effective behavioral treatment of focal hand dystonia in musicians alters somatosensory cortical organization. *Proc Natl Acad Sci U S A.* 2003;100:7942-7946.

38. Jankovic J. Can peripheral trauma induce dystonia and other movement disorders? Yes! *Mov Disord.* 2001;16:7-12.

39. Murase N, Rothwell JC, Kaji R, Urushihara R, Nakamura K, Murayama N, et al. Subthreshold low-frequency repetitive transcranial magnetic stimulation over the premotor cortex modulates writer's cramp. *Brain.* 2005;128(Pt 1):104-115.

40. Taira T, Harashima S, Hori T. Neurosurgical treatment for writer's cramp. *Acta Neurochir Suppl.* 2003;87: 129-131.

41. Goto S, Tsuiki H, Soyama N, Okamura A, Yamada K, Yoshikawa M, et al. Stereotactic selective Vo-complex thalamotomy in a patient with dystonic writer's cramp. *Neurology.* 1997;49:1173-1174.

42. Shibata T, Hirashima Y, Ikeda H, Asahi T, Hayashi N, Endo S. Stereotactic Voa-Vop complex cramp. *Eur Neurol.* 2005;5338-39.

43. Jedynak PC, Tranchant C, de Beyl DZ. Prospective clinical study of writer's cramp. *Mov Disord.* 2001;16: 494-499.

44. Sitburana O, Jankovic J. Focal hand dystonia, mirror dystonia and motor overflow. *J Neurol.* Sci 2007. In press.

45. Cohen LG, Hallett M. Hand cramps: clinical features and electromyographic patterns in a focal dystonia. *Neurology.* 1988;38:1005-1012.

46. Molloy FM, Shill HA, Kaelin-Lang A, Karp BI. Accuracy of muscle localization without EMG: implications for treatment of limb dystonia. *Neurology.* 2002;58:805-807.

47. Karp BI, Cohen LG, Cole R, Grill S, Lou JS, Hallett M. Long-term botulinum toxin treatment of focal hand dystonia. *Neurology.* 1994;44:70-76.

48. Hsiung GY, Das SK, Ranawaya R, Lafontaine AL, Suchowersky O. Long-term efficacy of botulinum toxin A in treatment of various movement disorders over a 10-year period. *Mov Disord.* 2002;17:1288-1293.

49. Yoshimura DM, Aminoff MJ, Olney RK. Botulinum toxin therapy for limb dystonias. *Neurology.* 1992;42:627-630.

50. Kruisdijk JJ, Koelman JH, Ongerboer de Visser BW, de Haan RJ, Speelman JD. Botulinum toxin for writer's cramp: a randomised, placebo-controlled trial and 1-year follow-up. *J Neurol Neurosurg Psychiatry.* 2007; 78(3):264-270.

51. Cole R, Hallett M, Cohen LG. Double-blind trial of botulinum toxin for treatment of focal hand dystonia. *Mov Disord.* 1995;10:466-471.

52. Behari M. Botulinum toxin in the treatment of writer's cramp. *J Assoc Physicians India.* 1999;47:694-698.

53. Cohen LG, Hallett M, Geller BD, Hochberg FH. Treatment of focal dystonias of the hand with botulinum toxin injections. *J Neurol Neurosurg Psychiatry.* 1989;52:355-363.

54. Rivest J, Lees AJ, Marsden CD. Writer's cramp: treatment with botulinum toxin injections. *Mov Disord.* 1991;6:55-59.

55. Wissel J, Kabus C, Wenzel R, Klepsch S, Schwarz U, Nebe A, et al. Botulinum toxin in writer's cramp: objective response evaluation in 31 patients. *J Neurol Neurosurg Psychiatry.* 1996;61(2):172-175.

56. Spector JT, Brandfonbrener AG. Methods of evaluation of musician's dystonia: critique of measurement tools. *Mov Disord.* 2007;22:309-312.

57. Jankovic J, Schwartz K, Donovan DT. Botulinum toxin treatment of cranial-cervical dystonia, spasmodic dysphonia, other focal dystonias and hemifacial spasm. *J Neurol Neurosurg Psychiatry.* 1990;53:633-639.

58. Poungvarin N. Writer's cramp: the experience with botulinum toxin injections in 25 patients. *J Med Assoc Thai.* 1991;74:239-247.

59. Tsui JKC, Bhatt M, Calne S, Calne DB. Botulinum toxin in the treatment of writer's cramp: A double blind study. *Neurology.* 1993;43:183-185.

60. Schuele S, Jabusch HC, Lederman RJ, Altenmuller E. Botulinum toxin injections in the treatment of musician's dystonia. *Neurology.* 2005;64:341-343.

61. Scheuele SU, Lederman RJ. Long-term outcome of focal dystonia in instrumental musicians. *Adv Neurol.* 2004;94:261-266.

62. Singer C, Papapetropoulos S. Adult-onset primary focal foot dystonia. *Parkinsonism Relat Disord.* 2006;12:57-60.

Botulinum Neurotoxin 10 in Tremors, Tics, Hemifacial Spasm, Spasmodic Dysphonia, and Stuttering

Anna Rita Bentivoglio, Alfonso Fasano, and Alberto Albanese

INTRODUCTION

Therapeutic indications for the use of botulinum neurotoxins (BoNT) in movement disorders have steadily expanded since the first introduction in patients with dystonia in the 1980s.[1] The possibility of treating patients with hemifacial spasm (HFS) was identified early,[2] whereas the indications for tremors[3] and spasmodic dysphonia (SD)[4] were proposed later. BoNT treatment was also later proposed for the treatment of eyelid tics, usually manifested by bursts of blinking but, in some cases, becoming more sustained, resembling blepharospasm.[5] With the exception of HFS, the indications reviewed in the present chapter have remained outside the mainstream of BoNT use, partly because of the limited number of patients affected, difficulty and risk in performing the treatment (as in the case of SD, particularly of the abductor type), and uncertain outcomes (as in the case of tremors).

HEMIFACIAL SPASM

HFS typically presents with unilateral, involuntary, intermittent and irregular clonic or tonic contractions of the cranial muscles supplied by the facial nerve.[6] HFS is a sporadic disorder in most cases, but it can occasionally occur as a familial disorder. The twitching movements usually start in the orbicularis oculi, initially involving the lower eyelid, gradually spreading to other ipsilateral facial muscles, frequently involving also the frontalis muscle, producing the "other Babinski sign" manifested by ipsilateral eye brow elevation.[7] HFS spasm may also spread to involve the platysma. HFS is a chronic disorder, affecting women more than men.[8] It is frequently attributed to the compression of the facial nerve at the root exit zone by an ectopic anatomic or pathologic structure. resulting in axono-axonal "ephaptic" transmission and increased excitability of the facial motor nucleus.[8] Peripheral facial nerve injury or antecedent Bell palsy can also precede HFS; in such cases, the HFS often coexist with a mild ipsilateral facial weakness and synkinesis.[9] Patients without an history of Bell palsy may still have abnormal electromyographic (EMG) findings suggesting a preceding facial nerve damage and subsequent pathologic regeneration.[8] HFS is unilateral in most cases but may rarely occur bilaterally.[10] In our experience, of 296 patients with HFS, two presented with a bilateral form, in which the two sides contracted asynchronously, but otherwise the HFS was typical without evidence of blepharospasm.

Treatment Options

HFS may have a severe impact on the patient's appearance and causes social embarrassment.

Dr. Bentivoglio has received lecture fees and research grants from Allergen and Ipsen; Dr. Fasano does not report any conflicts of interest; and Dr. Albanese reports the following disclosures: The Neurotoxin Institute, Advisory boards for Allergen, Ipsen, and Merz.

Because it persists during sleep, it may lead to insomnia. Because spontaneous remissions are infrequent,[11] most patients need to be treated for many years, if not over their entire lifetime. Treatment options aim at reducing or stopping muscular twitches, and include BoNT injections, medications, neurosurgery and more recently, doxorubicin chemomyectomy.

Medications are often ineffective in the long-term management of HFS, although they may provide transient relief. Many drugs have been used, usually without substantial benefit. These include carbamazepine, a membrane-stabilizing drug that has been reported to alleviate HFS in approximately 50% of patients.[12] In addition, baclofen, clonazepam, phenytoin, orphenadrine, felbamate, gabapentin, latanoprost (a prostaglandin derivative), and levetiracetam have been reported to provide at least transient or mild symptom relief.

Surgical approach, using microvascular decompression, consists of placing surgical gauze or some other barrier, such as surgical or fibrin glue, between the facial nerve and the compressing vessel.[13,14] The success rate of microvascular decompression is high (from 88% to 97%), but symptoms recur in as many as 25% of patients within 2 years after the surgery.[15] Furthermore, complications occur in more than 20% of the patients, and sometimes are severe (e.g., permanent deafness or facial palsy).[16] In the majority of cases, there is a durable resolution of HFS for up to 17 years, supporting the indication for surgery in younger patients.[17-20]

Chemical myectomy or facial nerve block with doxorubicin is a possible alternative; the results reported so far are promising, and the most frequent adverse events consist in skin inflammation.[21,22]

During the last 2 decades, BoNT treatment has emerged as the first-choice option for HFS.[23,24] Two randomized controlled trials[25,26] and more than 30 open-label studies, encompassing more than 2200 patients, have been published. The majority of these studies report on small series of patients, but several long-term observations of large cohorts confirm the safety and efficacy of this treatment.[11,23,27-32] A recent evidence-based review by the Therapeutics and Technology Assessment Subcommittee of the American Academy of Neurology concluded that "BoNT is possibly effective with minimal side effects for the treatment of HFS (one Class II and one Class III study). Botox® and Dysport®, after dosage adjustment, are possibly equivalent in efficacy (one Class II study)" and recommended BoNT injection as a treatment option for HFS (Level C).[33]

Botulinum Neurotoxin Treatment

BoNT injections are performed with the patient lying supine. The toxin is diluted to a minimum concentration of 10 to 25 Botox U/mL (Allergan, Irvine, CA), 50 to 100 U/mL Dysport (Ipsen, Milford, MA), or 5000 to 10,000 U/mL Neurobloc/Myobloc (Solstice Neurosciences, Malvern, PA) to minimize diffusion. The injections are performed using a 1-mL syringe with a 30-gauge needle. BoNT injections are placed subcutaneously because the orbicularis oculi, which is a superficial muscle, is easily reached by the local diffusion. EMG guidance is not necessary. The injections are placed in proximity of the pretarsal portion of the orbicularis oculi muscle, divided in two to three sites; most commonly the injection sites are close to the medial and lateral epicanthi in the upper and lower eyelids, close to the orbital rim. The orbicularis oculi has two anatomic-functional divisions (Fig. 10-1): the palpebral portion that closes the eyelids and the orbital portion that squeezes the eyes shut. The palpebral portion is further subdivided in two parts: the preseptal and the pretarsal regions. It has been reported that ptosis is less frequent when BoNT is injected into the lateral portion of the pretarsal orbicularis oculi, and occurs more frequently when injections are performed into the preseptal or orbital divisions.[29,34]

The sites of injection are determined by the observation of the involuntary twitches, which can be triggered by instructing the patient to contract their muscles while smiling or pursing their lips. Usually, in the first treatment session, only the periocular regions are injected. Later, if required, additional sites are treated to control the spread of contractions: the medial eyebrow, the procerus, the corrugator, the frontalis muscle, or the paranasal portion of the zygomaticus major muscle. When HFS involves the lower face, at least in the first treatment session, BoNT injections are placed only in the upper face, because it has been recognized that this may be sufficient to control lower facial spasms.[11,23] However, if lower facial muscles are particularly active or if there is residual mouth contraction following periocular treatment, targeting the orbicularis oris, the levator anguli, risorius, buccinator, or depressor

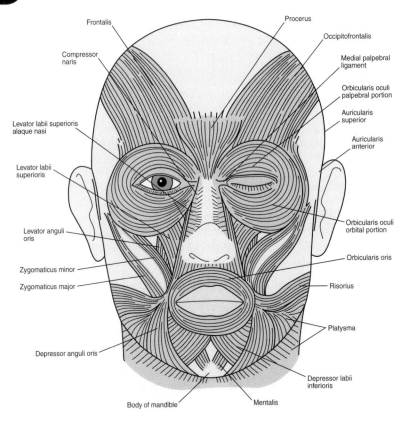

Frontalis
Procerus
Occipitofrontalis
Compressor naris
Medial palpebral ligament
Orbicularis oculi palpebral portion
Auricularis superior
Auricularis anterior
Levator labii superioris alaque nasi
Levator labii superioris
Levator anguli oris
Orbicularis oculi orbital portion
Zygomaticus minor
Orbicularis oris
Zygomaticus major
Risorius
Platysma
Depressor anguli oris
Depressor labii inferioris
Body of mandible
Mentalis

FIGURE 10-1. A number of facial muscles can be targeted with BoNT injections to reduce involuntary facial movements. Usually the muscles involved in the predominant involuntary movement are targeted during the first treatment session. The treatment can be refined and expanded in further sessions.

anguli oris may be considered, but only very small dosages should be used because injections into these areas can markedly distort facial expression, particularly when BoNT diffuses into the lips. The platysma muscles may also need to be injected if the HFS involves that part of the neck. The unaffected side of the face, mostly around the eye, may also require low doses of BoNT in order to avoid the appearance of asymmetric expressive facial lines.

The average dose used varies from 10 to 46 Botox U,[23,35] from 53 to 160 Dysport U,[36] or from 1250 to 9000 Myobloc/NeuroBloc U[37,38] (Table 10-1). Several reports indicate a lack of

correlation between the total dose injected and clinical outcome: the doses used in the "low-dose" Dysport protocol did not differ from standard dosages[39]; furthermore, no significant difference in the response rate and duration of improvement were found in patients receiving 15 or 25 Botox U.[40] Similar discrepancies were reported also by others.[41] In another paradigm, Botox doses were increased to provide a sustained effect with subsequent treatments.[31,32] Alternatively, a slight, albeit not significant (from 17.5 to 15.9 Botox U) dose reduction was reported after 10 years.[30] In two studies using Dysport,

TABLE 10-1 Suggested Doses for the Treatment of Hemifacial Spasm[36]

Drug Name	Orbicularis Oculi	Frontalis	Corrugator	Zygomaticus Major	Buccinator	Depressor Angolaris Oris
Botox U	15–20	10	1	1	2	1
Dysport U	45–60	30	3	3	6	3
Myobloc/ NeuroBloc U	1000	500	50	50	100	50

a dose reduction was observed after the seventh consecutive treatment[29] and a 25% reduction was reported after 5 years.[39]

In patients with HFS, improvement occurs soon after the first treatment,[39] with a latency varying from 2.6[42] to 5.4 days.[8] The clinical benefit generally lasts longer than in patients treated with BoNT for focal dystonia despite the use of smaller doses.[31,35,42-44] This longer lasting improvement may be due to a subclinical denervation present in HFS.

The success rate of BoNT treatment has been estimatedto be between 75%[28] and 100%,[23,45] with a truly reliable estimate around 95%, as reported in two long-term studies.[30,31] Patients with HFS have the lowest incidence of resistance to treatment, probably due to the low dosages used.[46] No secondary failures were reported in one series,[47] and an incidence of 0.9% per year was reported in another series[31]; furthermore, no evidence of immunoresistance was reported in a series of 110 patients.[8] Primary failures were estimated to be 0.02%[29] or 1.4% per year,[31] the lowest among different movement disorders treated with BoNT.

The mean duration of benefit was estimated between 75[48] and 196 days,[49] with a mean duration of approximately 90 days; this may increase,[30,32,50] decrease[41] or remain unchanged[27,29,43,47,51] with repeated treatments. It has been hypothesized that disuse atrophy may occur in the facial muscles with repeated BoNT injections; but histologic studies failed to provide evidence to support this possibility.[52]

Spontaneous prolonged remissions (up to 10 years) have been reported in a small number of patients treated with BoNT: 3% of patients in two series,[30,40] 4% in another.[11] These remissions occurred after a variable number of treatment sessions (from 1 to 6).

Side effects occur in approximately 30% of patients and consist of erythema or ecchymosis of the injected region, dry eyes, mouth droop, ptosis, edema, or facial weakness. These complications are transient and usually resolve within 1 to 4 weeks. Earlier studies reported a high frequency of ptosis (up to 53%) with an overall mean of approximately 12%,[43,51,53] likely due to diffusion of the toxin to the levator palpebrae superioris muscle. Mild symptoms of exposure keratitis (lacrimation and irritation of conjunctiva, occurring respectively in 3.6% and 2.3% of all treatments) are presumably an aftermath of decreased blink rate and incomplete eye closure from a partial

paralysis of the orbicularis oculi muscles. In several series, the most frequently reported side effect was facial weakness, involving 75%,[48] 95%,[40] or 97% of cases.[26] Facial weakness is more common when BoNT injections are placed in mid and low facial sites.[54] In a published series on blepharospasm,[43] 11.6% of the patients with facial weakness had received injections in the lower face, whereas a negligible portion of patients treated in the orbicularis oculi muscle had this complication. Because most patients report marked improvement of peribuccal spasms even when lower facial muscles are not directly injected,[44,47] which is probably due to local diffusion of the drug, caution must be taken before injecting these sites. A positive correlation between dose and occurrence of side effects has been reported.[30,39,40]

In our series of 665 BoNT treatments in 108 patients with HFS over the past 10 years, an average of 6.2 ± 5.5 (1–30) injections were performed in each patient. Botox was injected in 492 occasions and Dysport in 173 (unpublished data). The patients had a mean disease duration of 7.9 ± 5.4 years (1–26 years) with a mean follow up of 4.7 ± 3.0 years (0–11 years). At the last medical evaluation, the mean age of patients was 65.4 ± 14 years (29–92 years). The mean dose used per session was 11.2 ± 4.9 Botox U (1–50 U) and 46.5 ± 18.9 Dysport U (8–130 U). The analysis of repeated consecutive treatment revealed an increase of dose for either Botox ($\beta = 0.35$, $P < 0.001$) or Dysport ($\beta = 0.16$, not significant [n.s.]). Mean latency of clinical effect after the injection was 5.4 ± 5.3 days (0–40 days) for Botox and 4.9 ± 4.6 days (0–30 days) for Dysport, with no between-treatment differences. The duration of effect was longer for Dysport than for Botox: 105.9 ± 54.2 days (0–480 days) compared with 85.4 ± 41.6 days (0–330 days; $P < 0.001$). With repeated treatments, the duration of clinical benefit slightly increased with Botox ($\beta = 0.12$; $P < 0.01$), but remained constant for Dysport (Fig. 10-2).

A successful outcome was reported in 94% of treatment sessions (93.5% with Botox, 95.4% with Dysport, n.s.). There were no cases of primary or secondary resistance to BoNT. Side effects occurred in 116 of 665 sessions (17.4%), with comparable incidence with the two toxins. The most common side effects were palpebral ptosis and lacrimation. No correlation was found between the dose injected and the occurrence of side effects, either with Botox or with Dysport. No patient

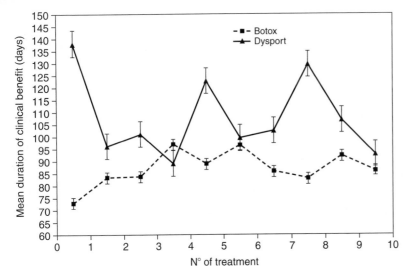

FIGURE 10-2. A series of 665 BoNT treatments in 108 patients with hemifacial spasm over 10 years. Longitudinal analysis of the mean duration of clinical benefit shows that the duration of clinical benefit is more predictable with Botox than with Dysport, probably due to variations in toxin diffusion.

discontinued treatment because of side effects, suggesting that the treatment was well tolerated.

New Botulinum Toxins

A new BoNT/A has been recently introduced in China (Prosigne, Lanzhou Institute of Biological Products, Shanghai, China), but the experience with this product is still limited. Its equivalency in terms of efficacy and safety with Botox has been suggested by a retrospective clinical study[55] and in a double-blind crossover trial in which 18 patients with HFS were randomized to Botox or Prosigne at a ratio of 1:1.[56] No data is currently available on the efficacy of Xeomin in HFS, but a controlled study is currently ongoing. BoNT/B has also been used for the treatment of HFS: clinical effects lasted about 8.5 weeks in the two patients treated with Myobloc over six sessions.[37] BoNT/C has also proven efficacious in two patients with HFS.[57]

SPASMODIC DYSPHONIA

SD is a focal laryngeal dystonia characterized by action-induced spasms of the vocal folds, which are normal at rest, but during phonation develop contractions that cause abnormal movements and muscle spasms and typically result in dysphonia while speaking.[58] Historically SD was wrongly called "spastic dysphonia" and considered a disorder of uncertain origin, often classified as psychogenic in nature. The dystonic nature of SD is suggested by its frequent occurrence in patients with cranial-cervical dystonia and by the improvement with "sensory tricks" such as yawn, laugh, cough, whisper, hum, or use of falsetto when starting to speak or while singing. Patients commonly report that their symptoms are worse when they are under emotional stress and are often better upon waking in the morning or after an alcoholic drink. Many can laugh and sing normally and, if able to speak different idioms, they find that their voice is better when speaking one language versus another. Symptoms usually worsen when the patients speak on the telephone.

The categorization of SD as a form of focal, laryngeal dystonia, was suggested by Marsden and Sheehy, who noted that "all evidence points to the conclusion that blepharospasm and oromandibular dystonia seen in Meige disease is another manifestation of adult-onset torsion dystonia, [and] since dysphonia may occur in the same syndrome, it is quite likely that dysphonia itself may be the sole manifestation of dystonia."[59] Later it was recognized that the characteristics of "spastic dysphonia" were similar to the dysphonia found in some patients with generalized and multifocal dystonia, and the clinical and EMG features of these patients revealed that most cases of dysphonia clinically diagnosed as "spastic dysphonia" were in fact focal forms of cranial dystonia.[60] Later, it became accepted that laryngeal dystonia may occur as a focal form of dystonia or in association with other affected sites in the context of a segmental or more widespread dystonia.

Different types of SD have been recognized.

1. The **adductor type** is the most common (more than 80% of cases published in large series) and presents spasms of the vocal muscle (thyroarytenoid muscle) (Fig. 10-3). This causes a strain-strangled voice that is harsh, often tremulous, with inappropriate pitch or pitch breaks, breathiness, and glottal fry. The intermittent voice stoppage or breaks (phonatory breaks) is due to overadduction of the vocal folds, which results in a staccato-like voice.

2. The **abductor type** is less common and is due to involuntary spasms of the posterior cricoarytenoid muscles (see Fig. 10-3), causing a prolonged abduction of vocal folds during voiceless consonants. This produces a breathy, effortful, hypophonic voice with abrupt termination of voicing, or whispered speech.

3. The **mixed adductor-abductor type** presents with an admixture of breathy breaks and tight harsh sounds.

It has been proposed that adductor and abductor features coexist in all patients and that the symptoms depend on whether there is more adductor or abductor activity.[61] Three other clinical variants have been reported[62]:

1. The **compensatory abductor dysphonia is** occasionally present in patients with the adductor form of SD that produces a breathy voice by whispering or not contracting the vocal folds to prevent spasms and broken speech patterns.

2. The **compensatory adductor dysphonia** is much rarer, seen in patients with abductor SD who try to prevent breathiness by attempting to speak with their vocal folds tightly contracted.

3. In **adductor breathing dystonia**, the patients develop adductor spasms during breathing, producing paradoxical vocal fold motion.

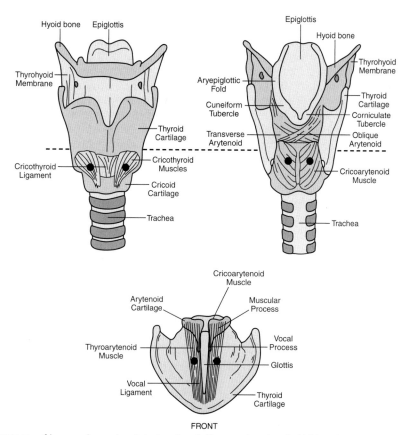

FIGURE 10-3. Anatomy of laryngeal muscles. Anterior view (*left*); posterior view (*middle*) and transverse section (*right*) of the larynx at the level of the dotted line. The *closed circles* indicate the muscles injected with BoNT in different forms of spasmodic dysphonia.

Symptoms of SD develop gradually over several months to years. SD typically affects patients in their mid-40s and is more common in women.[63,64]

Clinical and Instrumental Evaluation

All patients with SD should undergo a detailed head and neck examination, particularly focusing on any presence of dystonia in the head or neck.

The Unified Spasmodic Dysphonia Rating Scale is a standardized, validated, vocal rating scale that includes two sections, one for reading and conversational speech and the other for voice and speech tasks.[65] Another scale, the Global Rating Scale, has also been used to evaluate voice function, scored as a percentage of normal from 0 (maximum degree of impairment) to 100% (normal voice).[66]

Fiber optic laryngoscopy and stroboscopy allow to observe glottal function during phonation and to look for disruptions, spasms, breathy breaks, and tremor while the patient speaks. These movements can be video recorded and analyzed with slow speed and stop-action. Such examination cannot be reliably performed with indirect laryngoscopy, because anterior tongue traction limits speaking ability. Laryngostroboscopic examination of vocal function during speech segments is important for the diagnosis. The stroboscope can help define the nature of the associated tremor. Sometimes, a speech pathologist also makes acoustic and aerodynamic measures to evaluate for tremor, fundamental frequency, pitch and amplitude perturbation, harshness, fluency breaks, and breathiness. In patients with abductor dysphonia, laryngostroboscopic examination reveals a synchronous abduction of the true vocal fold that causes an extremely wide open glottic chink. Abductor spasms are triggered by consonant sounds, particularly when they are in the initial position in words. Having a patient say "taxi" or "Harry's hat" will often lead to an abnormal breathy break in speech. Laryngeal EMG helps evaluate tremor and areas of hyperactivity.

Treatment Options

Speech therapy has limited benefit and does not yield marked improvement in voice quality. When combined with BoNT, speech therapy may be useful in developing coping strategies treat the compensatory behaviors superimposed on SD.[67] Psychotherapy may help patients manage the associated problems with social interactions and other activities requiring voice, which can be considerable, and thereby minimize the stress-related deterioration of voice. There is no evidence, however, that psychotherapy or psychological intervention can relieve the symptoms of SD.

Occasionally, the patients may improve with benzodiazepines (i.e., clonazepam, lorazepam), or with baclofen and those with superimposed voice tremor may benefit from anticonvulsants (i.e., gabapentin, primidone), or beta-adrenergic antagonists (i.e., propranolol).

Until the introduction of BoNT, surgical interventions have been the only truly efficacious options, but side effects and disappointing long-term results limited its applicability.[68] Surgical interventions included unilateral recurrent nerve resection, unilateral superior laryngeal nerve resection, and anterior laryngoplasty. EMG and clinical evidence suggests that recurrence of symptoms is due to reinnervation following these surgical ablations. Recurrent laryngeal nerve avulsion is a technique introduced as a modification of standard nerve section to prevent neural regrowth to the hemiparalyzed larynx and subsequent recurrence of SD.[69] An alternative surgical approach aimed at preventing reinnervation is the selective section of the distal branches of the recurrent nerve, leading to the thyroarytenoid and sometimes the lateral cricoarytenoid muscle, followed by immediate reinnervation using a non laryngeal nerve, generally the sternohyoid branch of the ansa cervicalis.[70,71] There are other variants of these surgical procedures, including the use of transoral bilateral laser myoneurectomy of thyroarytenoid muscles.[72]

Notwithstanding all these surgical options, BoNT is currently recognized as the first-choice treatment for SD,[73] and surgery is recommended in cases in which BoNT is not efficacious. There are also reports of patients treated with both BoNT and surgery, in order to obtain maximal benefit.[74,75] A recent report, however, suggests caution on the use of this combined treatment.[76]

Botulinum Neurotoxin Treatment

The first BoNT treatment for SD was performed in 1984 on a patient with adductor SD[77]; patients with abductor SD were treated starting from 1988.[74] These observations were later confirmed by a double-blind study.[78]

A meta-analysis of 30 series (uncontrolled trials in most cases) indicated a moderate overall improvement of adductor dysphonia following BoNT treatment.[79] The Cochrane Collaboration concluded that, although only one double-blind trial was available, most studies reported comparable successful outcome on the length of treatment effect, degree of improvement, patient satisfaction, and observed side effects.[80] Furthermore, a systematic review on the diagnosis and treatment of dystonia concluded that BoNT/A (or BoNT/B if there is resistance to type A) are the first-line treatment for SD.[81] A recent evidence-based review recommended BoNT as a treatment option for adductor-type SD with a level B evidence, whereas the data was considered to be insufficient to evaluate the efficacy and safety of BoNT in the other variants of SD.[33]

Adductor Spasmodic Dysphonia

The most commonly used technique is the percutaneous injection of the laryngeal adductor muscles. The patient lies in the supine position with the neck extended. The needle is curved slightly to allow for a more anterior placement, and is inserted through the space between the cricoid and thyroid cartilages, pointing toward the thyroarytenoid muscle (Fig. 10-4). BoNT is injected using an insulated needle connected to an EMG recorder. The patient is asked to phonate, and EMG activity is recorded; the toxin is injected when the needle tip is located in an active area of the muscle. The patient is instructed to try not to cough or swallow when the needle is in the airway or in the thyroarytenoid muscle. Patients with uncontrollable cough can be treated with 0.3 mL of 1% lidocaine injected through the cricothyroid membrane into the subglottic space or into the underneath airway. The anesthetic is not given routinely because it diminishes the EMG interference pattern, reducing the precision of muscle targeting.

Other approaches have also been proposed.

- The indirect laryngoscopic technique uses the transoral approach, which is more familiar to the otolaryngologists and requires no EMG equipment. The vocal folds are visualized directly and the injections are performed using an L-shaped syringe, a device originally designed for collagen injections. The advantage of the this approach is the visual individuation of the target area that reduces soft tissue traumas; a drawback is the waste of the

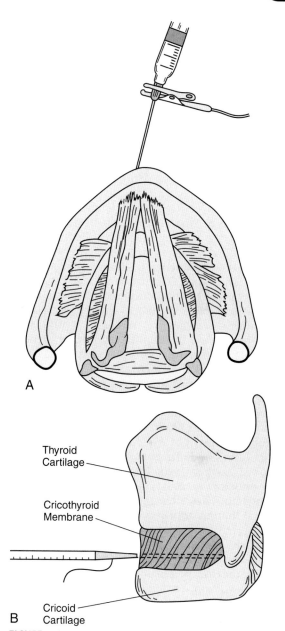

FIGURE 10-4. Percutaneous injection of the laryngeal adductor muscles: schematic view from above (**A**) and lateral view (**B**).

toxin due to the large dead volume in the long L-shaped needle.[82]

- The injection can be performed using a needle placed into the operative channel of a flexible fiber optic laryngoscope (transnasal approach).[83]

- The point-touch injection uses a needle inserted through the surface of the thyroid cartilage halfway between the thyroid notch and inferior edge of the thyroid cartilage. The toxin is then given once the needle is passed into the thyroarytenoid muscle.[84]

There are no comparative data on the efficacy and tolerability of these different techniques; however, EMG-guided percutaneous injections are considered the method of preference.

Unilateral or bilateral protocols have been proposed for BoNT injections into the thyroarytenoid muscle. Some authors have proposed to treat patients with relatively large doses (20–30 Botox U) given unilaterally, to simulate the effects of the recurrent nerve section, avoiding adverse events, such as breathiness or hoarseness.[85,86] A comparison of outcome between 16 patients treated with unilateral injections and 33 patients who received bilateral injections concluded that unilateral injections have a better efficacy/tolerability profile[87]: patients receiving unilateral injections had a significantly longer benefit and a higher rate of successful sessions. Others found that bilateral injections significantly prolonged the duration of benefit in men but not in women,[88] whereas others did not find substantial differences between the two techniques.[89] Blitzer and colleagues[75] suggested to use from 2.5 U to 7.5 Botox U in just one vocal fold. This would cause a vocal fold paresis, a period of breathy dysphonia, and eventually a 90% improvement in vocal function. Thereafter, the same authors considered that dystonia would exacerbate in the untreated vocal fold after unilateral paresis and shifted toward a bilateral injection protocol. They considered that such technique permits the use of smaller doses and produces better voicing. Yet another paradigm has been proposed for those patients who are exquisitely sensitive to BoNT injections and do not have benefit from small bilateral doses but who have unacceptable breathiness at larger doses. In such patients, it has been proposed to stagger larger BoNT doses, by performing a unilateral injection, and then give a contralateral injection 2 weeks apart. Finally, some patients prefer more frequent, smaller (0.1–0.5 Botox U) unilateral doses. Although the duration of benefit in these patients is only from 6 to 8 weeks, it avoids the risk of breathiness. Frequent injections, however, increase the exposure to the immune system and potentially increase the risk of formation of blocking antibodies. Although this is much more of a concern in patients receiving higher doses for other indications, such as cervical dystonia, nevertheless frequent, "booster," injections should be avoided whenever possible. It has been estimated that up to 20% of patients obtain no benefit from injection nor its side effects, suggesting the possibility that BoNT does not reach the appropriate vocal muscles in these cases.[90]

BoNT injections can be placed just into the thyroarytenoid muscles or also in the lateral cricoarytenoid and interarytenoid muscles.[91] It has been reported that simultaneous unilateral injections into both the thyroarytenoid and the lateral cricoarytenoid muscles gives the best overall improvement, the longest lasting benefit, and the shortest duration for undesirable breathiness.[92]

The BoNT doses used in SD vary depending on the toxin brand and the technique used (Table 10-2). In the earlier series, the total doses varied from 3.75 to 7.5 Botox U for bilateral injections,[78,93-95] and up to 15 U for unilateral injections.[85,86] Remarkably, much larger doses (up to 50 Botox U in each vocal cord) have also been used.[35] More recent data,

TABLE 10-2 Suggested Doses in the Treatment of Adductor-Type Spasmodic Dysphonia

Drug Name	Muscle Injection type	Vocal Cord (Thyroarytenoid Muscle) Unilateral	Bilateral	Lateral Cricoarytenoid Bilateral
Botox	Starting dose (U)	5–10	1.25–2.5	2.5–5
	Dilution	50 U/mL	25 U/mL	50 U/mL
Dysport	Starting dose (U)	20	5	10–20
	Dilution	200 U/mL	100 U/mL	100 U/mL
Myobloc/ Neurobloc	Starting dose (U)	200–500	50–100	100–200

however, recommended the use of lower doses.[96] In the 12-year experience reported by Blitzer and colleagues,[75] the dose range was between 0.005 and 30 Botox U (average: 3.09 U ±3.1). The average starting dose was 1 Botox U in each thyroarytenoid muscle. Others injected between 0.6 and 2.5 Botox U bilaterally and then adjusted the dose according to the clinical improvement; alternatively, 5 o Botox U were injected unilaterally. Truong and colleagues[68] suggested to start with 0.5 Botox U or 1.5 Dysport U when injecting bilaterally; then to adjust the dose as needed (the estimated average dose being 0.75–1 Botox U or 2–3 Dysport U).

The clinical effects become visible from 1 hour to 3 days after the injection, and the patients may then experience transient breathiness for up to 2 weeks. On average, patients treated with BoNT experience a 97% improvement of voice.[95] After few months, as the clinical effect of BoNT wears off, SD slowly recurs. The duration of improvement is dose related. In a long-term series of 747 patients, the average latency of effect was 2.4 days, with the peak effect at 9.0 days and a duration of benefit of 15.1 weeks.[75]

The treatment is generally well tolerated. In a double-blind controlled trial, it was reported that breathiness has higher incidence in the active drug-treated group.[78] A retrospective study reported mild breathiness in 35% and choking in 15% of the patients treated.[93] Compared with bilateral injections, alternating unilateral injections cause a significantly less breathy voice[87,97] and stronger voice intervals. A slightly higher incidence of aspiration, dysphagia, and breathiness was reported in the bilaterally injected group of patients, who required significantly lower doses of toxin to attain benefit.[88]

Abductor Spasmodic Dysphonia

Abductor SD is less frequent and more difficult to treat than the adductor form of SD. The posterior cricoarytenoid muscles, the cricothyroid muscles, or both, are usually injected in these patients. Using the EMG-guided percutaneous technique, the injections are performed by manually rotating the larynx away from the side of the intended injection. The posterior cricoarytenoid muscle is identified by EMG recording, using a needle inserted posterior to the posterior edge of the thyroid lamina. The needle is advanced through the inferior constrictor muscle to the cricoid cartilage and then moved out under EMG guidance to find

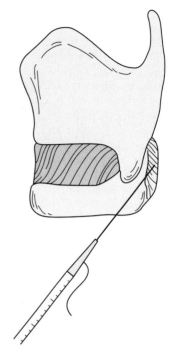

FIGURE 10-5. Percutaneous injection of the laryngeal abductor muscles (posterolateral approach) seen from a lateral view.

the posterior cricoarytenoid muscle (posterolateral approach) (Fig. 10-5). The patient is asked to sniff in order to activate this muscle and to swallow to stop its activity.[74]

An alternative technique includes the anterior approach, consisting of the supracricoid placement of the EMG needle under flexible transnasal laryngoscopic surveillance.[98] The needle is directed along the superior border of the posterior cricoid lamina and between the arytenoids. For anatomic reasons, the toxin is injected at the area above, to allow diffusion down into the muscle.

A refined simpler technique has the advantage of directing the injection into the muscle, and is particularly indicated in young individuals with soft cartilage. A small amount of 1% lidocaine is instilled in the subglottis before placing the EMG needle through the cricothyroid membrane just above the cricoid cartilage anteriorly. The needle is advanced along this plane and then directed laterally, until it hits the rostrum of the cricoid cartilage. The cartilage is impaled and, as the needle exits, there is often an appreciable burst of muscle activity from the posterior cricoarytenoid muscle (anterior transcricoid approach). In older patients, this approach is made difficult by the calcification of the cartilage.[99]

Bilateral injections are dangerous, because side effects include stridor and airway obstruction. Therefore, unilateral injections with 2.5 to 25 U of Botox are performed initially, by choosing the most active side of contraction, as determined by fiber optic laryngoscopy. A common technique is to inject 5 U Botox into the more active posterior cricoarytenoid muscle. If there is no subjective improvement in voice quality after 2 weeks, and if no airway symptoms have occurred, then the opposite muscle is injected with an additional Botox 5 U.[100,101] Another suggestion is: 2 to 4 U of Botox or 12 U of Dysport, with 1 U of Botox or 3 U of Dysport on the opposite side.[68] A lower dose protocol proposes 1.25 to 1.75 U of Botox in one muscle and 0.9 U on the opposite side (Table 10-3).[99] Generally, if a high dose is required on both sides, the second side can be injected with a delay of 2 weeks to avoid compromising the airway.

A review of the safety of simultaneous bilateral posterior cricoarytenoid muscle injections in 21 patients treated over 6 years demonstrated that this treatment is safe. The total BoNT dose injected bilaterally in each session was between 2.5 and 7.5 U of Botox, with an average total dose per session of 4.7 U. There were no life-threatening complications (intubations, tracheotomies, or admissions for airway observation); minor complications were self limited and included a 5% incidence of significant dyspnea and a 2% incidence of dysphagia.[102]

In a 12-year experience on 154 patients, the overall improvement was around 70%, the average onset of improvement was 4.1 days, and the benefit lasted for 10.5 weeks.[75] In approximately 20% of patients, weakening or paralyzing just one posterior cricoarytenoid muscle produced significant voice improvement; 80% needed a dose of 0.625 to 2.5 U of Botox into the contralateral posterior cricoarytenoid. The highest percent improvement was in the group with focal laryngeal involvement without tremor.[75] Of 154 treated patients, adverse effects included exertional wheezing in four patients and dysphagia in 10 patients, none of them requiring being intubated or tracheotomized related to treatment.[75]

One additional issue to be considered in patients with abductor dysphonia is that spasmodic activity may also take place in the adductor muscle, explaining some cases of poor treatment outcome.[103]

The cricothyroid muscle can also be injected, under EMG guidance, by percutaneous access. This muscle bends the vocal fold, antagonizing the posterior cricoarytenoid muscle.[100] In one series of SD patients, nine received bilateral injections (2.5 U of Botox on each side) in the cricothyroid muscles in addition to the posterior cricoarytenoid.[75] These patients still had breathy breaks or tremor despite significant limitation of abduction. Five of the nine injected patients had benefit consisting in a louder voice with fewer breaks. One patient got worse after the additional injection.

Mixed-Type Spasmodic Dysphonia

In the mixed adductor-abductor type of SD there is an admixture of breathy breaks and tight harsh sounds. The treatment aims at improving the most disturbing features, which in most patients, is the adductor component; in such cases, the treatment is directed at weakening the thyroarytenoid muscles. Sometimes in the mixed type, there are compensatory contractions that do not require treatment. However, in the truly mixed type both components occur, and if isolated adductor or

TABLE 10-3 Suggested Doses in the Treatment of Abductor-Type Spasmodic Dysphonia

Drug Name	Muscle Injection	Posterior Cricoarytenoid Unilateral	Posterior Cricoarytenoid Bilateral (Lower Dose on the Less Active Side)	Lateral Cricoarytenoid Bilateral
Botox	Starting dose (U)	1.25–5 U	1.5–3.0 and 1 U	2.5–5
	Dilution	25 U/mL	20 U/mL	50 U/mL
Dysport	Starting dose (U)	20 U	10 and 5	10–20
	Dilution	200/mL	100/mL	100 U/mL
Myobloc/Neurobloc	Starting dose (U)	50–200	50–150 and 50	100–200

abductor type of treatment is performed, the untreated component gets much worse. In such cases, adductor and abductor muscles both require treatment.

Botulinum Neurotoxin Type B

Resistance to BoNT injections for SD is uncommon, and there are no reported cases of secondary resistance to BoNT/A in a large series (901 patients treated with 6300 injections for more than ten years).[75] Secondary resistance has been reported in 2 patients after several years of regular treatments for SD, who failed to have the expected voice improvement after receiving their standard treatment.[104] In one of them, antibodies to BoNT/A were detected by mouse neutralization bioassay. It is conceivable that repeating injections at close intervals, as in the case of shortly spaced unilateral injections, may favor the development of immune response to BoNT.

BoNT/B stands as an alternative to BoNT/A in immunologically resistant patients. The experience with BoNT/B in SD is limited to the treatment of adductor type SD. In two patients who failed to respond to BoNT/A, 250 to 1000 U of Myobloc were injected in each vocal fold, with beneficial effects lasting for 4 months.[105] It has been reported that eight out of 10 treated patients who received 200 U of Myobloc on each side had a clinical improvement lasting for 8 weeks.[106] Three patients, who failed to respond to BoNT/A and subsequently received BoNT/B (up to 1000 U Myobloc on each side), were reported to improve for approximately 2 months.[68]

A direct comparison of BoNT/A and BoNT/B was performed on 32 patients with adductor SD who had been treated with stable doses of BoNT/A and were followed for 1 year with BoNT/B.[107] The conversion rate for laryngeal injections was 52.3:1 (B:A). BoNT-B was associated with more rapid onset of action (2.09 vs. 3.2 days) and a shorter duration of benefit (10.8 vs. 17 weeks) but no difference in safety profile.

SPASMODIC LARYNGEAL DYSPNEA

Spasmodic laryngeal dyspnea (SLD), or adductor breathing dystonia, causes a dystonic stridor. SLD has been typically described in the context of neurodegenerative disorders, such as multiple system atrophy, but it also occurs as a primary disorder in some patients. In SLD, the spasmodic vocal fold contraction is activated by breathing (primarily inspiration) rather than by speaking (as in the case of SD). SLD causes dyspnea by intermittently obstructing the glottic and supraglottic airway due to laryngeal and supralaryngeal pharyngeal muscle spasms. The patients present with stridor and tirage and, albeit rarely, may develop hypoxia. SLD abates during sleep and may improve with speaking.[108,109] Some of these patients may also have dystonic movements in other body districts or respiratory or breathing incoordination, with paradoxical movements of the diaphragm or of the chest wall.[110]

The treatment is generally similar to that of adductor SD. Localized unilateral injections are placed into the thyroarytenoid muscle and, if necessary, into the ventricular folds. The clinical improvement lasts from 9 weeks to 6 months.[111]

In a series of 12 patients a dose of 0.625 to 3.75 U, Botox was injected into each thyroarytenoid muscle, depending on the severity of the spasms.[75] The average preinjection function was 27% of normal, and pulmonary function tests showed abnormal flow volume loops with intermittent interruptions of airflow during inspiration or expiration in 20 of 24 patients. The average best postinjection function was 82% of normal. The mean duration of relief from the stridor was 14 weeks. A breathy voice lasting for 1 to 2 weeks was reported in 50% of the patients. Mild choking on fluids also occurred in five patients and lasted for 1 week. In 3 of 4 patients with severe stridor and multiple system atrophy (MSA), treated with 10 U of Botox injected into the right thyroarythenoid muscle, an improvement was documented one month after the injection.[76]

STUTTERING

Stuttering is an action-induced speech disorder with involuntary, audible, or silent repetitions or prolongations in the utterance of short speech elements (sounds, syllables) and words. Symptomatic treatment programs frequently have initial success; persistent benefit is variable and many patients remain disabled. Stuttering has many characteristics similar to SD, often including the presence of adductor laryngeal spasms that obstruct airflow (glottal block).

On this basis, it has been proposed that relief of the spasmodic dysphonic glottal blocks in stutterers would modify the stuttering phenomenon and increase fluency. Unilateral BoNT injections (doses ranging from 10 to 78 U of Botox) into the vocal fold improved fluency and speech in seven stuttering patients.[112] Fourteen adult patients were treated with 1.25 U of Botox injected into each thyroarytenoid muscle.[113] Improvement in fluency was documented at 2 and 6 weeks, with a functional relapse around 12 weeks. BoNT injections could be useful in the management of stuttering with glottal block after failure of speech interventional therapy.

VOCAL TREMORS

Patients with vocal tremor have a tremulous sound of their voice, which is especially audible while they pronounce prolonged vocals. There are different types of vocal tremors. SD may be associated with a tremor of the vocal folds: EMG studies found that almost 25% of patients with SD have an irregular 4- to 8-Hz tremor on phonation, whereas another 6% has a regular tremor similar to that of essential tremor (ET).[60] Vocal tremor in SD may be similar to that found in patients with ET, being synchronous with pharyngeal, lingual, velar, mandibular, facial, thoracic, and diaphragmatic tremor.[114]

The involvement of the thyroarytenoid muscle is predominant in SD cases without tremor, whereas the lateral cricoarytenoid muscle is equally involved when tremor is a relevant feature. It has been shown that the interarytenoid muscle may be involved in rare cases of tremulous SD.[91] In the majority of patients, the thyroarytenoid muscle alone has been injected and this may explain the poorer response rate to BoNT treatment of patients with SD and associated vocal tremor compared with patients with isolated SD. In a series of 81 patients with tremulous SD, the best outcome was achieved when the lateral cricoarytenoid muscle was also injected.[115]

Some patients with ET affecting the head and hands also present with voice tremor. Rarely, patients with Parkinson's disease may also display low-frequency (4–6 Hz) voice tremor. Many of these patients benefit from beta-adrenergic antagonists or other drugs used to treat ET, but sometimes this benefit is partial, particularly when high doses cannot be used. Objective acoustic measures have shown efficacy of BoNT in only a small number of treated patients, although the majority of them reported a subjective reduction in vocal effort.[116] Subjective evaluations reported a benefit in 67% of patients with essential voice tremor treated with BoNT/A, whereas acoustic analysis showed a nonsignificant decrease in the fundamental frequency and a decrease in the fundamental frequency during sustained vowel phonation.[117] An improvement in voice tremor was reported in another study following BoNT/A injection into the vocal cord.[118] The average doses used in each vocal muscle are 1.25 to 3.75 U of Botox or 4 to 12 of U Dysport. No experience with BoNT/B has been reported in the treatment of essential voice tremor.

TREMOR

Tremor is defined as a rhythmic, involuntary oscillatory movement of a body part; it is etiologically and physiologically heterogeneous.[119] BoNT has been tested on various tremor disorders in open-label and small controlled studies, and it has been proposed as a treatment for essential hand tremor.[3,20] Intramuscular BoNT injections may reduce tremor by weakening the muscles or by blocking gamma motor efferents and muscle spindle afferents.

In open-label trials of BoNT-A for ET affecting the hands, an improvement was reported in 6 of 10 patients and unwanted hand weakness was reported.[3] In a study of 16 patients followed for more than 6 weeks, a significant improvement occurred on the Webster tremor scale and on a global disability scale.[120] However, tremor amplitude decreased by no more than 25% and weakness of the digit extensors was a common side effect. A single-masked placebo-controlled study found that the treatment was better than placebo in more than half the patients; many had clinically significant weakness of the hands, which resolved over time.[121]

In a controlled study, 25 patients were randomized to receive 50 U of Botox or placebo into wrist extensors and flexors.[123] If patients did not respond, they were eligible to receive another injection of 100 U 4 weeks later. A significant improvement was observed after 4 to 16 weeks in the tremor severity rating scale. However, there were no significant changes in the functional rating scales. Patients treated with the active drug reported finger weakness.

Evidence of efficacy was observed in a multicenter, randomized, controlled study in which

133 ET patients were randomized to a low-dose (50 U of Botox) or a high-dose (100 U of Botox) regimen or to placebo treatment.[124] Injections were made under EMG guidance into the wrist flexors (flexor carpi radialis and ulnaris) and extensors (extensor carpi radialis and ulnaris). The study showed improvement of postural, but not kinetic, hand tremor, providing an explanation for limited functional improvement, since it is accepted that kinetic rather than postural tremor causes disability. A dose-dependent hand weakness was the most reported side effect. As a result of the extensor muscle weakness, which was observed in both controlled trials, injections into the wrist extensor muscles are now only rarely employed, and as a result, the frequency of extensor hand or finger weakness has disappeared without a compromise in the efficacy. BoNT should be considered as a treatment option for essential hand tremor in those patients in whom treatment with oral agents (Level B) has failed.[33]

A recent open-label trial enrolled five patients with primary writing tremor, a form of dystonic hand tremor. Four patients had significant improvement of symptoms after receiving low doses of BoNT/A for at least 1 year. The treatment schedule was flexible and involved the flexor carpi ulnaris, the extensor carpi ulnaris or radialis, the extensor digitorum communis, and the abductor pollicis longus. Each muscle was injected with a dose ranging from 10 to 12.5 U of Botox.[125]

Jaw tremor in Parkinson disease does not respond well to conventional antiparkinsonian medication and causes social embarrassment. It has been reported that BoNT injections may improve jaw tremor without relevant side effects. Three patients received injections into both masseter muscles with a mean dose of 53 U of Dysport (range: 30–100 U).[126]

Palatal tremor with associated ear click may also be treated with BoNT.[127] A recent review concluded that BoNT should not be reserved for refractory cases but should be considered a safe and effective first-line therapy.[128] The tensor veli palatini, levator veli palatine, or both have been injected with doses ranging from 5 to 20 U of Botox or from 5 to 60 U of Dysport. The treatment is generally safe; rarely have velopharyngeal insufficiency or nasal speech been recorded. In the rare cases of hereditary chin tremor and isolated high-frequenc jaw tremor, BoNT/A can be injected into the active muscles with marked reduction in the amplitude of the tremor.[129,130]

The evidence collected is insufficient to indicate a primary role of BoNT in the symptomatic treatment of tremors; however, there may be an indication for some specific forms or individual patients that cannot be adequately treated with systemic drugs or accepted surgical procedures, such as deep brain stimulation. BoNT can be helpful particularly with atypical presentations or when the tremor is confined to few muscles (Table 10-4). In the authors' experience head tremors are particularly suitable for BoNT treatment, which usually results in a satisfying outcome. The treatment paradigms follow the wide experience collected for cervical dystonia. Finally, very scanty data are available on BoNT-B treatment of tremors.[37]

TABLE 10-4 Suggested Doses in the Treatment of Upper Limb Tremor

Injection Site	Botox Dose (U)	Dysport Dose (U)	Myobloc/Neurobloc Dose (U)
Pronator teres	25–75	80–100	1000–2500
Pronator quadratus	10–50	80–100	1000–2500
Flexor carpi radialis	25–100	150	1000–3000
Flexor carpi ulnaris	20–70	100–150	1000–3000
Flexor digitorum superficialis	20–60	150–300	1000–3000
Flexor digitorum profundus	20–60	150–200	1000–3000
Flexor pollicis longus	10–30	30–60	1000–2500

Modified from Albanese A, Bentivoglio AR. Botulinum toxin in movement disorders. In: Jankovic J, Tolosa E, eds. *Parkinson's Disease and Movement Disorders*. 5th ed. Philadelphia: Lippincott Williams & Wilkins; 2007:605-619.

TICS

BoNT/A has been used to treat motor or vocal tics in patients with chronic tic disorders. The first anecdotal observations were performed in patients with Tourette syndrome and dystonic tics affecting the eyelids and the neck.[5] BoNT treatment reduced the frequency and the intensity of tics and ameliorated the associated premonitory sensory urge; the benefit lasted for several weeks.

In another series, 35 patients (30 men, 5 women) were treated with BoNT in the sites of their most problematic tics[131]: cervical or upper thoracic area (17 patients), upper face (14), lower face (7), vocal cords (4), upper back and/or shoulder (3), scalp (1), forearm (1), leg (1), and rectus abdominis (1). The response to BoNT was scored on a 0 to 4 clinical rating scale (0, no improvement, to 4, marked improvement in both severity and function). The mean peak effect recorded in 115 sessions was 2.8; the mean duration of benefit was 14.4 weeks; and the mean latency of benefit onset was 3.8 days. Twenty-one (84%) of 25 patients who reported premonitory sensations reported a marked relief.

A controlled trial has confirmed the efficacy of BoNT/A for the treatment of simple motor tics, yielding a 39% reduction in their number (compared with a 6% increase in the placebo group) and a significant reduction of the urge score.[132] The patients, however, did not report a consistent subjective benefit.

BoNT can also be indicated for vocal tics thereby ameliorating quality of life.[133,134] A series of 30 patients received 2.5 U of Botox in both vocal cords and were followed up for 12 months.[135] Vocal tics improved after treatment in 93% patients, with 50% being tic free. The mean response time was 5.8 days, and the mean duration of response was 102 days. Quality of life improved, and premonitory experiences dropped from 53% to 20%. Hypophonia was the only side effect of note (80% of patients).

In summary, it is worth trying BoNT/A in patients who have simple and repetitive motor or vocal tics, particularly if systemic medication is contraindicated or inefficacious. However, the long-term outcome in patients with tic disorders remains to be established. According to the evidence-based evaluation criteria the clinical studies available so far allow to state that BoNT is possibly effective for the treatment of motor tics, with a level C evidence, whereas there are insufficient data to determine the effectiveness of BoNT in phonic tics.[33]

References

1. Frueh BR, Felt TH, Wojno TH, Musch DC. Treatment of blepharospasm with botulinum toxin: a preliminary report. *Arch Ophthalmol.* 1984;102:1464-1468.
2. Mauriello JA. Blepharospasm, Meige syndrome, and hemifacial spasm: treatment with botulinum toxin. *Neurology.* 1985;35:1499-1500.
3. Jankovic J, Schwartz K. Botulinum toxin treatment of tremors. *Neurology.* 1991;41:1185-1188.
4. Blitzer A, Brin MF. Laryngeal dystonia: a series with botulinum toxin therapy. *Ann Otol Rhinol Laryngol.* 1991;100:85-89.
5. Jankovic J. Botulinum toxin in the treatment of dystonic tics. *Mov Disord.* 1994;9:347-349.
6. Digre K, Corbett JJ. Hemifacial spasm: differential diagnosis, mechanism, and treatment. *Adv Neurol.* 1988;49:151-176.
7. Stamey W, Jankovic J. The other Babinski sign in hemifacial spasm. *Neurology.* 2007;69:402-404.
8. Wang A, Jankovic J. Hemifacial spasm: clinical findings and treatment. *Muscle Nerve.* 1998;21:1740-1747.
9. Martinelli P, Giuliani S, Ippoliti M. Hemifacial spasm due to peripheral injury of facial nerve: a nuclear syndrome? *Mov Disord.* 1992;7:181-184.
10. Tan EK, Jankovic J. Bilateral hemifacial spasm: a report of five cases and a literature review. *Mov Disord.* 1999;14:345-349.
11. Mauriello JA, Leone T, Dhillon S, Pakeman B, Mostafavi R, Yepez MC. Treatment choices of 119 patients with hemifacial spasm over 11 years. *Clin Neurol Neurosurg.* 1996;98:213-216.
12. Alexander GE, Moses H. Carbamazepine for hemifacial spasm. *Neurology.* 1982;32:286-287.
13. Ryu H, Yamamoto S. A simple technique for neurovascular decompression of the cranial nerves. *Br J Neurosurg.* 2000;14:132-134.
14. Kurokawa Y, Maeda Y, Toyooka T, Inaba K. Microvascular decompression for hemifacial spasm caused by the vertebral artery: a simple and effective transposition method using surgical glue. *Surg Neurol.* 2004;61:398-403.
15. Piatt JH, Wilkins RH. Microvascular decompression for tic douloureux. *Neurosurgery.* 1984;15:456.
16. Loeser JD, Chen J. Hemifacial spasm: treatment by microsurgical facial nerve decompression. *Neurosurgery.* 1983;13:141-146.
17. Chung SS, Chang JH, Choi JY, Chang JW, Park YG. Microvascular decompression for hemifacial spasm: a long-term follow-up of 1,169 consecutive cases. *Stereotact Funct Neurosurg.* 2001;77:190-193.
18. Badr-El-Dine M, El-Garem HF, Talaat AM, Magnan J. Endoscopically assisted minimally invasive microvascular decompression of hemifacial spasm. *Otol Neurotol.* 2002;23:122-128.
19. Goto Y, Matsushima T, Natori Y, Inamura T, Tobimatsu S. Delayed effects of the microvascular decompression on hemifacial spasm: a retrospective study of 131 consecutive operated cases. *Neurol Res.* 2002;24:296-300.
20. Samii M, Gunther T, Iaconetta G, Muehling M, Vorkapic P, Samii A. Microvascular decompression to treat hemifacial spasm: long-term results for a consecutive series of 143 patients. *Neurosurgery.* 2002;50:712-718.
21. Wirtschafter JD, McLoon LK. Long-term efficacy of local doxorubicin chemomyectomy in patients with

blepharospasm and hemifacial spasm. *Ophthalmology.* 1998;105:342-346.

22. Ito M, Hasegawa M, Hoshida S, Miwa T, Furukawa M. Successful treatment of hemifacial spasm with selective facial nerve block using doxorubicin (adriamycin) under local anesthesia. *Acta Otolaryngol.* 2004;124: 217-220.

23. Flanders M, Chin D, Boghen D. Botulinum toxin: preferred treatment for hemifacial spasm. *Eur Neurol.* 1993;33:316-319.

24. Jost WH, Kohl A. Botulinum toxin: evidence-based medicine criteria in blepharospasm and hemifacial spasm. *J Neurol.* 2001;248(Suppl 1):21-24.

25. Park YC, Lim JK, Lee DK, Yi SD. Botulinum a toxin treatment of hemifacial spasm and blepharospasm. *J Korean Med Sci.* 1993;8:334-340.

26. Yoshimura DM, Aminoff MJ, Tami TA, Scott AB. Treatment of hemifacial spasm with botulinum toxin. *Muscle Nerve.* 1992;15:1045-1049.

27. Taylor JD, Kraft SP, Kazdan MS, Flanders M, Cadera W, Orton RB. Treatment of blepharospasm and hemifacial spasm with botulinum A toxin: a Canadian multicentre study. *Can J Ophthalmol.* 1991;26:133-138.

28. Elston JS. The management of blepharospasm and hemifacial spasm. *J Neurol.* 1992;239:5-8.

29. Jitpimolmard S, Tiamkao S, Laopaiboon M. Long term results of botulinum toxin type A (Dysport) in the treatment of hemifacial spasm: a report of 175 cases. *J Neurol Neurosurg Psychiatry.* 1998;751-757.

30. Defazio G, Abbruzzese G, Girlanda P, Vacca L, Curra A, De Salvia R, et al. Botulinum toxin A treatment for primary hemifacial spasm: a 10-year multicenter study. *Arch Neurol.* 2002;59:418-420.

31. Hsiung GY, Das SK, Ranawaya R, Lafontaine AL, Suchowersky O. Long-term efficacy of botulinum toxin A in treatment of various movement disorders over a 10-year period. *Mov Disord.* 2002;17: 1288-1293.

32. Mejia NI, Vuong KD, Jankovic J. Long-term botulinum toxin efficacy, safety, and immunogenicity. *Mov Disord.* 2005;20:592-597.

33. Simpson DM, Blitzer A, Brashear A, Comella C, Dubinsky R, Hallett M, et al. Botulinum neurotoxin for the treatment of movement disorders: an evidence-based review. *Neurology.* 2008;70:1699-1706.

34. Cakmur R, Ozturk V, Uzunel F, Donmez B, Idiman F. Comparison of preseptal and pretarsal injections of botulinum toxin in the treatment of blepharospasm and hemifacial spasm. *J Neurol.* 2002;249:64-68.

35. Jankovic J, Schwartz K, Donovan DT. Botulinum toxin treatment of cranial-cervical dystonia, spasmodic dysphonia, other focal dystonias and hemifacial spasm. *J Neurol Neurosurg Psychiatry.* 1990;53:633-639.

36. Frei K, Truong DD, Dressler D. Botulinum toxin therapy of hemifacial spasm: comparing different therapeutic preparations. *Eur J Neurol.* 2006;13(Suppl. 1): 30-35.

37. Wan XH, Vuong KD, Jankovic J. Clinical application of botulinum toxin type B in movement disorders and autonomic symptoms. *Chin Med Sci J.* 2005;20: 44-47.

38. Tousi B, Perumal JS, Ahuja K, Ahmed A, Subramanian T. Effects of botulinum toxin-B (BTX-B) injections for hemifacial spasm. *Parkinsonism Relat Disord.* 2004;10:455-456.

39. Van den Bergh P, Francart J, Mourin S, Kollmann P, Laterre EC. Five-year experience in the treatment of focal movement disorders with low-dose Dysport botulinum toxin. *Muscle Nerve.* 1995;18:720-729.

40. Chen RS, Lu CS, Tsai CH. Botulinum toxin A injection in the treatment of hemifacial spasm. *Acta Neurol Scand.* 1996;94:207-211.

41. Ainsworth JR, Kraft SP. Long-term changes in duration of relief with botulinum toxin treatment of essential blepharospasm and hemifacial spasm. *Ophthalmology.* 1995;102:2036-2040.

42. Shorr N, Seiff SR, Kopelman J. The use of botulinum toxin in blepharospasm. *Am J Ophthalmol.* 1985;99:542-546.

43. Dutton JJ, Buckley EG. Long-term results and complications of botulinum A toxin in the treatment of blepharospasm. *Ophthalmology.* 1988;95:1529-1534.

44. Ruusuvaara P, Setala K. Long-term treatment of involuntary facial spasms using botulinum toxin. *Acta Ophthalmol (Copenh).* 1990;68:331-338.

45. Chong PN, Ong B, Chan R. Botulinum toxin in the treatment of facial dyskinesias. *Ann Acad Med Singapore.* 1991;20:223-227.

46. Biglan AW, May M. Treatment of facial spasm with Oculinum (C. botulinum toxin). *J Pediatr Ophthalmol Strabismus.* 1986;23:216-221.

47. Mauriello JA, Coniaris H, Haupt EJ. Use of botulinum toxin in the treatment of one hundred patients with facial dyskinesias. *Ophthalmology.* 1987;94: 976-979.

48. Yu YL, Fong KY, Chang CM. Treatment of idiopathic hemifacial spasm with botulinum toxin. *Acta Neurol Scand.* 1992;85:55-57.

49. Borodic GE. Hemifacial spasm: evaluation and therapy. In: Jankovic J, Hallett M, eds. *Textbook of Botulinum Toxin Therapy.* New York: Marcel Dekker; 1994:331-353.

50. Frueh BR, Musch DC. Treatment of facial spasm with botulinum toxin. An interim report. *Ophthalmology.* 1986;93:917-923.

51. Carruthers J, Stubbs HA. Botulinum toxin for benign essential blepharospasm, hemifacial spasm and age-related lower eyelid entropion. *Can J Neurol Sci.* 1987;14:42-45.

52. Borodic GE, Ferrante R, Pearce LB, Smith K. Histologic assessment of dose-related diffusion and muscle fiber response after therapeutic botulinum A toxin injections. *Mov Disord.* 1994;9:31-39.

53. Savino P, Sergott R, Bosley T, Schatz N. Hemifacial spasm treated with botulinum A toxin injection. *Arch Ophthalmol.* 1985;103:1305-1306.

54. Elston JS. Botulinum toxin treatment of hemifacial spasm. *J Neurol Neurosurg Psychiatry.* 1986;49:827-829.

55. Tang X, Wan X. Comparison of Botox with a Chinese type A botulinum toxin. *Chin Med J (Engl).* 2000;113: 794-798.

56. Rieder CR, Schestatsky P, Socal MP, Monte TL, Fricke D, Costa J, et al. A double-blind, randomized, crossover study of Prosigne versus Botox in patients with blepharospasm and hemifacial spasm. *Clin Neuropharmacol.* 2007;30:39-42.

57. Eleopra R, Tugnoli V, Rossetto O, Montecucco C, De Grandis D. Botulinum neurotoxin serotype C: a novel effective botulinum toxin therapy in human. *Neurosci Lett.* 1997;224:91-94.

58. Blitzer A, Brin MF, Fahn S, Lovelace RE. Localized injections of botulinum toxin for the treatment of focal laryngeal dystonia (spastic dysphonia). *Laryngoscope.* 1988;98:193-197.

59. Marsden CD, Sheehy MP. Spastic dysphonia, Meige disease and torsion dystonia. *Neurology.* 1982;32:1202-1203.

60. Blitzer A, Lovelace RE, Brin MF, Fahn S, Fink ME. Electromyographic findings in focal laryngeal dystonia. *Ann Otol Rhinol Laryngol.* 1985;94:591-594.

61. Cannito MP, Johnson JP. Spastic dysphonia: a continuum disorder. *J Commun Disord.* 1981;14:215-233.

62. Blitzer A, Brin MF, Fahn S, Lovelace RE. Clinical and laboratory characteristics of focal laryngeal dystonia: study of 110 cases. *Laryngoscope.* 1988;98: 636-640.

63. Adler CH, Edwards BW, Bansberg SF. Female predominance in spasmodic dysphonia. *J Neurol Neurosurg Psychiatry.* 1997;63:688.

64. Schweinfurth JM, Billante M, Courey MS. Risk factors and demographics in patients with spasmodic dysphonia. *Laryngoscope.* 2002;112:220-223.

65. Stewart CF, Allen EL, Tureen P, Diamond BE, Blitzer A, Brin MF. Adductor spasmodic dysphonia: standard evaluation of symptoms and severity. *J Voice.* 1997;11:95-103.

66. Brin MF, Fahn S, Blitzer A, Ramig LO, Stewart C. Movement disorders of the larynx. In: Blitzer A, Brin MF, Sasaki CT, Fahn S, Harris K, eds. *Neurological Disorders of the Larynx.* New York: Thieme; 1992: 240-248.

67. Murry T, Woodson GE. Combined-modality treatment of adductor spasmodic dysphonia with botulinum toxin and voice therapy. *J Voice.* 1995;9:460-465.

68. Truong DD, Bhidayasiri R. Botulinum toxin therapy of laryngeal muscle hyperactivity syndromes: comparing different botulinum toxin preparations. *Eur J Neurol.* 2006;13(Suppl 1):36-41.

69. Weed DT, Jewett BS, Rainey C, Zealear DL, Stone RE, Ossoff RH, et al. Long-term follow-up of recurrent laryngeal nerve avulsion for the treatment of spastic dysphonia. *Ann Otol Rhinol Laryngol.* 1996;105: 592-601.

70. Berke GS, Blackwell KE, Gerratt BR, Verneil A, Jackson KS, Sercarz JA. Selective laryngeal adductor denervation-reinnervation: a new surgical treatment for adductor spasmodic dysphonia. *Ann Otol Rhinol Laryngol.* 1999;108:227-231.

71. Allegretto M, Morrison M, Rammage L, Lau DP. Selective denervation: reinnervation for the control of adductor spasmodic dysphonia. *J Otolaryngol.* 2003;32:185-189.

72. Su CY, Chuang HC, Tsai SS, Chiu JF. Transoral approach to laser thyroarytenoid myoneurectomy for treatment of adductor spasmodic dysphonia: short-term results. *Ann Otol Rhinol Laryngol.* 2007;116:11-18.

73. Clinical use of botulinum toxin. *NIH Consensus Statement.* 1990;8:1-20.

74. Blitzer A, Brin MF, Stewart C, Aviv JE, Fahn S. Abductor laryngeal dystonia: a series treated with botulinum toxin. *Laryngoscope.* 1992;102:163-167.

75. Blitzer A, Brin MF, Stewart CF. Botulinum toxin management of spasmodic dysphonia (laryngeal dystonia): a 12-year experience in more than 900 patients. *Laryngoscope.* 1998;108:1435-1441.

76. Sulica L, Behrman A. Management of benign vocal fold lesions: a survey of current opinion and practice. *Ann Otol Rhinol Laryngol.* 2003;112:827-833.

77. Blitzer A, Brin MF, Fahn S, Lange D, Lovelace RE. Botulinum toxin for the treatment of spastic dysphonia. *Laryngoscope.* 1986;96:1300-1301.

78. Troung DD, Rontal M, Rolnick M, Aronson AE, Mistura K. Double-blind controlled study of botulinum toxin in adductor spasmodic dysphonia. *Laryngoscope.* 1991;101:630-634.

79. Boutsen F, Cannito MP, Taylor M, Bender B. Botox treatment in adductor spasmodic dysphonia: a meta-analysis. *J Speech Lang Hear Res.* 2002;45:469-481.

80. Watts C, Nye C, Whurr R. Botulinum toxin for treating spasmodic dysphonia (laryngeal dystonia): a systematic Cochrane review. *Clin Rehabil.* 2006;20: 112-122.

81. Albanese A, Barnes MP, Bhatia KP, Fernandez-Alvarez E, Filippini G, Gasser T, et al. A systematic review on the diagnosis and treatment of primary (idiopathic) dystonia and dystonia plus syndromes: report of an EFNS/MDS-ES Task Force. *Eur J Neurol.* 2006;13: 433-444.

82. Ford CM, Bless DM, Lowery JD. Indirect laryngoscopic approach for injection of botulinum in spasmodic dysphonia. *Otolaryngol Head Neck Surg.* 1990;103: 752-758.

83. Rhew K, Fiedler DA, Ludlow CL. Technique for injection of botulinum toxin through the flexible nasolaryngoscope. *Otolaryngol Head Neck Surg.* 1994;111: 787-794.

84. Green DC, Ward PH, Berke GS, Gerratt BR. Point-touch technique of botulinum toxin injection for the treatment of spasmodic dysphonia. *Ann Otol Rhinol Laryngol.* 1992;101:883-887.

85. Miller RH, Woodson GE, Jankovic J. Botulinum toxin injection in the vocal fold for spasmodic dysphonia. A preliminary report. *Arch Otolaryngol Head Neck Surg.* 1987;113:603-605.

86. Ludlow CL, Naunton RF, Sedory SE, Schulz GM, Hallett M. Effects of botulinum toxin injections on speech in adductor spasmodic dysphonia. *Neurology.* 1988;38:1220-1225.

87. Bielamowicz S, Stager SV, Badillo A, Godlewski A. Unilateral versus bilateral injections of botulinum toxin in patients with adductor spasmodic dysphonia. *J Voice.* 2002;16:117-123.

88. Maloney AP, Morrison MD. A comparison of the efficacy of unilateral versus bilateral botulinum toxin injections in the treatment of adductor spasmodic dysphonia. *J Otolaryngol.* 1994;23:160-164.

89. Zwirner P, Murry T, Woodson GE. A comparison of bilateral and unilateral botulinum toxin treatments for spasmodic dysphonia. *Eur Arch Otorhinolaryngol.* 1993;250:271-276.

90. Galardi G, Guerriero R, Amadio S, Leocani L, Teggi R, Melloni G, et al. Sporadic failure of botulinum toxin treatment in usually responsive patients with adductor spasmodic dysphonia. *Neurol Sci.* 2001;22: 303-306.

91. Klotz DA, Maronian NC, Waugh PF, Shahinfar A, Robinson L, Hillel AD. Findings of multiple muscle involvement in a study of 214 patients with laryngeal dystonia using fine-wire electromyography. *Ann Otol Rhinol Laryngol.* 2004;113:602-612.

92. Inagi K, Ford CN, Bless DM, Heisey D. Analysis of factors affecting botulinum toxin results in spasmodic dysphonia. *J Voice.* 1996;10:306-313.

93. Brin MF, Fahn S, Moskowitz C, Friedman A, Shale HM, Greene PE, et al. Localized injections of botulinum toxin for the treatment of focal dystonia and hemifacial spasm. In: Fahn S, Marsden CD, Calne DB, eds. *Dystonia 2.* New York: Raven; 1988:599-608.

94. Brin MF, Blitzer A, Fahn S, Gould W, Lovelace RE. Adductor laryngeal dystonia (spastic dysphonia): treatment with local injections of botulinum toxin (Botox). *Mov Disord.* 1989;4:287-296.

95. Whurr R, Nye C, Lorch M. Meta-analysis of botulinum toxin treatment of spasmodic dysphonia: a review

of 22 studies. *Int J Lang Commun Disord.* 1998;33(Suppl):327-329.

96. Blitzer A, Sulica L. Botulinum toxin: basic science and clinical uses in otolaryngology. *Laryngoscope.* 2001;111:218-226.

97. Koriwchak MJ, Netterville JL, Snowden T, Courey M, Ossoff RH. Alternating unilateral botulinum toxin type A (BOTOX) injections for spasmodic dysphonia. *Laryngoscope.* 1996;106:1476-1481.

98. Rontal M, Rontal E, Rolnick M, Merson R, Silverman B, Truong DD. A method for the treatment of abductor spasmodic dysphonia with botulinum toxin injections: a preliminary report. *Laryngoscope.* 1991;101:911-914.

99. Meleca RJ, Hogikyan ND, Bastian RW. A comparison of methods of botulinum toxin injection for abductory spasmodic dysphonia. *Otolaryngol Head Neck Surg.* 1997;117:487-492.

100. Ludlow CL, Naunton RF, Terada S, Anderson BJ. Successful treatment of selected cases of abductor spasmodic dysphonia using botulinum toxin injection. *Otolaryngol Head Neck Surg.* 1991;104:849-855.

101. Bielamowicz S, Squire S, Bidus K, Ludlow CL. Assessment of posterior cricoarytenoid botulinum toxin injections in patients with abductor spasmodic dysphonia. *Ann Otol Rhinol Laryngol.* 2001;110: 406-412.

102. Stong BC, DelGaudio JM, Hapner ER, Johns MM, III. Safety of simultaneous bilateral botulinum toxin injections for abductor spasmodic dysphonia. *Arch Otolaryngol Head Neck Surg.* 2005;131:793-795.

103. Cyrus CB, Bielamowicz S, Evans FJ, Ludlow CL. Adductor muscle activity abnormalities in abductor spasmodic dysphonia. *Otolaryngol Head Neck Surg.* 2001;124:23-30.

104. Smith ME, Ford CN. Resistance to botulinum toxin injections for spasmodic dysphonia. *Arch Otolaryngol Head Neck Surg.* 2000;126:533-535.

105. Guntinas-Lichius O. Injection of botulinum toxin type B for the treatment of otolaryngology patients with secondary treatment failure of botulinum toxin type A. *Laryngoscope.* 2003;113:743-745.

106. Adler CH, Bansberg SF, Krein-Jones K, Hentz JG. Safety and efficacy of botulinum toxin type B (Myobloc) in adductor spasmodic dysphonia. *Mov Disord.* 2004;19:1075-1079.

107. Blitzer A. Botulinum toxin A and B: a comparative dosing study for spasmodic dysphonia. *Otolaryngol Head Neck Surg.* 2005;133:836-838.

108. Grillone GA, Blitzer A, Brin MF, Annino DJ Jr., Saint-Hilaire MH. Treatment of adductor laryngeal breathing dystonia with botulinum toxin type A. *Laryngoscope.* 1994;104:30-32.

109. Zwirner P, Dressler D, Kruse E. Spasmodic laryngeal dyspnea: a rare manifestation of laryngeal dystonia. *Eur Arch Otorhinolaryngol.* 1997;254:242-245.

110. Braun N, Abd A, Baer J, Blitzer A, Stewart C, Brin M. Dyspnea in dystonia: a functional evaluation. *Chest.* 1995;107:1309-1316.

111. Zwirner P, Murry T, Woodson GE. Effects of botulinum toxin on vocal tract steadiness in patients with spasmodic dysphonia. *Eur Arch Otorhinolaryngol.* 1997;254:391-395.

112. Ludlow CL. Treatment of speech and voice disorders with botulinum toxin. *JAMA.* 1990;264: 2671-2675.

113. Brin MF, Stewart C, Blitzer A, Diamond B. Laryngeal botulinum toxin injections for disabling stuttering in adults. *Neurology.* 1994;44:2262-2266.

114. Aronson AE, Brown JR, Litin EM, Pearson JS. Spastic dysphonia. II. Comparison with essential (voice) tremor and other neurologic and psychogenic dysphonias. *J Speech Hear Disord.* 1968;33:219-231.

115. Maronian NC, Waugh PF, Robinson L, Hillel AD. Tremor laryngeal dystonia: treatment of the lateral cricoarytenoid muscle. *Ann Otol Rhinol Laryngol.* 2004;113:349-355.

116. Warrick P, Dromey C, Irish JC, Durkin L, Pakiam A, Lang A. Botulinum toxin for essential tremor of the voice with multiple anatomical sites of tremor: a crossover design study of unilateral versus bilateral injection. *Laryngoscope.* 2000;110: 1366-1374.

117. Hertegard S, Granqvist S, Lindestad PA. Botulinum toxin injections for essential voice tremor. *Ann Otol Rhinol Laryngol.* 2000;109:204-209.

118. Adler CH, Bansberg SF, Hentz JG, Ramig LO, Buder EH, Witt K, et al. Botulinum toxin type A for treating voice tremor. *Arch Neurol.* 2004;61:1416-1420.

119. Deuschl G, Bain P, Brin M. Consensus statement of the Movement Disorder Society on Tremor. Ad Hoc Scientific Committee. *Mov Disord.* 1998;13(Suppl. 3):2-23.

120. Trosch RM, Pullman SL. Botulinum toxin A injections for the treatment of hand tremors. *Mov Disord.* 1994;9:601-609.

121. Henderson JM, Ghika JA, Van Melle G, Haller E, Einstein R. Botulinum toxin A in non-dystonic tremors. *Eur Neurol.* 1996;36:29-35.

122. Pullman S, Greene PF, Fahn S. Approach to the treatment of limb disorders with botulinum toxin A. Experience with 187 patients. *Arch Neurol.* 1996;53:617-624.

123. Jankovic J, Schwartz K, Clemence W, Aswad A, Mordaunt J. A randomized, double-blind, placebo-controlled study to evaluate botulinum toxin type A in essential hand tremor. *Mov Disord.* 1996;11: 250-256.

124. Brin MF, Lyons KE, Doucette J, Adler CH, Caviness JN, Comella CL, et al. A randomized, double masked, controlled trial of botulinum toxin type A in essential hand tremor. *Neurology.* 2001;56:1523-1528.

125. Papapetropoulos S, Singer C. Treatment of primary writing tremor with botulinum toxin type a injections: report of a case series. *Clin Neuropharmacol.* 2006;29:364-367.

126. Schneider SA, Edwards MJ, Cordivari C, Macleod WN, Bhatia KP. Botulinum toxin A may be efficacious as treatment for jaw tremor in Parkinson's disease. *Mov Disord.* 2006;21:1722-1724.

127. Deuschl G, Lohle E, Heinen F, Lucking C. Ear click in palatal tremor: its origin and treatment with botulinum toxin. *Neurology.* 1991;41:1677-1679.

128. Penney SE, Bruce IA, Saeed SR. Botulinum toxin is effective and safe for palatal tremor: a report of five cases and a review of the literature. *J Neurol.* 2006;253:857-860.

129. Gordon K, Cadera W, Hinton G. Successful treatment of hereditary trembling chin with botulinum toxin. *J Child Neurol.* 1993;8:154-156.

130. Gonzalez-Alegre P, Kelkar P, Rodnitzky RL. Isolated high-frequency jaw tremor relieved by botulinum toxin injections. *Mov Disord.* 2006;21: 1049-1050.

131. Kwak CH, Hanna PA, Jankovic J. Botulinum toxin in the treatment of tics. *Arch Neurol.* 2000;57:1190-1193.

132. Marras C, Andrews D, Sime E, Lang AE. Botulinum toxin for simple motor tics: a randomized,

double-blind, controlled clinical trial. *Neurology*. 2001;56:605-610.

133. Scott BL, Jankovic J, Donovan DT. Botulinum toxin injection into vocal cord in the treatment of malignant coprolalia associated with Tourette's syndrome. *Mov Disord*. 1996;11:431-433.

134. Salloway S, Stewart CF, Israeli L, Morales X, Rasmussen S, Blitzer A, et al. Botulinum toxin for refractory vocal tics. *Mov Disord*. 1996;11:746-748.

135. Porta M, Maggioni G, Ottaviani F, Schindler A. Treatment of phonic tics in patients with Tourette's syndrome using botulinum toxin type A. *Neurol Sci*. 2004;24:420-423.

136. Albanese A, Bentivoglio AR. Botulinum toxin in movement disorders. In: Jankovic J, Tolosa E, eds. *Parkinson's Disease and Movement Disorders*. ed 5th. Philadelphia: Lippincott Williams & Wilkins; 2007:605-619.

Upper Limb Skin and **11** Musculoskeletal Consequences of the Upper Motor Neuron Syndrome

Nathaniel H. Mayer and Alberto Esquenazi

INTRODUCTION

This chapter discusses the upper motor neuron (UMN) phenomena in the upper limb and how they lead to maladaptive skin and musculoskeletal consequences that affect health and function. The chapter begins with a clinical discussion of UMN phenomena, followed by a description of six problematic skin and musculoskeletal consequences. Treatment strategies with an emphasis on neurotoxin therapy will be identified where appropriate.

COMBINED EFFECTS OF POSITIVE AND NEGATIVE SIGNS: THE NET TORQUE IMBALANCE CONCEPT

Classically, UMN findings have included negative and positive signs including paresis, impaired dexterity, associated reactions, released flexor reflexes, hyperactive stretch reflexes, spastic co-contraction, and spastic dystonia.[1] Negative signs such as weakness are phenomena of *muscle underactivity*.[2] Positive signs take on a general characteristic of *muscle overactivity*[3] and are often untimely in their occurrence and problematic in their manifestations, although impairment of voluntary movement may be more disabling.[4]

In response to efferent neural activity from the central nervous system (CNS), skeletal muscle develops torque, a force acting through a bony lever arm about a joint's axis of rotation, For any given degree of freedom of joint motion, voluntary movement in everyday life is *bidirectional*, meaning that agonist and antagonist torques are freely intermixed. A task that starts with elbow flexion may soon generate elbow extension. An abducted shoulder may soon adduct, a supinated forearm may soon pronate. Fixed positions are not maintained for extended periods of time. A UMN lesion impairs voluntary control over individual degrees of freedom. As a consequence, positive sign activity promotes *unidirectional* movements that often persist as postures because voluntary two-way motion is impaired (Fig. 11-1). The combined effects of recurring chronically recurring positive and negative signs leads to a persistent net balance of muscle torques around individual joints with chronic effects on soft tissue and bone (Fig. 11-2). By forcing joints into undesired static positions or into uncontrolled dynamic movements, the combined effects of voluntary muscle underactivity and involuntary muscle overactivity may lead to maladaptive skin and musculoskeletal consequences. From this perspective, individual muscles may be considered units of structure and function in the production of limb segment

Both Dr. Mayer and Dr. Esquenazi have received unrestricted research funding from Allergan, Inc. Dr. Mayer is also a member of the Spasticity Advisory Board of Allergan and of the Neurotoxin Institute, which receives educational grant support from Allergan.

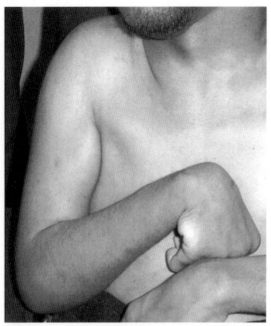

FIGURE 11-1. This patient with upper motor neuron syndrome has an adducted/internally rotated shoulder, flexed elbow, pronated forearm, flexed wrist and clenched fist. Positive signs promote *unidirectional* movements that often persist as postures when voluntary two-way motion of limb segments is impaired.

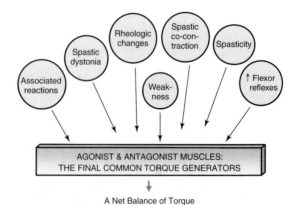

FIGURE 11-2. The combined effects of *chronically recurring* positive and negative signs leads to a net balance of muscle torque across individual joints that promotes chronic effects on muscle, other soft tissues and bone.

torques—a concept that can be exploited therapeutically with neurotoxins.

ASSOCIATED REACTIONS

Walshe[5] first described associated reactions as "released postural reactions deprived of voluntary control." Synkinesis is a term used by Bourbonnais more recently.[6] An associated reaction is linked (or associated) with a voluntary movement made in another limb. It may be due to disinhibited spread of voluntary motor activity into the affected UMN limb, and its intensity may depend on the intensity of the voluntary effort. Dewald and Rymer[7] thought that impaired descending supraspinal commands generated associated reactions. They hypothesized that unaffected bulbospinal motor pathways may have taken over the role of damaged UMN tracts when descending voluntary commands were transmitted.

Figure 11-3A and B reveal the everyday circumstances that can trigger associated reactions. The patient, a woman who sustained a hemorrhagic stroke involving the internal capsule and thalamus 5 months earlier, had

limited upper limb recovery with a Fugl-Meyer score of 29%. She reported that her right arm pulled in toward her chest spontaneously and that her elbow flexed upward. These annoying episodes occurred many times during an ordinary day, yet she was unable to identify any noteworthy triggers that made them happen. Examination revealed tight shoulder adductors and internal rotators, tight elbow flexors and forearm pronators. Dynamic surface electromyography (EMG) of pectoralis major, teres major and latissimus dorsi revealed activity during a variety of common motor behaviors such as standing up from a chair, coughing, laughing, waving or throwing a ball with the left hand, flexing the left elbow against resistance and weightbearing on her cane with the left hand. Associated reactions, as illustrated by this patient, occur in a variety of commonplace circumstances. Everyday voluntary efforts required for transfers, gait, and activities of daily living might be expected to provide many opportunities for associated reactions to develop in a UMN affected limb. The directionality of associated reaction behavior appears to be stereotyped, that is, different volitional efforts and contexts seem to recruit similar associated behaviors (as illustrated in Fig. 11-3A and B). Recurrent stereotypic movements, not reversed by voluntary contraction, may be a precursor to increased muscle stiffness and contracture. Severe impairment of voluntary movement yields a lack of movement production in directions opposite that of the motor behaviors of associated reactions. The net effect over time is the development of unidirectional limb attitudes that can lead to skin and musculoskeletal consequences.

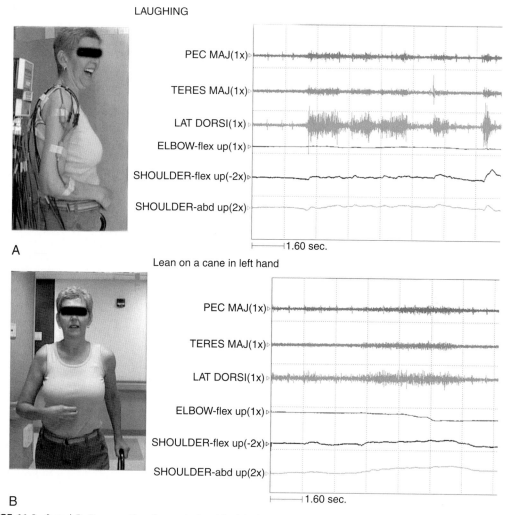

FIGURE 11-3. A and **B,** Five months after a stroke, this right hemiparetic patient reported that her right arm involuntarily pulled in toward her chest and her elbow flexed up. Dynamic surface electromyographic recordings revealed activity in pectoralis major, teres major, and latissimus dorsi during laughing (**A**) and *left* hand weight bearing on a cane (**B**). Associated reactions occur in a variety of commonplace everyday circumstances and contribute to chronically recurrent muscle activations that lead to unidirectional postures with persistent features.

FLEXOR AND EXTENSOR REFLEXES

The flexor reflex is a polysynaptic reflex that results in flexor muscle contraction.[8-10] It is elicited by afferent stimuli collectively known as flexor reflex afferents (FRAs). These afferents include cutaneous receptors (touch, temperature, pressure), nociceptors, group II afferents from muscle spindles, and free nerve endings that are scattered ubiquitously in and around skeletal muscles.[11] After entering the spinal cord, FRA activity ascends and descends a number of cord levels, making synapses in the internuncial pool, a system of spinal interneurons that is influenced by peripheral and central inputs including the brain stem.[12] The time course of polysynaptic flexor reflexes is slower than stretch reflexes and represents coordinated activity of motoneuron pools spanning many cord segments. By recruiting flexor muscles across several joints, the flexor reflex is an example of an interjoint reflex that has tissue protective value such as generating quick withdrawal from a noxious stimulus. Extensor reflexes are similarly polysynaptic and interjoint, and may subserve support functions. Flexor and extensor reflexes may play a role in complex coordinated patterns such as locomotor stepping generators and forward reach.

After a UMN lesion, FRA activity is enhanced.[13] When patients report spasm, it likely represents increased FRA activity.[14] Flexor spasms are more common in patients with spinal cord lesions including spinal forms of multiple sclerosis.[15] Herman[16] found reduced reciprocal inhibition in patients with spinal lesions. The manner in which afferent activity was transmitted within the spinal cord also differed in paraplegic and hemiplegic patients.[16] Flexor and extensor spasms may be triggered by overt stimuli or "spontaneously" by covert stimuli such as a full bladder, a stool-distended bowel, unnoticed skin ischemia from being in one position too long and many others. Clinically, flexor reflexes can range from the familiar Babinski sign to mass interjoint flexion movements that interrupt a wheelchair-to-bed transfer. Mass flexor movements involving many proximal and distal muscles are less suitable for treatment with focal agents such as botulinum toxin (BoNT). Oral agents and newer intrathecal pump technologies may be more apt.[17,18]

STRETCH-SENSITIVE SPASTICITY

The defining characteristic of clinical spasticity is excessive resistance of muscle to passive stretch, a resistance that increases as the examiner increases the rate of stretch.[1,19] In routine practice, however, clinicians also include tendon jerk hyperreflexia and clonus under spasticity.[20] The term spastic has been a popular adjective for describing clinical attributes, for example, spastic hemiparesis, spastic hand, spastic gait. The term spastic may be phenomenologic but it is not explanatory. The term spastic gait does not describe what is problematic about a patient's gait, and treatment of the phenomenon of spasticity may contribute little or nothing toward improving gait function.[21]

Spasticity is primarily a segmental reflex, afferent activity, elicited by muscle stretch, being abnormally processed in related cord segments, ultimately generating excessive drive on segmental alpha motor neurons innervating the very muscles being stretched.[1] Increased resistance correlates with increased EMG activity in the stretched muscle. Figure 11-4A illustrates spasticity of elbow flexors in an adult with cerebral palsy. EMG responses to stretch of elbow flexors at different rates of stretch are displayed. Velocity sensitivity is noted on the left side of the figure, the amount of EMG increasing as slow, moderate and rapid rates of stretch are applied. As the rate of stretch increases, EMG activity begins sooner with respect to the movement trace, as seen on the right side of the figure. Hence, resistance is felt at a smaller joint angle when the rate of stretch is faster. When spastic restraint of active movement is potentially present, patients frequently learn to slow their movement to minimize spastic antagonism to movement. Although they are not shown, similar EMG findings were observed for two other flexors of the elbow, biceps and brachialis, indicating that all three flexors were similarly spastic. This is not always the case because muscles within a group can be differentially spastic (see Fig. 11-4B). When using BoNT, it is important to identify which muscles of a group warrant injection. When a spastic muscle is stretched, reflex EMG activity, once triggered, continues throughout the period of dynamic stretch. If the muscle continues to be held at end range of stretch, some patients will continue to generate activity. Such persistent activity has been described as a static stretch reflex.[8,10] Primary endings of the muscle spindle are known to be rate sensitive, but secondary spindle endings have static length sensitivity.[22] The presence of static stretch reflex activity at end range helps inform the decision regarding a nerve block before applying a serial cast to relieve contracture.

A finding of spasticity by a clinician is not an object of treatment per se, in our opinion, although it is often identified as such.[21] If spasticity is felt as resistance to passive movement by clinicians, spasticity for patients may also be experienced as resistance to manipulation of a limb segment, but the resistance is experienced in the context of activities of daily living.[23,24] Spastic resistance may be encountered in many daily situations that require limb manipulation. In the clenched fist, for example, fingers must be opened passively, by the patient or by a caregiver, during activities such as hand washing, gloving, donning a splint, or cleaning and polishing fingernails. One of our patients complained that she could not do a one-handed glucose finger stick on the pad of her long finger because it was curled completely into the palm. Resistance to passive extension under these circumstances is a source of task restriction that ranges from hindrance to impossibility for many patients with upper motor neuron syndrome (UMNS).

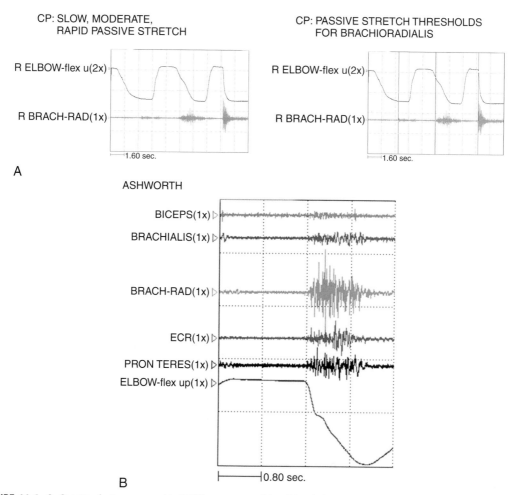

FIGURE 11-4. A, Spastic electromyographic (EMG) responses of brachioradialis to different rates of stretch in an adult with cerebral palsy. The top trace represents passive joint motion (flexion up, extension down). The bottom trace represents EMG of brachioradialis. Before each stretch, the muscle has no EMG activity. (Spastic muscle is classically silent at rest.) When slow, moderate, and rapid rates of stretch are applied, velocity sensitivity is demonstrated by increasing intensification of EMG activity as the rate of stretch increases. In addition, the onset threshold of EMG activity occurs at a smaller angle of joint displacement when velocity of stretch increases, as illustrated by the vertical lines linking EMG onsets to motion traces on the right side of the figure. Hence, when the rate of stretch is faster, an examiner is likely to feel resistance at smaller amplitudes of stretch. **B,** Passive stretch of five elbow flexors reveals differential spastic responses. The biceps appears to be least active in this patient. The examiner was performing an Ashworth maneuver, namely, complete passive extension of the elbow in about a second. An Ashworth score of 3 was assigned by the examiner to this record.

Others ascribe these problems of passive function to the phenomenon of spastic dystonia.[21]

It is important to realize that resistance to passive stretch, often referred to as muscle "tone," has neural and non-neural components.[25-27] The neural component of spastic muscle comes from its stretch reflex activity. The non-neural component comes from rheologic or physical properties intrinsic to muscle and other soft tissues. Many patients with UMNS have a large degree of non-neural resistance whose source is altered viscoelastic and

plastic properties of muscle tissue itself.[25,28-31] When spasticity emerges after a UMN lesion, increased muscle tone may be attributed primarily to its neural component. In time, muscle tone receives an enhanced contribution from its non-neural component when rheologic properties of muscle become stiffer. Often, as time from lesion increases, what passes for spastic resistance is, in large part, non-neural tissue stiffness, not spasticity. Distinguishing neural from non-neural components of muscle tone has important therapeutic implications for the use of BoNT, a treatment affecting the neural component of tone. Treatment of non-neural stiffness, particularly contracture, typically requires physical strategies such as aggressive stretching, serial casting or surgery.[32-35]

SPASTIC CO-CONTRACTION

Unlike spasticity, a phenomenon elicited at rest, co-contraction appears when the patient makes a voluntary effort with the affected limb. Co-contraction is described as excessive or inappropriate simultaneous activation of antagonist muscles during voluntary activation of agonists.[36-38] Overactive antagonist muscles create unbalanced torque that restrains movement, even causing movement reversal. The effect of antagonist restraint on agonist driven movement is much like stepping on the gas pedal and brake of a car simultaneously. Co-contraction produces unsmooth, effortful movements in a UMNS patient who must struggle to overcome the braking action of excessive antagonist contraction. Figure 11-5 illustrates alternating flexion and extension movements performed by an adult with hemiparesis due to stroke. EMG activity was recorded with surface electrodes from flexors (biceps, brachialis, brachioradialis) and extensors (medial, lateral, long head triceps). Figure 11-5 shows composite group activity, obtained by superimposing individual EMG records of flexors and extensors, respectively. During flexion phase, the elbow flexors

are active as agonists and during extension phase the extensors are active as agonists. However, during extension phase, the figure also shows co-contraction of flexors and the movement trace reveals that extension phase is irregular and prolonged with respect to the duration of flexion phase. The patient, with strain evident on his face, clearly struggles to extend his elbow (see photo insert of Fig. 11-5).

Co-contraction may represent an impairment of supraspinal control of reciprocal inhibition because abnormalities of Ia reciprocal inhibition have been reported in patients with UMNS.[39,40] Humphrey and Reed[41] have indicated that co-contraction can be activated and deactivated at a cortical level. Co-contraction is not necessarily related to muscle stretch because it can occur during isometric effort, but for isotonic movements, antagonist muscle lengthening (stretch) does occur during movement. Also, stretch sensitivity, if present, may generate a spastic contribution to antagonist muscle contraction under these conditions.[36] When patients are spastic, parsing antagonist overactivity into supraspinal co-contraction and stretch-sensitive spasticity during voluntary effort is not possible clinically. Hence, many authors use the term spastic co-contraction to denote the overall phenomenon. Technically, in co-contraction, the onset of antagonist EMG activity should begin before movement begins, indicating that supraspinal mechanisms are at work. As movement proceeds and antagonist muscles

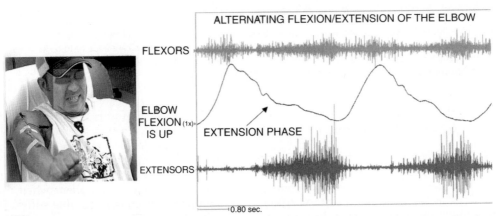

FIGURE 11-5. Voluntary alternating flexion and extension movements in an adult with hemiparesis. Composite electromyographic (EMG) activity from flexor and extensor groups was obtained by superimposing individual EMG records of flexors (biceps, brachialis and brachioradialis, top trace) and extensors (medial, lateral and long head triceps, bottom trace) respectively. Co-contraction of flexors is noted during extension phase, and the motion trace reveals irregular motion that is prolonged compared with the quicker and smoother flexion phase. The patient, with strain evident on his face, clearly struggles to extend his elbow against the braking action of the flexors.

are lengthened, a stretch reflex contribution may occur. Nevertheless, voluntary effort activates the defining feature of spastic co-contraction, namely, simultaneous activation of agonist and antagonist muscles.[42] BoNT injection of co-contracting antagonists is a potentially useful strategy to mitigate movement restraint.[43]

SPASTIC DYSTONIA

The term spastic dystonia originated in the work of Denny-Brown.[44,45] He noted that monkeys adopted persistent postures after a variety of cerebral cortex ablations. Any attempt by the examiner to pull the limb away from its persistent position was met by an increasing resistance of spring-like quality. The limb would fly back to its original position when let go. Denny-Brown used the term dystonia to describe persistent postures maintained by *active muscle contraction.* Active contraction underlying dystonia was verified by tonic EMG activity recorded at rest. In addition, muscle contraction was present without limb movement and was not abolished by cutting the dorsal roots, implying that dystonia was mediated efferently from supraspinal sources. Denny-Brown thought dystonia reflected a released motor mechanism having direct access to α-motor neurons.

In the absence of voluntary effort or passive stretch, patients with UMNS with demonstrable tonic muscle activity underlying a persistent posture have been called dystonic, consistent with Denny-Brown's original construct. Patients with UMNS with dystonic activity also appear to have stretch sensitivity and, hence, have been described as having spastic dystonia. Stretch sensitivity in UMNS patients can result not only in an increase but also a *lessening* of dystonic activity, which is especially true after prolonged stretch, a finding that has implications for therapeutic exercise and patient self-management. However, it is noted that rheologic changes in muscle compliance can also account for fixed postures in patients with chronic UMNS. Moreover, muscle contraction induced by other positive signs can bring thixotropic factors into play as well.[46,47] Before using a focal agent such as BoNT, it may be useful to know which muscles are dystonic. EMG recording equipment, if available, can help identify the distribution of persistent muscle activity at rest (Fig. 11-6). Without using such a method, it may be premature to assume that all patients with sustained limb postures have underlying tonic activity as their basis. Static tissue tension, contracture, and end positions of joints after an associated reaction may be sufficient to generate a net balance of torques mimicking postures of spastic dystonia.

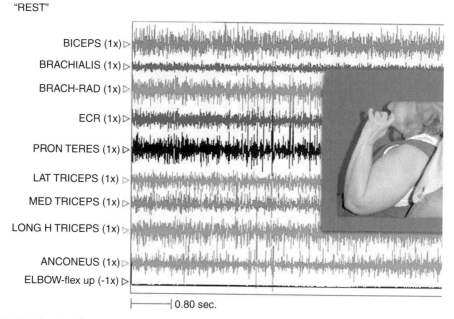

"REST"

BICEPS (1x) ▷
BRACHIALIS (1x) ▷
BRACH-RAD (1x) ▷
ECR (1x) ▷
PRON TERES (1x) ▷
LAT TRICEPS (1x) ▷
MED TRICEPS (1x) ▷
LONG H TRICEPS (1x) ▷
ANCONEUS (1x) ▷
ELBOW-flex up (-1x) ▷

├────────┤ 0.80 sec.

FIGURE 11-6. Distribution of persistent muscle activity at rest. The patient was unable to relax her elbow; it flexed involuntarily. Stretch sensitivity was present.

RHEOLOGIC TISSUE CHANGES AND CONTRACTURE

Muscle contracture refers to physical shortening of muscle length, and it is often accompanied by physical shortening of other soft tissues such as fascia, nerves, blood vessels, and skin. Muscle *contracture*, an invariant physical state of fixed shortening, is not to be confused with muscle *contraction*, a dynamic, variable state of internal shortening produced by sliding action of actin and myosin filaments. Contracture is promoted by processes that begin with the acute onset of a UMN lesion.[48] Acute paresis impairs cycles of shortening and lengthening of agonist and antagonist muscles during everyday voluntary usage; the force of gravity generates positional effects on limb segments and joints; positional effects are also created by a net balance of static rheologic forces across joints, and as preferential overactivity develops in particular muscle groups, a net balance of contractile forces promotes unidirectional effects on joint position that set the stage for the fixed shortening of contracture. In the upper limb, muscles that typically shorten include shoulder adductors and internal rotators, elbow flexors, forearm pronators, wrist, finger and thumb flexors, and thumb adductors. Familiar UMN patterns of deformity develop in the upper limb (see Fig. 11-1 above) and in the lower limb (see Chapter 15).[49]

The concept of rheologic change after a UMN lesion has literature support from many studies. Herman[25] described changes in the rheologic properties of spastic muscles in a study of 220 hemiplegic patients. Patients with contracture often had *reduced* reflex activity, yet resistance to passive stretch was high because of increased tissue stiffness and contracture.[50] His study indicated that an understanding of muscle tone should consider the complex interaction between rheologic and spastic properties of muscle because stretch reflexes themselves may be influenced by alterations in the physical properties of muscle. Along similar lines, Dietz and associates[29] in stroke and cerebral palsy and Thilmann and coworkers[31] have argued that hypertonia might not be related to exaggerated reflexes but rather to decreased compliance of soft tissues. O'Dwyer and colleagues suggested that what appears clinically as spasticity after stroke is actually increased muscle stiffness

and contracture. They suggested, as others earlier, that mechanical and biologic changes in soft tissues played a major role in resistance to both passive and active movements. Hufschmidt and Mauritz[28] proposed that abnormal cross-bridge connections between actin and myosin filaments could contribute to increased resistance to passive stretch and that these changes would very likely occur in muscles subjected to prolonged fixed positioning. Animal studies of Akeson and coworkers[52] demonstrated that immobility led to stiffness associated with water loss and collagen deposition. Gossman and associates,[53] Herbert,[30] and Carey and Burghardt[54] suggested, in various ways, that immobility imposed on a patient by the negative signs of UMN can result in soft tissue contracture. Other animal studies have indicated that some sarcomeres are lost and others become shorter and stiffer when muscles are immobilized in a shortened position[55-57] (but see Chapter 13). Soft tissues other than muscle also become less compliant in chronically shortened positions. For this reason, surgical correction of a severe contracture is limited to about half the lost range for fear of snapping contractured nerves and occluding blood vessels. After surgery, these soft tissues require progressive stretching to accomplish reversal of the residual contracture. Severe muscle contracture may also be accompanied by skin contracture that requires corrective plastic procedures. A clinical picture dominated by contracture will not respond to central muscle relaxants such as tizanidine and baclofen, peripheral relaxants such as dantrolene sodium, phenol neurolysis, or chemodenervation with BoNT. Although physical therapy and surgical methods have been the mainstay of contracture management, studies of children with cerebral palsy by Friden and Lieber[58,59] point to a process of structural remodeling of contracted muscle that may require new management techniques (see Chapter 13).

SKIN AND MUSCULOSKELETAL COMPLICATIONS IN THE UPPER LIMB

Two broad approaches have emerged in treating the consequences of maladaptive net torques: central strategy and peripheral strategy. The central strategy attempts to inhibit CNS circuitry that generates muscle overactivity. Clinical use of central muscle relaxants illustrates this approach. The peripheral strategy focuses more directly on specific muscles as offending torque generators, and treatment aims at reducing focal muscle torques. Examples of peripheral strategy include orthopaedic procedures such as muscle lengthening and transfers that rebalance or reroute muscle forces across joints, and neurotomies and phenol that denervate, causing focal muscle weakness in a specific motor nerve distribution. In recent years, BoNT has gained clinical traction as a treatment for muscle overactivity in patients with UMNS.[60] BoNT treatment is a good example of peripheral strategy, but for success, it requires specific identification of offending muscles that create maladaptive torques and consequences.[61] In the next section, we describe these consequences, and when appropriate, we will identify potentially offending muscles that may be considered for focal BoNT therapy.

SKIN INTEGRITY

Chronic limb postures, generated by positive phenomena and the failure of voluntary movement to relieve such postures, can lead to redundant skin folds that promote moisture accumulation, bacterial and fungal overgrowth with resulting malodor, skin irritation, infection, skin breakdown and ulceration (Fig. 11-7A). Skin of the axilla, elbow, palm and interdigital spaces is most often involved. At the shoulder, tight shoulder adductors promote a reddened, irritated axilla (see Fig. 11-7B). Malodor is often present, but skin breakdown is uncommon. The pectoralis major and teres major muscles are most typically involved, and chemodenervation with BoNT is a useful strategy. The latissimus dorsi may also contribute. Neurolysis with phenol is an alternative approach when BoNT, subject to a current ceiling dose of 600 U, requires conservation for muscles elsewhere. At the elbow, redness and irritation begin in the crease and spread outward to the edge of skin fold redundancy. Skin breakdown, less common in the axilla, is more common at the elbow. Stage IV ulceration with visible muscle and tendon can be seen and is commonly associated with severe contracture (see Fig. 11-7A). Five muscles can flex the elbow: biceps, brachialis, brachioradialis, pronator teres, and extensor carpi radialis. The brachioradialis, pronator teres and biceps

are typical offenders, but the brachialis is less of a problem in our opinion. When the forearm is fixed in pronation, particularly by a combination of overactive pronator quadratus and paretic supinators, the pronator teres can exert flexion torque across the elbow by reverse origin-insertion action. The extensor carpi radialis can exert similar flexor torque on a similar basis of tenodesis when the wrist is fixed in

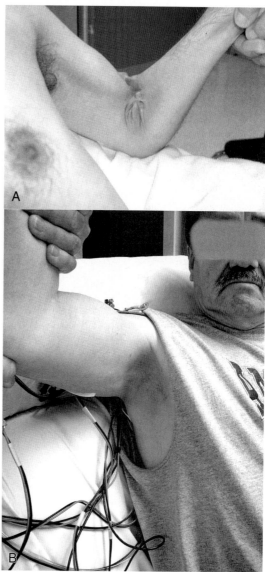

FIGURE 11-7. A, Redundant skin folds lead to moisture accumulation, bacterial overgrowth, skin irritation, skin breakdown, and ulceration. Note contracted skin folds, a result of many cycles of skin breakdown and healing against a background of severe elbow flexion contracture. **B,** A hemiparetic patient with shoulder adductor muscle overactivity and a reddened, irritated axilla.

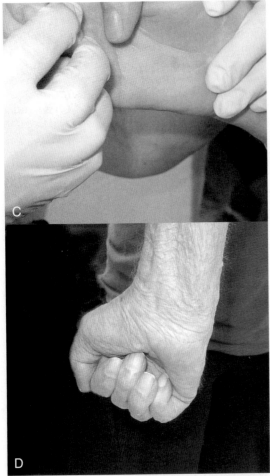

FIGURE 11-7 cont'd. C, Patients are examined for interdigital and palmer accumulations of moisture, irritation and breakdown. Note moisture in palm creases. **D,** Flexor digitorum profundus can drive fingernails into palmer skin and cause skin laceration.

malodor is particularly offensive, easily transferred to the examiner's skin, and not so quickly removed with washing. Patients are examined for interdigital and palmer accumulations of moisture, irritation, and breakdown. (see Fig. 11-7C). Nailbed infections including paronychia can occur. Infection of a fingernail bed can drive muscle overactivity, presumably through enhanced FRA activity, exacerbating clenching. When fingernails are burrowed into the palm and not easily visible, the flexor digitorum profundus (FDP) is involved. FDP can drive fingernails into palmer skin and cause laceration (see Fig. 11-7D). When the flexor digitorum sublimis (FDS) is involved, the fist may be clenched but the fingernails are visible because the distal interphalangeal joint (DIP) joints are extended. Both groups are often simultaneously involved but individual finger variation is surprisingly common. Electrical stimulation helps identify individual muscle fascicles of FDS and FDP prior to focal injection. At the thumb, metacarpophalangeal (MP) and interphalangeal joint (IP) skin folds can become macerated and reddened. IP flexion originates in overactivity of the flexor pollicis longus (FPL), and the thumb's fingernail can dig into index finger or palmer skin. MP flexion could be the result of FPL overactivity, but the flexor pollicis brevis (FPB) may also be involved. Pressure of a flexed thumb sometimes blanches and irritates the skin on the radial side of the index finger. The adductor pollicis (AP), FPB, and FPL may be involved.

flexion by overactive wrist and finger flexors. Midposition elbows are more typical of the brachioradialis and biceps, not pronator teres. A supinated flexed elbow is more typical of the biceps and brachialis, not the pronator teres and brachioradialis.

At the wrist, it is uncommon to see frank skin breakdown at the crease. Nevertheless, extreme flexor torque at the wrist can lead to skin maceration and irritation. Skin of the proximal palm, particularly when the wrist is flexed and ulnarly deviated, combined with tenting of the volar skin of the distal forearm can produce skin folds overhanging the wrist crease that trap moisture and become macerated. At the fingers, a clenched fist leads to a damp palm with skin irritation and malodor. The examiner should wear gloves because

BONE AND JOINT INTEGRITY

Before the emergence of positive signs, the negative sign of shoulder muscle paresis often results in gravity-driven stretch of the shoulder capsule. This produces inferior subluxation, which is usually self-limited and typically improving when activity in supraspinatus and the deltoids returns during antigravity standing. Occasionally, subluxation becomes chronic, especially when neurologic recovery is poor, causing pain when the arm is not supported during standing or sitting. Pain may be due to chronic stretch on the shoulder capsule, upper trapezius muscle, or from traction on the brachial plexus.[62] If pain improves with manual reduction and support of the subluxation, a mechanical pain mechanism can be assumed and treatment focuses on reducing the subluxation. Conservative approaches have included electrical stimulation to the deltoid and supraspinatus muscles or the use of a shoulder orthosis, but for practical reasons, a sling is commonly used. A sling relieves pain by supporting the humeral head in the glenoid and minimizing traction on shoulder structures. If the pain does not remit without a sling, some patients do not accept wearing the sling indefinitely and they can opt for surgical solutions that have included suspension procedures using ligaments[63] or the tendon of the long head of the biceps.[64]

Adhesive capsulitis can occur in patients with UMNS and also in those who develop a complex regional pain syndrome.[62] Glenohumeral motion becomes limited and painful. A painful stage is followed by an adhesive stage and a recovery stage; the course of the condition can extend for many months. Nonsteroidal anti-inflammatory drugs, physical therapy, and intra-articular injections are typical treatments. Selected cases may benefit from manipulation under anesthesia. Shoulder pain originating in bone and joint structures is often misinterpreted as painful spasticity, and treatment with BoNT is often requested. When shoulder muscle overactivity is present, we believe that BoNT treatment may be reasonable, not for treating painful spasticity, but for facilitating physical therapy. Weakening the contractile tension of large overactive muscles such as the pectoralis major, latissimus dorsi, and teres major will aid a physical therapy approach that needs to be aggressive in order to restore the severe loss of motion of adhesive capsulitis. The ability to wash the axilla and apply deodorant is very much hindered by lost, painful range of motion. When adhesive capsulitis has not responded adequately to nonoperative treatment, fluid expansion of the capsule or arthroscopic capsular release may be considered.[65]

Subluxation of the wrist can occur when there is excessive flexor overactivity and marked wrist extensor weakness (Fig. 11-8). Although the palmaris longus is missing in a small percentage of normal individuals, when present, this muscle contributes to wrist flexor torque along with flexor carpi radialis (FCR) and flexor carpi ulnaris (FCU).[66] The extrinsic finger flexors also promote wrist flexor torque. A severely subluxed wrist hampers donning a shirt, jacket sleeve, or winter gloves; prevents range-of-motion exercises; and facilitates carpal tunnel syndrome.

When bones of paretic limbs are deprived of muscular tension, osteoporosis can develop,

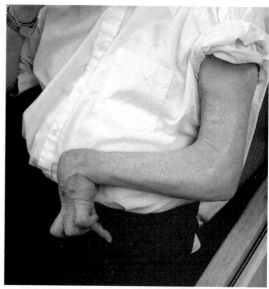

FIGURE 11-8. Subluxation of the wrist can occur when there is excessive flexor overactivity and marked wrist extensor weakness.

making a patient more prone to fracture.[67] Falls are a common mechanism of fracture in patients with central neurologic disease, but stress fractures, especially of the humerus, may occur when paralyzed patients are subjected to twisting, torsion, and pressure on the upper limbs during physical lift of the patient from bed to chair. Transfer by means of a Hoyer lift is preferable. From time to time, orthopaedic procedures such as hip dislocation interventions or joint replacement may be required in a patient with UMNS. In the postoperative period, intense muscle overactivity, triggered by FRA activity in tissues of the operative site, may disrupt soft tissue healing and threaten dislocation of hardware. Postoperative spasm can be painful and prolongs hospitalization.[68] The use of BoNT pre-emptively has been recommended in such patients.[69] It has been our practice to deliver BoNT to potentially offending muscles 2 to 3 weeks before surgery.

PHYSICAL PRESSURE AND INJURY

A variety of pressure phenomena may be attributed to muscle overactivity that leads to persistent postural attitudes. When the FDP is excessively active, fingernails dig into palmer skin, causing pressure marks, frank laceration,

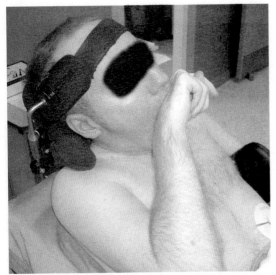

FIGURE 11-9. A flexed elbow and adducted, internally rotated shoulder can combine to press a fist into the chest, throat or face.

after chemodenervation to reduce the inevitable flexion contracture of the elbow is also a consideration. Ulnar nerve transposition may be needed.

In addition to median nerve fibers and blood vessels, the contents of the carpal tunnel also include tendons of the FDS, FDP, and FPL. Carpal tunnel syndrome (median neuropathy at the wrist) can develop in the presence of wrist flexion deformity caused by overactive finger and wrist flexors (Fig. 11-10). The tendons of overactive muscles coursing through the tunnel may increase pressure within the tunnel or cause compression or ischemia of the contents of the tunnel. The median nerve is often compressed against the leading or proximal edge of the transverse carpal ligament. Complaints of tingling, dysesthesia, and thenar atrophy should raise suspicion of carpal tunnel syndrome. The pain of carpal tunnel syndrome can exacerbate muscle overactivity elsewhere.

and infection (see Fig. 11-7D). A flexed elbow and an adducted, internally rotated shoulder can combine to press a fist into the chest, throat, or face (Fig. 11-9). Patients have complained of phasic flexor spasms in the upper limb that strike the upper chest, throat or jaw. At night, such spasms interfere with sleep. Prolonged posturing can lead to peripheral nerve injury. Persistent elbow flexion produces stretch and traction on the ulnar nerve, which wraps around the elbow in the cubital tunnel (see Fig. 11-8). Ulnar nerve injury can also be caused by chronic nerve pressure from a wheelchair's armrest when a patient with UMNS has little voluntary ability to unload the pressure. A patient with chronic elbow flexion who develops an intrinsic minus claw hand deformity hand (see Fig. 11-8) should be suspected of having ulnar nerve involvement at the elbow. Ulnar innervated intrinsic muscles of the hand flex the MP joints and extend the proximal interphalangeal (PIP) joints. Ulnar neuropathy produces an intrinsic minus deformity, featured as extension of the MP joints along with flexion at the PIP joints (see Fig. 11-8). The resulting unsightly claw hand affects the integrity of body image and gets hooked annoyingly on sleeves, coats, and sweaters. In the presence of chronic elbow flexion at 90 degrees or more, chemodenervation of elbow flexors (biceps, brachioradialis, brachialis and pronator teres) may be considered pre-emptively to reduce the degree of flexion. Serial casting several weeks

SOFT TISSUE INTEGRITY

Lost range of motion associated with muscle contracture is commonly seen after UMNS.[34,70,71] In the presence of high stretch sensitivity, determining the amount of lost motion and contracture can be confounded by dynamic stretch reflex activity. A temporary local anesthetic block often unmasks additional range of motion. The loss of range of

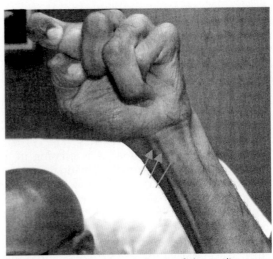

FIGURE 11-10. Pressure or ischemia of the median nerve by overactive finger and wrist flexors can produce carpal tunnel syndrome. Arrows point to bowstringing tendons of flexor carpi radialis, palmaris longus, and superficial finger flexor mass.

motion created by a contracture impairs or exacerbates the following: loss of skin integrity, stretch neuropathy, the effectiveness of residual voluntary movement, dressing, hygiene and grooming functions, and appearance of disfigurement. At the shoulder, adduction and internal rotation contracture limits access to the axilla necessary for dressing, washing, shaving axillary hair, and applying deodorant. A lack of abduction is more important for activities of daily living (ADLs) than a lack of external rotation. In addition to contracture, muscle overactivity may be present in some or all of the adductors/internal rotators including the pectoralis major, teres major, and latissimus dorsi.[61] Clinical palpation during elicitation of positive signs may help the examiner identify muscle contraction suitable for BoNT intervention. Dynamic EMG studies and local anesthetic blocks may also be of help to predict potential effects of longer term blocks. Phenol block of the thoracodorsal nerve, the medial and lateral pectoral nerves, and motor point of the teres major facilitates physical therapy within a few days. BoNT treatment is followed by aggressive physical stretching approximately 2 weeks after injection, when clinical blocking action should be well under way.

At the elbow, severe flexion contracture promotes tissue redundancy in the elbow crease, leading to maceration, redness, and skin breakdown (see Fig. 11-7). Washing the crease and dressing around the bend of the elbow is hampered by fixed deformity. Elbow flexion contracture greater than 90 degrees promotes ulnar nerve stretch neuropathy. In addition to contracture, muscle overactivity may be present in some or all of the following elbow flexors: biceps, brachialis, brachioradialis, and pronator teres. Clinical palpation during elicitation of positive signs may help the examiner identify muscle contraction suitable for BoNT intervention. Dynamic EMG studies and local anesthetic blocks may also be of help to predict potential effects of longer term blocks. Reduction of elbow flexion contracture, in the presence of muscle overactivity, is handled with blocks followed by serial casting.[70,72] Casting may proceed immediately after blocking with phenol, a drug with local anesthetic properties. Casting after BoNT is initiated about 2 weeks after injection, when clinical blocking action should be well under way. At the forearm, pronation contracture orients the palm and fingers away from the patient's field of vision, hindering such functions as hand washing, fingernail grooming, donning of gloves and splints, and

for diabetics, performing blood glucose finger sticks. Pronator teres and pronator quadratus may be involved. If these muscles are overactive, BoNT can reduce their neural contribution to muscle tone and facilitate contracture lessening physical techniques.[70]

At the wrist, flexion contracture can lead to maceration, irritation, and breakdown in the wrist crease. Sleeve openings may need to be made larger to accommodate a severely flexed wrist. Carpal tunnel syndrome occurs. Patients have a particular dislike of wrist flexion and clenched fist deformities, neither of which may be covered up by clothing. The wrist flexors and extrinsic finger flexors pass in front of the wrist's axis of rotation; hence, both of these muscle groups can contribute to wrist flexion deformity. Tightness of each group is tested separately. When fingers are held flexed, passive extension of the wrist tests wrist flexor tightness. Fully extending the fingers before extending the wrist adds the finger flexor contribution to flexor resistance across the wrist. Serial casting preceded by BoNT injection of overactive wrist flexors and finger flexors is a useful strategy. A hyperextended wrist is seen less frequently than a flexed wrist but can cause greater hand problems. The hyperextended wrist promotes a clenched fist because of finger flexor tenodesis. Lengthening of finger flexors passing ventral to the axis of rotation of the wrist generates more passive tension according to their tension-length curve, causing the fingers to flex into the palm. Positive signs also may add input to finger flexors, enhancing the clenching behavior. BoNT injection of overactive wrist extensors (extensor carpi radialis [ECR], extensor carpi radialis brevis [ECRB], and extensor carpi ulnaris [ECU]) helps promote a more neutral position of the wrist, lessening the tenodesis effect of wrist hyperextension.

For the fingers, a tight FDS is characterized by severe flexion of the MCP and PIP joints but not of the DIP joints.[61] Although the fist is clenched, the fingernails are visible and the pads of the fingers typically touch the palm. If FDP is involved, the fingernails are buried into the palm, often indenting or even lacerating the palmer skin. Contracture of the finger flexors is likely when the fingers cannot be extended unless the wrist is flexed. Dynamic EMG studies of FDS and FDP with intramuscular wire electrodes can provide information about the neural component. Local anesthetic blocks of selective median branches to FDS and FDP may provide similar information. Extrinsic finger flexor contracture of nonneural origin may be treated with serial casting. If a strong neural contribution is also present, BoNT can be a helpful adjunct to serial casting, initiated about 2 weeks after injection. Contracture of the intrinsic muscles results in a roof top hand. The MCP joints are flexed about 90 degrees, whereas the PIP and DIP joints are fully extended. When the MCP joints are flexed, the PIP joints cannot be flexed because of intrinsic muscle contracture. Swan neck deformity is found when FDP is overactive. The DIP joint is flexed (head of the Swan), whereas the long neck of the Swan is a PIP joint that is extended or abnormally hyperextended 15 degrees or more. The intrinsic plus deformity narrows the space between the fingers, making these slit-like areas vulnerable to maceration, malodor and ulceration. BoNT for overactivity combined with stretch splinting techniques is a potentially useful strategy.

For the thumb, contracture of FPL produces a thumb-in-palm deformity.[73] The thumbnail may notch the index finger or the nail may dig into the palm. Redundant skin over the crease of the IP joint attracts moisture. Flexion contracture of the intrinsic FPB exacerbates redundant skin, especially the larger fold of the MP joint, which macerates easily. Contracture of the AP narrows the web space and makes insertion of objects into the palm through the web space difficult or impossible, preventing the hand from being used as a holder. BoNT for the neural component combined with serial casting for the nonneural component is a potentially useful strategy. Tendon lengthenings, transfers, capsuloplasties, plastic skin procedures, and joint fusions are alternative peripheral strategies for upper limb joints with contracture.

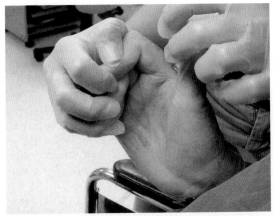

FIGURE 11-11. Tight finger flexors impede access to hand and fingers, and make thorough hand washing difficult. Frequent washing and drying is required to keep the hand free of malodor.

across the palm may counter maceration and malodor. Resting hand splints, meant to maintain wrist and finger position, are not always popular with patients because torque exerted by clenched fingers against a hard splint surface can cause pain and skin blanching. A proper and comfortable fit is not always predictable when the intensity of positive signs varies throughout the day and their effectiveness has been questioned.[76] A clenched fist often makes cutting, cleaning, and polishing fingernails difficult. A pronated forearm compounds the problem because it causes the palm to be down and away from the patient, making one-handed nail care impossible to do. Someone else has to supinate the forearm if the patient wants to do the care. If someone else provides nail care, a combined clenched fist and flexed wrist can be very problematic for them.

PERSONAL CARE INTEGRITY

UMNS patterns of deformity can hinder hygiene, dressing, and grooming and reducing positive signs such as arm spasticity has been associated with improved arm function.[74,75] Patients and caregivers often have to struggle against hypertonic muscles to perform personal care. For example, tight adductors reduce access to the axilla making ADLs and personal care difficult. Tight finger flexors impede access to the hand and fingers, and make thorough hand washing difficult (Fig. 11-11). More time and more frequent washing and drying are required to keep the hand free of malodor. Hand splints that prop fingers open and allow air to circulate

BODY IMAGE INTEGRITY

Integrity of body image is a normal psychological desire and is important for emotional balance. Patients react negatively to the appearance of various UMNS deformities such as a flexed elbow, bent wrist, clenched fist, and thumb-in-palm deformity.[77] They complain that their postures are ugly and unsightly. (see Figs. 11-1, 11-3B, 11-6, and 11-7A).[78] Patients with deformity may intuitively feel that their appearance signals a lessening of their value as an individual, a sign of their imperfection for socialization, sexuality, and vocational pursuits.[79,80] Medical treatment to redress the grievance of a body image deformity is wrongly understood if such treatment is construed as cosmetic and not as an important part of a patient's rehabilitation treatment, both physical and psychological, after sustaining a severe neurologic insult. In the context of UMNS, the psychological distress of altered body image is intimately bound up with how a person feels about himself or herself, distressed feelings that truly serve as a barrier to the rehabilitation process.[81,82]

CONCLUSION

UMNS has classically been described in terms of positive and negative signs. The combined effects of chronically recurring positive and negative signs produces a net balance of muscle torques around individual upper limb joints that lead to maladaptive skin and musculoskeletal consequences. Two broad approaches, central strategy and peripheral strategy, have emerged to treat the consequences of maladaptive torques. Central strategy attempts to modify CNS pathways that generate muscle overactivity. Peripheral strategy directs treatment toward specific muscles and other soft tissues that generate maladaptive torques. Peripheral strategy serves as a basis for many orthopaedic procedures, physical and occupational therapy techniques, neurotomies, and neurolysis. In recent years, BoNT has become a good example of a useful peripheral strategy, but its success requires specific identification of offending muscles that create maladaptive skin and musculoskeletal consequences.

References

1. Sheean G. The pathophysiology of spasticity. *Eur J Neurol.* 2002;9(suppl 1):3-9.
2. Mayer NH, Herman RM. Phenomenology of muscle overactivity in the upper motor neuron syndrome. *Eura Medicophys.* 2004;40:85-110.
3. Gracies JM, Elovic E, Zorowitz R, McGuire J, Simpson D. Traditional pharmacologic treatments for spasticity part I: Local treatments. In: Brashear A, Mayer NH, eds. *Spasticity and Other Forms of Muscle Overactivity in the Upper Motor Neuron Syndrome: Etiology, Evaluation, Management and the Role of Botulinum Toxin.* New York: WE MOVE; 2008:57-79.
4. Burke D. Spasticity as an adaptation to pyramidal tract injury. In Waxman SG, ed. *Functional recovery in neurological disease, advances in neurology.* New York: Raven Press; 1988:401-423.
5. Walshe FMR. On certain tonic or postural reflexes in hemiplegia, with special reference to the so-called 'associated movements'. *Brain.* 1923;46:1-37.
6. Bourbonnais D. Quantification of upper limb synkinesis in hemiparetic subjects. *Rehabilitation R & D Progress Report 1994.* Dept of Veterans Affairs 32, 1995:118-119.
7. Dewald JPA, Rymer WZ. Factors underlying abnormal posture and movement in spastic hemiparesis. In: Thilmann AF, Burke DJ, Rymer WZ, eds. *Spasticity: mechanisms and management.* Berlin: Springer-Verlag; 1993. p. 123-138.
8. Sheean G. Neurophysiology of spasticity. In: Barnes MP, Johnson GR, eds. *Upper Motor Neurone Syndrome and Spasticity, Clinical Management and Neurophysiology.* Cambridge, UK: Cambridge University Press; 2001:12-78.
9. Palmeri A, Weisendanger M. Concomitant depression of locus coerulus neurons and of flexor reflexes by an alpha-2 adrenergic agonist in rats: A possible mechanism for an alpha-2 mediated muscle relaxation. *Neuroscience.* 1990;34:177-187.
10. Whitlock JA. Neurophysiology of spasticity. In: Glen MB, Whyte J, eds. *The Practical Management of Spasticity in Children and Adults.* Philadelphia: Lea & Febiger; 1990:8-33.
11. Jankowska E, Lackberg ZS, Dyrehag LE. Effects of monoamines on transmission from group II muscle afferents in sacral segments in the cat. *Eur J Neurosci.* 1994;6:1058-1061.
12. Baldissera F, Hultborn H, Illert M. Integration in spinal neuronal systems. *Handbook of Physiology.* Bethesda: American Physiological Society; 1981:509.
13. Lance JW. Pyramidal and extrapyramidal disorders. In: Shahani DT, ed. *Electromyography in CNS Disorders: Central EMG.* Boston: Butterworth; 1984:1-19.
14. Benecke R. Spasticity/spasms: clinical aspects and treatment. In: Berardelli A, Benecke R, Manfield M, Marsden C, eds. *Motor Disturbances.* London: Academic Press; 1990:169-177.
15. Smith C, Birnbaum G, et al, US Tizanidine Study Group. Tizanidine treatment of spasticity caused by multiple sclerosis: results of a double-blind, placebo-controlled trial. *Neurology.* 1994;44(suppl 9):34-44.
16. Herman R, Freedman W, Meeks SM. Physiological aspects of hemiplegic and paraplegic spasticity. In: Desmedt JE, ed. *New Developments in Electromyography and Clinical Neurophysiology,* Basel: Karger; 1973: 579-588.
17. Coffey R, Cahill D, Steers W. Intrathecal baclofen for intractable spasticity of spinal origin: results of a long-term multicenter study. *J Neurosurg.* 1993;45: 833-837.
18. Meythaler JM, Guin-Renfroe S, Brunner RC, Johnson A, Hadley MN. Intrathecal baclofen for spastic hypertonia from stroke. *Stroke.* 2001;32:2099-2109.
19. Lance JW. Symposium synopsis. In Feldman RG, Young RR, Koella WP, eds. *Spasticity: Disordered Motor Control.* Chicago: Yearbook Medical; 1980:485-494.
20. Nathan P. Some comments on spasticity and rigidity. In: Desmedt JE, ed. *New Developments an Electromyography and Clinical Neurophysiology.* Basel: Karger; 1973:13-14.
21. Gracies JM, Elovic E, Zorowitz R, McGuire J, Simpson D. Traditional pharmacologic treatments for spasticity part II: Systemic treatments. In: Brashear A, Mayer NH, eds. *Spasticity and Other Forms of Muscle Overactivity in the Upper Motor Neuron Syndrome: Etiology, Evaluation. Management and the Role of Botulinum Toxin.* New York: WE MOVE; 2008:79-109.
22. Matthews PBC. Muscle spindles: their messages and their fusimotor supply. In: Brooks VB, ed. *Handbook of Physiology.* Vol. II. Bethesda: American Physiological Society; 1981:189.

23. Bergfeldt U, Borg K, Kullander K, Julin P. Focal spasticity therapy with botulinum toxin: effects on function, activities of daily living and pain in 100 adult patients. *J Rehabil Med.* 2006;38:166-171.

24. Bhakta BB, Couzens JA, Chamberlain MA, Bamford JM. Impact of botulinum toxin type A on disability and carer burden due to arm spasticity after stroke: a randomized double blind placebo controlled trial. *J Neurol Neurosurg Psychiatry.* 2000;69:217-221.

25. Herman R. The myotatic reflex. Clinico-physiological aspects of spasticity and contracture. *Brain.* 1970;93:273-312.

26. Katz RT, Rymer WZ. Spastic hypertonia: mechanisms and measurement. *Arch Phys Med Rehabil.* 1989;70:144-155.

27. Powers RK, Marder-Meyer J, Rymer WZ. Quantitative relations between hypertonia and stretch reflex threshold in spastic hemiparesis. *Ann Neurol.* 1988;23:115.

28. Hufschmidt A, Mauritz KH. Chronic transformation of muscle in spasticity: A peripheral contribution to increased tone. *J Neurol Neurosurg Psychiatry.* 1985;48:676-685.

29. Dietz V, Trippel M, Burger W. Reflex activity and muscle tone during elbow movements in patients with spastic paresis. *Ann Neurol.* 1991;30:767-779.

30. Herbert R. The passive mechanical properties of muscle and their adaptations to altered pattern of use. *Aust J Physiother.* 1988;34:141-149.

31. Thilmann AF, Fellows SJ, Ross HF. Biomechanical changes at the ankle joint after stroke. *J Neurol Neurosurg Psychiatry.* 1991;54:134-139.

32. Graham H, Selber P. Musculoskeletal aspects of cerebral palsy. *J Bone Joint Surg.* 2003;85-B:157-166.

33. Zablotny C, Andric MF, Gowland C. Serial casting: Clinical applications for the adult head-injured patient. *J Head Trauma Rehabil.* 1987;2(2):46-52.

34. Keenan MAE, Mayer NH, Esquenazi A, Pelensky JA. Neuro-orthopaedic approach to the management of common patterns of upper motoneuron dysfunction after brain injury. *NeuroRehabilitation.* 1999;12:119-144.

35. Keenan M. Upper extremity orthoses for the brain injured patient. In: Goldberg B, Hsu JD, eds. *Atlas of Orthoses and Assistive Devices.* St. Louis: Mosby-Year Book, Inc.; 1997:95-112.

36. Damiano DL. Reviewing muscle co-contraction: is it a developmental, pathological, or motor control issue. *Phys Occup Ther Pediatr.* 1993;12:3-20.

37. Gracies J. Pathophysiology of spastic paresis. II: Emergence of muscle overactivity. *Muscle Nerve.* 2005;31:552-571.

38. Delwaide PJ, Oliver E. Pathophysiological aspects of spasticity in man. In: Benecke R, Marsden CD, eds. *Motor Disturbances.* London: Academic Press; 1987:153-168.

39. Okuma Y, Lee RG. Reciprocal inhibition in hemiplegia: Correlation with clinical features in recovery. *Can J Neurol Sci.* 1996;23:15-23.

40. Fellows SJ, Klaus C, Ross HF, Thilmann AF. Agonist and antagonist EMG activation during isometric torque development at the elbow and spastic hemiparesis. *Electroencephalogr Clin Neurophysiol.* 1994;93:106-112.

41. Humphrey DR, Reed DJ. Separate cortical systems for control of joint movement and joint stiffness: reciprocal activation and co-activation of antagonist muscles. In: Desmedt JE, ed. *Motor control mechanisms in health and disease.* New York: Raven Press; 1983: 347-372.

42. Gracies JM, Wilson L, Gandevia SC, Burke D. Stretch position of spastic muscles aggravates their co-contraction in hemiplegic patients. *Ann Neurol.* 1997;42: 438-439.

43. Gracies JM. Physiological effects of botulinum toxin in spasticity. *Mov Disord.* 2004;19(Suppl 8): S120-128.

44. Denny-Brown D. *The Cerebral Control of Movement,* Liverpool: University Press; 1966.

45. Denny-Brown D. Historical aspects of the relation of spasticity to movement. In: Feldman RG, Young RR, Koella WP, eds. *Spasticity: Disordered Movement Control.* Chicago: Year Book Medical Publishers; 1980:1-15.

46. Axelson HW. Signs of muscle thixotropy during human ballistic wrist joint movements. *J Appl Physiol.* 2005;99:1922-1929.

47. Vattanasilp W, Ada L, Crosbie J. Contribution of thixotropy, spasticity, and contracture to ankle stiffness after stroke. *J Neurol Neurosurg Psychiatry.* 2006;69: 34-39.

48. Gracies J. Pathophysiology of spastic paresis. I: Paresis and soft tissue changes. *Muscle Nerve.* 2005;31: 535-551.

49. Mayer NH, Esquenazi A, Childers MK. Common patterns of clinical motor dysfunction. In: Mayer NH, Simpson DM, eds. *Spasticity: Etiology, Evaluation, Management and the Role of Botulinum Toxin.* New York: WE MOVE; 2002:16-26.

50. Pohl M, Mehrholz J, Rockstroh G, Ruckriem S, Koch R. Contractures and involuntary muscle overactivity in severe brain injury. *Brain Inj.* 2007;21:421-432.

51. O'Dwyer N, Ada L, Neilson PD. Spasticity and muscle contracture following stroke. *Brain.* 1996;119: 1737-1749.

52. Akeson WH, Woo SLY, Amiel D, Coutts RD, Daniel D. The connective tissue response to immobility: Biochemical changes in periarticular connective tissue of the immobilized rabbit knee. *Clin Orthop.* 1973; 93:356.

53. Gossman MR, Rose SJ, Sahrmann SA, Katholi CR. Length and circumference measurement in one-joint and multijoint muscles in rabbits after immobilization. *Phys Ther.* 1986;66:516-520.

54. Carey JR, Burghardt DT. Movement dysfunction following CNS lesions: a problem of neurologic or muscular impairment. *Phys Ther.* 1993;73:538-547.

55. Tabary JC, Tabary C, Tardieu C, Tardieu G, Goldspink G. Physiological and structural changes in the cat soleus muscle due to immobilization at different lengths by plaster casts. *J Physiol.* (Lond) 1972; 224:231-244.

56. Williams PE, Goldspink G. Changes in sarcomere length and physiological properties in immobilized muscle. *J Anat.* 1978;127:459-468.

57. Witzmann FA, Kim DH, Fitts RH. Hindlimb immobilization: length-tension and contractile properties of skeletal muscle. *J Applied Physiol.* 1982;53: 335-345.

58. Friden J, Lieber RL. Spastic muscle cells are shorter and stiffer than normal cells. *Muscle Nerve.* 2003; 26:157-164.

59. Ponten E, Gantelius S, Lieber RL. Intraoperative muscle measurments reveal a relationship between contracture formation and muscle remodeling. *Muscle Nerve.* 2007;36:47-54.

60. Sheean G. Botulinum toxin treatment of adult spasticity: A benefit-risk assessment. *Drug Safety.* 2006; 29:31-48.

61. Mayer N. Choosing upper limb muscles for focal intervention after traumatic brain injury. *J Head Trauma Rehabil.* 2004;19:119-142.

62. Keenan MAE, Mehta S. Neuro-Orthopedic management of shoulder deformity and dysfunction in brain-injured patients. *J Head Trauma Rehabil.* 2004;19:143-154.

63. Braun RM, Botte MJ. Treatment of shoulder deformity in acquired spasticity. *Clin Orthop Rel Res.* 1999;368:54-65.

64. McDaid PK, Keenan MAE. Management of upper extremity dysfunction following stroke and brain injury. In: Chapman M, ed. *Chapman's Orthopaedic Surgery,* Philadelphia: Lippincott Williams & Wilkins; 2001:1809-1854.

65. Ogilvie-Harris DJ, Biggs DJ, Fitsialos DP, MacKay M. The resistant frozen shoulder: Manipulation versus arfthroscopic release. *Clin Orthop Rel Res.* 1995;319:238-248.

66. Thompson NW, Mockford BJ, Cran GW. Absence of palmaris longus muscle:a population study. *Ulster Med J.* 2001;70:22-24.

67. Lloyd M, Spector TD, Howard R. Osteoporosis in neurological disorders. *J Neurol Neurosurg Psychiatry.* 2000;68:543-547.

68. Nolan J, Chalkiadis GA, Low J, Olesch CA, Brown TC. Anaesthesia and pain management in cerebral palsy. *Anaesthesia.* 2000;55(1):32-41.

69. Barwood S, Baillieu C, Boyd R, Brereton K, Low J, Nattress G, et al. Analgesic effects of botulinum toxin A: a randomized, placebo-controlled clinical trial. *Dev Med Child Neurol.* 2000;42:116-121.

70. Mayer NH, Esquenazi A, Keenan MAE. Assessing and treating muscle overactivity in the upper motoneuron syndrome. In: Zasler ND, Katz D, Zafonte RD, eds. *Brain Injury Medicine.* New York: Demos; 2007:615-653.

71. Ada L, O'Dwyer N, O'Neill E. Relation between spasticity, weakness and contracture of the elbow flexors and upper limb activity after stroke: an observational study. *Disabil Rehabil.* 2006;28:891-897.

72. Lannin NA, Novak I, Cusick A. A systematic review of upper extremity casting for children and adults with central nervous system motor disorders. *Clin Rehabil.* 2007;21:963-976.

73. Mayer NH, Esquenazi A. Muscle overactivity and movement dysfunction in the upper motoneuron syndrome. *Phys Med Clin North Am.* 2003;14:855-863.

74. Francis HP, Wade DT, Turner-Stokes L, Kingswell RS, Dott CS, Coxon EA. Does reducing spasticity translate into functional benefit? An exploratory meta-analysis. *J Neurol Neurosurg Psychiatry.* 2004;75:1547-1551.

75. Rousseaux M, Kozlowski O, Froger J. Efficacy of botulinum toxin A in upper limb function of hemiplegic patients. *J Neurol.* 2002;249:76-84.

76. Lannin NA, Cusick A, McCluskey A, Herbert RD. Effects of splinting on wrist contracture after stroke: a randomized controlled trial. *Stroke.* 2007;38:111-116.

77. Kvigne K, Kirkevold M. Living with bodily strangeness: women's experiences of their changing and unpredictable body following a stroke. *Qual Health Res.* 2003;13(9):1291-1310.

78. Piotrowski MM. Body image after a stroke. *Rehabil Nurs.* 1982;7:11-13.

79. Carleton V. Sexuality after a stroke. *Nurs N Z.* 1995;1:13-15.

80. O'Connell B, Hanna B, Penney W, Pearce J, Owen M, Warelow P. Recovery after stroke: a qualitative perspective. *J Qual Clin Pract.* 2001;21:120-125.

81. Ellis-Hill C, Payne S, Ward C. Using stroke to explore the Life Thread Model: An alternative approach to understanding rehabilitation following acquired disability. *Disabil Rehabil.* 2007;29:1-10.

82. White MA, Johnstone AS. Recovery from stroke: does rehabilitation counselling have a role to play? *Disabil Rehabil.* 2000;22:140-143.

Clinical Trials of Botulinum Toxin in Adult Spasticity

12

Antonio E. Elia, Filippini Graziella, and Alberto Albanese

INTRODUCTION

Spasticity is defined as a velocity-dependent increase in stretch reflex activity and is one of the forms of muscle overactivity that may affect patients with damage to the central nervous system (CNS), particularly either the brain or the spinal cord.[1] Spasticity is a sign of the upper motor neuron syndrome that is characterized by a combination of positive and negative signs, including hypertonia, involuntary movements (spasms, clonus), decreased range of motion (ROM), contractures, and spasm-related pain (Table 12-1). The most common causes of spasticity are acute CNS lesions, such as stroke or traumatic spinal cord and brain injuries. In addition, spasticity can be caused by neurodegenerative (such as amyotrophic lateral sclerosis) or inflammatory (such as multiple sclerosis) CNS disorder. Spasticity predisposes to the development of contractures, leading to further functional impairment.

Spastic features normally establish gradually, also following an acute CNS lesion, then improve spontaneously during the months following onset and stabilize. The relationship between the clinical features of spasticity and the ensuing disability has not been completely established. In clinical trials on antispasticity drugs, the observed reduction in spasticity has not been unequivocally associated with clear functional gains in daily living activities. There are possible ways to explain the failure to observe functional gain in patients treated with antispastic agents that are efficacious in reducing spasticity. First, it is possible that spasticity does not contribute as much as the associated weakness to the observed limitation of function.[2] Second, the published studies may have been inadequately powered to detect functional gain or, third, the outcome measures used were insufficiently sensitive.[3]

Rehabilitation programs for patients with spasticity must take into account several variables in addition to changes of excitability within spinal neural networks. Considerable intrinsic muscular changes may contribute to a continuous rigidity while muscles are stretched, a phenomenon that, in turn, enhances stretch reflex responses.[4] The spastic posture and deformity of the affected limb often prove to be particularly disabling. Patients suffering from stroke frequently develop flexor spasticity of the upper limb that impairs motor usage of the hand; their caregivers, therefore, have to face problems such as maintaining hygiene and dressing. On the other hand ability to stand or walk usually relies on a certain degree of residual spasticity, and treatment plans often involve a trade-off between spasticity reduction and preservation of residual motor function.[5]

A number of spasticity treatments are available, such as physical therapy, oral antispastic medication (e.g., baclofen and tizanidine) and intrathecal agents (e.g., baclofen). Oral medications often provide limited relief and frequently lead to side effects. Intrathecal baclofen, instead, provides a significant reduction of muscle tone and some ensuing functional gain; however, this is an invasive

Drs. Elia and Graziella do not report any conflicts of interest. Dr. Albanese is disclosing that he is associated with NTI, and has worked on advisory boards for Allergan, Ipsen, and Merz.

TABLE 12-1 Upper Motor Neuron Syndrome: Positive and Negative Signs

Positive Signs	Negative Signs
Phasic and tonic stretch reflexes[51,52]	Muscle weakness[52]
Co-contraction[52]	Loss of finger dexterity[52]
Released flexor reflexes[52,53]	Loss of selective control of limb movement
Associated reactions (synkinesia)[52]	
Spastic dystonia[52]	
Increased muscle stiffness that may contribute to contracture[52,53]	

treatment that requires an implantation procedure and can lead to adverse reactions such as headache, nausea, and excessive weakness. Neuromuscular blockade by local injections of phenol or alcohol effectively reduce spasticity but are limited mainly by the occurrence of severe pain. In this scenario, focal injections of botulinum neurotoxin (BoNT) provide a simple and effective tool for the management of spasticity in specific body regions.

The management of spasticity aims at reducing disability and improving residual motor function based on clinical evaluation independent of the etiology. However, cases of spasticity secondary to an acute event (such as trauma or stroke) that is likely to have a unique occurrence provide ideal conditions to perform clinical evaluations of antispasticity treatments. By contrast, in cases with progressive or remitting clinical phenomenology, the outcome of antispasticity therapies is difficult to evaluate. The same is true for children who suffer from spasticity. Developmental changes significantly affect outcome in addition to antispastic treatments.

Outcome measures of spasticity evaluate variations of muscle tone, ROM, and limb posture. Measures of disability evaluate function in activities of daily living, hygiene, dressing, limb position, and pain interfering with daily activities. The relationship between spasticity and disability measures has not been ascertained, and this limitation provides uncertainty on the functional value of antispasticity treatments. A correlation with spasticity scores has been demonstrated only for the Disability Assessment Scale (DAS), which varies linearly with the Ashworth scale (AS).[6]

The present chapter reviews the available evidence on the use of BoNT/A and /B in managing spasticity in adult patients and differentiates between outcome on spasticity and on disability.

AVAILABLE OUTCOME MEASURES

In order to identify appropriate treatment objectives, it has been proposed to distinguish between active and passive function.[2] Active function is impaired when spasticity interferes directly with voluntary movement, whereas passive function is impaired when there is little or no residual voluntary movement, due to severe weakness, and spasticity does not contribute to the motor impairment. As far as active function is concerned, the goal of spasticity treatment is to reduce motor overactivity in order to improve movement; for passive function, instead, the goal is to reduce painful spasms and pain during mobilization, attain better hygiene or prevent contractures.

Measures of Spasticity

The most widely used spasticity measure is the AS, which was initially developed as a simple clinical tool to test the efficacy of antispastic drugs in patients with multiple sclerosis by evaluating the resistance perceived while moving a joint through its full range.[7] Later, the 1+ rating (falling between 1 and 2) was added with the aim to increase sensitivity (thus, yielding to the modified Ashworth Scale [MAS]).[8] The AS and the MAS can be used as an ordinal level measure, based on a five-point rating of muscle tone from zero ("no increase in tone") to four ("limb rigid in flexion or extension"). A study found that the scale is more reproducible in the upper than in the lower limb and that the AS is overall more reliable than the MAS.[9] The use of AS and MAS as outcome measures has been questioned because they evaluate resistance to passive movements rather than spasticity[10]; however, these scales remain the most widely used outcome measures in clinical trials, and have high inter-rater reliability.[11]

Other available measures of spasticity include the spasm frequency scale and indirect measures, such as goniometric assessment of ROM or analysis of postures.

The original Penn spasm frequency scale[12] was created to assess the antispastic effect of intrathecal baclofen and is based on the evaluation of the number of spasms per hour. Another scale measuring daily spasm frequency was used to evaluate the effect of BoNT injections in multiple sclerosis patients.[13] In this study, a "spasticity score" was created by multiplying ASs and spasm frequency.

Goniometric ROM assessment has good intra- and inter-rater reliability when applied to children with cerebral palsy.[14] ROM scores have been used for status and follow-up assessments of spasticity changes and correlate with ASs.[15] It has also been shown that ROM changes are sensitive to antispastic treatment in stroke patients.[16]

Analysis of body postures can also be used to monitor the effects of antispastic treatments in given clinical settings. The maximal distance between the knees can help monitoring the effects of treatment for hip adductor spasticity. Finger curl at rest and ankle position at rest can reflect antispastic therapeutic effects in patients with severe spasticity. These various clinical scales correlate poorly with each other, suggesting that each of them assesses different aspects of the spasticity syndrome.[17]

Measures of Disability

The selection of outcome measures to assess the functional impact of spasticity is not straightforward, and this is probably the reason why that in most spasticity studies, disability and functioning were not evaluated using comparable outcome measures. Furthermore, functional improvement has been rarely considered a primary outcome measure in studies evaluating spasticity treatments. Earlier studies have mainly assessed activities of daily living, which primarily measure the ability of an individual to perform activities required in daily chores, such as bathing, dressing, using the toilet, moving around the house, and eating. These are generic measures that estimate the patients' functional status regardless of the specific underlying impairment[18]; many spasticity studies have used other generic measures of disability, such as the functional independence measure (FIM) or the Barthel index, and generally they have not demonstrated changes directly related to variations of spasticity.[19] The lack of validated functional outcome measures is surprising, particularly because functional recovery is the primary goal of spasticity treatment in clinical practice.

Global Disability Scales

The FIM is an 18-item, seven-level, ordinal scale intended to be sensitive to changes over the course of a comprehensive inpatient medical rehabilitation program. It was designed to assess areas of dysfunction in activities that commonly occur in subjects with any progressive, reversible or stable neurologic, musculoskeletal, or other disorder. This scale encompasses few cognitive, behavioral, and communication-related functional items and is not specific to any diagnosis. The Barthel ADL index is the most widely used scale for activities of daily living. It measures 10 elementary aspects of activity related to self-care and mobility, such as walking, dressing, going to the toilet, and being continent. The validity and reliability of this nonspecific scale are supported by a number of studies.[20] The Fugl-Meyer physical performance scale assesses five dimensions of impairment, including three aspects of motor control: amplitude of joint movement, pain, sensitivity, motor impairment of the upper and lower extremities and balance. Each item is scored in an ordinal 3-point scale. The DAS assesses disability in four areas of daily living activities: personal hygiene (including the presence of palm maceration or infection), dressing, limb position (with psychological and social interference in patient's life) and pain interfering with daily activities. This is the only scale of functional impairment that correlates with variations of spasticity measured by the AS.[6]

Tests of Limb Dexterity

The nine-hole peg test is a simple and quick test of manual dexterity. The patient takes nine pegs out of their holes and returns them to their original position. The score measures the maximum time (up to 50 seconds) and the mean time per peg. This scale is both valid and reliable,[21] and is particularly sensitive to changes in performance in the upper range; it is less useful in patients with severe impairment who are unable to pick the pegs.

In addition, it is not sensitive to detect proximal weakness. The Jebsen test was developed to evaluate the patient's functional capabilities in commonly used activities in a standardized fashion. The test items include a range of fine motor, weighted and nonweighted, timed hand functions: (1) writing (copying) a 24-letter sentence; (2) turning over 3-×-5" cards; (3) picking up small common objects such as a paper clip, bottle cap and coin; (4) simulated feeding using a teaspoon and five kidney beans; (5) stacking checkers; (6) picking up large light objects (empty tin can); and (7) picking up large heavy objects (full tin can weighing 1 lb). The "action research arm test" is a modification of a battery of tests first introduced in 1965, which was designed to assess proximal and distal strength, as well as dexterity. Although the original test has been shortened,[22] it retains good validity and reliability. The Frenchay arm test consists of a five pass/fail tasks like picking up a glass of water, drinking, and combing one's hair. The score varies from 0 (poor) to 5 (better hand function).

Other Measures Used in Spasticity Trials

The SF-36 is a multipurpose, short-form, health survey with 36 questions providing an eight-scale profile of physical and mental health measures. This generic measure is irrespective of age, disease, or treatment; it has been used to evaluate the disease burden relative to specific populations, and to differentiate health benefits produced by a wide range of different treatments.

The global assessment scale is a generic measure used to evaluate the clinical effects of a treatment. The overall response to treatment is evaluated with a score from −4 (indicating very marked worsening) to 0 (no change) and up to +4 (very marked improvement).[23]

The Rivermead motor assessment is a well-validated instrument used to assess motor impairment in functions frequently affected by stroke. This is a 13-point measure of gross function; each function is scored on a two-point ordinal scale (0, cannot perform; 1 performs fully).[24]

The Visual Analog Scale was originally used to measure mood state and was later applied to measure the severity of pain experiences. It provides a very simple and intuitive rating between two possible extremes ("I do not have any pain," "my pain could not be worse"). By using a 10-cm scale graded from 0 to 100 (or from 0 to 10), a visual quantification of the severity of pain is obtained. The pain score is obtained by measuring from the left-hand end of the line to the patient's mark in millimeters. The intensity of pain can also be assessed by indicating a number from 0 (no pain) to 10 (maximal pain).[25]

POST-STROKE SPASTICITY

There are 13 randomized placebo-controlled trials (RCTs) on the use of BoNT/A in adult spasticity due to stroke, three with Botox (Allergan, Irvine, CA) and 10 with Dysport (Ipsen, Milford, MA). There is only one published RCT of BoNT/B (with Neurobloc/Myobloc [Solstice Neurosciences, Malvern, PA]) in this indication. Eleven of the BoNT/A trials studied the upper limb and two studied the lower limb. The single BoNT/B study was of poststroke upper limb spasticity.

Studies Using Botox

Trials using Botox examined changes in elbow, wrist, or finger flexor spasticity.[3,26,27] In these trials, patients with at least moderate or severe spasticity, as measured by the AS, were recruited and the primary outcome goal was a reduction in spasticity (Table 12-2). These trials found a significant effect of BoNT/A in reducing muscle tone measured at elbow, wrist and finger flexors. In dose-ranging studies,[26,27] the biggest effect was seen at the highest dose used for each joint examined. Elbow spasticity was examined in two studies[26,27] that found a significant reduction of the AS after injection of 200 U in the biceps. The overall effect was significantly in favor of BoNT/A compared with placebo and lasted 4 weeks in one study[26] and 9 weeks in the other.[27] Wrist spasticity was examined in three studies[3,26,27] that found a significant effect in favor of BoNT/A compared with placebo after injection of 100 U in the flexors carpi. The overall effect lasted for 6 weeks,[26] 9 weeks,[27] and 12 weeks,[3] respectively. Finger flexor spasticity was examined in two studies[3,27] that found a significant reduction of AS scores after injection into the finger flexors. The overall effect lasted for 12 weeks after injection of a cumulative dose of 100 U,[3] and for 3 weeks after injection of a

TABLE 12-2 Summary of Randomized Placebo-Controlled Botox® Trials in Poststroke Spasticity

Design	Dose (U)	Patients	Eligibility	Etiology	Max. Follow-Up (Weeks)	Muscles Injected (Dose Range Per Muscle)	Main Outcome Measures Reported	Reference
Randomized double-blind dose-ranging study	75 150 300	39 (37 included in analysis) Placebo: 10 75 U: 9 150 U: 9 300 U: 9	At least 9 months poststroke spasticity. An average elbow and wrist flexor tone of grade 2.5 or higher as measured by NAS.	Data available for 35 patients: thrombotic stroke in 22; embolic stroke in 5; hemorrhagic stroke in 8.	16	Bi (50-200 U); FCR (15-60 U); FCU (10-40 U)	NAS, FIM, R36V1, FMS, CDS, PA, FRS, GAS	26
Randomized double-blind parallel group study	200 to 240	126 (122 included in analysis) Placebo: 62 200–240 U: 64	Stroke at least six months earlier. NAS of 3 or 4 for wrist flexor and 2 or higher for finger flexor tone.	Stroke for all patients. Causes not reported.	12	FCR (75–225 U); FCU (70–225 U); FDS (75–225 U)	NAS, GAS, DAS	3
Randomized double-blind dose-ranging study	90 180 360	91 (77 included in analysis) Placebo: 26 90 U: 21 180 U: 23 360 U: 21	Stroke at least six months earlier. MAS of 2 or higher for elbow, and 3 or higher for wrist flexors.	Data available for 86 patients: thrombotic stroke in 51; embolic stroke in 16; hemorrhagic stroke in 19.	24	Bi (50–200 U); FCR (15–60 U); FCU (10–40 U); FDs (7.5–30 U); FDP (7.5–30 U)	EAS, GAS, 5FSP, FIM	27

CDS, caregiver dependency scale; DAS, Disability Assessment Scale; EAS, expanded Ashworth scale; FCR, flexor carpi radialis; FIM, functional independence measure; FMS, Fugl-Meyer scale; 5FSP, five-point frequency and severity of pain scale; GAS, global assessment scale; NAS, normal Ashworth scale; R36V1, Rand 36-item health survey 1.0.

cumulative dose of 60 U.[27] These trials also included secondary outcome measures of disability. BoNT/A treatment improved the global assessment scale without evidence of a dose-dependent response.[26,27] One study reported an increase in the number of patients with reduced disability in the BoNT/A group compared with placebo.[3] Other studies did not find an improvement of disability or pain reduction.[26,27] In one study, global motor function, assessed by the Fugl-Meyer scale, was unchanged.[26] Health-related quality of life was assessed in two trials[26,27]: there was a nonsignificant improvement on the Rand 36-item health survey[26] and a significant improvement on the SF-36 in patients receiving the lowest doses (90 U).[27]

Studies Using Dysport

Trials using Dysport have evaluated upper limb or lower limb spasticity. Trials on the upper limb evaluated treatments of elbow, wrist, or finger flexor spasticity; trials on the lower limb evaluated ankle plantar flexor spasticity (Table 12-3). Three studies evaluated the number of patients who had a reduction of ASs in the upper limb joints.[28-30] It resulted in a significant effect in favor of BoNT/A compared with placebo at Week 4 in two trials[28,29], and at week 8 in another.[30] The dosage varied between 200 and 600 U in the biceps and 75 and 225 U in finger or wrist flexors. Dose-ranging studies did not reveal a dose-dependent response to treatment.[28,30]

Three trials evaluated the mean changes in ASs. One study reported that BoNT could not reduce the AS 2, 6, or 12 weeks after a total injection of 1000 U in the elbow, wrist, and finger flexors.[31] Another trial reported improvement of finger flexor spasticity 2, 6, or 12 weeks after a total injection of 1000 U.[32] Elbow spasticity was reduced only 2 weeks after treatment, but not 6 or 12 weeks after administration of BoNT/A. A dose-ranging study in the arm reported no improvement of AS with the highest doses employed (1500 U), but suggested that BoNT/A treatment was overall better than placebo.[33]

Functional measures showed inconsistent results. One study reported an improvement in the action research arm test and the Barthel's index following treatment with 500 U, but a worsening following treatment with 1000 U.[30] Other studies did not find an improvement of disability assessed by the Barthel's index[28,29] or of global motor function assessed by the Rivermead motor assessment[28] or of the time required for dressing and the Frenchay arm test.[33] In one of these studies, there was a significant improvement in the ability to clean the palm of the affected hand, but this effect occurred only in patients who received a combined treatment with BoNT/A and electrical stimulation.[31]

Information on the frequency and severity of pain was available for six studies, which used different methods to assess and score pain.[26-30,32,34] In two trials, patients with hemiplegic shoulder pain were recruited to evaluate reduction of pain as the primary outcome. One study of failed to identify a significant reduction in the Visual Analog Scale after injections of 250 U in the pectoralis major and the biceps.[35] Another study found a significant reduction in a 10-point pain scale 4 weeks after the injection of 500 U in the subscapularis muscle.[25] In the remaining four studies, pain reduction was analyzed as secondary outcome: one study reported a significant decrease of pain in patients receiving BoNT/A, which was more evident at doses higher than 500 U,[30] whereas the other studies reported no pain reduction.[28,29,32]

Two studies assessed the effect of BoNT/A on the lower limb. In a dose-ranging study, the gastrocnemius muscle was injected with 500, 1000, or 1500 U.[34] A significant reduction of spasticity occurred throughout the 12-week observation period, as measured by the number of patients who had a reduction of the AS, and a dose-dependent response to treatment was observed. Functional outcomes (distance walked in 2 minutes, stepping rate, Rivermead motor assessment) did not improve in this trial, but a dose-dependent reduction of pain perception was reported. A crossover trial was also performed in the lower limb to evaluate the effect of injecting 1000 U in various distal muscles.[36] This study showed a reduction of the mean AS and improvement of the Fugl-Meyer score after 1 month, but no improvement in gait velocity. Muscle tone was reduced in ankle extensors, ankle invertors, and ankle dorsiflexors for about 3 months.

Studies Using MyoBloc/Neurobloc

One small trial only evaluated BoNT/B in upper limb spasticity.[37] This was a two-phase clinical trial characterized by a double-blind

TABLE 12-3 Summary of Randomized Placebo-Controlled Dysport Trials in Poststroke Spasticity

Design	Dose (U)	Patients	Eligibility	Etiology	Max. Follow-Up (Weeks)	Muscles Injected (Dose Range per Muscle)	Main Outcome Measures Reported	Reference
Randomized double-blind cross-over study	1000	23 (23 included in analysis) Placebo first: 13	Chronic hemiparetic patients	Stroke due to ischemia in 14 patients and hemorrhage in 5. Traumatic hemiparesis in 4 patients.	17	TS (500-1000 U) So (200-400 U) TP (200-350 U) FDL (150-300 U)	AS, FM	36
Randomized double-blind comparison with four treatment arms	1000	24 (24 included in analysis) Placebo: 6 Placebo and electrical stimulation: 6 1000 U: 6	Hemiplegic patients. At least six and not more than 12 months after stroke. Upper limb spasticity of at least grade 3 as measured by MAS	Supratentorial lesion due to ischemia in 18 patients or hemorrhage in 6 patients.	12	Bi (250 U); B (250 U); FCU (125 U); FCR (125 U); FDS (125 U); FDP (125 U)	MAS, LPR, ADL	31
Randomized double-blind dose-ranging study	500 1000 1500	21 (25 randomizations, 25 included in analysis) Placebo: 6 500 U: 6 1000 U: 7	Hemiplegic patients. Significant disabling spasticity.	Spastic hemiplegia due to stroke in 19 patients and traumatic brain injury in 2 patients.	12	Bi (330-1000) FCR/FCU (80-250) FDS/FDP (80-250)	ROM, MAS, TD, FAT, FC, GCAS, WT	33
Randomized double-blind parallel group study	1000	40 (38 included in analysis) Placebo: 20 1000 U: 20	Hemiplegic patients with finger flexor or elbow flexor spasticity of grade higher than 2 as measured by MAS.	Stroke for all patients. Causes not reported.	12	Bi (100-400 U); BR (100-200 U); FCU (100-200 U); FDS (200-500 U); FDP (100-300 U)	MAS, ROM, RP, BI	32
Randomized double-blind dose-ranging study	500 1000 1500	83 (82 included in analysis) Placebo: 20 500 U: 22 1000 U: 22 1500 U: 19	Hemiplegic stroke at least 3 months before recruitment. MAS ≥ 2 in the wrist, elbow and finger flexor.	Data available for 73 patients: ischemic stroke in 44; embolic stroke in 14; hemorrhagic stroke in 15.	16	Bi (200-600 U); FCR (75-225 U); FCU (70-225 U); FDS (75-225 U); FDP (75-225 U)	MAS, ROM, SP, RMA, BI	28

Study design	Dose	N (included in analysis)	Patient criteria	Stroke data	No.	BTX (units)	Outcomes	Ref.
Randomized double-blind parallel group study	1000	59 (59 included in analysis) Placebo: 32 1000 U: 27	Hemiplegic stroke at least 3 months before recruitment. MAS ≥ 2 in at least two of the wrist, elbow and finger flexor and 1+ in the remaining area.	Data available for 53 patients: ischemic stroke in 29; embolic stroke in 13; hemorrhagic stroke in 11.	16	Bi (300-400 U); FCR (150 U); FCU (150 U); FDS (150-250 U); FDP (150 U)	MAS, ROM, SP, BI	29
Randomized double-blind dose-ranging study	500 1000 1500	234 (228 included in analysis) Placebo: 55 500 U: 59 1000 U: 60 1500 U: 60	Hemiplegic stroke at least 3 months before recruitment. Spastic equinovarus deformity of the ankle.	Data available for 221 patients: thrombotic stroke in 125; embolic stroke in 25; intracerebral hemorrhage in 63; subarachnoid hemorrhage in 8.	12	GC: (500-1500 U)	MAS, ROM, RMA, SAP	34
Randomized double-blind parallel group study	350 500 1000	50 (50 included in analysis) Placebo: 15 350 U: 15 500 U: 15 1000 U: 5	Upper limb spasticity, medically and neurologically stable.	Ischemic stroke in 28; embolic stroke in 2; hemorrhagic stroke in 20.	24	Bi (150-400 U); FCR (50-150 U); FCU (50-150 U); FDS (50-150 U); FDP (50-150 U)	MAS, ARA, BI, VAS	30
Randomized double-blind parallel group study	500	17 (16 included in analysis) Placebo: 9 500 U: 8	Hemiplegic shoulder pain of 2 weeks duration or more and shoulder adductor and elbow flexor spasticity.	Stroke for all patients. Causes not reported.	12	Bi (250 U); PM (250 U)	VAS, AS, ROM	35
Randomized double-blind parallel group study	500	20 (20 included in analysis) Placebo: 10 500 U: 10	Hemiplegic patients presenting with upper limb spasticity related to cerebral stroke.	Ischemic stroke in 11; hemorrhagic stroke in 9.	4	SCa (500 U)	10vPS, AS, MAS	25

10vPS, 10-point pain verbal scale; ADL, customized activities of daily living scale; ARA; action research arm test; AS, Ashworth scale; BI, Barthel index; FAT, Frenchay arm test; FC, finger curl; FCR, flexor carpi radialis; FCU, flexor carpi ulnaris; FDL, flexor digitorum longus; FDP, flexor digitorum profundus; FDS, flexor digitorum superficialis; GC, gastrocnemius; GCAS, global clinical assessment scale; LPR, limb position at rest; MAS, modified Ashworth scale; PM, pectoralis major; RP, 0-10 rating of pain; RMA, Rivermead motor assessment: ROM, range of motion; SAP, subjective assessment of pain; SCa, subscapularis muscle; So, soleus; TP, tibialis posterior; TS, triceps surae; VAS, visual analog scale.

phase, followed by an open phase. The primary outcome was to assess muscle tone by the AS at the elbow, wrist, finger, and thumb flexors. Fifteen patients (10 in the BoNT-B group and five in the placebo group) were treated with injections into the biceps, the flexor carpi ulnaris, the flexor carpi radialis, the flexor digitorum sublimis, and the flexor digitorum profundus. In the group receiving BoNT/B, the total dose injected was of 10000 U for each patient. The results did not show any significant effect on upper limb spasticity either during the 16-week double blind phase or during the 12-week open phase. Furthermore, the assessment of pain and disability, as measured by the Jebsen or nine-hole peg test, did not show differences in the BoNT/B-treated group compared with placebo.

SPASTICITY IN MULTIPLE SCLEROSIS

Treatment of spasticity in multiple sclerosis is a difficult endeavor in view of the complex clinical picture. The advantage of BoNT rests in its focal use, its lasting action over many weeks, and the complete reversibility of effect. Apart from focal spasticity, BoNT can of course also be used as an additive in patients with systemic treatment. Therapeutic objectives are the reduction of muscle tone and pain, the prevention of fixed contractures, the improvement of disability, and the relief of symptoms secondary to spasticity, for example, in dislocations. Furthermore, treatment of specific "trigger muscles" can block the action-triggered overflow of spasticity, for instance, from distal to proximal muscles in the lower limbs.[38]

Three studies[13,39,40] and a systematic review[41] evaluated the use of BoNT/A in multiple sclerosis. Two of them[13,39] evaluated patients with thigh adductor spasticity and one[40] evaluated four patients with lower limb spasticity and one with upper limb spasticity.

In the first study,[39] the number of patients with improvement in adductor spasticity score was significant higher in the Botox group than in the placebo group. Furthermore, seven out of nine participants had improvement in hygiene scores in the BoNT/A group, compared with two in the placebo group. In the study of Grazko and colleagues,[40] all the patients in the Botox group had a two-point AS improvement that persisted for 1 to 3 months. No placebo effect was observed.

A dose-ranging study compared 500, 1000, and 1500 Dysport U to placebo.[13] There was a significant improvement (greater than placebo) only for the maximum between-knees distance in the 1500 U group 4 weeks after treatment, without any significant difference in ASs. In all BoNT groups, the duration of effect, which was measured as the time required for re-treatment, was significantly greater than placebo. There were more frequent reports of weakness in the BoNT groups (especially the 1500 U group) than in placebo.

SPASTICITY IN OTHER DISORDERS

Clinical data on the treatment of spasticity in patients with motor neuron disease are scanty. A systematic review failed to identify any BoNT trial.[42] The use of BoNT in amyotrophic lateral sclerosis is probably hampered by the presence of muscle atrophy, whereas the treatment could be helpful in primary lateral sclerosis. In keeping with this view, a recent retrospective study showed that the base width is reduced in patients with upper motor neuron syndrome who receive treatment in calf muscles.[43]

SAFETY OF BoNT IN SPASTICITY

BoNT/A is well tolerated and must be regarded as a safe treatment, because no study reported significantly more adverse events in the treated groups than in placebo arms. One study reported excessive weakness after injections of high doses (1500 Dysport U) in the upper limb,[30] which is consistent with reports of similar weakness after upper limb treatment of patients with multiple sclerosis[13] and cerebral palsy.[44] Published data on the safety of BoNT/A in patients with dystonia and other movement disorders also indicate a good safety profile.[45] A recent pooled analysis of BoNT/A safety in patients with poststroke spasticity concluded that nausea was the most frequent problem in those treated with BoNT/A, however it affected only 2.2% of cases.[46] BoNT/B may have more side effects than BoNT/A, particularly on autonomic function. In the BoNT/B trial on poststroke spasticity, dry mouth was more common in the treated group than in controls.[37] A special tropism for autonomic nerve terminals has been suggested by trials with BoNT/B for other indications.[47]

CONCLUSIONS AND OUTLOOK

BoNT injections are employed as focal antispastic agents usually as part of complex rehabilitation protocols.[48] Ability to stand or walk usually relies on a certain degree of residual spasticity, and treatment plans often involve a trade-off between spasticity reduction and preservation of residual motor function.[5] Therefore, functional outcome is not necessarily directly related to the reduction of spasticity and to the doses of BoNT injected.

This systematic review provides evidence that BoNT/A treatment reduces hypertonia associated with poststroke spasticity in elbow, wrist, and finger flexors and also foot flexors. A significant effect on spasticity is demonstrated by the reduction of mean ASs and by the number of patients with MAS improvement. In most trials, the peak muscle tone reduction occurred about 4 weeks after injection and lasted for up to 3 months, which is consistent with the duration of BoNT effect seen in dystonia.[49,50] In patients with dystonia, BoNT injections are usually repeated at regular intervals. The efficacy and outcome of repeated treatments in patients with spasticity remains unsettled. The available data on BoNT-B are insufficient to assess its effect on spasticity.

Most studies did not support an effect of BoNT/A on patients' disability.[26-29,34] However, in most cases, assessment of disability is inadequate to identify changes due to reduced upper limb spasticity, particularly improved hand function. Further controlled studies need to address the effects of repeated BoNT treatments in patients with spasticity and the efficacy of BoNT treatment on the resulting functional disability.

References

1. Lance JW. The control of muscle tone, reflexes, and movement: Robert Wartenberg Lecture. *Neurology*. 1980;30:1303-1313.
2. Sheean GL. Botulinum treatment of spasticity: why is it so difficult to show a functional benefit? *Curr Opin Neurol*. 2001;14:771-776.
3. Brashear A, Gordon MF, Elovic E, Kassicieh VD, Marciniak C, Do M, et al. Intramuscular injection of botulinum toxin for the treatment of wrist and finger spasticity after a stroke. *N Engl J Med*. 2002;347:395-400.
4. O'Dwyer NJ, Ada L, Neilson PD. Spasticity and muscle contracture following stroke. *Brain*. 1996;119:1737-1749.
5. Woldag H, Hummelsheim H. Is the reduction of spasticity by botulinum toxin a beneficial for the recovery of motor function of arm and hand in stroke patients? *Eur Neurol*. 2003;50:165-171.
6. Brashear A, Zafonte R, Corcoran M, Galvez-Jimenez N, Gracies JM, Gordon MF, et al. Inter- and intrarater reliability of the Ashworth Scale and the Disability Assessment Scale in patients with upper-limb poststroke spasticity. *Arch Phys Med Rehabil*. 2002;83:1349-1354.
7. Ashworth B. Preliminary trial of carisoprodol in multiple sclerosis. *Practitioner*. 1964;192:540-542.
8. Bohannon RW, Smith MB. Interrater reliability of a modified Ashworth scale of muscle spasticity. *Phys Ther*. 1987;67:206-207.
9. Pandyan AD, Johnson GR, Price CI, Curless RH, Barnes MP, Rodgers H. A review of the properties and limitations of the Ashworth and modified Ashworth Scales as measures of spasticity. *Clin Rehabil*. 1999;13:373-383.
10. Pandyan AD, Van Wijck FM, Stark S, Vuadens P, Johnson GR, Barnes MP. The construct validity of a spasticity measurement device for clinical practice: an alternative to the Ashworth scales. *Disabil Rehabil*. 2006;28:579-585.
11. Platz T, Eickhof C, Nuyens G, Vuadens P. Clinical scales for the assessment of spasticity, associated phenomena, and function: a systematic review of the literature. *Disabil Rehabil*. 2005;27:7-18.
12. Penn RD, Savoy SM, Corcos D, Latash M, Gottlieb G, Parke B, et al. Intrathecal baclofen for severe spinal spasticity. *N Engl J Med*. 1989;320:1517-1521.
13. Hyman N, Barnes M, Bhakta B, Cozens A, Bakheit M, Kreczy-Kleedorfer B, et al. Botulinum toxin (Dysport) treatment of hip adductor spasticity in multiple sclerosis: a prospective, randomised, double blind, placebo controlled, dose ranging study. *J Neurol Neurosurg Psychiatry*. 2000;707-712.
14. Mutlu A, Livanelioglu A, Gunel MK. Reliability of goniometric measurements in children with spastic cerebral palsy. *Med Sci Monit*. 2007;13:CR323-CR329.
15. Chung SG, Van Rey E, Bai Z, Roth EJ, Zhang LQ. Biomechanic changes in passive properties of hemiplegic ankles with spastic hypertonia. *Arch Phys Med Rehabil*. 2004;85:1638-1646.
16. de Jong LD, Nieuwboer A, Aufdemkampe G. The hemiplegic arm: interrater reliability and concurrent validity of passive range of motion measurements. *Disabil Rehabil*. 2007;29:1442-1448.
17. Biering-Sorensen F, Nielsen JB, Klinge K. Spasticity-assessment: a review. *Spinal Cord*. 2006;44:708-722.
18. Cohen ME, Marino RJ. The tools of disability outcomes research functional status measures. *Arch Phys Med Rehabil*. 2000;81(suppl 2):S21-S29.
19. Hinderer SR, Gupta S. Functional outcome measures to assess interventions for spasticity. *Arch Phys Med Rehabil*. 1996;77:1083-1089.
20. Wade DT, Collin C. The Barthel ADL Index: a standard measure of physical disability? *Int Disabil Stud*. 1988;10:64-67.
21. Heller A, Wade DT, Wood VA, Sunderland A, Hewer RL, Ward E. Arm function after stroke: measurement and recovery over the first three months. *J Neurol Neurosurg Psychiatry*. 1987;50:714-719.
22. Lyle RC. A performance test for assessment of upper limb function in physical rehabilitation treatment and research. *Int J Rehabil Res*. 1981;4:483-492.

23. Naumann M, Yakovleff A, Durif F. A randomized, double-masked, crossover comparison of the efficacy and safety of botulinum toxin type A produced from the original bulk toxin source and current bulk toxin source for the treatment of cervical dystonia. *J Neurol.* 2002;249:57-63.

24. Lincoln N, Leadbitter D. Assessment of motor function in stroke patients. *Physiotherapy.* 1979;65:48-51.

25. Yelnik AP, Colle FM, Bonan IV, Vicaut E. Treatment of shoulder pain in spastic hemiplegia by reducing spasticity of the subscapular muscle: a randomised, double blind, placebo controlled study of botulinum toxin A. *J Neurol Neurosurg Psychiatry.* 2007;78:845-848.

26. Simpson DM, Alexander DN, O'Brien CF, Tagliati M, Aswad AS, Leon JM, et al. Botulinum toxin type A in the treatment of upper extremity spasticity: a randomized, double-blind, placebo-controlled trial. *Neurology.* 1996;46:1306-1310.

27. Childers MK, Brashear A, Jozefczyk P, Reding M, Alexander D, Good D, et al. Dose-dependent response to intramuscular botulinum toxin type A for upper-limb spasticity in patients after a stroke. *Arch Phys Med Rehabil.* 2004;85:1063-1069.

28. Bakheit AM, Thilmann AF, Ward AB, Poewe W, Wissel J, Muller J, et al. A randomized, double-blind, placebo-controlled, dose-ranging study to compare the efficacy and safety of three doses of botulinum toxin type A (Dysport) with placebo in upper limb spasticity after stroke. *Stroke.* 2000;31:2402-2406.

29. Bakheit AM, Pittock S, Moore AP, Wurker M, Otto S, Erbguth F, et al. A randomized, double-blind, placebo-controlled study of the efficacy and safety of botulinum toxin type A in upper limb spasticity in patients with stroke. *Eur J Neurol.* 2001;8:559-565.

30. Suputtitada A, Suwanwela NC. The lowest effective dose of botulinum A toxin in adult patients with upper limb spasticity. *Disabil Rehabil.* 2005;27:176-184.

31. Hesse S, Reiter F, Konrad M, Jahnke MT. Botulinum toxin type A and short-term electrical stimulation in the treatment of upper limb flexor spasticity after stroke: a randomized, double-blind, placebo-controlled trial. *Clin Rehabil.* 1998;12:381-388.

32. Bhakta BB, Cozens JA, Chamberlain MA, Bamford JM. Impact of botulinum toxin type A on disability and carer burden due to arm spasticity after stroke: a randomised double blind placebo controlled trial. *J Neurol Neurosurg Psychiatry.* 2000;69:217-221.

33. Smith SJ, Ellis E, White S, Moore AP. A double-blind placebo-controlled study of botulinum toxin in upper limb spasticity after stroke or head injury. *Clin Rehabil.* 2000;14:5-13.

34. Pittock SJ, Moore AP, Hardiman O, Ehler E, Kovac M, Bojakowski J, et al. A double-blind randomised placebo-controlled evaluation of three doses of botulinum toxin type A (Dysport) in the treatment of spastic equinovarus deformity after stroke. *Cerebrovasc Dis.* 2003;15:289-300.

35. Kong KH, Neo JJ, Chua KS. A randomized controlled study of botulinum toxin A in the treatment of hemiplegic shoulder pain associated with spasticity. *Clin Rehabil.* 2007;21:28-35.

36. Burbaud P, Wiart L, Dubos JL, Gaujard E, Debelleix X, Joseph PA, et al. A randomised, double blind, placebo controlled trial of botulinum toxin in the treatment of spastic foot in hemiparetic patients. *J Neurol Neurosurg Psychiatry.* 1996;61:265-269.

37. Brashear A, McAfee AL, Kuhn ER, Fyffe J. Botulinum toxin type B in upper-limb poststroke spasticity: a double-blind, placebo-controlled trial. *Arch Phys Med Rehabil.* 2004;85:705-709.

38. Kabus C, Hecht M, Japp G, Jost WH, Pohlau D, Stuckrad-Barre S, et al. Botulinum toxin in patients with multiple sclerosis. *J Neurol.* 2006;253(suppl. 1): I26-I28.

39. Snow BJ, Tsui JK, Bhatt MH. Treatment of spasticity with botulinum toxin: a double-blind study. *Ann Neurol.* 1990;28:512-515.

40. Grazko MA, Polo KB, Jabbari B. Botulinum toxin A for spasticity, muscle spasms, and rigidity. *Neurology.* 1995;45:712-717.

41. Shakespeare DT, Boggild M, Young C. Anti-spasticity agents for multiple sclerosis. *Cochrane Database Syst Rev.* 2003;(4):CD001332.

42. Ashworth NL, Satkunam LE, Deforge D. Treatment for spasticity in amyotrophic lateral sclerosis/motor neuron disease. *Cochrane Database Syst Rev.* 2006;(1):CD004156.

43. Cioni M, Esquenazi A, Hirai B. Effects of botulinum toxin-A on gait velocity, step length, and base of support of patients with dynamic equinovarus foot. *Am J Phys Med Rehabil.* 2006;85:600-606.

44. Wasiak J, Hoare B, Wallen M. Botulinum toxin A as an adjunct to treatment in the management of the upper limb in children with spastic cerebral palsy. *Cochrane Database Syst Rev.* 2004;(4):CD003469.

45. Naumann M, Jankovic J. Safety of botulinum toxin type A: a systematic review and meta-analysis. *Curr Med Res Opin.* 2004;20:981-990.

46. Turkel CC, Bowen B, Liu J, Brin MF. Pooled analysis of the safety of botulinum toxin type A in the treatment of poststroke spasticity. *Arch Phys Med Rehabil.* 2006;87:786-792.

47. Dressler D, Eleopra R. Clinical use of non-A botulinum toxins: botulinum toxin type B. *Neurotox Res.* 2006;9:121-125.

48. Esquenazi A. Improvements in healthcare and cost benefits associated with botulinum toxin treatment of spasticity and muscle overactivity. *Eur J Neurol.* 2006;13(suppl 4):27-34.

49. Jankovic J, Schwartz K. Botulinum toxin injections for cervical dystonia. *Neurology.* 1990;40:277-280.

50. Bentivoglio AR, Albanese A. Botulinum toxin in motor disorders. *Curr Opin Neurol.* 1999;12:447-456.

51. Gracies JM. Pathophysiology of impairment in patients with spasticity and use of stretch as a treatment of spastic hypertonia. *Phys Med Rehabil Clin N Am.* 2001;12:747-768.

52. Mayer NH, Esquenazi A. Muscle overactivity and movement dysfunction in the upper motoneuron syndrome. *Phys Med Rehabil Clin N Am.* 2003;14: 855, viii.

53. Mayer NH. Clinicophysiologic concepts of spasticity and motor dysfunction in adults with an upper motoneuron lesion. *Muscle Nerve.* 1997;20(Suppl.6): S1-S13.

Biological and Mechanical Pathologies in Spastic Skeletal Muscle: The Functional Implications of Therapeutic Neurotoxins **13**

Samuel R. Ward and Richard L. Lieber

INTRODUCTION

Spasticity, a neurologic problem secondary to an upper motor neuron (UMN) lesion, has a significant effect on skeletal muscle. The UMN lesions may be secondary to a cerebral vascular accident, head injury, spinal cord injury, or degenerative diseases such as multiple sclerosis, or perinatal brain injuries such as cerebral palsy. Functional ability in these patients can be severely compromised due to abnormal neuromuscular activity and abnormal muscle mechanics, but the basic mechanisms underlying these deficits are not clearly understood. The therapeutic use of neurotoxins has allowed these patients to functionally improve, but even less is known about the interaction between neurotoxins and the neuromuscular system. In this review, we evaluate the current evidence in the literature suggesting that skeletal muscle tissue itself is altered in UMN conditions and when neurotoxins are used therapeutically on muscle. Experimental studies were evaluated that included a variety of methods encompassing joint mechanics, tissue mechanics, and muscle morphology. Taken together, the literature strongly supports the assertion that spastic muscles are altered in a way that is unique among muscle plasticity models and therapeutic use of neurotoxin may temporarily improve these tissue level changes. Further studies are required to detail the intra- and extracellular modifications of skeletal muscle that occur secondary to UMN syndrome, optimize neurotoxin dosing requirements, and make functional changes predictable.

UMN lesions can cause severe impairment of voluntary movement. Dystonia, paresis, and spasticity are a few of the serious complications that affect movement in these individuals. As a result, these patients suffer from decreased range of motion, decreased voluntary strength, and increased joint stiffness, but the basic mechanisms underlying the functional deficits that occur after the development of UMN syndrome are not clearly understood. At this point, it is important to note that,

Dr. Ward has received grant support from the National Institutes of Health. Dr. Lieber has received grant support from the National Institutes of Health, the Department of Veteran's Affairs, Defense Advance Research Projects Agency (DARPA), and the United Cerebral Palsy Foundation. He also acts as a consultant to Allergan, Inc. (Irvine, CA).

159

in general, we are attempting to discuss the skeletal muscle problems associated with UMN syndrome, which we appreciate are a constellation of problems. One of those problems is spasticity, which although present in many patients with UMN, is difficult to uncouple from dystonia, contracture, or paresis. As a result, much of the literature in the area, including our own, suggests that muscular findings are directly attributable to spasticity per se, yet this may be a simplistic view. Given these points, it should become obvious that careful subsetting of spastic patients may be highly beneficial for future work in this area.

Although the etiology of UMN problems is central, many therapies are directed toward the peripheral nerves and muscles. As a result, therapeutic interventions involving stretching, casting, splinting, botulinum toxin injection, and electrical stimulation of the muscles are not completely effective.[1-5] It is estimated that the complications of cerebral palsy alone can cost nearly $500,000 over the lifetime of a single individual.[6] Consequently, UMN syndromes and their sequelae, represent significant scientific and economic challenges.

Considerable scientific and medical literature exists regarding the etiology and treatment of spasticity specifically. However, because spasticity is only one of many symptoms associated with UMN syndrome, most research has focused on the nervous system. This is certainly reasonable because the primary lesion leading to spasticity is located in the central nervous system. Thus, many studies measure skeletal muscle electromyographic activity, lesion size and shape, and patient gait characteristics. In addition, there is wide discussion of the various surgical procedures used to correct spastic deformities.[7] Far less attention has been directed toward understanding the structural and functional changes in skeletal muscle that occur secondary to spasticity and UMN syndrome. With a few notable exceptions,[8-10] the properties of skeletal muscle have largely been ignored. Yet, with recent technical advances, it is now possible to characterize many properties of skeletal muscle from patients with UMN syndrome, and it is becoming increasingly clear that there are dramatic changes in the skeletal muscle in these patients.

Muscle and neural changes are usually related,[11] but recent data have revealed certain changes in muscle that are not easily explained by classic interpretations of the effects of neural changes alone.[12-14] It is, therefore, important to improve our understanding of the structural and functional changes that occur in the muscle of those with UMN syndrome. Understanding muscle plasticity will thereby improve, because the spasticity model appears to be unlike any other plasticity model previously studied. In addition, increased understanding will lend insight into the nature of spasticity itself, because muscles respond in stereotypical fashion to altered neural and mechanical input. Finally, because most of the interventions related to spasticity revolve around treatment of the musculoskeletal system, improved understanding of muscle-tendon unit properties may lead to the development of more rational interventions to treat these patients.

The purpose of this review is to provide a focused presentation of the structural and mechanical changes that occur within skeletal muscles secondary to UMN syndrome. Although spasticity is cited specifically, we appreciate that this is only one of many complications related to UMN syndrome that may be affecting skeletal muscle. This literature is limited, and among these studies, complete agreement is lacking; this emphasizes the need for a constructive review of the topic.

SKELETAL MUSCLE PLASTICITY

It is reasonable to study skeletal muscle properties even though the primary lesion is neural, because muscles respond in a fairly stereotypical manner to the amount and type of activity imposed on them. For example, the classic studies of the 1960s and 1970s revealed that chronic electrical stimulation of skeletal muscle can progressively transform skeletal muscle cells into a slower phenotype.[15-18] Although there are subtle differences among muscles in terms of the nature, extent, and time-course of the transformation, the results are surprisingly consistent. There is general agreement that chronic electrical stimulation produces increased capillary density, increased percentage of type I muscle fibers, decreased fiber size (if the stimulation duration is long enough), increased endurance, and decreased strength. This serves as a template that describes the changes that occur in skeletal muscle with increased use. Voluntary exercise, especially when performed for long durations, results in many of the same muscle changes.[19]

Spasticity is often thought to result in changes typically seen in increased use models, as the following discussion will highlight.

The opposite model, chronic decreased use of skeletal muscle, which can be studied using models of simulated weightlessness,[20] tenotomy,[21] immobilization in a shortened position,[22,23] or spinal cord isolation,[24,25] causes muscle fibers to decrease their size and transform toward faster phenotypes. One of the most extreme examples of such a transformation was reported in a rat spinal cord injury model in which the rats lived about half their lifespan with UMN lesions and, as a result, converted almost all of their muscle fibers to the fastest phenotype, even in the very slow soleus muscle.[26,27] Similar results have been reported for humans[28] and in other animals[24,29-31] after traumatic spinal cord injury. It is clear that an analysis of fiber-type distribution of skeletal muscle can be a useful indicator of the amount and type of activity that a muscle has received over an extended period of time. In addition to fiber-type distribution, fiber size provides insights into the extent of fiber use. Increased use of skeletal muscle at high loads produces muscle fiber hypertrophy, whereas decreased use leads to muscle cell atrophy. Both responses appear to be load dependent. Thus, fiber size is typically interpreted as an indirect indicator of the amount of force imposed on a muscle.

Taken together, muscle fiber-type distribution and muscle fiber size distribution provide insight into the overall type and amount of use imposed on a muscle. Therefore, these parameters are often studied in spastic muscle in an attempt to determine its use pattern. However, in spite of the ease of measuring these parameters, they are not very specific and probably provide only a general indicator of muscle use. Excellent reviews of skeletal muscle plasticity and monographs on the subject are widely available in the literature.[11,19,32,33]

MUSCLE FIBER TYPE AND FIBER SIZE CHANGES WITH SPASTICITY

Because measurement of muscle fiber size and type is commonly used in the diagnosis of neuromuscular diseases[34] and also because such studies are relatively easy to perform, it is not surprising that biopsy studies are the most prevalent type of study performed on spastic muscle. Despite their apparent ease, there are methodologic concerns that make these studies difficult to interpret definitively. Specific issues that must be addressed in any biopsy study are the fraction of the muscle actually being sampled, the gradient of fiber type and fiber size distribution across and along the muscle, the variability in fiber type and fiber size between muscles, whether different muscles or muscle groups are being used to compare normal subjects and diseased patients, and the variability in clinical presentation of patients.

Most of these issues were not addressed by any of the studies reviewed. For example, it was extremely rare to find a study in which the same muscle was measured in populations of individuals with and without spasticity. In most studies, owing to practical and ethical considerations, data were reported from different muscles for the two experimental groups, and individuals with and without spasticity were almost always of different age—this was especially true in studies of spasticity secondary to static perinatal encephalopathy (cerebral palsy), in which it is almost impossible to obtain normal tissue from children. In at least one study, the investigators endeavored to match the age groups by using historical pathologic specimens from children (which turned out to be normal), but these biopsies were from different muscles as compared with the spastic patients.[35] These factors obviously confound the study of muscle spasticity and make it difficult to generalize results across either age groups or diagnoses.

In spite of such limitations, one common finding in biopsy studies is that fiber size variability is increased in muscles from patients with spasticity. When sectioned, normal skeletal muscle biopsies have tightly packed fibers that form polygons juxtaposed to one another. However, most published micrographs of muscle from spastic patients showed abnormalities such as increased fiber size variability, increased numbers of rounded fibers, moth-eaten fibers, and in some cases, increased extracellular space.[35-40] When fiber size is measured and expressed as coefficient of variation, the value is always higher for spastic muscle samples compared with normal samples. Fiber size variability is characteristic of numerous neuromuscular disorders as well as occurring in spasticity, so such findings are not very specific.[41] The mechanistic basis for this response is not known. It should be noted that muscle fiber tapering occurs near the end of some fibers and may result in fiber size variation, but this is not considered a pathologic state.[42-44]

It would be convenient if fiber-type distribution changes were consistent among studies, but this is not the case. Because many investigators were predisposed to the idea that spastic muscles were chronically active, it may have been tempting to interpret an increase in type I fiber percentage from spastic patients as evidence of muscle fiber-type transformation. Unfortunately, whereas a few studies have indeed reported an increased percentage of type I fibers,[38,39,45] others reported an increased percentage of type II fibers[46] or no change in fiber-type distribution.[35-37,40] There is thus no agreement that spasticity represents either an increased- or decreased-use model, perhaps in part due to the sampling problems inherent to the biopsy procedure itself.[41,47] For example, when fiber-type percentages were measured from vastus lateralis biopsies and compared with the fiber-type distributions within the entire human vastus lateralis,[48,49] such values were notoriously inaccurate. However, considering the literature as a whole, the results probably indicate that spastic muscle is not simply subjected to chronic increased or decreased activation. This is likely due, in part, to the fact that spasticity is often not observed in isolation. For example, patients may also have dystonia, paresis, or contracture associated with their disease process.

MECHANICAL CHANGES IN SPASTIC MUSCLE

Indirect biomechanical studies have demonstrated that spastic muscles have altered intrinsic mechanical stiffness.[14,50] What structures might be responsible for this altered stiffness? Comprehensive answers cannot be provided at this time. However, two recent studies[14,50] indicated that the passive mechanical properties of isolated muscle cells and small muscle fiber bundles were altered secondary to spasticity. It is important to note, that spasticity was directly assessed in these patients and is therefore cited specifically, but these patients generally suffered from UMN syndrome. These two studies provide a view of the complex interactions between muscle cells and the extracellular matrix that may result from spasticity.

To compare directly the intrinsic passive mechanical properties of normal and spastic muscle cells (i.e., muscle cells obtained from biopsies of patients with spastic limbs), a novel method was developed in which muscle biopsies were removed from patients at the time of reconstructive surgery (secondary to cerebral palsy for the spastic muscle) or during surgical repair (radial nerve injury or trauma for the normal muscle) and were placed in a relaxing solution designed to prevent hypercontraction of the muscle fibers.[51] Then, using high-powered microscopic illumination, segments of individual cells were dissected free of the surrounding connective tissue and placed into a micromechanical testing apparatus that enabled passive elongation of the muscle cell with simultaneous measurement of intracellular sarcomere length.[12] Muscle cells were elongated in 250-μm increments, and the relationship between muscle passive stress and sarcomere length was quantified. The slope of the single cell stress-strain curve was then used to calculate fiber elastic modulus as previously described in detail.[12] Interestingly, the tensile modulus of muscle cells from spastic patients was more than twice that of patients who had an intact neuromuscular system (Fig. 13-1),[13] demonstrating that the intrinsic passive stiffness of individual spastic muscle cells was increased. In addition,

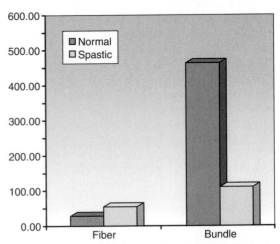

FIGURE 13-1. The tangent modulus (stiffness) of spastic single muscle fibers is higher ($P < 0.05$) than normal single fibers (*left*). However, spastic muscle fiber bundles are less ($P < 0.05$) stiff than normal fiber bundles (*right*). These data suggest that the increased resistance to passive stretch observed in spastic skeletal muscle is due, in part, to muscle level intracellular changes. (Adapted from Lieber RL, Runesson E, Einarsson F, Fridén J. Inferior mechanical properties of spastic muscle bundles due to hypertrophic but compromised extracellular matrix material. *Muscle Nerve.* 2003;28:464-471. Reprinted with permission of John Wiley & Sons, Inc.)

the resting sarcomere length of spastic cells (i.e., the length of the sarcomeres when the muscle cell was completely unloaded), was significantly shorter in spastic muscle cells compared with normal cells. Internal cytoskeletal structures set resting sarcomere length in muscle cells.[52] These two findings demonstrate that the structures within the muscle cell responsible for setting resting sarcomere length and determining cellular elastic modulus are altered in spastic muscle. The most obvious candidate for this structure is the giant intracellular cytoskeletal protein titin.[53] Titin has been demonstrated in frog skeletal muscles to bear almost the entire elastic load during passive elongation and is a significant component that bears the passive load in human muscle.[54] Can the titin protein be altered secondary to spasticity? There are no definitive data, but there is circumstantial evidence to suggest that it is possible. For example, it has been demonstrated, based on the differences in cDNA sequences, that titin can exist in multiple isoforms between heart and skeletal muscle and even among various skeletal muscles.[53] It is known that the titin isoform in heart muscle is much stiffer and much shorter than the titin isoforms in most skeletal muscles. Furthermore, it has also been demonstrated that the titin isoform can change within heart muscle under pathologic conditions, specifically in ischemia-induced cardiomyopathy. This condition is usually accompanied by elevated left ventricular end-diastolic pressure, which follows from increased myocardial stiffness resulting from upregulated collagen expression. However, in addition to collagen proliferation, a switch from a stiff to a more compliant isoform of titin was documented.[55] In skeletal muscle, it has been shown that relative titin concentrations (titin/MHC and titin/actin) decline in a rat model of denervation[56]; however, this model does not fully characterize spasticity as we have previously noted. In humans with spinal cord injuries, the it has been reported that titin isoforms are not altered.[57] However, myofibrillar passive tension was also not altered in the muscles of these patients.[57] Therefore, it remains possible that titin isoforms may be altered in spastic skeletal muscles that have elevated passive tensions on the single fiber level, although definitive evidence of this change has not been reported.

Because surgical reconstructive procedures are often performed on spastic muscles to restore or augment function, it is of interest to know whether the increased resistance to stretch that is "felt" by surgeons in the operating room may be explained by differences in the elastic properties of muscle cells within spastic muscle. To investigate this point, small bundles of muscle cells were subjected to the same procedure as described earlier for single cells and their elastic moduli were measured.[13] These small bundles of cells (5–50 fibers) contained the same types of muscle cells that were tested previously, but they were also ensheathed by the connective tissue matrix of the muscle tissue. Several interesting findings emerged. First, the tangent modulus measured in bundles was significantly greater than the same modulus measured in single cells (see Fig. 13-1).[13] However, the difference was much more pronounced for normal muscle bundles than for spastic muscle bundles. Whereas spastic muscle bundle modulus was increased by only about twofold over the single fiber modulus, in normal muscle, the modulus was increased more than 16 times compared with the modulus of the normal isolated muscle cell. These data demonstrate a clear difference in the mechanical properties of spastic muscle tissue bundles compared with normal muscle fiber bundles. The differences were even more impressive when the structural differences between the two bundle types are considered—only 40% of the spastic muscle bundle cross-sectional area was occupied by muscle fibers, whereas 95% of normal muscle bundle was occupied by muscle fibers. Morphologically, there was a large amount of poorly organized extracellular material in spastic bundles compared with normal bundles. One can calculate the mechanical properties of the extracellular matrix material in the bundles by subtracting the single cell modulus from whole bundle modulus. When this is done, it is seen that the extracellular matrix of the spastic muscle has a modulus of ~0.2 GPa, whereas normal muscle has a modulus of ~8 GPa—about 40 times greater. These data demonstrate that although spastic muscle contains a larger amount of extracellular matrix material, the quality of that material is compromised compared with that of normal muscles. It is of interest that the spastic muscle model with high fiber stiffness in a compliant extracellular matrix shows the opposite adaptation as the ischemic heart muscle, which possesses a very stiff extracellular matrix and compliant fibers. The only other explicit description of extracellular matrix changes in spastic muscle was based on biochemical measurement of collagen concentration, which increased dramatically in spastic muscle.[36]

MUSCLE FUNCTIONAL RESPONSES TO NEUROTOXIN THERAPY

Despite the widespread use of neurotoxins for the treatment of neuromuscular diseases, few studies directly measure muscle function or document tissue level changes in muscle. The relevant literature in this area is limited to studies documenting qualitative movement improvements,[58] measuring kinematic and kinetic changes during gait,[58-60] or quantifying changes in joint torque.[61] Recently, we have developed an animal model of neuromuscular paralysis that allows us to study system level changes (i.e., gait and joint torques), but also to study muscle at the tissue and biologic levels.[62] In this model, the tibialis anterior muscle is maximally activated via direct stimulation of the peroneal nerve. In these experiments, the tibialis anterior muscles of Sprague-Dawley rats are injected unilaterally with 6 units/kg of botulinum neurotoxin type A (BoNT/A), normal saline, or any other drug of interest. Using BoNT/A, we have demonstrated that injected muscles are profoundly

weak at 1 week and 1 month, but were recovering by 1 month (Fig. 13-2A). This, in itself is not surprising, but perhaps more interesting, when the contralateral BoNT/A muscle was tested, dorsiflexion torque was significantly less than the contralateral saline control muscle (see Fig. 13-2B) despite no difference in animal mass. The absence of growth-associated torque increases in the contralateral limb suggests that there may be a systemic effect of BoNT/A on muscle remote from the site of injection. Systemic effects have also been demonstrated in humans,[63] but the mechanism of such changes has not been documented.

SPASTIC MUSCLE FIBER TYPE SIZE CHANGES IN RESPONSE TO NEUROTOXIN THERAPY

Recently, we were able to study the muscles of children who have been injected with BoNT/A to relieve spasticity in various muscles of the forearm and hand.[64] These children were undergoing surgical lengthening of spastic muscles 5 to 14 months postinjection to relieve joint contracture. The most surprising result was that the average fiber area of muscles that were injected with BoNT/A was significantly

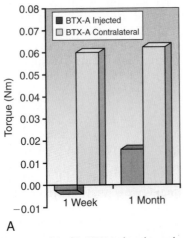

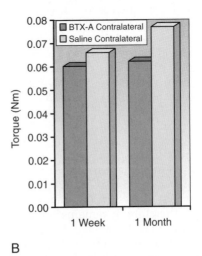

A   B

FIGURE 13-2. A, In a rat model of BoNT/A-induced muscle paralysis, dorsiflexion torque is severely compromised at 1 week ($P < 0.05$) and 1 month ($P < 0.05$) but begins to recover by 1 month. Notice that dorsiflexion torque is actually negative at 1 week, which is likely due to peroneal muscle activation through the peroneal nerve. **B,** Comparison of the contralateral limb in the botulinum neurotoxin type A (BoNT/A)–injected animals with the contralateral limb in the saline-injected animals reveals that there is some weakness in the BoNT/A injected animals at sites distant to the original injection at one month ($P < 0.05$). Data are presented as mean ± SE and n=6-8 per group.

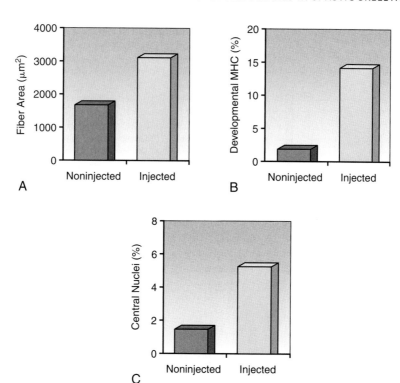

FIGURE 13-3. Comparison between groups injected with botulinum toxin (injected) and groups that were not injected (noninjected). **A,** Fiber area was significantly greater in injected compared with noninjected muscles ($P < 0.005$). **B,** Percentage of central nuclei was significantly greater in injected compared with noninjected muscles ($P < 0.01$). **C,** Percentage of muscle cells expressing both fast and slow myosin heavy chain isoforms. (Adapted from Runesson E, Ward SR, Stankovic N, Friden J, Lieber RL. Spastic muscles injected with botulinum toxin (type A) show intriguing signs of growth and pathology. *Muscle Nerve.* 2007. In press. Reprinted with permission of John Wiley & Sons, Inc.)

larger compared with that of muscles from subjects who had never received a BoNT/A injection (Fig. 13-3A). This is an important finding because decreased fiber area was also observed in spastic muscles (which never received BoNT/A).[12,13] Another significant difference between experimental groups was the increased capillarity of the injected muscles. The number of capillaries per fiber in the injected muscles was twice that of the noninjected muscles. Numerous pathologic signs were observed in the BoNT/A-injected tissue. For example, although the noninjected muscles had a normal internal nuclear percentage of $1.90 \pm 0.41\%$,[34,65] there was a threefold increase of central nuclei in injected versus noninjected muscles (see Fig. 13-3B). This result indicates that the injection process induced a degeneration-regeneration cycle that did not simply occur secondary to chronic spasticity. This abnormality is consistent with the fact that the injected muscles showed many other pathologic signs including increased numbers of angular fibers, an increased

percentage of fibers expressing both fast and slow myosin heavy chain isoforms, and an increased percentage of fibers expressing developmental MHC isoforms (see Fig. 13-3C). Taken together, these data suggest that BoNT/A-injected muscles likely undergo a degeneration-regeneration cycle. From this finding, it is possible to postulate that BoNT/A may be beneficial to muscle function, although further research is needed to explore this idea.

PRACTICAL CONSIDERATIONS IN NEUROTOXIN DELIVERY

Dose-Volume Interactions

One of the most important aspects of developing a high-resolution animal model of neurotoxin therapy is the ability to experimentally address clinically important questions. One such consideration is the relationship between

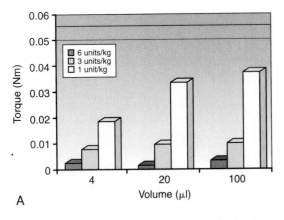

A

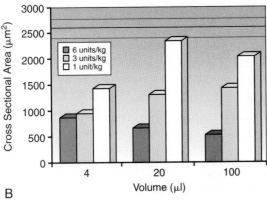

B

FIGURE 13-4. A, Dorsiflexion torque of botulinum neurotoxin type A (BoNT/A) 6 unit–, 3 unit–, and 1 unit–injected limbs 1 month post injection. Comparative values for saline controls are represented by three horizontal lines (mean ± SEM). **B,** Muscle fiber cross-sectional area of BoNT/A 6 unit–, 3 unit–, and 1 unit–injected limbs 1 month post injection. Comparative values for saline controls are represented by three horizontal lines (mean ± SEM). (Adapted from Hulst JB, Minatomo VB, Lim MJ, Bremner SN, Ward SR, Lieber RL. *The Effects of Dose and Volume on Muscle Structure and Function After Botulinum Toxin Injection* San Francisco, CA: Transactions of the Othopaedic Research Society; 2008.)

the injection concentrations and muscle paralysis. To address this question, we injected the tibialis anterior muscle of rats (unguided) with 6 units, 4 units, or 1 unit of toxin diluted in 100 μL, 20 μL, or 4 μL of normal saline (n = 6/group, 9 groups).[66] Animals were injected under anesthesia and returned to cage activity for 1 month. At the time of sacrifice, maximum isometric dorsiflexion torque was tested using a custom-made dynamometer and direct stimulation of the fibular nerve. The results of this study demonstrated that progressive increases in the dose of BoNT/A, and not volume, were associated with progressive muscle weakness (Fig. 13-4A). When muscle fiber cross-sectional area was quantified from histologic sections of the muscle (laminin immunohistochemistry), it became obvious that there was an interaction between dose and volume (see Fig. 13-4B). Although these fiber level changes could not be measured at the functional level, low and intermediate doses of the toxin at relatively high dilutions spared the fiber cross-sectional area.

Exercise as an Adjunct to Neurotoxin Delivery

One attempt to increase the efficacy of BoNT/A treatment involved activation of the affected muscle. Hughes and Whaler[67] hypothesized that the NT is most efficient in blocking neuromuscular junction activity when muscles are activated. This is reasonable in light of the report that nerve stimulation accelerates toxin internalization into the nerve terminal.[68] Although there are reports that both electrical stimulation[69-71] and voluntary exercise[72] do enhance the effects of toxin injection, none of these studies directly measured systemic muscle function. Rather, outcomes were judged based on subjective rating scales and voluntary strength estimates. Observed functional changes may thus be due to voluntary activation changes, neuromuscular junction functional changes, muscle fiber size changes, muscle fiber–type changes, or a combination of all of these factors.

To determine whether physical manipulation such as electrical stimulation and passive manipulation can alter the efficacy of BoNT/A treatment, we developed a high-resolution functional model of muscle torque generation that enables serial strength testing after treatment.[62] In addition, because the muscle tissue is accessible at the end of the experiment, functional changes can be directly interpreted in light of the structural properties of the muscle itself. We have been able to demonstrate that isometric exercise and passive stretch significantly improved the paralytic effect of BoNT/A in injected muscles.[62] In this experiment, Sprague-Dawley rats were divided into four experimental groups: BoNT/A (BT, n = 8), BoNT/A + isometric contraction (IC; n = 7), BoNT/A + passive stretch (PS; n = 7), and saline control (n=4). Animals were injected under anesthesia and returned to cage activity for 1 month before sacrifice. In the exercise groups, 10 maximum isometric contractions (via direct nerve stimulation) or 10 passive stretches were performed after the injection. At the time of sacrifice, maximum isometric dorsiflexion torque was tested using a custom-made dynamometer and direct stimulation of the fibular nerve. These data demonstrate that BoNT/A injection efficacy is increased (i.e., muscle force is decreased) after exercise regardless of whether the muscle manipulation is active (IC) or passive (PS) (Fig. 13-5A). Additionally, this exercise effect appears to be protective to the contralateral extremity in terms of torque and fiber cross-sectional area (see Fig. 13-5B). However, the mechanism of this effect was not clear.

Certainly, neural activity is not necessary since the PS groups were completely passive, and the angular velocity of plantarflexion was too slow to elicit a stretch reflex. The effect may have been as simple as distributing the injectate among the muscles' neuromuscular junctions, in which case almost any physical manipulation of the muscle would suffice. However, these questions will require further experimental work.

Passive Mechanical Changes in Response to Neurotoxin Therapy

Based on previous data suggesting that spastic muscles are more stiff in young humans with static encephalopathy[12,13] and that the passive mechanical properties of muscle can change with altered use,[73] we are currently investigating the affects of BoNT/A treatment on the passive mechanical properties of muscle. In this

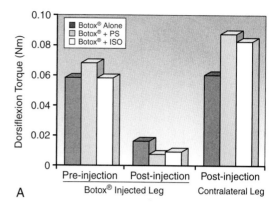

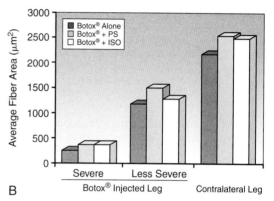

FIGURE 13-5. A, Dorsiflexion torque measured from botulinum toxin type A (BoNT/A)–injected leg (*two left groups of bars*) and the contralateral leg (*rightmost bars*) for the three treatments. Note that the two groups receiving manipulation (either passive stretch [PS] or isometric [ISO]) showed the greatest weakness. **B,** Fiber area measured in BoNT/A-injected muscles (*left two groups of bars*) and contralateral muscles (*rightmost bars*) for the three experimental treatments. Area is shown for the two different regions of the BoNT/A-injected muscles. (Adapted from Minamoto VB, Hulst JB, Lim MJ, Peace WJ, Bremner SN, Ward SR, Lieber, RL. Increased efficacy and decreased systemic-effects of neurotoxin injection after active and passive muscle manipulation. *Develop Med Child Neurol.* 2007;49:907-914.)

model, the tibialis anterior muscles of rats are injected with 6 units/Kg of BoNT/A and animals are returned to cage activity for 1 month. After this time, muscles are harvested and single muscle cells are extracted for mechanical testing. Our preliminary data suggest that injected muscles have 30% less stiffness than normal cells (Fig. 13-6).[74] It is important to note that this stiffness measurement, from a mechanical perspective, is insensitive to fiber area. Therefore, the reduction in stiffness we observed is not related to the decrease in area seen in these fibers. These data are promising because they suggest that

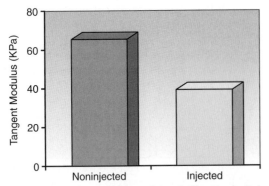

FIGURE 13-6. The tangent modulus (stiffness) of single muscle fibers is lower ($P < 0.05$) than normal muscle fibers 1 month after a single dose of botulinum neurotoxin type A (Botox, Allergan, Inc., Irvine, CA). (Adapted from Thacker BE, Tomiya A, Hulst JB, Bremner SN, Lieber RL, Ward SR. *Muscle Fiber Atrophy and Decreased Elastic Modulus in Response to Botulinum Toxin Injection.* San Francisco, CA: Transactions of the Orthopaedic Research Society; 2008.)

some of the tissue level changes associated with muscle spasticity may be reversible.

IMAGING AND NEUROTOXIN DELIVERY

In the process of acquiring the dose-volume and injections plus exercise data, we developed an assay for tracking intramuscular injections. Using a 7T high-resolution magnetic resonance imaging system, we were able to exploit the differences between muscle and injection T2 relaxation times. This imaging modality is capable of tracking injections as small as 100 µl (60 µm in-plane resolution) at 7-minute time intervals (Fig. 13-7A to C). The quantitative portion of the imaging technique is achieved by sampling each pixel in the image at 11 equally spaced echo times and fitting the signal decays as a function of time. The result of fitting the exponential decay is an absolute T2 time constant for each pixel. These data are then superimposed onto the structural image revealing 10 fold longer T2 times in the injected region compared with surrounding muscle. When this process is repeated in 7-minute increments, measurable diffusion (decreasing T2 relaxation times and increasing area within the muscle) can be seen in as little as 20 minutes. Using these methods in preliminary experimental work, we have been able to demonstrate that fluid is readily distributed and diffuses between muscle fascicles. Additionally, large injection volumes often separate fascicles and propagate between muscle boundaries (see Fig. 13-7B).

SUMMARY AND FUTURE DIRECTIONS

Although the primary lesion leading to spasticity lies within the central nervous system, muscle in patients with spasticity is also dramatically altered. This conclusion is based on results from studies using a variety of experimental methods in a number of diseases, across a wide range of patient ages. To summarize, we have made the case for the following alterations in spastic muscle: (1) altered muscle fiber size and fiber-type distribution; (2) proliferation of extracellular matrix material, measured morphologically and biochemically; (3) increased muscle cell stiffness, and (4) inferior mechanical properties of extracellular material compared with normal muscle. Improvement of the quality of life of patients with UMN syndrome depends on creating a new understanding of muscular changes that occur secondary to their syndrome process, and the development of rational interventions to either prevent these changes or reverse them. One such intervention is the therapeutic application of neurotoxins. We have presented the evidence from the literature and our own

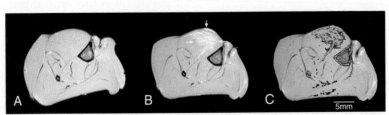

FIGURE 13-7. T2-weighted, multiecho magnetc resonance images of rat lower extremities before (**A**) and after (**B**) 100-µl injections of botulinum neurotoxin type A (BoNT/A) (*arrows*). The multiecho sequences allow a quantitative map of the T2 times to be superimposed on the injection region (**C**).

laboratory that muscles injected with BoNT/A (1) immediately have dramatically reduced force generating capacity, and (2) may have reduced mechanical stiffness. Relative to the injection itself, we have shown that (1) muscle weakness may not be isolated to the injected muscle in the small muscles of a rat, (2) the injection concentration is an important determinant of local and systemic weakness, and (3) exercise may augment the efficiency of paresis in neurotoxin therapy. Details of the structural changes that occur in spastic muscle and spastic muscle treated with neurotoxins are lacking. Basic questions that must be addressed in this field follow logically from the material presented herein. What are the proteins that are altered within spastic muscle cells and the extracellular matrix of spastic muscle tissue? What are the signaling events that lead to protein level changes in spastic muscle? How does neurotoxin therapy change muscle at the protein level over time? What are the important characteristics of optimal neurotoxin treatment? Specifically, what is the interaction between muscle structure and injection concentration? What are the important constraints to neurotoxin delivery within a muscle? Are there adjuncts to neurotoxin therapy (e.g., exercise) that improve efficiency and reduce side effects. These are the types of questions that must ultimately be answered to develop rational surgical and rehabilitation strategies to treat patients who suffer from this devastating malady.

References

1. Cadenhead SL, McEwen IR, Thompson DM. Effect of passive range of motion exercises on low goniometric measurements of adults with cerebral palsy. *Phys Ther*. 2002;82:658-669.
2. DeDeyne PG. Application of passive stretch and its implications for muscle fibers. *Phys Ther*. 2001;81:819-827.
3. Moseley AM. The effect of casting combined with stretching on passive ankle dorsiflexion in adults with traumatic injuries. *Phys Ther*. 1997;77:240-247.
4. Pohl M, Ruckriem S, Mehrholz J, Ritschel C, Strik H, Pause MR. Effectiveness of serial casting in patients with severe cerebral spasticity: a comparison study. *Arch Phys Med Rehabil*. 2002;83:784-790.
5. Steffen TM, Mollinger LA. Low-load, prolonged stretch in the treatment of knee flexion contractures in nursing home residents. *Phys Ther*. 1995;10:886-896.
6. Waitzman NJ, Romano PS, Scheffler RM. Estimates of the economic costs of birth defects. *Inquiry*. 1994;31:188-205.
7. Keenan ME. The orthopaedic management of spasticity. *J Head Trauma Rehabil*. 1987;12:62-71.
8. Dietz V, Quintern J, Berger W. Electrophysiological studies of gait in spasticity and rigidity. *Brain*. 1981;104:431-449.
9. Dietz V, Trippel M, Berger W. Reflex activity and muscle tone during elbow movements in patients with spastic paresis. *Ann Neurol*. 1991;30:767-779.
10. Herman R. The myotatic reflex. Clinico-physiological aspects of spasticity and contracture. *Brain*. 1970;93:273-312.
11. Salmons S, Henriksson J. The adaptive response of skeletal muscle to increased use. *Muscle Nerve*. 1981;4:94-105.
12. Fridén J, Lieber RL. Spastic muscle cells are shorter and stiffer than normal cells. *Muscle Nerve*. 2003;27:157-164.
13. Lieber RL, Runesson E, Einarsson F, Fridén J. Inferior mechanical properties of spastic muscle bundles due to hypertrophic but compromised extracellular matrix material. *Muscle Nerve*. 2003;28:464-471.
14. Sinkjaer T, Magnussen I. Passive, intrinsic and reflex-mediated stiffness in the ankle extensors of hemiparetic patients. *Brain*. 1994;117:355-363.
15. Eisenberg BR, Salmons S. The reorganization of subcellular structure in muscle undergoing fast-to-slow type transformation. A stereological study. *Cell Tissue Res*. 1981;220:449-471.
16. Pette D, Smith M, Staudte H, Vrbova G. Effects of long-term electrical stimulation on some contractile and metabolic characteristics of fast rabbit muscles. *Pflugers Arch*. 1973;338:257-272.
17. Salmons S, Streter FA. Significance of impulse activity in the transformation of skeletal muscle type. *Nature*. 1976;263:30-34.
18. Salmons S, Vrbova G. The influence of activity on some contractile characteristics of mammalian fast and slow muscles. *J Physiol (London)*. 1969;201:535-549.
19. Saltin B, Gollnick PD. Skeletal muscle adaptability: significance for metabolism and performance. XXX, ed. *Handbook of Physiology*. Baltimore: American Physiological Society; 1983:539-554.
20. Roy RR, Bello M, Bouissou P, Edgerton R. Size and metabolic properties of fibers in rat fast-twitch muscles after hindlimb suspension. *J Appl Physiol*. 1987;62:2348-2357.
21. Buller AJ, Lewis DM. Some observations on the effects of tenotomy in the rabbit. *J Physiol (London)*. 1965;178:326-342.
22. Booth FW, Kelso JR. Effect of hind-limb immobilization on contractile and histochemical properties of skeletal muscle. *Pflugers Arch*. 1973;342:123-238.
23. Maier A, Cocket JL, Simpson DR, Saubert CI, Edgerton VR. Properties of immobilized guinea pig hindlimb muscles. *Am J Physiol*. 1976;231:1520-1526.
24. Roy RR, Pierotti DJ, Flores V, Rudolph W, Edgerton VR. Fibre size and type adaptations to spinal isolation and cyclical passive stretch in cat hindlimb. *J Anat*. 1992;180:491-499.
25. Roy RR, Sacks RD, Baldwin KM, Short M, Edgerton VR. Interrelationships of contraction time, Vmax, and myosin ATPase after spinal transection. *J Appl Physiol*. 1984;56:1594-1601.
26. Lieber RL, Johansson CB, Vahlsing HL, Hargens AR, Feringa ER. Long-term effects of spinal cord transection on fast and slow rat skeletal muscle. I. Contractile properties. *Exp Neurol*. 1986;91:423-434.
27. Lieber RL, Fridén JO, Hargens AR, Feringa ER. Long-term effects of spinal cord transection of fast and slow rat skeletal muscle. II. Morphometric properties. *Exp Neurol*. 1986;91:435-448.
28. Grimby G, Broberg C, Krotkiewska I, Krotkiewski M. Muscle fiber composition in patients with traumatic cord lesion. *Scand J Rehabil Med*. 1976;8:37-42.

29. Jiang B, Roy R, Edgerton R. Expression of a fast fiber enzyme profile in the cat soleus after spinalization. *Muscle Nerve.* 1990;13:1037-1049.

30. Jiang B, Roy RR, Edgerton VR. Enzymatic plasticity of medial gastrocnemius fibers in the adult chronic spinal cat. *Am J Physiol.* 1990;259:C507-C14.

31. Roy RR, Talmadge RJ, Hodgson JA, Oishi Y, Baldwin KM, Edgerton VR. Differential response of fast hind-limb extensor and flexor muscles to exercise in adult spinalized cats. *Muscle Nerve.* 1999;22:230-241.

32. Pette D. *Plasticity of Muscle.* New York: Walter de Gruyter & Company 1980.

33. Pette D. *The Dynamic State of Muscle Fibers*, Berlin: Walter de Gruyter & Company 1990.

34. Carpenter S, Karpati G. *Pathology of Skeletal Muscle.* New York: Churchill Livingstone 1984.

35. Rose J, Haskell WL, Gamble JG, Hamilton RL, Brown DA, Rinsky L. Muscle pathology and clinical measures of disability in children with cerebral palsy. *J Orthop Res.* 1994;12:758-768.

36. Booth CM, Cortina-Borja MJ, Theologis TN. Collagen accumulation in muscles of children with cerebral palsy and correlation with severity of spasticity. *Dev Med Child Neurol.* 2001;43:314-320.

37. Castle ME, Reyman TA, Schneider M. Pathology of spastic muscle in cerebral palsy. *Clin Orthop Relat Res.* 1979;142:223-233.

38. Dietz V, Ketelsen UP, Berger W, Quintern J. Motor unit involvement in spastic paresis. Relationship between leg muscle activation and histochemistry. *J Neurol Sci.* 1986;75:89-103.

39. Ito M, Araki A, Tanaka H, Tasaki T, Cho K, Yamazaki R. Muscle histopathology in spastic cerebral palsy. *Brain Dev.* 1996;18:299-303.

40. Romanini L, Villani C, Meloni C, Calvisi V. Histological and morphological aspects of muscle in infantile cerebral palsy. *Ital J Orthop Traumatol.* 1989;15:87-93.

41. Dubowitz V, Brooke MH. *Muscle Biopsy: A Modern Approach.* Philadelphia: W.B. Saunders, Ltd; 1973.

42. Ounjian M, Roy RR, Eldred E, Garfinkel A, Payne JR, Armstrong A, et al. Physiological and developmental implications of motor unit anatomy. *J Neurobiol.* 1991;22:547-559.

43. Trotter JA. Dynamic shape of tapered skeletal muscle fibers. *J Morphol.* 1991;207:211-223.

44. Trotter JA, Purslow PP. Functional morphology of the endomysium in series fibered muscles. *J Morphol.* 1992;212:109-122.

45. Marbini A, Ferrari A, Cioni G, Bellanova MF, Fusco C, Gemignani F. Immunohistochemical study of muscle biopsy in children with cerebral palsy. *Brain Dev.* 2002;24:63-66.

46. Sjöström M, Fugl-Meyer AR, Nordin G, Wahlby L. Post-stroke hemiplegia; crural muscle strength and structure. *Scand J Rheumatol.* 1980;7:53-67.

47. Bergstrom J. Percutaneous needle biopsy of skeletal muscle in physiological and clinical research. *Scand J Clin Lab Invest.* 1975;35:609-616.

48. Lexell J, Downham D, Sjostrom M. Distribution of different fiber types in human skeletal muscles. A statistical and computational study of the fiber type arrangement in m. vastus lateralis of young, healthy males. *J Neurol Sci.* 1984;65:353-365.

49. Lexell J, Downham D, Sjostrom M. Distribution of different fibre types in human skeletal muscles. Fibre type arrangement in m. vastus lateralis from three groups of healthy men between 15 and 83 years. *J Neurol Sci.* 1986;72:211-222.

50. Mirbagheri MM, Barbeau H, Ladouceur M, Kearney RE. Intrinsic and reflex stiffness in normal and spastic, spinal cord injured subjects. *Exp Brain Res.* 2001;141:446-459.

51. Wood DJ, Zollman J, Reuban JP, Brandt PW. Human skeletal muscle: properties of the "chemically skinned" fiber. *Science* (Washington DC). 1975;187:1075-1076.

52. Wang K, McCarter R, Wright J, Beverly J, Ramirez-Mitchell R. Viscoelasticity of the sarcomere matrix of skeletal muscles. The titin-myosin composite filament is a dual-stage molecular spring. *Biophys J.* 1993;64:1161-1177.

53. Labeit S, Kolmerer B. Titins: Giant proteins in charge of muscle ultrastructure and elasticity. *Science* (Washington DC). 1995;270:293-296.

54. Magid A, Law DJ. Myofibrils bear most of the resting tension in frog skeletal muscle. *Science* (Washington DC). 1985;230:1280-1282.

55. Neagoe C, Kulke M, del Monte F, Gwathmey JK, de Tombe PP, Hajjar RJ, et al. Titin isoform switch in ischemic human heart disease. *Circulation.* 2002;106:1333-1341.

56. Chen SP, Sheu JR, Lin AC, Hsiao G, Fong TH. Decline in titin content in rat skeletal muscle after denervation. *Muscle Nerve.* 2005;32:798-807.

57. Olsson MC, Kruger M, Meyer LH, Ahnlund L, Gransberg L, Linke WA, et al. Fibre type-specific increase in passive muscle tension in spinal cord-injured subjects with spasticity. *J Physiol.* 2006;577(Pt 1):339-352.

58. Galli M, Cimolin V, Valente EM, Crivellini M, Ialongo T, Albertini G. Computerized gait analysis of botulinum toxin treatment in children with cerebral palsy. *Disabil Rehabil.* 2007;29:659-664.

59. Desloovere K, Molenaers G, De Cat J, Pauwels P, Van Campenhout A, Ortibus E, et al. Motor function following multilevel botulinum toxin type A treatment in children with cerebral palsy. *Dev Med Child Neurol.* 2007;49:56-61.

60. Papadonikolakis AS, Vekris MD, Korompilias AV, Kostas JP, Ristanis SE, Soucacos PN. Botulinum A toxin for treatment of lower limb spasticity in cerebral palsy: gait analysis in 49 patients. *Acta Orthop Scand.* 2003;74:749-755.

61. Longino D, Butterfield TA, Herzog W. Frequency and length-dependent effects of Botulinum toxin-induced muscle weakness. *J Biomech.* 2005;38:609-613.

62. Minamoto VB, Hulst JB, Lim MJ, Peace WJ, Bremner SN, Ward SR, Lieber RL. Increased efficacy and decreased systemic-effects of neurotoxin injection after active and passive muscle manipulation. *Develop Med Child Neurol.* 2007;49:907-914.

63. Racette BA, Lopate G, Good L, Sagitto S, Perlmutter JS. Ptosis as a remote effect of therapeutic botulinum toxin B injection. *Neurology.* 2002;59:1445-1447.

64. Runesson E, Ward SR, Stankovic N, Friden J, Lieber RL. Spastic muscles injected with botulinum toxin (type A) show intriguing signs of growth and pathology. *Muscle Nerve.* 2007;In press.

65. Engel AG, Banker AQ, eds. *Myology.* New York, NY: McGraw-Hill Book Company; 1986.

66. Hulst JB, Minatomo VB, Lim MJ, Bremner SN, Ward SR, Lieber RL. *The Effects of Dose and Volume on Muscle Structure and Function After Botulinum Toxin Injection.* San Francisco, CA: Transactions of the Othopaedic Research Society; 2008.

67. Hughes R, Whaler B. Influence of nerve-ending activity and of drugs on the rate or paralysis of rat diaphragm

preparation by *Cl. Botulinum* type A toxin. *J Physiol.* 1962;160:221-233.

68. Black JD, Dolly JO. Interaction of 125I-labeled botulinum neurotoxins with nerve terminals. II. Autoradiographic evidence for its uptake into motor nerves by acceptor-mediated endocytosis. *J Cell Biol.* 1986;103:535-544.

69. Bayram S, Sivrioglu K, Karli N, Ozcan O. Low-dose botulinum toxin with short-term electrical stimulation in poststroke spastic drop foot: a preliminary study. *Am J Phys Med Rehabil.* 2006;85:75-81.

70. Frasson E, Priori A, Ruzzante B, Didone G, Bertolasi L. Nerve stimulation boosts botulinum toxin action in spasticity. *Mov Disord.* 2005;20:624-629.

71. Eleopra R, Tugnoli V, Caniatti L, De Grandis D. Botulinum toxin treatment in the facial muscles of humans: evidence of an action in untreated near muscles by peripheral local diffusion. *Neurology.* 1996;46: 1158-1160.

72. Chen R, Karp BI, Hallett M. Botulinum toxin type F for treatment of dystonia: long-term experience. *Neurology.* 1998;51:1494-1496.

73. Toursel T, Stevens L, Granzier H, Mounier Y. Passive tension of rat skeletal soleus muscle fibers: effects of unloading conditions. *J Appl Physiol.* 2002;92: 1465-1472.

74. Thacker BE, Tomiya A, Hulst JB, Bremner SN, Lieber RL, Ward SR. *Muscle Fiber Atrophy and Decreased Elastic Modulus in Response to Botulinum Toxin Injection.* San Francisco. CA: Transactions of the Orthopaedic Research Society; 2008.

Treatment of Motor Disorders in Cerebral Palsy with Botulinum Neurotoxin

14

Jane Leonard and H. Kerr Graham

INTRODUCTION

Botulinum neurotoxins have been used in the management of movement disorders associated with cerebral palsy (CP) for the past 15 years. This has led to the development of sophisticated multidisciplinary management programs for such diverse problems as spastic equinus, hemiplegic posturing in the upper limb, excessive drooling, and pain management. In the interests of an improved understanding of these new management approaches, it is necessary to review current ideas on the definition, classification, and rehabilitation paradigms in CP.

CEREBRAL PALSY: DEFINITIONS

CP was first described in 1861 by William Little, an English physician who later introduced tenotomy for the correction of deformity to the practice of medicine in England. He proposed a link between abnormal parturition, difficult labor, premature birth, asphyxia neonatorum, and physical deformities.[1] The term CP was also used by Sir William Osler in 1889 in a book titled *The Cerebral Palsies of Children*.[2] Freud considered CP to be caused not just at parturition but also earlier in pregnancy because of "deeper effects that influenced the development of the foetus."[3]

Mac Keith and Polani of the Little Club in the UK defined CP as 'a persisting but not unchanging disorder of movement and posture, appearing in the early years of life and due to a non-progressive disorder of the brain, the result of interference during its development.'[4] Bax redefined this as 'a disorder of movement and posture due to a defect or lesion of the immature brain' and recommended that description should be based on clinical features, and that attempts to define certain syndromes combining clinical etiologic and pathologic features should be avoided.[5] He hoped for a simple definition that could be translated universally. A revised definition, emphasizing the underlying heterogeneity of the condition, was introduced in 1992 as "an umbrella term covering a group of non-progressive, but often changing, motor impairment syndromes secondary to lesions or anomalies of the brain arising in the early stages of development."[6]

The definition of CP was revised again in 2005 by an international committee as "a group of permanent disorders of the development of movement and posture, causing activity limitation, that are attributed to non-progressive disturbances that occurred in the developing fetal or infant brain.[7] The motor disorders of CP are often accompanied by disturbances of sensation, perception, cognition, communication, and behavior, by epilepsy, and by secondary musculoskeletal problems."[8]

Dr. Leonard does not report any conflicts of interest. Professor Kerr Graham discloses that he receives research support from Allergan and is a consultant for the Neurotoxin Institute.

CLASSIFYING CEREBRAL PALSY

CP is the most common cause of physical disability affecting children in developed countries, with a prevalence of 2 to 2.5/1000 live births.[8] It affects about 764,000 children and adults in the United States of America, with an economic burden approaching $1.18 billion in direct medical costs and $1.105 billion in direct nonmedical costs and an additional $9.24 billion in indirect costs, for a total cost of $11.5 billion or an average of $921,000 per individual.[9]

Spastic CP is the most common type of movement disorder, accounting for approximately 60% to 85% of all CP in developed countries.[8] Spasticity can be defined as a velocity-dependent resistance to passive movement of a joint and its associated musculature.[10] Spasticity, among other features of an upper motor neuron syndrome, leads to a loss of ability of muscle to stretch in a relaxed state. This is important because such stretch of the relaxed muscle is a stimulus to longitudinal growth.[11] Dyskinetic CP accounts for approximately 10% to 25% of cases, and is characterized by involuntary movements and fluctuating muscle tone, which result in an inability to execute and coordinate simple tasks.[12] Dyskinetic movement disorders may be athetoid, dystonic, or choreic. Ataxic CP accounts for less than 5% of cases.[8]

The classification of CP, which encompasses heterogeneous clinical phenotypes, has provoked controversy in recent years.[13] The heterogeneity of disorders covered by the term CP may severely compromise communication.[14] Common ground for communication about the child with CP is crucial for aspects such as diagnosis, management, and research.

Traditionally, CP has been classified according to motor type and topographic distribution (limb distribution).[15,16] Motor classification is according to the movement disorders listed earlier. Topographic distribution includes terms such as hemiplegia, diplegia and quadriplegia, and the less frequently used terms monoplegia and triplegia, indicating number of limbs involved. Classifications based on motor type and topographic distribution have poor reliability, even when observers are experienced and undergo special training.[17] However, they are familiar, widely used, and clinically significant.[18]

A simplification of the above-mentioned limb distributions to either unilateral involvement or bilateral involvement has been suggested to improve the agreement of this type of classification.[19]

It has become apparent that additional characteristics must be taken into account for a classification scheme to contribute further to the understanding and management of CP. The World Health Organization's (WHO's) International Classification of Functioning (ICF) describes health conditions in several domains, including body structure and function, activities and participation, as noted in Figure 14-1.

These are modified by environmental factors and personal factors.[20] Various tools exist to measure parameters relevant to CP in the ICF domains, and new measurement tools are being developed.

Perhaps the most important domain relevant to management is "body structure and function." Fortunately, there are now valid and reliable tools to classify and measure gross motor function in both the upper and lower limbs.

The Gross Motor Function Classification System (GMFCS) is a five-level ordinal grading system based on the assessment of self-initiated

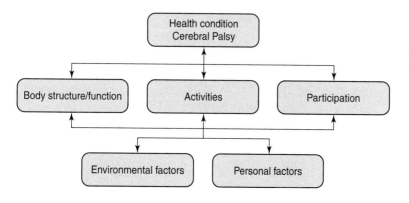

FIGURE 14-1. The World Health Organization International Classification of Functioning as applied to cerebral palsy.

movement with emphasis on function during sitting, standing, and walking.[21] It has been shown to be a valid, reliable, stable, and clinically relevant method for the classification and prediction of motor function in children with CP between the ages of 2 and 12 years (Fig. 14-2).

The Manual Activity Classification System (MACS) was styled on the GMFCS, with five ordinal levels that are intended to differentiate between levels of manual ability in a clinically meaningful way. Interobserver reliability between health professionals has been shown to be very high.[22] The revised definition and classification of CP in 2005 and the development of the GMFCS and the MACS have dramatically improved communication about the child with CP.

GMFCS E & R between 6th and 12th birthday: Descriptors and illustrations

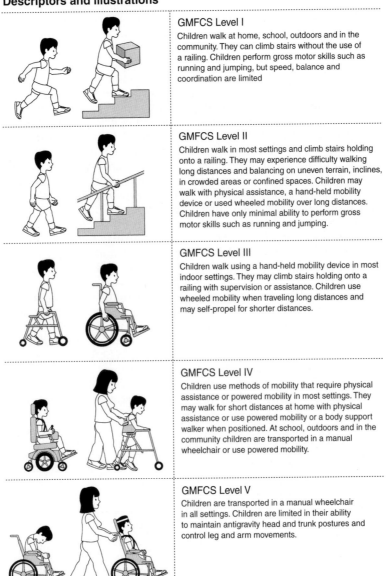

GMFCS Level I

Children walk at home, school, outdoors and in the community. They can climb stairs without the use of a railing. Children perform gross motor skills such as running and jumping, but speed, balance and coordination are limited

GMFCS Level II

Children walk in most settings and climb stairs holding onto a railing. They may experience difficulty walking long distances and balancing on uneven terrain, inclines, in crowded areas or confined spaces. Children may walk with physical assistance, a hand-held mobility device or used wheeled mobility over long distances. Children have only minimal ability to perform gross motor skills such as running and jumping.

GMFCS Level III

Children walk using a hand-held mobility device in most indoor settings. They may climb stairs holding onto a railing with supervision or assistance. Children use wheeled mobility when traveling long distances and may self-propel for shorter distances.

GMFCS Level IV

Children use methods of mobility that require physical assistance or powered mobility in most settings. They may walk for short distances at home with physical assistance or use powered mobility or a body support walker when positioned. At school, outdoors and in the community children are transported in a manual wheelchair or use powered mobility.

GMFCS Level V

Children are transported in a manual wheelchair in all settings. Children are limited in their ability to maintain antigravity head and trunk postures and control leg and arm movements.

FIGURE 14-2. Illustrations and descriptors for the Gross Motor Function Classification System in children with cerebral palsy aged 6 to 12 years. (Illustrations copyright © Kerr G, Reid B, Harvey A. The Royal Children's Hospital, Melbourne, Australia.)

CEREBRAL PALSY AND THE UPPER MOTOR NEURON SYNDROME

CP is the most common cause in childhood of upper motor neuron syndrome, which has positive and negative features. Positive effects include phenomena such as spastic hypertonia, co-contraction, associated reactions, and hyper-reflexia. The negative effects include weakness, deficient motor control, and impaired sensation. Although clinicians may emphasize the positive effects, the negative effects may have a greater impact on gross motor function. In essence, weakness and deficient motor control are greater barriers to function than spasticity and other positive features. However, positive features such as spasticity are pivotal in establishing a chain of events that lead to progressive musculoskeletal pathology, including fixed contractures of muscle-tendon units, torsional deformities of long bones, joint instability, and degenerative arthritis. In the growing child, intervention to ameliorate spastic hypertonia and other positive features may delay or prevent the cascade effect leading to progressive musculoskeletal pathology (Fig. 14-3).

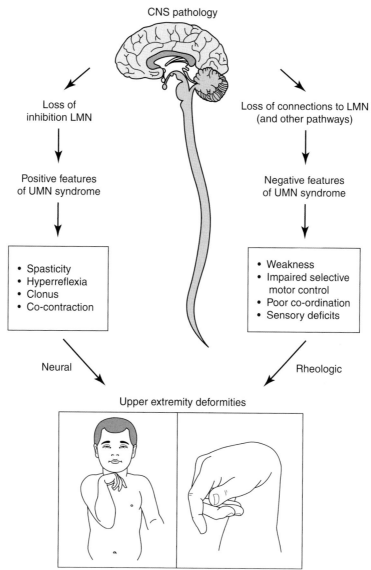

FIGURE 14-3. Neuromuscular skeletal pathology of the upper extremity in hemiplegic cerebral palsy. (Modified from Chin TYP, Duncan JA, Johnstone BR, Graham HK. Management of the upper limb in cerebral palsy. J Pediatr Orthop 2005;14:389-404.)

CEREBRAL PALSY AND PROGRESSIVE MUSCULOSKELETAL PATHOLOGY

Fixed musculoskeletal pathology in CP is acquired during childhood. Children with CP do not have contractures, dislocated hips, or scoliosis at birth. These common deformities are acquired during childhood. Muscle growth in children is a race between the pacemakers, that is, the physes of the long bones, and the muscle-tendon units, in which the muscles are doomed to second place.[23] Frequent stretching of relaxed muscle is a prerequisite for normal muscle growth. In children with CP, the muscles do not readily relax because of their positive features, and they are stretched infrequently because of reduced voluntary activity of their opposite counterparts. Muscle hyperactivity generated by positive signs on one side of a joint plus reduced voluntary activity on the other side of the joint leads to failure of longitudinal muscle growth, contractures, and fixed deformities.[24,25] The limb pathology can be considered in three stages:

Stage 1: Typically, deformities in the younger child with CP are all dynamic or reversible. This is the phase when positive sign management, gait training, and the use of orthoses may be most useful. Orthopedic surgery is not indicated.

Stage 2: There are fixed contractures, which may require surgical lengthening of muscles or tendons.

Stage 3: There are changes in bones and joints, including torsion of the long bones and joint instability. The most common torsional problems are medial femoral torsion and lateral tibial torsion. Joint instability problems include hip subluxation and subtalar collapse in the hindfoot[23] (Fig. 14-4).

MEASUREMENT OF SPASTICITY IN CEREBRAL PALSY

Of the few clinical measures of spasticity that exist, none are validated for use in children. The Ashworth and modified Ashworth scales are blunt and unresponsive tools in the assessment of the child with CP.[26,27] Their evaluations are subjective, and reliability between investigators is often a problem. Of much greater utility is the measurement of dynamic joint range, which can be used across most major joints as a quantitative measure of spasticity.[28,29]

The range of motion (ROM) of joints in both the upper and lower limbs is classically used as a proxy measure of the length of muscles crossing that joint. In the upper limb, the range of elbow extension is taken to be a

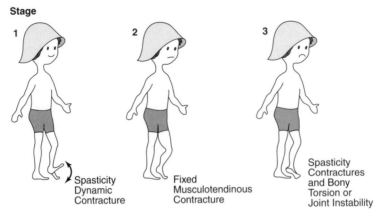

Stage

1 Spasticity
Dynamic
Contracture

2 Fixed
Musculotendinous
Contracture

3 Spasticity
Contractures
and Bony
Torsion or
Joint Instability

- Physical Therapy
- Orthotics
- Botulinum Neurotoxin A

- Tendon Lengthening

- Tendon Lengthening
- Rotational Osteotomies
- Arthrodeses

FIGURE 14-4. The three principal stages in the transition of dynamic gait dysfunction to fixed musculoskeletal pathology in children with cerebral palsy. (Modified from Hutchinson R, Graham HK. Management of spasticity in children. In Barnes MP, Johnson GR, eds. Upper Motor Neurone Syndrome and Spasticity. Clinical Management and Neurophysiology, 2nd ed. Cambridge, UK: Cambridge University Press; 2008.)

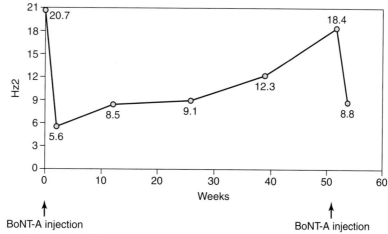

FIGURE 14-5. Resonant frequency in the hemiplegic upper limb and response to injection of botulinum toxin type A. Note the dramatic fall in resonant frequency from 20.7 Hz² to 5.6 Hz² immediately after injection, followed by a slow increase in resonant frequency back to 18.4 Hz² at 1 year after injection. At this point, a second injection is given with a further fall in resonant frequency from 18.4 Hz² to 8.8 Hz². (From Corry IS, Cosgrave AP, Walsh EG, et al. Botulinum toxin A in the hemiplegic upper limb: a double blind trial. Dev Med Child Neurol 1997;39:185-193, with permission.)

measure of the length of the elbow flexors, the biceps and brachialis. Loss of elbow extension (fixed flexion deformity) is taken to mean shortening of the elbow flexors, although it should be noted that other factors such as intrinsic joint contractures must be excluded.

The Tardieu scale grades the quality of the reaction of the muscle to passive stretch and measures the dynamic component of muscle spasticity. To measure the dynamic component the joint is moved as fast as possible through its full range of movement.[28] The angle when the muscles first catch (when the stretch reflex is elicited) is measured as R1, and the angle of full passive range of movement (ROM) of the joint is R2. The difference between these angles (R2-R1) reflects the potential ROM available to the child if spasticity could be eliminated (dynamic component). The quality of the muscle reaction is rated from 0 (no resistance through the range of passive movement) to 5 (joint immovable).

The measurement of R2 and R1 is of great practical relevance in the management of spasticity because it helps to

- differentiate between spasticity and contracture
- quantify the degree of spasticity present
- select which muscles might respond to spasticity management
- serve to monitor the response to spasticity management

Resonant frequency[30] is an objective assessment of joint stiffness that is altered by muscle tone. It has been used to describe mechanical stiffness in the wrist and ankle for children with CP. It has been defined as the frequency of movement of a joint at which the maximum speed and amplitude are produced from a given preset force.[31] It has been described in the hemiplegic upper limb spasticity and also been used in assessment of muscle tone at the ankle in lower limb spasticity,[32] showing a significant increase in resonant frequency comparing the spastic limb with the normal one in hemiplegic CP (Fig. 14-5).

INTERNATIONAL CLASSIFICATION OF FUNCTIONING AND QUALITY OF LIFE

The concept of disability is giving way to a health status construct in which biologic, social, and personal attributes determine activity and participation in society. These concepts are embodied in the ICF developed by the World Health Organization. The ICF is linked to causes of impairments and disabilities through the International Classification of Diseases. It provides a useful framework for understanding the impact of physical or structural deficits (impairments) on the performance of tasks (activities) and engagement in activities at home, school, and in the community (participation).[20] It also considers the effect of environmental and personal factors on function and disability, whether assistive devices can be used to enhance performance, and quantifies the severity of impairments. The use of concepts embodied in the ICF helps clinicians gain a comprehensive understanding of a child's physical impairment and its impact on function. This forms a basis for establishing treatment goals and developing treatment plans (see Fig. 14-1).

Traditional outcome measures used in medicine, especially survival or reduction of symptoms, do not capture the whole range of ways in which a patient may be affected by illness or treatment.[33] The inclusion of more holistic outcomes, such as measures of quality of life (QoL) and health-related quality of life (HRQoL), is gaining increasing interest. Despite ongoing discussions of health measurement, researchers have yet to decide upon a universal definition of QoL and HRQoL. What has become clear, however, is that QoL refers to the notion of holistic well-being,[34] whereas HRQoL focuses on the health-related components of life satisfaction,[35] such as self-care, mobility, and communication.

CEREBRAL PALSY AND MULTIDISCIPLINARY MANAGEMENT

The physical management of CP in childhood is complex and best provided in a multidisciplinary team approach with input from developmental pediatricians, pediatric neurologists, occupational therapists, physiotherapists, orthotists, orthopedic surgeons, pediatric physiatrists, and plastic surgeons.

The motor impairment in CP is often accompanied by associated impairments, as noted in the 2005 revised definition.[7] These associated impairments may include epilepsy, hearing and visual problems, cognitive and attentional deficits, and emotional and behavioral issues and later developing musculoskeletal problems.[13] Multidisciplinary management ensures that the child is seen as an individual within a family and a community, and decisions are based on comprehensive evaluation. Relevant assessments may include standardized physical examination, video recording of gait, and instrumented gait analysis. Three-dimensional gait analysis usually includes kinematics,

kinetics, electromyography, and physiological testing.[23]

CEREBRAL PALSY AND THE SPASTICITY COMPASS

The choice of interventions for the management of the movement disorders associated with CP in children is extensive and varied. It can be difficult at first sight to determine on what criteria the choice should be made between many competing options. The concept of the "spasticity compass" can be a useful template with which to compare some of the characteristics of the principal intervention, in terms of whether they are focal or generalized in their effect and to whether they are temporary or permanent. It is then possible to construct a compass with 'general-focal' on the north-south axis and 'reversible-permanent' on the east-west axis (Fig. 14-6). Each intervention can then be located in the appropriate quadrant or area of the grid, as defined by the two axes. For example, oral medications are general (all nerves or all muscles in all body areas) but clearly temporary in effect. When oral medications are stopped, their effects stop after an interval determined by the pharmacokinetics of the drug in question. Selective dorsal rhizotomy (SDR) is a neurosurgical procedure in which 30% to 50% of the dorsal rootlets between L1 and S1 are transected for the permanent relief of spasticity in a highly selective group of children with spastic diplegia.[36-38] The principal effects are on the lower limbs, although there may be minor effects on the upper limbs. Therefore, the position on the grid is permanent and halfway between general and focal.

Oral medications used for the management of spasticity in children with CP include benzodiazepines, especially diazepam, baclofen, dantrolene sodium and tizanidine.[9] Artane and L-dopa are used in dystonia. All are limited in usefulness by a combination of limited benefit and side effects. They have been extensively reviewed in several recent publications and will not be considered further here.[9,39,40]

The limited lipid solubility of baclofen when administered orally can be overcome by intrathecal administration using a programmable, battery-operated implantable pump connected to a catheter and delivery system to the intrathecal space. This is an invasive procedure with the potential for serious adverse events including mortality. However, it is the most effective

FIGURE 14-6. The spasticity compass and spasticity management in children with cerebral palsy. The north-south axis is general-focal and the west-east axis is permanent-reversible.

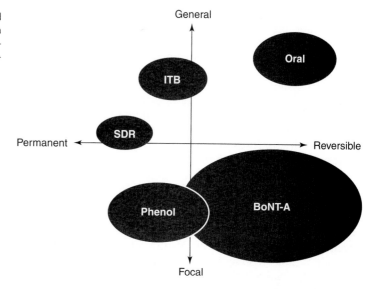

current method available for the management of severe spasticity, dystonia, and mixed movement disorders in CP and a number of other conditions, including spasticity of spinal origin and acquired brain injury. The role of intrathecal baclofen (ITB) has been reviewed extensively in several recent publications.[9,41]

Chemodenervation is invaluable in the management of focal spasticity and dystonia.[42] Phenol neurolysis was much more widely used before the introduction of botulinum neurotoxin A (BoNT/A).[43,44] The principal limitation on its use is pain at the site of injection and postinjection paresthesia. This is because phenol is not selective and has the same effect on sensory nerve fibers as motor fibers. Hence its use in mixed nerves in children with CP is very limited.[43]

Phenol can be used in various concentrations and administered by a variety of routes to nerves of all sizes. In CP the principal indications are neurolysis of the musculocutaneous nerve in the management of elbow flexor spasticity. In the lower limb, the principal application is neurolysis of the obturator nerve for adductor spasticity.[44] These nerves have such limited sensory distribution that the usual strictures in respect of sensory disturbance and paresthesia do not apply.

BOTULINUM NEUROTOXIN IN CEREBRAL PALSY

Clinical experience with BoNT/A) in treatment of spasticity in children spans more than a decade with the pioneering trials from Koman and colleagues in the United States of America[45] and Graham and colleagues in the United Kingdom.[46,47] There are seven Botulinum toxin serotypes (A-F) of which only types A and B have been reported in children with CP. The differences in serotypes have been described in detail elsewhere in this volume.

Botulinum neurotoxin type B has a shorter duration of action than type A and a less satisfactory adverse event profile, in children with CP.[48,49] The majority of clinical applications to date, in CP have therefore been with botulinum neurotoxin A (BoNT/A). BoNT/A is a potent neurotoxin produced by the bacterium *Clostridium botulinum* under anaerobic conditions. It produces a dose-dependent, reversible chemodenervation of the injected muscle by blocking presynaptic release of acetylcholine at the neuromuscular junctions. Because of rapid and high-affinity binding to receptors at the neuromuscular junctions of the target muscle, little systemic spread of toxin occurs.[50] Neural transmission is restored initially by the sprouting of new nerve endings, but these are finally eliminated at about three months, when the original nerve endings regain their ability to release acetylcholine. A reduction in muscle strength and spasticity is seen, with the effect usually lasting 3 to 6 months. Careful biomechanical studies show reduced muscle stiffness for up to 12 months after a single injection of BoNT/A.[42]

Effective management of children with CP requires understanding of the pathophysiology and natural history of each subtype or classification of the movement disorders, careful individualized assessment of abilities and limitations, and a broad knowledge of the appropriate applications and limitations of treatment modalities. The predictable movement patterns and postures that are characteristic of spasticity enable a systematic clinical rationale to be developed to determine the role of BoNT/A to manage the spasticity and improve function. The management of dystonia with BoNT/A is more complex, particularly when spasticity and dystonia are present in combination.

Although the principle of BoNT/A therapy in children is remarkably simple, the application can be challenging in the presence of a complex, changing movement disorder. BoNT/A injections result in a localized, temporary, reversible chemodenervation of the injected muscles, thus converting weakness with muscle hyperactivity to weakness with muscle hypoactivity. Although CP is not a focal disorder, it may be appropriate to treat identified focal problems, as long as the intervention is goal directed. Muscle hyperactivity in children, while being a common problem that impairs voluntary movement, can, on occasion, be valuable for maintenance of trunk posture or weight bearing on a weak limb or for ambulation.[51] Spasticity and other positive signs should not be treated just because they are present. Hence the prime goal of muscle hyperactivity management must be improved function. Muscle "balancing" in the growing, changing child requires a range of complementary and carefully timed intervention options.[51] There are other impairments that commonly coexist with the spastic movement disorder in children with CP that may influence treatment decisions: cognition; motivation; vision and hearing impairments; behavior disorders, and epilepsy.[51]

The use of BoNT/A addresses only part of the overall management of movement disorder, and the therapeutic indications for the role of BoNT/A therapy need to take account of the following principles:

- The movement problem is focal or regional, that is, only a few muscles are impeding the goal. This is often the case, that is, treating a focal problem within a generalized condition.
- The movement problem is dynamic or hyperkinetic, that is, due to muscle overactivity or hyperactivity.
- Identification and management of other contributions to the movement problem and dysfunction are critical

- It is essential to identify individual treatment goals that are meaningful, motivational, and useful to the child.[51]

Botulinum toxin may prove to be a useful adjuvant in conservative management of the muscle hyperactivity of CP. Successful management with these injections may allow delay of surgical intervention until the child is older and at less risk of possible complications, including the need for repeated surgical procedures.[52]

Reduced muscle tone provides a window of opportunity for therapeutic intervention. The denervation temporarily reduces unwanted muscle contraction and provides an opportunity for the spastic muscles to be stretched and the usual dominating involuntary patterns to be controlled. The antagonist muscles can be strengthened, which provides the opportunity to develop better muscle balance and control in some children.[53] Physical interventions such as casting and the use of orthoses can be used to guide and direct children's responses to altered muscle states and to assist them to learn new and more functional motor patterns.[54-56] The need for an individualized, coordinated multidisciplinary approach to the use of BoNT/A in the management of children with CP is evident. The popularity of BoNT/A as a treatment method in CP may have grown too fast, with popular use outstripping intelligent and effective application. The variation in functional outcomes is unsurprisingly vast.

MANAGEMENT OF MUSCLE HYPERACTIVITY IN THE LOWER LIMBS WITH BOTULINUM NEUROTOXIN A

Spastic Equinus

The most common dynamic deformity in children with CP is spastic equinus, which affects about 60% to 80% of children, in population based studies.[18]

Injection of the gastrocsoleus muscle is by far the most common and most important indication for BoNT/A therapy in children with CP. This is not only because BoNT/A is moderately effective but because the alternative, early muscle-tendon surgery is so very harmful.[57] The introduction of BoNT/A to the management of equinus in children with CP has dramatically changed the functional outcome of these children to a degree that those who have not worked in the pre-BoNT/A era can scarcely appreciate. Before widespread use of BoNT/A for spastic equinus, the majority of children with CP who walked on their toes had a lengthening of their Achilles' tendons by the age of 5 or 6 years.[58] This resulted in complete correction of equinus and set the scene for the progressive development of crouch gait, which was much more disabling than the original equinus gait. This could only be partially salvaged by complex, invasive orthopedic surgery repeated at intervals throughout childhood.[59] Now children with spastic equinus usually commence BoNT/A therapy aged between 1 and 3 years, in conjunction with physical therapy and the use of appropriate ankle-foot orthoses (AFOs). They receive injections every 6 to 12 months for several years until gross motor function plateaus at 4 to 6 years of age. Residual contractures and bony torsion can then be dealt with as "single event, multilevel surgery." The functional outcomes of this sequential nonoperative, BoNT/A-based program followed by one episode of multilevel reconstructive surgery, is an order of magnitude better than the piecemeal surgery of the past. Hence a nonoperative program of care using BoNT/A should be viewed as complementary to orthopedic surgical reconstruction and not as an alternative.

Upper motor neuron gait patterns in early childhood are dominated by "true equinus," although other muscles may be hyperactive and contribute to gait dysfunction.[60,61] It is the safe and effective correction of spastic equinus that results in the most significant improvements in gait and gains in gross motor function. Injection protocols for the gastrocsoleus have been developed by pooling experience gained from several studies and are now well established and fully described.[45,47,62-65]

Selection of target muscles for injection should be based on a combination of observation of gait and posture, standardized physical examination, and appreciation of the child, parent's, and therapist's functional goals and current limitations. It is very important to identify the child's sagittal gait pattern, whether the child has spastic hemiplegia or spastic diplegia (Figs. 14-7 to 14-9).[60,61,66]

Doses and dilution of BoNT/A for the management of spastic equinus depend on the preparation used and have been published elsewhere.[9,67] The majority of experienced clinicians are now using higher doses and greater dilutions than were employed in earlier

Spastic hemiplegia (right)

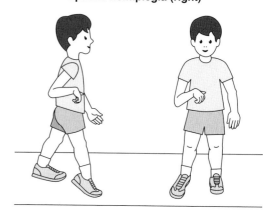

Target muscles

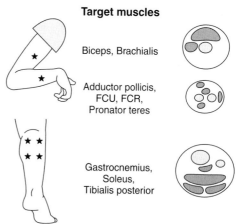

Biceps, Brachialis

Adductor pollicis,
FCU, FCR,
Pronator teres

Gastrocnemius,
Soleus,
Tibialis posterior

FIGURE 14-7. Posturing in spastic hemiplegia in children with cerebral palsy and the usual target muscles in the upper and lower limb, which are commonly injected with botulinum neurotoxin type A. (From Gibson N, Graham HK, Love S. Botulinum toxin A in the management of focal muscle overactivity in children with cerebral palsy. *Disabil Rehabil.* 2007;29:1813-1822, with permission.)

studies.[43,68] This has improved the efficacy of injection without a significant increase in systemic spread and adverse events.

Identification of the target muscle has traditionally been based on anatomic landmarks and palpation. However, biomechanical tests may be helpful, but it should be noted that the accuracy of injection based on palpation is very poor, except for the gastrocsoleus.[69] Electrical stimulation and ultrasound have dramatically improved the accuracy of injection of target muscles in children with CP. It has been more difficult to determine if improved accuracy of injection has improved outcomes.[70,71]

Injection of BoNT/A for spastic equinus increases the dynamic length of the gastrocsoleus and also provides improvements in ankle

Spastic diplegia

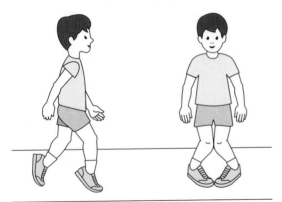

Spastic quadriplegia

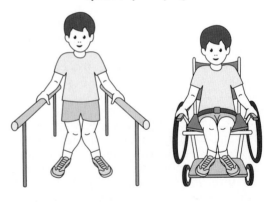

Target muscles

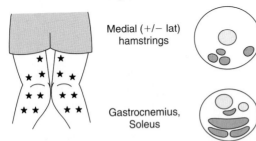

Medial (+/− lat) hamstrings

Gastrocnemius, Soleus

FIGURE 14-8. Spastic diplegia typical posturing in the child with spastic diplegia and the most frequently injected target muscles in the lower limbs. (From Gibson N, Graham HK, Love S. Botulinum toxin A in the management of focal muscle overactivity in children with cerebral palsy. *Disabil Rehabil.* 2007;29:1813-1822, with permission.)

Target muscles

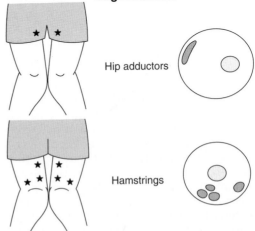

Hip adductors

Hamstrings

FIGURE 14-9. Posture in a child with spastic quadriplegia and the commonly injected target muscles with botulinum neurotoxin type A. (From Gibson N, Graham HK, Love S. Botulinum toxin A in the management of focal muscle overactivity in children with cerebral palsy. *Disabil Rehabil.* 2007;29:1813-1822, with permission.)

dorsiflexion during gait. Koman and colleagues[55] reported improvements in gait as determined by the Physician Rating Scale. Many authors have reported gait improvements using instrumented gait analysis, including kinematics, kinetics, and electromyography.[72-74] This usually leads to small but important gains in gross motor function. There is evidence that this delays the onset of fixed equinus, which delays the need for orthopedic surgery until the optimum age. There is less need for repeat surgery, and surgical outcomes and overall gross motor function and gait are improved.

Spastic Equinovarus and Equinovalgus

Spastic equinovarus is the result of muscle hyperactivity in the gastrocsoleus, tibialis posterior and/or tibialis anterior muscles. One third of cases are caused by the tibialis posterior muscle, one third by the tibialis anterior muscle, and one third by overactivity

in both the tibialis posterior and tibialis anterior muscles.[75] In spastic equinovarus the most effective strategy is to inject the gastrocsoleus and the tibialis posterior muscles. Injection of tibialis anterior muscle is not advised on the basis that this would weaken ankle dorsiflexion.

Equinovalgus is not usually the result of muscle imbalance but altered biomechanics. It is best managed by injection of the gastrocsoleus muscle and provision of an appropriate AFO.[76]

The management of spastic equinus by BoNT/A has had a very positive impact on the overall management of CP in childhood. Early surgical lengthening of the gastrocsoleus muscle can be avoided, and about 40% of children will not require calf lengthening surgery. For those who do progress to surgery,

surgery need only be performed once and can be performed at the optimum age.

Injection of the Hamstrings and Adductor Muscles in Cerebral Palsy

The indications, techniques and outcomes of injecting the hamstring and adductor muscles were first described by Corry et al[46] and subsequently by others. Muscle hyperactivity in the hamstring and adductor muscles is more prevalent in the more severely involved child and may result in scissoring postures and crouch gait. Although there is evidence for improved function and reduced improved ease of care in some studies, the goal of preventing spastic hip displacement has not been realized. In a large multicenter randomized trial, Graham and colleagues[77] studied the effects of injection of the adductor and hamstring muscles with BoNT/A every 6 months, combined with a hip abduction brace, during a 3-year randomized clinical trial. The rate of hip displacement was reduced slightly in the treatment group, but most children required surgical stabilization of their hips either during the study or soon after the study concluded.

Multilevel Injections of Botulinum Neurotoxin A in Cerebral Palsy

Molenaers and colleagues[78,79] developed practical approaches to multilevel hyperactivity management in children with CP, basing their approach on the model of multilevel surgery. They developed techniques for injecting the iliopsoas muscle and established the safety of high-dose administration of BoNT/A in children.[80] Their approach emphasizes the role of instrumented gait analysis to design the intervention, injection of multiple target muscles under mask anesthesia, and supplemental casting, orthoses, and intensive rehabilitation.[81] They have reported significant improvements in gait and function in a number of well-designed studies.[80,82,83]

Botulinum Toxin A and Phenol Neurolysis in Cerebral Palsy

Given the disappointing effects of BoNT/A injection in the hip adductors, Graham and colleagues[44] have described combining phenol neurolysis for adductor spasticity with BoNT/A chemodenervation of the hamstring and calf muscles in a pilot study. The principal indication is the younger child in whom multilevel spasticity and spastic hip displacement are combined. They found that the intervention was effective in managing hip displacement and in improving gait and function.[44]

Practical Aspects of Administration of Botulinum Neurotoxin A in Cerebral Palsy

There are currently three commercially available preparations of BoNT/A and one of BoNT/B. All have different characteristics,[84] potency, and dose ranges.[9] There have been several guides to dosing and administration of the various preparations in children.[9,67]

Injection of the gastrocsoleus muscle is the simplest and most widely used technique. A variety of techniques may be used to facilitate injection, including conscious sedation, topical anesthetic creams applied to the skin over the proposed injection sites, administration of nitrous oxide, and various combinations of these approaches.[85]

The control afforded by mask anesthesia permits injection of multiple sites in multiple target muscles, using electrical stimulation. The use of multiple injection sites is probably safer and possibly more effective than fewer sites. A suggested method is injecting four sites in the calf and two sites in the adductors and hamstrings.[40] Muscle stimulation is advised for all target muscles, except the gastrocsoleus.[69]

BOTULINUM NEUROTOXIN A IN THE UPPER LIMB IN CEREBRAL PALSY

Upper limb dysfunction is a common and disabling consequence of CP, particularly in children with spastic hemiplegia who have generally achieved independent walking. Impairment of upper limb function can have an impact on self-care abilities in activities of daily living, access to education, leisure activities, and eventually vocational outcomes (participation). Children may not be able to reach for objects, manipulate toys, feed themselves, or use assistive communication devices. A modest improvement in reaching function could have tremendous benefits.[49]

In spastic hemiplegia, the upper limb deformities typically include internal rotation and adduction at the shoulder, and this may progress in a small minority of patients to anterior migration of the humeral head.[86] The pectoralis major and the subscapularis muscles are usually the main deforming forces. At the elbow, flexion deformity is common, initially dynamic, progressing to a fixed deformity with variable degrees of joint contracture. In the forearm, pronation deformities are ubiquitous and are the result of muscle imbalance between spastic pronators (pronator teres and pronator quadratus) and weak supinators. Loss of active supination results in a contracture in the interosseous membrane and may predispose to subluxation or dislocation of the radial head. Flexion deformities of the wrist and fingers are the most common deformities in the upper limb, because the spastic flexors overpower the weaker extensors. Wrist flexion deformity usually is accompanied by ulnar deviation, because the ulnar deviators are more powerful than the radial deviators.[86] The "thumb-in-palm" deformity is common and is associated with significant functional impairment.[86-88]

As with all deformities, there is a postural-dynamic phase with gradual development of fixed contracture of the muscle-tendon units caused by muscle imbalance. Eventually, this leads to the phase of decompensation, which may include fixed joint contractures and joint subluxation. Different muscles develop fixed contractures at different speeds. The pronator teres is invariably the first muscle in the hemiplegic upper limb to develop a contracture. This is not because it is more hyperactive than other muscles but because it is never stretched by antagonist action.[86-89] Loss of active supination is present to some degree in all children with hemiplegia. Prevention of pronation contracture is simple in principle but difficult in practice. The pronator teres must be stretched out fully to its maximum length by the parent or therapist because the child is unable to do this for himself.[86]

Conventional therapeutic management of upper limb hyperactivity in children with CP has involved use of splinting and casting, passive stretching, the facilitation of posture and movement, medication, or surgery. The use of BoNT/A in the lower limbs of children with CP is well established, and more recently, it has been used in the upper limbs. The principal aim of treatment using BoNT/A injections to the upper limb of children with CP is to enhance function by allowing children to employ their treated arm in daily activities more efficiently and effectively. Further aims are to decrease hypertonicity and increase ROM, thus preventing contracture formation and delaying the need for surgery.[90] It is usually the nondominant arm that is being treated as an assisting hand. However in children with quadriplegia whose function is more limited, it may well be the function of the dominant arm (or both) that one seeks to improve. Intramuscular injection of BoNT/A alone is not guaranteed to enable a child to use the hemiplegic limb, and it is recommended that it be used in conjunction with physiotherapy and occupational therapy training.

Most of the children who are treated have hemiplegic CP and may lack compliance with rehabilitation following BoNT/A treatment because they have such a high level of function in their contralateral, noninvolved upper limb. In addition to this learned nonuse, retraining upper limb movements is intrinsically more difficult than for the lower extremities because it lacks the repetitive motor task characteristic of walking. Part of the problem also relates to the higher incidence of dystonia, weakness, sensory impairment, and poor selective motor control coexisting with spasticity in the upper extremity compared with the lower extremity in these children. These negative features may reduce any benefit gained from BoNT/A injections and lead to more limited results in clinical studies.

Fehlings et al[53] used strict criteria to ensure that only children with pure upper limb spastic type hemiplegia were included in their study. Of 50 children screened initially for the study, 20 were excluded because they were unable to initiate voluntary movement of the digits or had fixed joint contractures. The suitable candidates for BoNT/A therapy should be able to initiate finger movements, and to activate and strengthen antagonist muscles to take advantage of the BoNT/A weakened agonists. They should have good grip strength, because grip strength may be reduced by BoNT/A injection.[53] Family-identified limitations, problems, and goals should be analyzed. The movement disorder including selective motor control and characteristic posturing at rest and during functional activities should be assessed, as should active and passive joint ROM. A functional assessment should be performed, and video recordings can also be useful.

In typical hemiplegic posturing, the most common target muscles are the biceps, brachialis, pronator teres, flexor carpi ulnaris, flexor carpi radialis, and adductor pollicis.[86] The long finger flexors should usually be avoided to prevent weakening grip strength. When the aim is improved palmar hygiene, injection of the finger flexors is always required.

The larger muscles are injected in one or two sites, with the smaller ones being injected in one site. Small volume–high concentration injections are usually advised in the upper limb, to reduce diffusion to important antagonist muscles or unwanted targets, such as the long finger flexors. Precise targeting with electrical stimulation, electromyography, or ultrasound is mandatory.[69] Use of palpation for targeting the injection is much too inaccurate.[86] Upper limb dose guides have been published elsewhere.[9,86]

There is increasing evidence recently of the benefit of BoNT/A on upper limb function. Wall et al[91] were the first to report use of BoNT/A in the upper limbs of five children with CP in 1993. Injection of adductor pollicis muscle was coupled with rigid splinting in children with a thumb-in-hand deformity, and led to improvements in hand function (key grip, precision grip) precision pinch, palmar grip, and the performance of bimanual tasks. Corry et al[42] conducted a double-blind randomized placebo-controlled study involving multiple injections into the spastic upper extremity of children with CP. The main results were that intramuscular injection of BoNT/A resulted in consistent reduction in spasticity and muscle stiffness as measured by a torque motor. The torque motor was used to measure the resonant frequency of the wrist as an objective and quantifiable measure of forearm muscle stiffness. Although improvements were found in tone, ROM, grasp, and cosmesis, there was little effect on functional ability in a coin pick-up test.

Fehlings et al[53] conducted a single-blind randomized study involving 30 participants with hemiplegia. There were significant improvements in function in the BoNT/A group as measured by the Quality of Upper Extremity Skills Test (QUEST) at 1 month. Kawamura et al[92] compared the effects of low- and high-dose BoNT/A to improve upper extremity function. There was no difference in hand and arm function between a low dose and a high dose, supporting the lower dose intervention. Wallen et al[93] demonstrated that the dynamic joint ranges in the upper limb respond to BoNT/A, and that there is a

significant improvement in activities and participation at 3 and 6 months following the injections.

In a randomized, single-blind trial of BoNT/A and occupational therapy, it was reported that children who have BoNT/A in addition to therapy had greater improvements, and that this gain was sustained at 6 months.[94] A recent study used the WHO ICF model as a study template and a single-blind, randomized controlled study design, to investigate the effects of BoNT/A and low-intensity occupational therapy, in the upper limbs of children with hemiplegic CP. The authors reported significant improvements in body structure, activity, participation, and self-perception.[95] Another recent study reported that repeated use of BoNT/A is safe and effective in the upper limbs of children with CP. Injections at 6-month intervals may be worthwhile, when combined with appropriate occupational therapy.[94] These studies have focused on spastic movement disorders and the use of BoNT/A. To date, only one study has focused on dystonic upper limb movement disorder, in CP and the use of BoNT/B.[49] Seven children with CP and upper extremity dystonia were enrolled in a clinical trial of BoNT/B, which was injected into the biceps and brachioradialis muscles of one or both arms. The primary outcome measure was the change in maximum speed of hand movement during attempted forward reaching. Reaching speed improved in response to injection, and dystonia scores on the Burke-Fahn-Marsden dystonia scale, the Unified Dystonia Rating Scale, and the Unified Parkinson's Disease Rating Scale improved. Larger controlled trials are needed to confirm these interesting, preliminary results.[49]

Objective evaluation of upper limb function using a standardized, validated instrument is strongly recommended to document baseline function and also to assess changes following treatment. There is a variety of established instruments that can be used as outcome measures for upper limb interventions: QUEST,[96] Melbourne Assessment of Unilateral Upper Limb Function (Melbourne assessment[97]) and Assisting Hand Assessment (AHA[98]). However, most of these studies have failed to find sustained improvements with these tools.

Treatment goals must be individualized for each child, according to the type of movement disorder, limb distribution, abnormal postures, and functional goals. Children with spastic hemiplegia function at a high level and may require interventions aimed at developing more sophisticated fine motor control for bimanual hand activities. In contrast, a child with spastic quadriplegia have a more severe global problem of upper limb spasticity, making any useful function or even hygiene difficult. Simpler hand activities such as grasping and releasing assistive walking devices are the main objectives of treatment in some of these children. In those still more severely affected, ease of dressing and hygiene are the primary reasons for correcting upper limb deformities.

Functional goals should be realistic. Ranked in order of importance, the most significant prognostic factors in relation to function in the hemiplegic upper limb are sensory impairment, loss of selective motor control, and weakness, followed by spasticity.[86] When function cannot be improved or the gains are marginal, the cosmetic problems of the hemiplegic upper limb must not be forgotten. These children are in mainstream schooling and the majority will enter employment. In one upper limb trial, the single most reported benefit was the reduction in elbow flexion posturing when walking rapidly.[42] This had little to do with function but everything to do with cosmesis. Spasticity trials in the hemiplegic upper limb should incorporate a measure of satisfaction with the appearance of the upper limb.

There is much more work to be done in the upper limb including combining BoNT/A injection with surgery and exploiting the muscular relaxation achieved by BoNT/A with targeted splinting and therapy programs. In particular, the emerging role of constraint-induced movement therapy (CIMT), in combination with injections of botulinum toxin is an exciting direction for further research.[99-101]

ADVERSE EVENTS OF BOTULINUM NEUROTOXIN THERAPY IN CEREBRAL PALSY

BoNT/A is remarkably safe in children with CP, as reported in many large studies.[63,68,102,103] Most adverse events have been minor and self-limiting. Neither permanent neurovascular injury nor deep infection has been reported as complications of intramuscular injection. Remote side effects including incontinence and dysphagia have occasionally been reported. Incontinence is of great concern to

parents but usually resolves very quickly. Dysphagia, aspiration, and chest infection are the most serious complications after injection of BoNT/A and, if unrecognized or inadequately treated, could lead to death from asphyxia. In particular, a subgroup of children with spastic quadriplegia with pseudobulbar palsy seems to be much more sensitive to systemic spread after focal injection of BoNT/A.[104] Such children have a relative contraindication to the use of BoNT/A. They should either not have injections of BoNT/A or the doses should be significantly reduced.

Drooling

Pathologic drooling (sialorrhea) affects 10% to 40% of children with CP and may be socially incapacitating.[105-108] As well as psychosocial and hygiene problems, drooling may interfere with speech, eating, and quality of life.

The submandibular glands produce 60% to 70% of resting saliva, and the parotid glands provide most of the peri-prandial increase. BoNT/A may be injected into the salivary glands, to reduce cholinergic mediated secretion and reduce drooling.[109]

Studies of salivary gland injection in children with BoNT/A have shown encouraging results, with a reduction in drooling and few side effects.[110-113] Sedation and analgesia with a combination of topical anaesthetic cream, oral midazolam, and nitrous oxide gas are sufficient to allow the procedure to be tolerated by children.

The appropriate dose of BoNT/A for use in intraglandular injections has not been clarified but have been similar to those suggested for the treatment of spasticity. Jongerius et al[109] have cited 1-1.5 mL of saline as an appropriate volume in children, achieving adequate spreading while diminishing the risk of diffusion. It has been reported that injecting both the submandibular and parotid glands is superior to injecting either gland alone.[114] Ultrasound guidance enables precise targeting of the salivary glands and more accurate injection.

Injection of BoNT/A for drooling has fewer reported side effects than oral anticholinergic medications. Minor side effects of BoNT/A injection include chewing difficulties, dry mouth, and transient weakness of mouth closure.

Intrasalivary injections can be considered when oral medications have not been tolerated before considering more invasive surgical procedures.

BOTULINUM NEUROTOXIN A AS AN ANALGESIC AGENT IN CEREBRAL PALSY

The analgesic role of BoNT/A is complex and is currently under intense evaluation in animal models and in many clinical trials.[115] Clinical applications include migraine, painful muscle spasms in a wide range of conditions, and the management of pain associated with arthritis and various musculoskeletal problems.[116,117] Pain is a major clinical problem in the many older children and adolescents with CP. There are many possible causes, but degenerative joint disease compounded by spastic hypertonia may be the most common. In CP there is frequently a vicious circle of pain and spasm, in which pain provokes muscle spasm, which further increase pain. The pain-spasm cycle may be most effectively broken by injection of BoNT/A.[114]

BoNT/A can also be used to treat muscle spasm following operative procedures, for example, following adductor-release surgery. This improved pain control can accelerate recovery.[118]

CONCLUSION

Treatment challenges in children with CP include deciding when to start with intervention such as injection of botulinum toxin A, as well as establishing a maintenance therapy and deciding when to conclude the therapy. Measuring functional outcomes in motor disabled children remains challenging, especially across the domains of the ICF. The age at which BoNT/A is approved for use in children with CP varies from country to country. Off-label use is common but ideally should be in the context of approved clinical trials. There is reasonable clinical evidence to suggest that younger children respond more fully and for longer periods of time than do older children. This may be the result of the progression from dynamic posturing to fixed contracture.

The hyperactive muscles in children with spastic hemiplegia and spastic diplegia can be safely injected from age 18 to 24 months. Treatment seems to be most effective between the ages of 2 and 6 years in the context of a global management program including the use of orthoses, serial casting, and physical therapy. By age 6 to 10 years children will have reached plateau in terms of physical functioning, and many no longer require injection therapy. Some develop fixed contractures and are more effectively managed by orthopedic surgical procedures. BoNT/A can be used effectively to manage focal hyperactivity in the context of a nonfocal disorder such as CP. It is important to highlight that in this context, focal muscle hyperactivity does not exist alone, and in many cases, it may be weakness, contracture, and selective motor control that may have the biggest impact on function. Careful classification of the type of muscle hyperactivity, its contribution to overall disability, and assessment of the contribution of other coexistent features of the movement disorder is important to determine an effective management strategy.

References

1. Little WJ. On the incidence of abnormal parturition, difficult labour, premature birth and asphyxia neonatorum on the mental and physical condition of the child, especially in relation to deformities. *Trans Obstet Soc London.* 1862;3:293.
2. Osler W. *The Cerebral Palsies of Children. A Clinical Study for the Infirmary for Nervous Diseases.* Philadelphia: Blakiston; 1889.
3. Freud S. Die infantile Cerebrallahmung. In: Northnagel H, ed. *Specielle Pathologie und Therapie. Bd IX, Teil III*, Vienna: Holder; 1897:1-327.
4. Mac Keith RC, MacKenzie ICK, Polani PE, eds. The Little Club Memorandum on terminology and classification of 'cerebral palsy.' *Cereb Palsy Bull.* 1959;1:27-35.
5. Bax MCO. Terminology and classification of cerebral palsy. *Dev Med Child Neurol.* 1964;6:295-307.
6. Mutch L, Alberman E, Hagberg B, Kodama K, Perat MV. Cerebral palsy epidemiology: Where are we now and where are we going? *Dev Med Child Neurol.* 1992;34:547-551.
7. Bax M, Goldstein M, Rosenbaum P, Leviton A, Paneth N. Proposed definition and classification of cerebral palsy. Review. *Dev Med Child Neurol.* 2005;47:571-572.
8. Stanley FJ, Blair E, Alberman E. What are the cerebral palsies? In: Bax M, Hart HM, eds. *Cerebral Palsies: Epidemiology and Causal Pathways*, London, UK: MacKeith Press; 2000:8-13.
9. M.E.N.T.O.R.S. (Methodologies for Experts in Neurotoxin Therapy: Outreach, Resources and Support). Focus on Cerebral Palsy. *Monograph: A Continuing Medical Education DVD Activity.* New York, NY: The Institute for Medical Studies; 2004.
10. Lance JW. Symposium Synopsis. In: Feldman RG, Young RR, Koella WP, eds. *Spasticity: Disordered Motor Control.* Chicago: Year Book Publishers; 1980:485-494.

11. Holly RG, Barnett JG, Ashmore RG, Mole PA, Molé PA. Stretch induced growth in chicken wing muscles: a new model of stretch hypertrophy. *Am J Physiol.* 1980;238:C62-C71.

12. Delgado MR, Albright AL. Movement disorders in children: Definitions, classifications, and Grading systems. *J Child Neurol.* 2003;18:1.

13. Rosenbaum P, Paneth N, Leviton A, Goldstein M, Bax M, Bax M, et al. A report: the definition and classification of cerebral palsy April 2006. *Dev Med Child Neurol.* 2007;109(suppl):8-14.

14. Steenbergen B. Using the MACS to facilitate communication about manual abilities of children with cerebral palsy. *Dev Med Child Neurol.* 2006;48:948.

15. Fay T. Cerebral palsy; medical considerations and classification. *Am J Psychiatry.* 1950;107:180.

16. Balf CL, Ingram TTS. Problems in the classification of cerebral palsy in childhood. *BMJ.* 1955;2:163.

17. Blair E, Stanley F. Interobserver agreement in the classification of cerebral palsy. *Dev Med Child Neurol.* 1985;27:615-622.

18. Howard J, Soo B, Graham HK, Boyd RN, Reid S, Lanigan A, et al. Cerebral palsy in Victoria: motor types, topography and gross motor function. *J Pediatr Child Health.* 2005;41:479-483.

19. Surveillance of cerebral palsy in Europe (SCPE): a collaboration of cerebral palsy surveys and registers. *Dev Med Child Neurol.* 2000;42:816-824.

20. World Health Organization: *International Classification of Functioning, Disability and Health (ICF).* Geneva, Switzerland: World Health Organization; 2001.

21. Palisano R, Rosenbaum P, Walter S, Russell D, Wood E, Galuppi B. Development and reliability of a system to classify gross motor function in children with cerebral palsy. *Dev Med Child Neurol.* 1997;39:214-223.

22. Eliasson A-C, Krumlinde-Sundholm L, Rosblad B, Beckung E, Arner M, Ohrvall A-M, et al. The Manual Ability Classification System (MACS) for children with cerebral palsy: scale development and evidence of validity and reliability. *Dev Med Child Neurol.* 2006;48:549-554.

23. Graham HK, Selber P. Musculoskeletal aspects of cerebral palsy. *J Bone Joint Surg.* 2003;85-B:157-166.

24. Ziv I, Blackburn N, Rang M, Koreska J. Muscle growth in the normal and spastic mouse. *Dev Med Child Neurol.* 1984;26:94-99.

25. Cosgrove AP, Graham HK. Botulinum toxin A prevents the development of contractures in the hereditary spastic mouse. *Dev Med Child Neurol.* 1994;36:379-385.

26. Ashworth B. Preliminary trial of carisoprodol in multiple sclerosis. *Practitioner.* 1964;192:540-542.

27. Bohannon RW, Smith MB. Interrater reliability of a modified Ashworth scale of muscle spasticity. *Phys Ther.* 1987;67:206-207.

28. Tardieu G, Shentoub S, Delarue R. A la recherché d'une technique de mesure de la spasticite. *Rev Neurol.* 1954;91:143-144.

29. Fosang AL, Galea MP, McCoy AT, Reddihough DS, Story I. Measures of muscle and joint performance in the lower limb of children with cerebral palsy. *Dev Med Child Neurol.* 2003;45:664-670.

30. Corry IS. *Use of a Motion Analysis Laboratory in Assessing the Effects of Botulinum Toxin in Cerebral Palsy [thesis] Belfast:* Northern Ireland: The Queens University of Belfast, 1995.

31. Lakie M, Walsh EG, Wright GE. Resonance at the wrist demonstrated by the use of a torque motor: an instrumented analysis of muscle tone in man. *J Physiol.* 1984;353:265-285.

32. Brown JK, Walsh EG, Bell E, Wright GV. The use of resonant frequency measurement in assessment of muscle tone. *J Pediatr Orthop.* 1991;11:405.

33. Waters EB, Maher E. Assessing quality of life. In: Moyer Y, ed. *Evidence Based Paediatrics and Child Health.* London, UK: British Medical Journal Books; 2004: 99-110.

34. Albrecht GL, Devlieger PJ. The disability paradox: high quality of life against all odds. *Soc Sci Med.* 1999;48:977-988.

35. Guyatt GH, Feeny DH, Patrick DL. Measuring health-related quality of life. *Ann Intern Med.* 1993;118: 622-629.

36. Peacock WJ, Staudt LA. Spasticity in cerebral palsy and the selective posterior rhizotomy procedure. *J Child Neurol.* 1990;5:174-178.

37. McLaughlin JF, Bjornson KF, Astley SJ, Graubert C, Hays RM, Roberts TS, et al. Selective dorsal rhizotomy: efficacy and safety in an investigator-masked randomised clinical trial. *Dev Med Child Neurol.* 1998;40:220-232.

38. Steinbok P, Reiner A, Beauchamp RD, Cochrane DD, Keyes R. Selective functional posterior rhizotomy for treatment of spastic cerebral palsy in children. *Pediatr Neurosurg.* 1992;18:34-42.

39. O'Flaherty S, Waugh M-C. Pharmacologic management of the spastic and dystonic upper limb in children with cerebral palsy. *Hand Clin.* 2003;19:585-589.

40. Hutchinson R, Graham HK. Management of spasticity in children. In: Barnes MP, Johnson GR, eds. *Upper Motor Neurone Syndrome and Spasticity. Clinical Management and Neurophysiology.* 2nd ed. Cambridge, UK: Cambridge University Press; 2008, pp 214-239.

41. Albright AL, Ferson SS. Intrathecal Baclofen therapy in children. *Neurosurg Focus.* 2006;21:e3.

42. Corry IS, Cosgrove AP, Walsh EG, McClean D, Graham HK. Botulinum toxin A in the hemiplegic upper limb: a double-blind trial. *Dev Med Child Neurol.* 1997;39:185-193.

43. Gracies J-M, Elovic E, McGuire J, Simpson D. Traditional pharmacological treatments for spasticity. Part 1: Local treatments. *Muscle Nerve.* 1997; 20(suppl 6):S61-S91.

44. Khot A, Sloan S, Desai S, Harvey A, Wolfe R, Graham HK. Adductor release and chemodenervation in children with cerebral palsy: A pilot study in 16 children. *J Child Orthop.* 2008;2:293-299.

45. Koman LA, Mooney JF, Smith B, Goodman A, Mulvaney T. Management of cerebral palsy with botulinum-A toxin: preliminary investigation. *J Pediatr Orthop.* 1993;13:489-495.

46. Corry IS, Cosgrove AP, Duffy CM, Taylor TC, Graham HK. Botulinum toxin A in hamstring spasticity. *Gait Posture.* 1999;10:206-210.

47. Cosgrove AP, Corry IS, Graham HK. Botulinum toxin in the management of the lower limb in cerebral palsy. *Dev Med Child Neurol.* 1994;36:386-396.

48. Gormley M, Pries G, Kawiecki J, Quigley S, Deshpande S. Adverse events in CP children receiving botulinum toxin type B. Abstract. Basic and Therapeutic Aspects of Botulinum and Tetanus Toxin Meeting 23-25 June 2005, Denver, Colorado, USA.

49. Sanger TD, Kukke SN, Sherman-Levine S. Botulinum toxin type B improves the speed of reaching in children with cerebral palsy and arm dystonia: an open-label, dose-escalation pilot study. *J Child Neurol.* 2007;22:116-122.

50. de Paiva A, Meunier FA, Molgo J, Aoki KR, Dolly JO. Functional repair of motor endplates after botulinum neurotoxin type A poisoning: Biphasic switch of synaptic activity between nerve sprouts and their parent terminals. *Proc Natl Acad Sci U S A*. 1999;96: 3200-3205.

51. Gibson N, Graham HK, Love S. Botulinum toxin A in the management of focal muscle overactivity in children with cerebral palsy. *Disabil Rehabil*. 2007;29:1813-1822.

52. Koman LA, Mooney JF, Smith BP, Goodman A, Mulvaney T. Management of spasticity in cerebral palsy with botulinum toxin-A toxin: report of a preliminary, randomized, double-blind trial. *J Pediatr Orthop*. 1994;14:299-303.

53. Fehlings D, Rang M, Glazier J, Steele C. An evaluation of botulinum-A toxin injections to improve upper extremity function in children with hemiplegic cerebral palsy. *J Pediatr*. 2000;137:331-337.

54. Graham HK. Botulinum toxin A in cerebral palsy: Functional outcomes. Invited editorial. *J Pediatr*. 2000;137:300-303.

55. Koman LA, Brashear A, Rosenfeld S, Chambers H, Russman B, Rang M, et al. Botulinum toxin type A neuromuscular blockade in the treatment of equinus foot deformity in cerebral palsy: A multicentre, open-label clinical trial. *Pediatrics*. 2001;108: 1062-1071.

56. Hoare BJ, Imms C. Upper-Limb injections of botulinum toxin-A in children with cerebral palsy: A critical review of the literature and clinical implications for occupational therapists. *Am J Occup Ther*. 2004;58:389-397.

57. Borton DC, Walker K, Pirpiris M, Nattrass GR, Graham HK. Isolated calf lengthening in cerebral palsy. Outcome analysis of risk factors. *J Bone Joint Surg*. 2001;83-B:364-370.

58. Rang M. Cerebral palsy. In: Morrissey RT, ed. *Lovell and Winter's Paediatric Orthopaedics*. 3rd ed. Vol.1. Philadelphia: J.B. Lippincott; 1990:465-506.

59. Rodda JM, Graham HK, Galea MP, Baker R, Nattrass GR, Wolfe R. Correction of severe crouch gait in spastic diplegia by multilevel orthopaedic surgery: Outcome at one and five years. *J Bone Joint Surg*. 2006;88-A: 2653-2664.

60. Rodda J, Graham HK. Classification of gait patterns in spastic hemiplegia and spastic diplegia: A basis for a management algorithm. *Eur J Neurol*. 2001;8(suppl 5):S98-S108.

61. Rodda JM, Graham HK, Carson L, Galea MP, Wolfe R. Sagittal gait patterns in spastic diplegia. *J Bone Joint Surg*. 2004;86-B:251-258.

62. Metaxiotis D, Siebel A, Doederlein L. Repeated botulinum toxin A injections in the treatment of spastic equinus foot. *Clin Orthop Rel Res*. 2002;394: 177-185.

63. Bakheit AM, Severa S, Cosgrove A, Morton R, Roussounis SH, Doderlein L, et al. Safety profile and efficacy of botulinum toxin A (Dysport) in children with muscle spasticity. *Dev Med Child Neurol*. 2001;43:234-238.

64. Ubhi T, Bhakta BB, Ives HL, Allgar V, Roussounis SH. Randomised double blind placebo controlled trial of the effect of botulinum toxin on walking in cerebral palsy. *Arch Dis Child*. 2000;83:481-487.

65. Flett PJ, Stern LM, Waddy H, Connell TM, Seeger JD, Gibson SK. Botulinum toxin A versus fixed cast stretching for dynamic calf tightness in cerebral palsy. *J Paediatr Child Health*. 1999;35:71-77.

66. Winters T, Gage J, Hicks R. Gait patterns in spastic hemiplegia in children and adults. *J Bone Joint Surg*. 1987;69A:437-441.

67. Graham HK, Aoki KR, Autti-Ramo I, Boyd RN, Delgado MR, Gaebler-Spira DJ, et al. Recommendations for the use of botulinum toxin type A in the management of cerebral palsy. *Gait Posture*. 2000;11:67-79.

68. Goldstein EM. Safety of high-dose botulinum toxin type A therapy for the treatment of pediatric spasticity. *J Child Neurol*. 2006;21:189-192.

69. Chin TYP, Nattrass GR, Selber P, Graham HK. Accuracy of intramuscular injection of Botulinum toxin A in juvenile cerebral palsy. *J Pediatr Orthop*. 2005;25: 286-291.

70. Schroeder AS, Berweck S, Lee SH, Heinen F. Botulinum toxin treatment of children with cerebral palsy—a short review of different injection techniques. *Neurotox. Res*. 2006;9:189-196.

71. Berweck S, Feldkamp A, Francke A, Nehles J, Schwerin A, Heinen F. Sonography-guided injection of botulinum toxin A in children with cerebral palsy. *Neuropediatrics*. 2002;33:221-223.

72. Corry IS, Cosgrove AP, Duffy CM, McNeill S, Taylor TC, Graham HK. Botulinum toxin A compared with stretching casts in the treatment of spastic equinus: A randomised prospective trial. *J Pediatr Orthop*. 1998;18:304-311.

73. Sutherland DH, Kauffman KR, Wyatt MP, Chambers HG. Injection of botulinum toxin A into the gastrocnemius muscle of patients with cerebral palsy: a 3-dimensional motion analysis study. *Gait Posture*. 1996;4:269-279.

74. Boyd RN, Pliatsios V, Starr R, Wolfe R, Graham HK. Biomechanical transformation of the gastroc-soleus muscle with botulinum toxin A in children with cerebral palsy. *Dev Med Child Neurol*. 2000;42:32-41.

75. Michlitsch MG, Rethlefsen SA, Kay RM. The contributions of anterior and posterior tibialis dysfunction to varus foot deformity in patients with cerebral palsy. *J Bone Joint Surg*. 2006;88A:1764-1768.

76. Bennett GC, Rang M, Jones D. Varus and valgus deformities of the foot in cerebral palsy. *Dev Med Child Neurol*. 1982;24:499-503.

77. Graham HK, Boyd R, Carlin JB, Dobson F, Lowe K, Nattrass G, et al. Does Botulinum toxin A combined with hip bracing prevent hip displacement in children with cerebral palsy and "hips-at-risk"? A randomized controlled trial. *J Bone Joint Surg*. 2008;90-A:23-33.

78. Molenaers G, Desloovere K, Eyssen M, Decaf J, Jonkers I, De Cock P. Botulinum toxin type A treatment of cerebral palsy: an integrated approach. *Eur J Neurol*. 1999;6(suppl 4):S51-S57.

79. Molenaers G, Desloovere K, De Cat J, JonkersI, De Borre L, Pauwels P, et al. Single event multilevel botulinum toxin type A treatment and surgery: similarities and differences. *Eur J Neurol*. 2001;8(suppl 5):88-97.

80. Molenaers G, Eyssen M, Desloovere K, Jonkers I, De Cock P. A multilevel approach to botulinum toxin type A treatment of the (ilio)psoas in spasticity in cerebral palsy. *Eur J Neurol*. 1999;6(suppl 4):S59-S62.

81. Molenaers G, Desloovere K, Fabry G, De Cock P. The effects of quantitative gait assessment and botulinum toxin A on musculoskeletal surgery in children with cerebral palsy. *J Bone Joint Surg*. 2006;88-A: 161-170.

82. Desloovere K, Molenaers G, De Cat J, Pauwels P, Van Campenhout A, Ortibus E, et al. Motor function following multilevel botulinum toxin type A treatment

in children with cerebral palsy. *Dev Med Child Neurol.* 2007;49:56-61.

83. van Rhijn J, Molenaers G, Ceulemans B. Botulinum toxin type A in the treatment of children and adolescents with an acquired brain injury. Randomized controlled trial. *Brain Inj.* 2005;19:331-335.

84. Aoki KR. A compoarison of the safety margins of botulinum neurotoxin serotypes A, B, and F in mice. *Toxicon.* 2001;39:1815-1820.

85. *Treating Children with Botulinum Toxin.* The Rehabilitation Department, The Children's Hospital at Westmead, New South Wales, Australia

86. Chin T, Graham HK. Botulinum toxin in the management of upper limb spasticity in cerebral palsy. *Hand Clin.* 2003;19:591-600.

87. Graham HK. Botulinum toxin type A management of spasticity in the context of orthopaedic surgery for children with spastic cerebral palsy. *Eur J Neurol.* 2001;8:30-39.

88. Brown JK, Walsh EG. Neurology of the upper limb. Congenital hemiplegia. In: Neville B, Goodman R, eds. *Clinics in Developmental Medicine.* No 150. London, UK: MacKeith Press; 2000:113-149.

89. Boyd RN, Graham HK. Botulinum toxin A in the management of children with cerebral palsy: indications and outcome. *Eur J Neurol.* 1994;1:S15-S22.

90. Wallen M, O'Flaherty SJ, Waugh M-CA. Functional outcomes of intramuscular botulinum toxin type A and occupational therapy in the upper limbs of children with cerebral palsy: a randomized controlled trial. *Arch Phys Med Rehabil.* 2007;88:1-10.

91. Wall SA, Chait LA, Temlett JA, Perkins B, Hillen G, Becker P. Botulinum A chemodenervation: a new modality in cerebral palsied hands. *Br J Plast Surg.* 1993;46:703-706.

92. Kawamura A, Campbell K, Lam-Damji S, Fehlings D. A randomized controlled trial comparing botulinum toxin A dosage in the upper extremity of children with spasticity. *Dev Med Child Neurol.* 2007;49:331-337.

93. Wallen MA, O'Flaherty SJ, Waugh M-CA. Functional outcomes of intramuscular botulinum toxin type A in the upper limbs of children with cerebral palsy: a phase II trial. *Arch Phys Med Rehabil.* 2004;85:192-200.

94. Lowe K, Novak I, Cusick A. Repeat injection of botulinum toxin A is safe and effective for upper limb movement and function in children with cerebral palsy. *Dev Med Child Neurol.* 2007;49:823-829.

95. Russo RN, Crotty M, Miller MD, Murchland S, Flett P, Haan E. Upper-limb botulinum toxin A injection and occupational therapy in children with hemiplegic cerebral palsy identified from a population register: a single-blind, randomized, controlled trial. *Pediatrics.* 2007;119:e1149-e1158.

96. DeMatteo C, Law M, Russell D, Pollack N, Rosenbaum P, Walter S: *QUEST: Quality of Upper Extremity Skills Test Manual.* Hamilton, ON: Neurodevelopmental Research Unit, Chedoke Campus, Chedoke-McMasters Hospital; 2000.

97. Randall MJ, Carlin J, Reddihough DS, Chondros P. Reliability of the Melbourne Assessment of unilateral upper limb function—a quantitative test of quality of movement in children with neurological impairment. *Dev Med Child Neurol.* 2001;43:761-767.

98. Krumlinde-Sundholm L, Eliasson AC. Development of the Assisting Hand Assessment: A Rasch-built measure intended for children with unilateral upper limb impairments. *Scand J Occup Ther.* 2003;10:10-26.

99. Boyd RN, Morris ME, Graham HK. Management of upper limb dysfunction in children with cerebral palsy: a systematic review. *Eur J Neurol.* 2001;8(suppl 5):150-166.

100. Eliasson AC, Krumlinde-Sundholm L, Shaw K, Wang C. Effects of constraint-induced movement therapy in young children with hemiplegic cerebral palsy: an adapted model. *Dev Med Child Neurol.* 2005;47:266-275.

101. Hoare B, Imms C, Carey L, Wasiak J. Constraint-induced movement therapy in the treatment of the upper limb in children with hemiplegic cerebral palsy: a Cochrane systematic review. *Clin Rehabil.* 2007;21:675-685.

102. Delgado MR. The use of botulinum toxin type A in children with cerebral palsy: a retrospective study. *Eur J Neurol.* 1999;6(suppl 4):S11-S18.

103. Mohamed KA, Moore AP, Rosenbloom L. Adverse events following repeated injections with botulinum toxin A in children with spasticity. *Dev Med Child Neurol.* 2001;43:791.

104. Howell K, Selber P, Graham HK, Reddihough D. Botulinum neurotoxin A: An unusual systemic effect. *J Paediatr Child Health.* 2007;43:499-501.

105. Harris SR, Purdy AH. Drooling and its management in cerebral palsy. *Dev Med Child Neurol.* 1987;29:807-811.

106. Jongerius PH, Rotteveel JJ, Van den Hoogen F, Joosten F, van Hulst K, Gabreëls FJ. Botulinum toxin A: a new option for treatment of drooling in children with cerebral palsy. *Presentation of a case series. Eur J Pediatr.* 2001;160:509-512.

107. Suskind DL, Tilton A. Clinical study of botulinum-A toxin in the treatment of sialorrhea in children with cerebral palsy. *Laryngoscope.* 2002;112:73-81.

108. Bothwell JE, Clarke K, Dooley JM, Gordon KE, Anderson R, Wood EP, et al. Botulinum toxin A as a treatment for excessive drooling in children. *Pediatr Neurol.* 2002;27:18-22.

109. Jongerius PH, Joosten F, Hoogen FJ, Gabreels FJ, Rotteveel JJ. The treatment of drooling by ultrasound-guided intraglandular injections of botulinum toxin type A into the salivary glands. *Laryngoscope.* 2003;113:107-111.

110. Ellies M, Rohrbach-Volland S, Arglebe C, Wilken B, Laskawi R, Hanefeld F. Successful management of drooling with botulinum toxin A in neurologically disabled children. *Neuropediatrics.* 2002;33:327-330.

111. Savarese R, Diamond M, Elovic E, Millis SR. Intraparotid injection of botulinum toxin A as treatment to control sialorrhoea in children with cerebral palsy. *Am J Phys Med Rehabil.* 2004;83:304-311.

112. Jongerius PH, Van der Hoogen FJ, Van Limbeek J, Gabreëls FJ, van Hulst K, Rotteveel JJ. Effect of botulinum toxin in the treatment of drooling: a controlled clinical trial. *Pediatrics.* 2004;114:620-627.

113. Hassin-Baer S, Scheuer E, Buchman AS, Jacobson I, Ben-Zeev B. Botulinum toxin injections for children with excessive drooling. *J Child Neurol.* 2005;20:120-123.

114. Reid SM, Johnstone BR, Westbury C, Rawicki B, Reddihough DS. Randomized trial of botulinum toxin injections into the salivary glands to reduce drooling in children with neurological disorders. *Dev Med Child Neurol.* 2008;50:123-128.

115. Aoki KR, Childers MK. *Pharmacology in Pain Relief. The Use of Botulinum Toxin Type A in Pain Management.*

A Clinician's Guide, 2nd ed. Columbia, MO: Academic Information Systems Inc; 2002:32-61.

116. Childers MK, Simons DG. Myofascial pain syndromes. In: Childers MK, ed. *The Use of Botulinum Toxin Type A in Pain Management. A Clinician's Guide*, 2nd ed. Columbia, MO: Academic Information Systems Inc; 2002:77-100.

117. Childers MK. Pain and disordered motor control. In Childers MK, ed. *The Use of Botulinum Toxin Type A in*

Pain Management. A Clinician's Guide, 2nd ed. Santa Cruz, CA: Academic Information Systems Inc.; 2002:101-111.

118. Barwood S, Baillieu C, Boyd R, Brereton K, Low J, Nattrass G, et al. Analgesic effects of botulinum toxin A: a randomized, placebo-controlled clinical trial. *Dev Med Child Neurol*. 2000;42:116-121.

Clinical Experience 15
and Recent Advances
in the Management of
Gait Disorders with
Botulinum Neurotoxin

Alberto Esquenazi and Nathaniel H. Mayer

INTRODUCTION

Acquired brain injury produces focal but variable patterns of muscle dysfunction across upper and lower limb joints. Characteristics of the upper motor neuron syndrome (UMNS) include the presence of spasticity and other positive signs, weakness, and a variety of motor control abnormalities that impair the regulation of voluntary movement and interfere with activities of daily living, mobility, and communication. (see Chapter 11). The chief cause of this interference has to do with impairment of a patient's ability to produce and regulate voluntary movement brought on by corticospinal system damage that is also accompanied by muscle overactivity (spasticity and co-contraction). The latter may be defined as an unwanted, velocity-dependent stretch reflex phenomenon occurring when a patient attempts to move a limb actively or when an examiner moves the patient's limb passively.[1] Although the mechanisms of spasticity are largely unknown, current ideas favor the notion that afferent signals from the limbs and descending signals of supraspinal origin are mishandled at the level of the segmental spinal cord by one or more interneuronal systems. Clinicians have used the Ashworth scale[2] as a surrogate measure to assess the positive sign of spasticity, particularly as a measurement of change in resistance to stretch before and

after pharmacologic treatment interventions. The Tardieu scale has proven to be a better clinical assessment tool that truly measures the velocity component of spasticity, but it does require practice for it to be reliable.[3,4]

Most patients and clinicians will complain about spasticity, but no one means the same thing when they use the term. Lance published this frequently cited definition for the phenomenon: "a motor disorder characterized by a velocity dependent increase in tonic stretch reflexes (muscle tone) with exaggerated tendon jerks, resulting from hyperexcitability of the stretch reflex, as one component of the upper motoneuron syndrome."[5] Signs of spasticity are useful as a diagnostic indicator pointing to the presence of an upper motor neuron lesion, but in general, rehabilitation clinicians are more preoccupied with addressing the functional problems of their patients linked to the consequences of an upper motor neuron lesion. Common terminology, which reflects their clinical practice emphasis, includes spastic gait or spastic equinovarus. For these clinicians, evaluation and treatment of spasticity takes on broader dimensions, reflecting their interest in clinical patterns of motor dysfunction that produce functional impairment and can result in disability. The clinician must be able to see spastic phenomena within the larger context of impaired motor control in order to identify appropriate

Dr. Esquenazi is disclosing that he has received unrestricted research funding from Allergan, Inc. Dr. Mayer is disclosing that he has received unrestricted research funding from Allergan, Inc. Also he is a member of the Spasticity Advisory Board of Allergan and of the Neurotoxin Institute which receives educational grant support from Allergan.

treatment methods for a patient's functional problems resulting from a central nervous system injury. The National Center for Medical Rehabilitation Research (NCMRR) has suggested that new methods of treatment should be evaluated for effects on multiple dimensions of the disabling process, including not only the dimension of impairment (as exemplified by Ashworth scale measurements), but also other dimensions such as functional limitations and disabilities (i.e., difficulty fulfilling role functions).[6] Lower extremity posturing that affects gait and transfer dysfunctions represents a significant spectrum of functional limitations that are attributable to the positive signs of the UMNS.

In a broader sense and from our perspective, evaluation of spasticity focuses on three issues: (1) identifying the clinical pattern of motor dysfunction and its source; (2) identifying the patient's ability to control muscles involved in the clinical pattern; and (3) the differential role of muscle stiffness and contracture as it relates to a functional problem. From our collective clinical experience evaluating several thousand patients and for purposes of knowledge transfer and educational expediency, we have identified and published the six most common clinical patterns of motor dysfunction affecting the lower limbs during gait and six more for the upper limb that are typically found in patients with acquired brain injury and an upper motor neuron lesion.[7] For the purpose of this paper, we will focus on the lower limb patterns only (Table 15-1), but the reader is encouraged to review additional publications on the subject.[7-9]

A variety of muscles may contribute to these clinical patterns and the related motor dysfunction across joints and limb segments. When many muscles cross a joint, each muscle can vary in its characteristics. Because each muscle may contribute to motion and the movement of a specific joint, information about each muscle's contribution is useful to the assessment as a whole. Evaluation focuses on the characteristics of these muscles in terms of their voluntary or selective control, strength, spastic reactivity, rheologic stiffness, and contracture. Proper treatment depends on sorting out this information. These patterns of dysfunction are amenable to strategies of focal evaluation and localized treatment. Clinical examination supported by laboratory studies is the mainstays of evaluation and clinical questions of interest regarding a given muscle that might be targeted for localized intervention.

TABLE 15-1 Lower Limb Patterns of Motor Dysfunction in Upper Motor Neuron Syndrome
Equinus/equinovarus foot
Hyperextended (striatal) great toe
Stiff knee
Flexed knee
Adducted hip
Flexed hip

We use dynamic electromyography to help identify the voluntary and spastic characteristics of individual muscles during gait, and we use anesthetic nerve blocks to identify the properties of stiffness and contracture in particular muscle groups.[10,11]

The treatment algorithms for these problems are implemented by identifying (1) muscles that contribute to the deformity across a joint; (2) the stage of recovery from injury; and most importantly, (3) clinical goals agreed on and applicable to the patient. In Table 15-1, we itemize the frequently found patterns of motor dysfunction affecting gait after acquired brain injury and subsequently discuss them in detail.

Commonly these patterns do not present in isolation but usually present superimposed with others in the lower limb and frequently even with patterns affecting the upper limb.[12]

PATTERNS OF UPPER MOTOR NEURON DYSFUNCTION

The lower limb patterns of upper motor neuron dysfunction that affect walking are presented in this chapter in the order of their presentation frequency: (1) equinovarus foot, (2) hyperextended great toe, (3) stiff knee, (4) flexed knee, (5) adducted (scissoring) thighs, and (6) flexed hip.[6,7]

From a gait cycle perspective, patterns of equinovarus foot, hyperextended great toe and flexed knee are considered problematic throughout the swing and stance phase of the cycle. Stiff knee and adducted thigh are predominantly deviations of swing phase while the flexed hip is considered a stance-phase deviation. All patterns in some way potentially influence the two main functional

TABLE 15-2 Problem Categories

Category	Feature
Type I	Symptomatic
Type II	Passive Function
Type III	Active Function
Type IV	Mixed

outcomes of walking; translation of the center of gravity and support of the body's mass against gravity (i.e., upright stability). These patterns can also produce a variety of functional problems unrelated to walking that can affect many other activities of daily living by impairing access or interfering with limb positioning and producing pain. We have categorized these problems into four types, as listed in Table 15-2.

Type I—Symptomatic refers to pain, flexor spasms, extensor spasms, and clonus as some of the presenting problems.

Type II—Passive function refers to the passive manipulation of limbs to achieve functional ends, typically performed by caregivers, although patients may also manipulate their limbs passively with their noninvolved limbs.

Type III—Active functions, on the other hand, refer to patient's direct use of the limb to carry out a functional activity.

Type IV—Mixed, combines two or more of them.

We now describe each one of the patterns in more detail, as well as our assessment and treatment approach for them.

Equinovarus Foot

Equinovarus foot is the most common upper motor neuron posture seen in the lower limb and the one that can most impair walking. The foot and ankle are turned down and in (Fig. 15-1A and B). Toe curling or toe clawing may coexist in this deformity. The lateral border of the foot, particularly the fifth metatarsal head, is typically compressed against the floor during weight bearing or against the footrest of a wheelchair. Skin breakdown over the metatarsal head may develop from constant pressure.

Equinovarus foot is frequently sustained throughout stance phase, and inversion may worsen with weight bearing, causing ankle instability as the gait cycle progresses. Limited

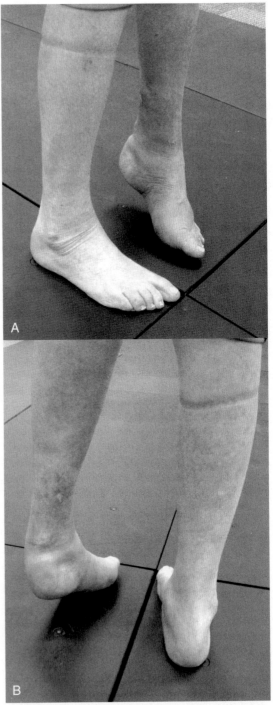

FIGURE 15-1. Equinovarus foot posture seen from (**A**) anterior medial and (**B**) posterior views. Note weight bearing on the anterior lateral border of the foot and lack of heel contact with the floor.

dorsiflexion during early and midstance restrains the appropriate forward rotation of the tibia over the stationary foot, frequently producing knee hyperextension and possibly resulting in compensatory hip flexion. Impairment of ankle dorsiflexion in late stance and preswing interferes with push-off and forward propulsion, resulting in significant reduction in ankle joint power generation. During swing phase, equinus posture of the foot may result in a limb clearance problem, whereas the abnormal posture of the foot in stance phase may result in instability of the body as a whole. Under these circumstances, correction of this particular problem is essential, even for individuals with limited ambulation capacity.

Because of functional redundancy, a number of muscles may generate the unbalanced forces resulting in equinovarus foot pattern. Muscles that can potentially contribute to the deforming forces of the equinovarus posture include the tibialis anterior, tibialis posterior, long toe flexors, gastrocnemius, soleus, extensor hallucis longus and intrinsics of the foot. Weakness of the peroneus longus and peroneus brevis in stance phase and the extensor digitorum longus in swing phase may also play a role.[11]

The clinical examination in combination with dynamic polyelectromyographic (poly-EMG) recordings of the above-mentioned muscles obtained during walking provide a more detailed understanding of the genesis of this deformity. Dynamic poly-EMG recordings often demonstrate prolonged activation of the gastrocnemius and soleus complex and the long toe flexors as the most common cause of plantar flexion. Occasionally, the gastrocnemius and soleus muscles may activate differentially, and treatment interventions must take this into consideration. Medial and lateral gastrocnemius rarely activate differentially.[13]

Inversion frequently is the result of the overactivation of the tibialis posterior and/or anterior in combination with the gastrocnemius and soleus and, at times, the extensor hallucis longus (Fig. 15-2). If the tibialis posterior and anterior are both contributing to the varus deformity as in the case presented for illustration, a decision has to be made about which one of the two muscles is the main contributor.[14,15] A diagnostic tibial nerve block with lidocaine to the posterior tibial or peroneal nerves to eliminate one of them and observe the resulting foot posture is a useful approach.

One has to be mindful that reducing activation of the gastrocsoleus complex will tend to increase dorsiflexion in the stance phase. When dorsiflexion increases, the long toe flexors

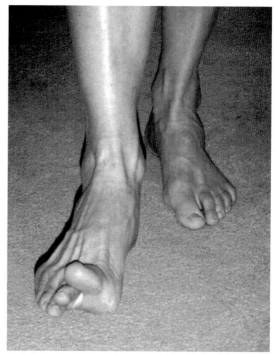

FIGURE 15-2. Hallux hyperextension caused by extensor hallucis longus overactivity. In stance phase, weight bearing is increased under the first metatarsal, and the patient may report pressure at the tip of the toe when wearing shoes.

tighten because of tenodesis effect, adding a new problem to the situation.

Based on the dynamic poly-EMG correlated with clinical findings, the treatment of choice can now be made to include injection of botulinum neurotoxin (BoNT) into the tibialis posterior, gastrocnemius, soleus, and long toe flexors. When a contracture is evident, serial casting or surgical intervention may be needed to address the physical shortening of soft tissues.[16]

Hyperextended Great Toe

Hyperextended great toe is a deformity that is characterized by extension of the big toe throughout the gait cycle, sometimes referred to as striated toe or hitchhiker's toe. Ankle varus may accompany this foot deformity because of the insertion of the extensor halucis longus, equinus may also be evident if other muscles are overactive (Fig. 15-3). When wearing shoes, the patient may complain of pain at the tip of the big toe and under the first metatarsal head during weight bearing in stance phase. During gait, toe extension in early and

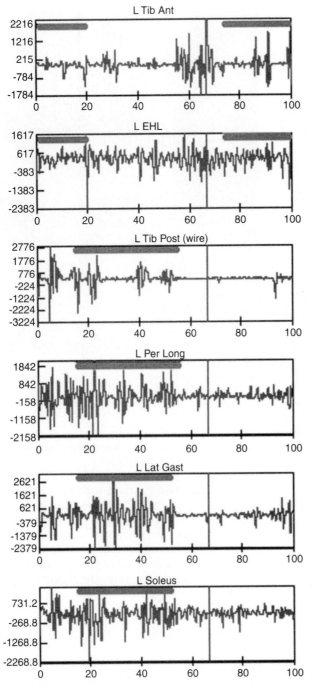

FIGURE 15-3. Dynamic electromyograph displayed with CODA MPX1 software during ambulation using Motion Lab surface electrodes, the tibialis posterior recording was obtained with an intramuscular wire. Data was normalized (0 = initial contact); the vertical line at 68% indicates the end of stance and beginning of swing phase. Note increase electromyographic activity for extensor hallucis longus and soleus throughout the gait cycle and the abnormal out-of-phase activation of the gastrocnemius muscle in the swing phase when compared with normal timing represented by the gray bar.

midstance complicates weight bearing. Thus, hyperextended great toe has an impact on translation of the center of gravity during the stance component of limb advancement. It also has an impact on center-of-gravity stability during stance phase loading and single-limb support.[17] A number of muscles may generate unbalanced forces with respect to the hyperextended great toe pattern. The extensor hallucis longus provides a deforming force, causing great toe hyperextension.

A weak flexor hallucis longus may not be able to compensate and offset the extension force generated by the extensor muscle. When equinovarus is present as well, analysis of the contributions of tibialis anterior, tibialis posterior, gastrocnemius, and soleus most be taken into account. Chemodenervation with BoNT/A or a motor point injection with phenol to the extensor hallucis longus can achieve an effective therapeutic intervention.

Flexed Knee

In the flexed knee deformity, the knee remains flexed throughout stance and swing phases. A flexed knee during stance phase requires compensatory hip flexion on the same side and increased contralateral hip and knee flexion during swing phase (to shorten the limb sufficiently for limb clearance). Bilateral knee flexion deformity results in a crouched gait pattern, as is frequently seen in congenital spastic diplegia.[18] The impact of a flexed knee on translation of the center of gravity may be observed during limb advancement of swing phase. Lack of full knee extension in terminal swing limits limb advancement and results in a shortened step length. The flexed knee also has an impact on stance phase advancement because knee extension from mid- to terminal stance is restricted, requiring excessive contralateral hip and knee flexion to achieve limb clearance and possibly affecting energy efficiency due to excessive vertical displacement of the center of mass[19] (Fig. 15-4).

Dynamic poly-EMG recordings obtained from medial and lateral hamstrings, quadriceps, gastrocnemius, and soleus should help clarify the contribution of each of these muscles to the deformity.[7,20]

EMG recordings frequently demonstrate overactivation of the hamstrings, medial more than lateral. Excessive activity in the gastrocnemius restrains knee extension, particularly during swing phase. Kinematic data demonstrate limited knee extension and, frequently, compensatory hip flexion.[7,20]

Interventions that may be considered to reduce overactive hamstrings include phenol neurolysis to the motor branches of the sciatic nerve, motor point blocks with phenol to the hamstrings, or the more advantageous chemodenervation with BoNT. Chemodenervation with BoNT to the gastrocnemius can easily be achieved. Patients who have large muscle mass and severe spasticity may require larger doses of the selected agent. In addition, a potential undesirable effect is gastrocnemius and soleus group weakness that may lead to the drop off gait pattern in terminal stance (i.e., sudden and simultaneous ankle dorsiflexion and knee flexion). An ankle-foot orthosis that controls

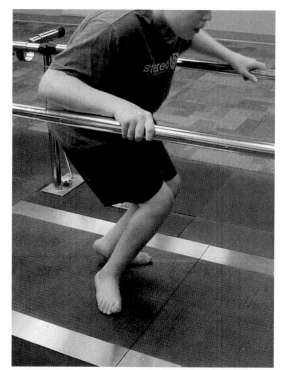

FIGURE 15-4. Crouched gait (flexed knees and hips) in a patient with upper motor neuron syndrome caused by perinatal brain injury.

dorsiflexion such as a ground reaction ankle-foot orthosis.

For those patients in whom surgery is indicated, a transfer of the long toe flexors into the os calcis can be used as a technique to increase plantarflexor muscle strength.[21] The approach is considered in combination with other surgical interventions such as distal hamstring lengthening or release followed by serial casting to gradually address any residual knee flexion deformity.[22]

Stiff Knee

The stiff knee is a swing-phase deformity. The knee is kept extended during preswing and initial swing, resulting in a reduction of the arc of motion, with its peak at less than 40 degrees (normal reference, 60 degrees). In addition, there may be delay in the timing of swing phase joint flexion and a concomitant reduction in hip flexion.[23] Knee flexion during walking at normal velocity is generated principally by the inertia-related pendulum effect resulting from hip flexion. Reduced hip flexion moment may result in decreased knee flexion

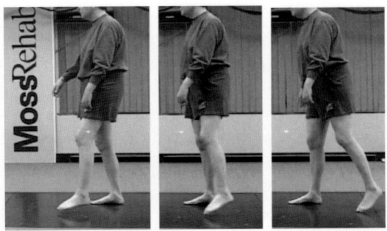

FIGURE 15-5. Stiff knee gait (lack of knee flexion in swing phase) in a patient with upper motor neuron syndrome after a stroke. The problem can interfere with limb clearance.

in swing phase (Fig. 15-5). A stiff knee functionally lengthens the limb and poses problems for clearance, particularly, during the preswing and swing phases of gait. This deviation may cause foot drag, tripping, and even falling for which the patient attempts to compensate by ipsilateral circumduction, hip hiking, or contralateral vaulting (early heel rise) that increases energy consumption. The effect of a stiff knee includes an increase in the inertial load of the swinging limb (by virtue of its longer moment arm when the knee is extended compared with the normally flexed knee of swing phase). The inertial load of a stiff knee influences translation of the center-of-gravity during limb advancement of swing phase.

Frequently, poly-EMG demonstrates a reduction in the activation of iliopsoas, along with excessive activation of the rectus femoris, vastus intermedius, vastus medialis, vastus lateralis, and at times, excessive activation of the gluteus maximus or even the hamstrings, working as hip extensors. If an ankle equinus deformity is also present, a reduction in joint power generation and plantarflexion moment may result in further reduction of knee flexion. Based on clinical and laboratory findings, chemodenervation with BoNT to individual heads of the quadriceps may be considered. Phenolization of the motor branch of the femoral nerve innervating the quadriceps mechanism is also an option, but this intervention requires more skill to perform and may result in undesirable excessive knee extensor weakness and instability in the stance phase of walking. Overactivity of the gluteus maximus in the

swing phase that restrains hip flexion and swing-limb advancement, can be managed with BoNT chemodenervation to the gluteus maximus as well.[24]

Adducted (Scissoring) Thigh

This deformity is characterized by adduction of the hip during the swing phase of locomotion. An adducted thigh results in a narrow base of support in the stance phase, potentially impairing balance.[25] It also can interfere with limb clearance and advancement because the adducting swing-phase limb may collide with the stance limb (Fig. 15-6). When adductor spasticity is complicated by hip flexor spasticity, toileting and perineal access for hygiene are markedly hampered, frequent repositioning of the patient sitting in a chair is required and often meets with limited success. It is essential to ascertain if the deformity is obligatory (the result of adductor spasticity) or compensatory (the result of weak hip flexors), because treatment will differ. A percutaneous temporary diagnostic obturator nerve block with lidocaine can be used to differentiate the role of hip adduction if the clinician is uncertain of the nature of the problem. Longer term interventions, such as percutaneous phenol nerve block, are easily carried out with excellent functional results.[25,26]

After the intervention, aggressive stretching of the hip adductors and strengthening of the hip flexors and abductors is pursued. Electrical stimulation to the hip abductors may be beneficial for this purpose.

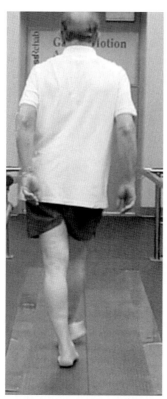

FIGURE 15-6. Adducted hip (scissoring gait) pattern with resulting narrow base of support in a patient with upper motor neuron syndrome caused by traumatic brain injury. Note position of the right foot crossing midline and promoting reduced balance similar to walking on a tight rope. The problem can also interfere with left limb advancement due to interference with the path of motion during the swing phase.

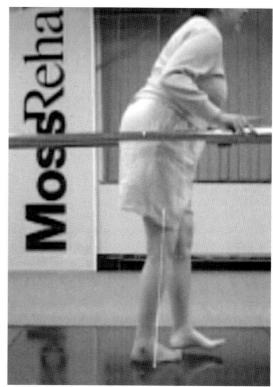

FIGURE 15-7. Flexed hip pattern with limited limb advancement and shortened step length in a patient with upper motor neuron syndrome caused by acquired brain injury. Note forward trunk lean and use of upper limb for support.

Flexed Hip

Excessive hip flexion causes a patient to experience difficulty when standing up from a seated position, may negatively affect both phases of the gait cycle, and may affect positioning efforts for perineal care and sexual intimacy. In normal gait, the hip is flexed at initial contact but, thereafter, extends throughout the stance phase, restricting forward advancement of the body over this limb. The result is a shortened contralateral step. Excessive hip flexion also affects stability of the center of gravity by influencing single-limb support during stance. Severe hip flexion deformity may promote development of a knee flexion deformity due to abnormal posture of the hip in the supine position[27,28] (Fig. 15-7).

Dynamic poly-EMG recordings of the iliopsoas, pectineus, gluteus maximus, hamstrings, rectus femoris, and lumbar paraspinals should help in determining the contribution of the different muscles in the gait cycle. Overactive iliopsoas, pectineus, rectus femoris, and hip adductors, or weakness of the hip extensors and paraspinals may be evident.[8] Interventions to reduce spasticity of the hip flexors (iliopsoas and rectus femoris), particularly chemodenervation with BoNT to the iliopsoas and rectus femoris or the use of phenol motor branch block to the rectus femoris can be easily performed and are followed by appropriate rehabilitation stretching techniques.[29]

BOTULINUM TOXIN

BoNT/A, currently available in the United States only under the brand name Botox (Allergan, Irvine, CA), has strong neuromuscular blocking properties. In Europe, Canada, and several countries in Latin America, it is also approved for the management of spasticity secondary to cerebral palsy and stroke and sold under the Dysport (Ipsen, Milford, MA) and Botox brand names. Serotype B toxin is also approved in the United States and Europe for cervical dystonia under the brand name Myobloc or Neurobloc (Solstice Neurosciences, Malvern, PA).[18,30]

The purpose of a BoNT block is to reduce force produced by a contracting overactive muscle or muscle group. A reduction in muscle tension can lead to improvement in passive and active range of motion and allow for more successful stretching of tight musculature. More subtly, and more importantly, too, a patient's improved control over movement and posture may allow for compensatory behaviors during functional activities (unmasking).[31] A reduction in spastic activity in one muscle or muscle group may have consequences for tone in other muscle groups of the limb or even in other limbs through a reduction in the overall effort required to perform movement or through changes in sensory information going to the central nervous system from that limb.[32,33] Identifying muscles with volitional capacity is important to the achievement of this goal. Another requirement is behavioral compliance and the ability to incorporate the newly gained increases in motion into the daily routine.

Also, the application of external devices such as braces, splints, casts, and even shoes can be facilitated by chemodenervation.[34]

BoNT is injected directly into an offending muscle. The major advantages in its use are the ease of application that permits its injection without anesthesia and its predictable effect. The most common adverse reaction is excessive weakness of injected muscles, but nausea, headache, and fatigue have also been reported. With some of the BoNT formulations, dysphagia has been reported when injecting muscles in close proximity to the neck structures, No adverse effect on the sensory system is evident with BoNT, but pain, when present before injection, may be improved.[35]

Even when a patient develops excessive weakness as a response to the paralytic effect of the toxin, no anaphylactic response has ever been reported for BoNT injection. Therapeutic doses of Botox for individual muscles have ranged between 10 and 300 units, depending on the size of the muscle being injected and the degree of spasticity.[35,36] Owing to the potential risk of migration out of the muscle and the possibility of antibody formation, usually not more than 50 units are injected in each site, with a maximum of 600 units administered in a single treatment session. This may be sufficient, however, to treat a number of muscles in that one session.[18,24,30]

To minimize the risk of immunoresistance with BoNT, physicians should use the smallest possible effective dose; extend the interval between treatments for at least 3 months or longer, if possible; and avoid the use of booster injections in between treatments.[35] Development of resistance to BoNT/A with the current formulation of Botox therapy does not appear to be an important clinical issue in the management of patients with UMNS-related muscle overactivity. Careful documentation of muscle selection, dose, number of sites, dilution, and effects is encouraged so that in the next treatment cycle, one may adjust the dose as necessary. In our practice, we limit dose per treatment to no more than 600 units of Botox, and if multiple large muscles are to be injected, increasing the dilution to improve diffusion as well as using techniques for localization of the endplate can extend the maximum dose for more muscles. The other option is to focus the available dose to a few muscles and consider using other interventions such as phenol to achieve a complete treatment strategy.[37]

With the currently available information, we recommend not injecting BoNT/A into patients who are pregnant or lactating. Before using BoNT/A in the clinical management of spasticity, the physician should be knowledgeable about the diagnosis and medical management of the condition producing spasticity and should be proficient in the relevant anatomy and kinesiology. The physician should have a clear understanding of the potential benefits of unmasking function and of the limitations of this therapeutic intervention. Because there is a several-day delay between injection of toxin and onset of action, a patient may require several sessions to optimize the dose that seems to be necessary for optimal treatment. Unlike dystonia, in which voluntary capacity is not an issue, spastic muscles may very well have voluntary capacity, which the clinician would like to preserve, and therefore, titration of the paralytic effect of the toxin becomes a much more critical factor in its administration because unmasking of function may occur. The duration of toxin effectiveness is usually 10 weeks to 4 months. In our experience, patients have received 400 to 600 units of Botox at 3-month intervals for more than 3 years without evidence of loss of effectiveness of the medication.

It would seem that the BoNT treatment might be most effective when used early as a temporizing management of spasticity, particularly in the period of expected neurologic recovery in which spasticity is changing as motor recovery occurs, or in patients with chronic conditions as an effective tool to simulate the potential effects of surgery, to the benefit of the surgeon and patient alike.

The strategy of performing a BoNT injection is as follows. The skin is prepared by cleaning it with alcohol before insertion of the Teflon-coated, 25-gauge stimulating injecting needle. The electrically conductive inner core of the tip of the needle is used to pass current to the tissues or to record EMG activity.[38] After injection, muscle activation should be encouraged to increase the uptake and internalization of the toxin, which, in turn, can prolong the duration of effect.[39] When the paralytic effect seems evident, aggressive stretching, muscle re-education, and functional training are performed (see Table 15-1).

PHENOL

Phenol, a benzene derivative, is also known as carbolic acid; it denatures the protein membrane of peripheral nerves in aqueous concentrations of 5%. When phenol is injected in or near a nerve bundle, phenol's neurolytic action on the myelin sheath or the cell membrane of axons with which it makes contact serves to reduce neural traffic along the nerve, reducing muscle overactivity.[40]

The onset of the destructive process with higher concentrations of phenol may begin to show effects several days after injection, but phenol also has a local anesthetic feature that allows a clinician and the patient to see partial results shortly after the phenol block is performed.[40] The denaturing process induced by phenol extends biologically on the order of weeks, perhaps months. Eventually regeneration occurs, so a phenol block is used clinically as a temporizing measure rather than a permanent intervention. In our clinical experience and in the experience of others, the effect of a phenol block typically lasts 2 to 5 months.[40] Histologically, it has been shown that phenol destroys axons of all sizes, probably in a patchy distribution, but moreso on the outer aspect of the nerve bundle, onto which phenol is dripped. In such a model, interior axons within a nerve bundle are theoretically spared moreso than their sibling axons located more peripherally, where phenol has access to them. When phenol is injected percutaneously, it is extremely likely that the nerve block will be incomplete. This is especially useful in situations in which a spastic muscle also has volitional capacity because, under these circumstances, it is desirable to reduce spasticity while still preserving the volitional capacity of that muscle.

The technique of phenol injection is based on electrical stimulation of motor nerves for localization of the injection site. Except for few circumstances, we generally inject motor branches close to the offending muscle or muscle group (motor point). This is necessary to avoid sensory dysesthesia. Several texts are available that identify muscles and their motor points. A surface stimulator is briefly used to approximate the percutaneous stimulation site in advance. The skin is prepared with alcohol, and a local anesthetic can be injected or rubbed onto the skin.

The purpose is to eliminate cutaneous motor reflexes that may cause the limb to jump when the blocking needle is subsequently inserted.[27] A 25-gauge, Teflon-coated hypodermic needle (which is the same needle used for BoNT injections) is advanced toward the motor nerve. Depth of penetration and directional orientation of the needle tip require a steady hand, a competent knowledge of anatomy, and a good assistant. Electrical stimulation is adjusted by noting whether muscle contraction of the desired muscle takes place. As one gets closer to the motor nerve, less current intensity is required to produce a contractile response. The motor nerve is injected when minimal current produces a visible or palpable contraction. We use a Duo Stim electrical stimulator with pulse frequencies of one per second; we typically inject when the milliampere reading on the unit reads 0.4 mA. We generally inject 2 to 7 mL of 5% to 7% aqueous solution of phenol. For longer effects, larger volumes, and longer distances between the site of injection and the distance to the neuromuscular junction of the muscle are used. The literature does report that phenol applied to sensory nerves may produce a dysesthesia that is troublesome.[41] For this reason, we do not recommend injection of mixed peripheral nerves except in a patient who is vegetative and indifferent to any sensory consequences. (Actually, sensory blockade may help reduce spasticity by reducing afferent input to a hyperexcitable motor system.) After the block, we recommend that ice be applied to the injection site for 10 to 15 minutes every 2 hours as needed to reduce local irritation or swelling. Because a certain amount of needling is required to find the best place for injecting the motor nerve, we prefer not to use phenol in patients receiving anticoagulation medication.[12]

The technique for BoNT injection (see above) may be preferable in this circumstance. As with any injection, care needs to be taken not to inject phenol into a blood vessel, and aspirating before the injection achieves this. We use the help of an assistant to perform the injection while the physician holds the needle still. In contrast, a physician can generally perform injection with BoNT without assistance. The literature has reported a range of injections between 1 and 10 mL of phenol in various concentrations, usually not exceeding 7%. The lethal range of phenol that gets into the central nervous system is approximately 8.5 g. Ten milliliters of a 7% solution of phenol contains 0.7 g of phenol, a 10-fold factor of safety. We generally do not inject more than 15 mL of 7% phenol in a session. If a phenol block seems ineffective after several weeks, it may be repeated. With repeated phenol injections, an increase in fibrous tissue at the site of injection may occur, and this may make repeat injections more difficult.

CONCLUSIONS

In summary, spasticity is a widespread, disabling form of muscle overactivity affecting patients with central nervous system damage resulting in upper motor neuron syndrome. There is a range of effective therapies for the treatment of spasticity (e.g., physical, anesthetic, chemodenervation, neurolytic injections, and surgery), but all therapies must be selected using an individualized, multidisciplinary treatment program targeted to achieve patient goals.[42] Using the classification scheme presented in this paper should facilitate goal selection and communication between patients, caretakers, and the clinical team. The identification of the muscles responsible for the presenting abnormal patterns of gait dysfunction is of particular importance when the treatment intervention selected is BoNT/A chemodenervation which is an effective selective agent without the adverse effects of other interventions.

References

1. Farmer SF, Swash M, Ingram DA, Stephens JA. Changes in motor unit synchronization following central nervous lesions in man. *J Physiol.* [London]. 1993;463:83-105.
2. Ashworth B. Preliminary trial of carisoprodal in multiple sclerosis. *Practitioner.* 1964;192:540.
3. Tardieu C, Huet de la Tour E, Bret MD, Tardieu G. Muscle hypoextensibility in children with cerebral palsy. I: Clinical and experimental observations. *Arch Phys Med Rehabil.* 1982;63:97-102.
4. Gracies JM, Marosszeky JE, Renton R, Sandanam J, Gandevia SC, Burke D. Short-term effects of dynamic lycra splints on upper limb in hemiplegic patients. *Arch Phys Med Rehabil.* 2000;81:1547-1555.
5. Lance JW. Symposium synopsis. In: Feldman RG, Young RR, Koella WP, eds. *Spasticity: Disordered Motor Control.* Chicago: Year Book Medical Publishers; 1980:485-494.
6. Campbell SK. Framework for the measurement of neurological impairment in disability. In: Wyster MJ, ed. *Contemporary Management of Motor Control Problems. Proceedings of the II Step Conference.* Alexandria VA: Foundation for Physical Therapy; 1991:146-147.
7. Mayer N, Esquenazi A, Childers M. Common patterns of clinical motor dysfunction. *Muscle Nerve.* 1997;6(suppl):S21-S35.
8. Mayer N, Esquenazi A. Muscle overactivity and movement dysfunction in the upper motoneuron syndrome. *Phys Med Rehabil Clin North Am.* 2003;14:855-883.
9. Esquenazi A, Mayer N. Instrumented assessment of muscle overactivity and spasticity with dynamic polyelectromyographic and motion analysis for treatment planning. *Am J Phys Med Rehabil.* 2004; 83(suppl):S19-S29.
10. Mayer NH, Esquenazi A, Keenan MAE. Patterns of upper motoneuron dysfunction in the lower limb. gait disorders. *Adv Neuroly.* 2001;87:311-319.
11. Esquenazi A. Evaluation and management of spastic gait in patients with traumatic brain injury. *J Head Trauma Rehabil.* 2004;19:109-118.
12. Mayer N. Choosing upper limb muscles for focal intervention after traumatic brain injury. *J Head Trauma Rehabil.* 2004;19:119-142.
13. Esquenazi A, Vachranukunkiet T, Hirai B. EMG activity of the medial and lateral gastrocnemius during pathological gait. *Arch Phys Med Rehabil.* 1988;69:778.
14. Fuller DA, Keenan MA, Esquenazi A, Whyte J, Mayer N, Fidler-Sheppard R: The impact of instrumented gait analysis on surgical planning: treatment of spastic equinovarus deformity of the foot and ankle. *Foot Ankle Int.* 2002;22:738-743.
15. Cionni M, Esquenazi A, Hirai B. Effects of botulinum toxin-A on gait velocity, step length and base of support of patients with dynamic equinovarus foot. *Am J Phys Med Rehabil.* 2006;85:600-606.
16. Mayer N, Esquenazi A, Keenan MAE. Analysis and management of spasticity, contracture and impaired motor control. medical rehabilitation of traumatic brain injury. In: Horn L, Zasler N, ed. *Medical Rehabilitation of Traumatic Brain Injury.* Philadelphia: Henley & Belfus; 1996; 411-458.
17. Esquenazi A. Falls and fractures in older post-stroke patients with spasticity: consequences and drug treatment considerations. *Clin Geriatr.* 2004;12:27-35.
18. Koman LA, Mooney J, Smith B, Goodman A. Cerebral palsy management by neuromuscular blockade with botulinum-A toxin. *NIH Consensus Development*

Conference on Clinical Use of Botulinum Toxin. November, 1990, Bethesda, MD.

19. Esquenazi A, Talaty M, Gait analysis: technology and clinical application. In: Braddom RL, ed. *Physical Medicine and Rehabilitation*, 3rd ed. Philadelphia: Elsevier Inc.; 2007:93-110.

20. Esquenazi A, Hirai B. Gait analysis in stroke and head injury. In: Craik RL, Oatis CA, eds. *Gait Analysis, Theory and Application*. St. Louis: Mosby; 1995:412-419.

21. Keenan MA, Lee GA, Tuckman SA, Esquenazi A. Improving calf muscle strength in patients with spastic equinovarus deformity by transfer of the long toe flexors to the os calcis. *J Head Trauma Rehabil*. 1999;14:163-175.

22. Esquenazi A. Assessment and orthotic management of gait dysfunction in individuals with traumatic brain injury. In: Hsu J, Michael J, Fisk J, eds. *Atlas of Orthotics*. Philadelphia: Elsevier; 2008:441-447.

23. Goldberg SR, Ounpuu S, Arnold AS, Gage JR, Delp SL. Kinematic and kinetic factors that correlate with improved knee flexion following treatment for stiff-knee gait. *J Biomech*. 2006;39:689-698.

24. Brin M. Dosing, administration, and a treatment algorithm for use of botulinum toxin a for adult-onset spasticity. Spasticity Study Group. *Muscle Nerve*. 1997;6(suppl):S208-S220.

25. Ofluoglu D, Esquenazi A, Hirai B. Temporospatial parameters of gait after obturator neurolysis in patients with spasticity. *Am J Phys Med Rehabil*. 2003;82: 832-836.

26. Gooch JL, Patton CP. Combining botulinum toxin and phenol to manage spasticity in children. *Arch Phys Med Rehabil*. 2004;85:1121-1124.

27. Mayer NH, Herman RM. Phenomenology of muscle overactivity in the upper motor neuron syndrome. *Eura Medicophys*. 2004;40:85-110.

28. O'Dwyer N, Ada L, Neilson PD. Spasticity and muscle contracture following stroke. *Brain*. 1996;119: 1737-1749.

29. Sheean G. Botulinum toxin treatment of adult spasticity: a benefit-risk assessment. *Drug Saf*. 2006;29: 31-48.

30. Ward AB, Aguilar M, De Beyl Z, Gedin S, Kanovsky P, Molteni F, et al. Use of botulinum toxin type A in management of adult spasticity—a european consensus statement. *J Rehabil Med*. 2003;35:98-99.

31. Jankovic J, Schwartz K. Clinical correlates of response to botulinum toxin injections. *Arch Neurol*. 1991;48:1253-1256.

32. Esquenazi A, Mayer N, Garreta R. Influence of botulinum toxin type A treatment of elbow flexor spasticity on hemiparetic gait. *Am J Phys Med Rehabil*. 2007;In press.

33. Fleuren JF, Nederhand MJ, Hermens HJ. Influence of posture and muscle length on stretch reflex activity in poststroke patients with spasticity. *Arch Phys Med Rehabil*. 2006;87:981-988.

34. Carda S, Molteni F. Selective neuromuscular blocks and chemoneurolysis in the localized treatment of spasticity. *Eura Medicophys*. 2004;40:123-130.

35. Dosing and administration of botulinum toxin for muscle overactivity in adults with an upper motor neuron syndrome. In: Brashear A, Mayer N, eds. *Spasticity and Other Forms of Muscle Overactivity in the Upper Motor Neuron Syndrome*. New York: We-Move; 2008:207-218.

36. Jankovic J, Esquenazi A, Fehlings D, Freitag F, Lang A, Naumann M. Evidence-based review of patient-reported outcomes with botulinum toxin type A. *Clin Neuropharmacol*. 2004;27:234-244.

37. Mayer N, Whyte J, Wannstedt G, Elis C. Comparative efficacy of two botulinum toxin injection techniques for elbow flexor hypertonia. *Arch Phys Med Rehabil*. 2008;89:982-987.

38. Chin TYP, Nattrass GR, Selber P, Graham HK. Accuracy of intramuscular injection of botulinum toxin A in juvenile cerebral palsy: A comparison between manual needle placement and placement guided by electrical stimulation. *J Pediatr Orthop*. 2005;25:286-291.

39. Esquenazi A, Mayer N. Electric stimulation to prolong the duration of botulinum toxin type A effect on spasticity: a double-blind, placebo-controlled study. *Arch Phys Med Rehabil*. 2007;88:E105.

40. Glenn M. Nerve blocks. In: Glen M, Whyte J, eds. *The Practical Management of Spasticity in Children and Adults*. Philadelphia: Lea & Febiger; 1990:227-258.

41. DeLateur BJ. A new technique of intramuscular phenol neurolysis. *Arch Phys Med Rehabil*. 1972;53:179-185.

42. Esquenazi A. Improvements in healthcare and cost benefits associated with botulinum toxin treatment of spasticity and muscle overactivity. State of the art publication 2006 on the use of botulinum toxin. *Europ J Neurol*. 2006;13:27-34.

Treatment of 16 Oromandibular Dystonia, Bruxism, and Temporomandibular Disorders with Botulinum Toxin

Nwanmegha Young and Andrew Blitzer

INTRODUCTION

Temporomandibular disorders (TMDs) are a collection of conditions affecting the temporomandibular joint (TMJ) and the muscles of mastication and contiguous tissue components. It is estimated that more than 10 million people suffer from this condition in the United States.[1-3] Owing to the complex relationship between the muscles of mastication and the TMJ, there are a wide variety of clinical presentations for these disorders. The term TMD as a clinical label is used primarily to designate conditions that present with pain in the face or jaw area. It also encompasses the clinical syndrome of headaches, earaches, trismus, masticatory muscle hypertrophy, and clicking and popping of the TMJ.[4-8] Traditional treatment of TMD has consisted of occlusal therapy, appliances, physical therapy, joint surgery, behavioral counseling, and medications.[9-12] Prospective, randomized clinical studies have demonstrated the effectiveness of using a biologic neuromuscular blocking agent, botulinum toxin (BoNT), for the treatment of neurologic disorders associated with hyperactivity of skeletal muscles.[13,14] More recently, BoNT has been increasingly used as an adjuvant treatment for head and neck pain such as tension-type and migraine headaches.[15,16] The pain relieving effects of BoNT were observed during clinical trials for the treatment of cervical and oromandibular dystonias (OMDs).[17-18] Recent scientific study has suggested that pain relief is caused by decreasing the release of inflammatory mediators (calcitonin gene–related peptide, substance P, glutamate, and so on) whose release is mediated by soluble N-ethylmaleimide–sensitive factor attachment receptor (SNARE) proteins.[19-22] Our experience in treating OMD with BoNT, led to the realization that not only did function improve in these patients, but there was also a significant reduction in pain. Therefore, we embarked on treating patients with TMD.

CLINICAL SYNDROMES

TMD is a nonspecific diagnosis describing pain related to jaw and masticatory muscles of unclear etiology. Our experience has demonstrated that a diverse group of TMDs involving the orofacial musculature are amenable to treatment with BoNT. These disorders include (1) bruxism, (2) OMDs, (3) myofascial pain,

Dr. Young does not report any conflicts of interest. Dr. Blitzer is reporting that he received research funding from Allergan, Inc and Merz. Also, he is a consultant to Myotech and is a minor share holder. He also receives royalty income from Zomed/Medtronics.

(4) trismus, (5) masseter and temporalis hypertrophy, and (6) headaches.

Bruxism

Bruxism, which includes clenching or grinding of the teeth, or both, affects from 50% to 95% of the adult population.[23-25] Bruxism is caused by the activation of reflex chewing activity. Various forms of bruxism have been described.[26,27] The etiology of this disorder is uncertain. Some experts believe that it is related to anxiety and stress. Other explanations include asymmetry of teeth, and digestive and sleep disturbances. Bruxism can affect the muscles solely or can act as a parafunction that is an initiating and/or perpetuating factor in more involved forms of TMD involving joint damage. The treatment of bruxism includes behavioral therapy, dental appliances, and medications.[28-30] Many characteristics of bruxism mimic those of dystonia, including similar epidemiology, pain, and exacerbation by external factors such as fatigue, stress, and emotional stress. Several experts have suggested that bruxism may itself be a form of focal dystonia.[31] If bruxism is a type of dystonia, it is possible that the success of the most common treatment of bruxism, with intraoral appliances or occlusal adjustments, may simply be a "sensory trick" that relieves dystonic symptoms. Regardless of the etiology of bruxism, successful use of BoNT for bruxism has been described.[32-35]

Oromandibular Dystonia

OMD can occur alone or with other focal or generalized dystonias.[36-38] Spasms of the muscles of mastication can lead to pain, abnormal jaw positioning, TMJ dysfunction, and trismus (Fig. 16-1). The diagnosis can be difficult. In addition to BoNT, treatments include anticholinergics, benzodiazepines, and other oral agents.[39-44] OMD is categorized as a focal dystonia that involves the musculature of the masticatory apparatus and lower face, and may involve the tongue. It manifests as distorted oral position and function, resulting in orofacial disfigurement, dysfunction, and often pain. Although it is commonly viewed as a neurologic disorder, there is no doubt of its inclusion as a subset of TMDs owing to the involvement of the masticatory apparatus.[45,46] We have demonstrated successful treatment

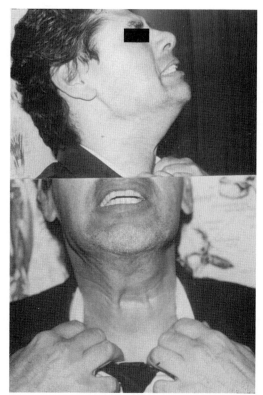

FIGURE 16-1. Demonstrates a man with oromandibular dystonia. Note the platysma banding indicating involvement of the neck musculature.

of this disorder with BoNT.[47,48] Even more significantly, early evidence of pain relief with BoNT in the treatment of OMD has been reported.[48,49]

Myofascial Pain

Myofascial pain syndrome (MPS) is one of the common causes of TMD.[50-52] It manifests as discomfort or pain in the muscles that control jaw function and neck and shoulder muscles. It does not have a uniformly accepted definition or a well-understood pathology.[53-56] It is estimated that 14% of the US population suffers from chronic musculoskeletal pain and that 21% to 93% of these patients have MPS.[57-61] The clinical hallmark of MPS is the "trigger point," a region of focal tenderness in a taut band of muscle fibers that, on compression, produces referred pain in characteristic areas for specific muscles. Conventional treatments emphasize muscle relaxation using physical and pharmacologic therapies.[62,63] Previous studies demonstrated that a reduction in bite strength, concomitant with BoNT,

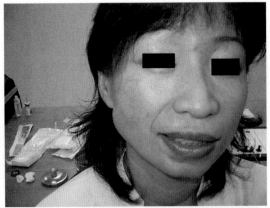

FIGURE 16-2. Unilateral masseter hypertrophy in a Korean woman.

resulted in pain relief.[64,65] In fact, the pain relief outlasts the weakening of the muscles treated. BoNT therapy can alleviate pain of myofascial origin and, indirectly, pain of arthrogenic origin from diminished joint loading.

Masseter and Temporalis Hypertrophy

The etiology of benign masseteric and temporalis hypertrophy is generally unknown (Fig. 16-2). Some believe it is due to work hypertrophy, such as in habitual jaw clenching or teeth grinding.[66-69] Interestingly, benign masseteric hypertrophy is frequently found among Korean persons who favor chewing dried squid, a tough and chewy delicacy.[70-72] Masseter hypertrophy is largely regarded as a cosmetic facial deformity, although some report pain associated with this condition.[73] Treatment with BoNT produces decreased force on chewing and clenching and a muscle atrophy[74,75] (Fig. 16-3).

Trismus

Trimus, or "lockjaw," is a limitation in jaw opening usually caused by a tonic contraction of the muscles of mastication of the muscle of mastication.[76] In the past, trismus was used to describe restriction of mouth opening seen in patients with tetanus, also called "lock-jaw," but trismus can be caused by a variety of conditions including stroke, head trauma, surgery, and radiation.[77,78] BoNT has been reported to relieve these conditions by reducing the involuntary contractions of the involved muscles.[79]

Tension Headaches

Although the pathophysiology of headaches is not clear, there is evidence that botulinum toxin type A (BoTX/A) may be beneficial in treating tension, migraine, cluster, and cervicogenic headaches.[80-82] By far the most

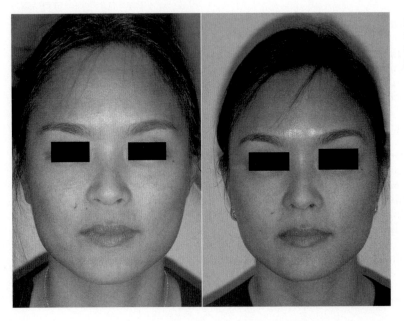

FIGURE 16-3. Before and after of multiple botulinum toxin treatment in a lady with benign masseter hypertrophy.

common headache types are tension and migraine. Many tension headaches involve the temporalis and/or masseter muscles. Tension headaches are generally characterized by aching, tenderness, or sensations of pressure or constriction. It is estimated that 38% of the population will experience tension headache in any given year.[83] Treatment for acute episodes include simple analgesics, nonsteroidal anti-inflammatory agents, and muscle relaxants.[84] Several small studies have demonstrated that treatment of tension headache with BoNT/A is effective.[85] The topic of headaches is reviewed elsewhere in this volume.

BOTULINUM TOXIN AND TREATMENT OF TEMPOROMANDIBULAR DISORDERS AND OROMANDIBULAR DYSTONIA

The initial treatment of TMD usually consists of physical therapy, occlusal appliances, and medications. If joint pathology is involved, surgery also may be beneficial. BoNT has been successfully used as primary therapy when other modes have failed. Over the past 12 years, we have developed a TMD algorithm for management with BoNT, based on more than 200 patients treated in our office for TMD. We usually treat patients after traditional conservative therapies were found to be ineffective and before surgery. At this time, we do not include patients with primary TMJ pathology. Therapy is directed toward the patient's specific symptoms. Sometimes the imbalance of the forces of the muscle of mastication can lead to pain in the surrounding neck musculature due to posturing. In our experience, this is usually relieved after treatment of the primary site.

Injection Methods

A thorough knowledge of the underlying anatomy of the muscles that may be involved in TMD is essential for both diagnosis and treatment. We typically divide target muscles into those that open the jaw and those that close it (Table 16-1). Injection of each of the muscles of mastication is typically performed under electromyographic (EMG) control.

TABLE 16-1 Muscles of Mastication

Jaw-Opening Muscles	Jaw-Closing Muscles
Anterior digastric	Masseter
External pterygoid	Temporalis
	Internal pterygoid

Ground and reference leads are placed on the skin and connected to an EMG machine. The skin of the injection site is then cleaned with alcohol. A hollow 27-gauge, Telfon-coated, monopolar EMG needle is placed on a 1-mL tuberculin syringe. The needle is then passed through the skin into the targeted muscle. Proper placement is confirmed by electrical signal.

Temporalis

The temporalis muscle is readily accessible superficially in the temple area. It is a fan-shaped muscle of variable expanse and depth. Multiple injection points, superficial and deep, are usually used to adequately weaken this muscle (Fig. 16-4). Superficial injections are performed into the thinner upper regions of the muscle in a fan shape. No special precautions are required, although advancing the needle too deeply engages bone and damages the needle. As one proceeds posteriorly, the muscle becomes thicker; therefore, deeper injections are required. For this injection, particular note must be taken of the split of the superficial temporalis fascia

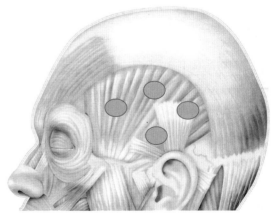

FIGURE 16-4. Injection sites for botulinum toxin in the temporalis muscle.

approximately 1.5 cm superior to the zygomatic arch. In this area, there are two superficial fascia layers with fat in between, where the muscle is deeper. If the operator uses the tactile sensation of penetration of the needle through fascia as a guide for injection, two penetrations are necessary in this area. This latter injection is probably very useful because the muscle in this area is the thickest before insertion on the coronoid process of the mandible. Aspiration before injection is critical because the superficial temporal artery and vein course through this field.

Masseter

The masseter muscle is readily accessible clinically. It is a thick muscle of trapezoidal shape extending from the zygomatic arch superiorly to the lower border of the mandible inferiorly and from the posterior border of the mandibular ramus posteriorly to midcheek anteriorly. Approximately five diffuse injections are recommended, preferably targeted to areas of highest activity on EMG, greatest muscle bulk, and greatest discomfort (Fig. 16-5). Care must be taken with anterior and superior injections of this muscle because diffusion of BoNT to the zygomaticus major muscle nearby may result in an adverse cosmetic effect, specifically preventing the patient from raising the corner of the mouth and thus causing an asymmetric smile.

Medial Pterygoid

The medial pterygoid muscle lies on the medial surface of the mandible and is somewhat difficult to reach (Fig. 16-6). The utility of injecting this muscle in most instances is questionable because adequate relaxation of the masseter and temporalis jaw-closing muscles appears to provide enough clinical effect to relieve pain relief and reduce joint loading. However, in some cases of OMD, in which opening of the mouth remains difficult, the internal pterygoid muscle may be treated. The muscle can be injected extraorally via a submandibular route. However, the angulation does not lend itself to good visibility or easy access to the superior aspect of the muscle. The intraoral approach allows palpation of the muscle before injection except when the patient has a sensitive gag reflex or limitation in oral opening. In either technique, care must be taken to stay within the muscle because superior medial injection can approach the infratemporal fossa and its contents. Branches of the external carotid artery, branches of the trigeminal nerve, and muscles of the pharynx can be adversely affected. Inferior medial injection outside the medial pterygoid can affect the submandibular gland as well as muscles of the floor of the mouth. Therefore, EMG guidance is required.

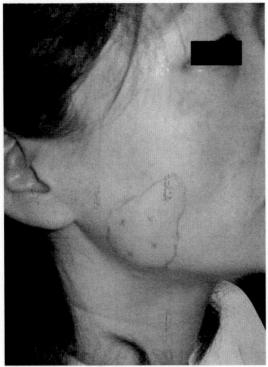

FIGURE 16-5. Markings are injection points for the masseter muscle.

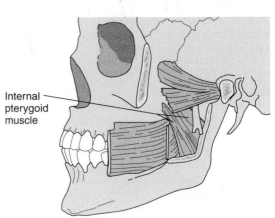

Internal pterygoid muscle

FIGURE 16-6. Anatomy of the medial pterygoid muscle.

Lateral Pterygoid

This small muscle requires EMG guidance for injection because of its size and location. The approach is operator dependent, either extra- or intraoral. Using an extraoral approach, one must establish the location of the condylar head by palpation as the patient demonstrates a full range of mandibular motion. The needle is inserted through the skin, through the coronoid notch area anteriorly, and slightly deeper. The patient is then asked to mobilize the mandible from side to side, listening for bursts of activity on the EMG. Aspiration and injection are performed once proper position is ascertained. This approach, however, engages the muscle perpendicularly and limits the amount of the muscle that can be treated. The intraoral approach engages the muscle in a parallel fashion. The intraoral approach involves palpation of the external pterygoid plate posterior to the maxillary tuberosity. Once the needle is inserted through mucosa, it is helpful to visualize the patient's ear (knowing that the TMJ is just anterior to the external auditory meatus) to guide the needle laterally and posteriorly. This is performed with EMG guidance to allow injection in several places along the length of the muscle. There are variations of these basic techniques. Considerable caution must be taken while injecting in this infratemporal fossa area, as noted previously. It is also important to note that the muscle is surrounded by the pterygoid plexus of veins.

Because the lateral pterygoid is a relatively small muscle and may not be the major contributor to jaw opening dystonia, Jankovic et al[86] first showed in 1990 that an injection of botulinum toxin into the submental muscle complex in such patients may be beneficial. Subsequent studies confirmed initial observation.[87-89] Our standard approach now is to inject the lateral pterygoids and the anterior belly of the digastric muscle bilaterally.

CLINICAL EXPERIENCE

Our first TMD patient was treated in 1989. The patient was a man who had severe daily headaches; huge, tender masseter muscles; TMJ clicking; and moderate trismus. Most treatments were ineffective, and he chewed through night guards each week. He required 75 units of Botox in each masseter and 25 units in each temporalis muscle every 3 to 4 months, but he had near-complete cessation of pain and dysfunction after each treatment.

We then embarked on an open-label study, treating patients with dose ranges of: masseter muscle, 15 to 75 units per muscle; temporalis muscle, 10 to 30 units; internal pterygoid muscle, 10 to 20 units; and external pterygoid muscle, 7.5 to 15 units. The muscles injected were determined by the patients reporting of location of pain, muscle tenderness to palpation, and observed functional abnormalities. We generally start with 25 units in each masseter and 12.5 to 25 units in each temporalis muscle (in patients who primarily clenched their teeth) and 7.5 units in each lateral pterygoid (for patients with bruxing and grinding). Additional muscles were added, depending on symptoms and clinical examination. The patient returned at 2 weeks for a re-evaluation. If he or she continued to have pain, a booster dose was given to the persistently painful muscles.

In reviewing the first 200 patients, we found a 70% response rate, with a response defined as 50% or more reduction in pain and/or frequency of pain. We noted that many of the patients who still had pain had both a decrease in resting pain and a decrease in the amount of daily medication to control the pain. After repeated injections, there was a trend for increased response and increased duration of benefit. This suggests a central increase in pain threshold.

The adverse events were minimal. Less than 10% of the patients (usually those with doses of 50 U or more in the masseter muscles) complained of a decreased ability to chew solid foods. A number of the patients could not chew food before treatment due to pain. Two patients reported a change in their smile, due to slight weakness from diffusion of toxin to the levator anguli oris and zygomaticus muscles. Slight tenderness at the site of injection and 3 patients with skin ecchymosis were also reported.

Based on the promsing results of the open-label study, we designed a multicenter study. It was a double-blind, placebo controlled dose comparison study with randomized treatment into 4 arms: placebo, 75 units (25 U each masseter muscle, 12.5 U each temporalis muscle), 100 units (25 U each masseter and temporalis), and 150 units (50 U each masseter, 25 U each temporalis). The study population consisted of male and female patients 18 years or older who had TMD pain and no primary joint disease, met other entry criteria, and gave written informed consent.

The primary objective of this study was to examine the efficacy of Botox (Allergan, Irvine, CA) relative to placebo in the management of TMD. The primary end point addressing this objective is the proportion of responders, defined as those patients who exhibit at least a 50% decrease in their maximum temporomandibular pain at rest measured by a Visual Analog Scale pain rating scale, from baseline to week 8. The results will be analyzed in the near future and published when available.

SIDE/ADVERSE EFFECTS

The most common side effects were temporary bruising and pain at the sites of injection. Less common adverse effects reported were difficulty chewing, dysphagia, and asymmetry of the face.

CONCLUSIONS

Pain related to the TMJ and the associated muscles of mastication is a very common report. TMDs are a common cause of chronic facial pain and headache. The disorder is thought to be secondary to hyperfunction of the muscles of mastication resulting in chronic inflammation and pain. TMD is considered a group of pathologies affecting the masticatory muscles, the TMJ, and related structures. TMD pain may be muscular pain or joint pain and can be associated with headache, myofascial pain of the back and shoulders and neck pain. There can be associated disorders within the TMJ such as ankylosis and arthritis; however, these disorders can often be present without any accompanying joint pathology. Associated complaints include earache, headache, neck pain, and facial swelling.

TMD is a widespread pain disorder of the head and neck. Chronic pain and associated symptoms significantly interfere with interpersonal relations, professional duties, and overall quality of life. Patients suffering from chronic pain have an increased risk of developing psychiatric disorders, particularly affective disorders such as depression.[90] A detailed examination with appropriate diagnostic testing often allows the physician to classify the specific disorder and initiate an effective therapeutic plan.

BoNT provides significant relief from facial pain in many of the patients, and reduces intensity, frequency, and duration of recurrent episodes when properly administered. The exact mechanism is still not completely understood. We suggest that BoNT therapy be instituted after standard conservative therapy failure and before surgical interventions. Injection protocols, including fixed-site and follow-the-pain techniques, have provided lasting relief in patients with TMD, idiopathic facial pain, trigeminal neuralgia, and headache. The adverse effects from BoNT are often mild, transient, and limited to adjacent muscle weakness, which can often be avoided through the use of proper injection technique. Further basic and clinical trials are necessary to fully elucidate the efficacy of this treatment, but BoNT therapy may provide a safe and effective means by which to treat TMD and other chronic pain disorders in the head and neck.

References

1. Dworkin SF, Huggins KH, LeResche L et al. Epidemiology of the signs and symptoms in temporomandibular disorders: clinical signs in cases and controls. *J Am Dent Assoc.* 1990;120:273-281.
2. McFarlane TV, Blinkhorn AS, Davies RM, Kincy J, Worthington HV. Orofacial pain in the community: prevalence and associated impact. *Community Dent Oral Epidemiol.* 2002;30:52-60.
3. Lipton JA, Ship JA, Larasch-Robinson D. Estimated prevalence and distribution of reported orofacial pain in the United States. *J Am Dent Assoc.* 1993;124:115-121.
4. McNeill C, ed. Epidemiology. In: *Temporomandibular Disorders: Guidelines for Clasification, Assessment, and Management.* Chicago: Quintessence Publishing Co; 1993:19-22.
5. Pow EHN, Leung KCM, McMillan AS. Prevalence of symptoms associated with temporomandibular disorders in Hong Kong Chinese. *J Orofac Pain.* 2001;15:228-234.
6. Kaplan AS. Classification. In: Kaplan AS, Assael LA, eds. *Temporomandibular Disorders; Diagnosis and Treatment,* 1st ed. Philadelphia, PA: WB Saunders; 1991:106-117.
7. Carlsson GE. Epidemiology and treatment need for temporomandibular disorders. *J Orofac Pain.* 1999;13:232-237.
8. Ohrbach R, Stohler C. Research diagnostic criteria for temporomandibular disorders: current diagnostic systems. *J Craniomandib Disord Facial Oral Pain.* 1992;6:307-317.
9. Magnusson T, Carlsson GE, Egermark-Eriksson I. An evaluation of the need and demand for treatment of craniomandibular disorders in a young Swedish population. *J Craniomandib Disord.* 1991;5:57-63.
10. Molin C. From bite to mind: TMD-a personal and literature review. *Int J Prosthodont.* 1999;12:279-288.
11. Dionne RA. Pharmacologic treatments for temporomandibular disorders. *Oral Surg Oral Med Oral Pathol Oral Radiol Endod.* 1997;83:134-142.

12. Murphy GJ. Physical medicine modalities and trigger point injections in the management of temporomandibular disorders and assessing outcome. *Oral Surg Oral Med Oral Pathol Oral Radiol Endod.* 1997;83: 118-122.

13. Jankovic J. Blepharospasm and oromandibular-laryngeal-cervical dystonia: a controlled trial of botulinum A toxin therapy. *Adv Neurol.* 1988;50: 583-591.

14. Brin MF. Advances in dystonia: genetics and treatment with botulinum toxin. In: Smith B, Adelman G, eds. *Neuroscience Year, Supplement to the Encyclopedia of Neuroscience.* Boston: Birkhauser, 1992;56-58.

15. Blumenfeld A, Binder WJ, Blitzer A, Katz H. The emerging role of botulinum toxin type A in headache prevention. *Op Tech Otolaryngol Head Neck Surg.* 2004;15: 90-96.

16. Binder WJ, Brin MJ, Blitzer A, Schoenrock LD, Pogoda JM. Botulinum toxin type A (BOROX) for treatment of migraine head headaches: an open label study. *Otolaryngol Head Neck Surg.* 2001;123: 669-676.

17. Blitzer A, Brin MF, Greene PE, Fahn S. Botulinum toxin injection for the treatment of oromandibular dystonia. *Ann Oto Rhinol Laryngol.* 1989;98:93-97.

18. Brin M, Blitzer A, Herman S, Steward C. Oromandibular dystonia: treatment of 96 cases with botulinum A. In: Jankovic J, Hallett M, eds. *Therapy with Botulinum Toxin.* New York: Marcel Dekker, 1994:429-435.

19. Ambalavanar R, Moritani M, Moutanni A, Gangula P, Yalampali C, Dessem D. Deep tissue inflammation upregulates neuropeptides and evokes nociceptive behaviors which are modulated antagonist. *Pain.* 2006;129:53-68.

20. Andrew D, Greenspan JD. Mechanical and heat sensitization of cutaneous nociceptors after peripheral inflammation in the rat. Nociceptors after peripheral inflammation in the rat. *J. Neurophysiol.* 1999;82: 2649-2656.

21. Akoki KR. Review of a proposed mechanism for the antinociceptive action of botulinum toxin type A. *Neurotooxicology.* 2005;26:785-793.

22. Beyak MJ, Ramji N, Krol KM, Kawaja MD, Vanner SJ. Two TTX-resistant A+ currents in mouse colonic forsal root ganglia neurons and their role in colitis-induced hyperexcitability. *Am J Physiol Gastrointest Liver Physiol.* 2004;287:G845-G855.

23. Tan E-K, Jankovic J. Bruxism in Huntington's disease. *Mov Disord.* 2000;15:171-173.

24. De Kanter RJ, Truin GJ, Burgersdijk RC, Van 't Hof MA, Battistuzzi PG, Kalsbeek H, et al. Prevalence in the Dutch adult population and a meta-analysis of signs and symptoms of temporomandibular disorder. *J Dent Res.* 1993;72:1509-1518.

25. Dworkin SF, Turner JA, Mancl L, Wilson L, Massoth D, Huggins KH, et al. A randomized clinical trial of a tailored comprehensive care treatment program for temporomandibular disorders. *J Orofac Pain.* 2002;16:259-276.

26. Dao TT, Lavigne GJ. Oral splints: the crutches for temporomandibular disorders and bruxism? *Crit Rev Oral Biol Med.* 1998;9:345-361.

27. Major PW, Nebbe B. Use and effectiveness of splint appliance therapy: review of the literature. *Cranio.* 1997;15:159-166.

28. De Wijer A, De Leeuw JR, Steenks MH, Bosnian F. Temporomandibular and cervical spine disorder: self-reported signs and symptoms. *Spine.* 1996;21: 1638-1646.

29. McMillan AS, Wong MCM, Zheng J, Lam CLK. Prevalence of orofacial pain and treatment seeking in Hong Kong Chinese. *J Orofac Pain.* 2006;20: 218-225.

30. Carlsson GE, Helkimo M. Epidemiologic studies of mandibular function. *J Prosthet Dent.* 1983;50: 134-135.

31. Wooten-Watts M, Tan E-K, Jankovic J. Bruxism and cranial-cervical dystonia: is there a relationship? *Cranio.* 1999;17:1-6.

32. Tan E-K, Jankovic J. Treating severe bruxism with botulinum toxin. *J Am Dent Assoc.* 2000;131:211-216.

33. Fillippi GM, Errico P, Santarelli R, Bagolini B, Manni E. Botulinum A. toxin effects on rat jaw muscle spindles. *Acta Otolaryngol.* 1993;113:400-404.

34. Freund B, Schwartz M. The use of botulimum toxin for the treatment of temporomandibular disorder. *Oral Health.* 1998;88:32-37.

35. Rosales RL, Arimura K, Takenaga S, Osame M. Extrafusal and intrafusal muscle effects in experimental botulinum toxin-A injection. *Muscle Nerve.* 1996;19:488-496.

36. Thompson PD, Obeso JA, Delgado G, Gallego J, Marsden CD. Focal dystonia of the jaw and the differential diagnosis of unilateral jaw and masticatory spasm. *J Neurol Neurosurg Psychiatry.* 1986;49:651-656.

37. Tolosa ES. Clinical features of Meige's disease (idiopathic orofacialo dystonia). A report of 17 cases. *Arch Neurol.* 1981;38:147-151.

38. Defazio G, Lamberti P, Lepore V, Livrea P, Ferrari E. Facial dystonia: clinical features, prognosis and pharmacology in 31 patients. *Ital J Neurol Sci.* 1989;10: 553-560.

39. Jordan DR, Patrinely JR, Anderson RL, Thiese AM. Essential blepharospasm and related dystonias. *Surv Ophthalmol.* 1989;34:123-132.

40. Klawans HL, Tanner CM. Cholinergic pharmacology of blepharospasm with oromandibular dystonia (Meige's syndrome). *Adv Neurol.* 1988;49:443-449.

41. Gimenez Roldan S, Mateo D, Orbe M, Munoz Blanco JL, Hipola D. Acute pharmacologic tests in cranial dystonia. *Adv Neurol.* 1988;49:451-465.

42. Greene P, Shale H, Fahn S. Analysis of open-label trials in torsion dystonia using high dosages of anicholinergics and other drugs. *Mov Discord.* 1988;3: 46-60.

43. Gollomp SM, Fahn S, Burke RE, Reches A, Illson J. Therapeutic trials in Meige syndrome. *Adv Neurol.* 1983;37:207-213.

44. Jankovic J, Orman J. Tetrabenazine therapy of dystonia, chorea, tics, and other dyskensias. *Neurology.* 1988;38:391-394.

45. Sutcher HD, Underwood RB, Beatty RA, Sugar O. Orofacial dyskinesia: a dental dimension. *JAMA.* 1971;216:1459-1463.

46. Tolosa E, Marti MJ. Blepharospasm-oromandibular dystonia syndrome (Meige's syndrome): clinical aspects. *Adv Neurol.* 1988;49:73-84.

47. Blitzer A, Brin MF, Greene PE, Fahn S. Botulinum toxin injection for the treatment of oromandibular dystonia. *Ann Otol Rhinol Laryngol.* 1989;98:93-97.

48. Brin MF, Fahn S, Moskowitz C, Friedman A, Shale HM, Greene PE, et al. Localized injections of botulinum toxin for the treatment of focal dystonia and hemifacial spasm. *Mov Disord.* 1987;2:237-254.

49. Brin MF. Interventional neurology: treatment of neurological conditions with local injections of botulinum toxin. *Arch Neurobiol.* 1991;54(suppl 3): 7-23.

50. Block SL. Differential diagnosis of masticatory muscle pain and dysfunction. *Oral Maxillofac Clin North Am.* 1995;7:29-49.

51. De Kanter RJ, Truin GJ, Burgersdijk RC, Van 't Hof MA, Battistuzzi PG, Kalsbeek H, et al. Prevalence in the Dutch population and a meta-analysis of signs and symptoms of temporomandibular disorder. *J Dent Res.* 1993;72:1509-1518.

52. Carlsson GE, LeResche L. Epidemiology of temporomandibular disorders in temporomandibular disorders and related pain conditions. In: Sessle BJ, Bryant PS, Dionne RA, eds. *Progress In Pain Research and Management.* Vol. 4. Seattle, WA: IASP Press. 1995:211-226.

53. Austin DG. Special considerations in orofacial pain and headache. *Dent Clin North Am.* 1997;41:325-339.

54. Rugh JD, Solberg WK. Oral health status in the United States: temporomandibular disorders. *J Dent Educ.* 1985;49:398-406.

55. Locker D, Slade G. Prevalence of symptoms associated with temporomandibular disorders in a Canadian population. *Community Dent Oral Epidemiol.* 1988;16:313-320.

56. Schiffman EL, Fricton JR, Haley DP, et al. The prevalence and treatments needs of subjects with temporomandibular disorders. *J Am Dent Assoc.* 1990;120:295-303.

57. Von Korff M. Health services research and temporomandibular disorders. In: Sessle BJ, Bryant PS, Dionne RA, eds. *Progress in pain research and management.* Vol. 4. Seattle, WA: IASP Press. 1995:227-236.

58. Dworkin SF, Huggins K, Wilson LE, Mancl L, Turner J, Massoth D, et al. A randomized clinical trial using research diagnostic criteria for temporomandibular disorders: axis I to target clinic cases for a tailored self care TMD program. *J Orofac Pain.* 2002;16:48-63.

59. Gremillion HA. The prevalence and etiology of temporomandibular disorders and orofacial pain. *Tex Dent J.* 2000;117:30-39.

60. Greene CS. The etiology of temporomandibular disorders: implications for treatment. *J Orofac Pain.* 2001;15:93-105.

61. Kamisaka M, Yatani H, Kuboki T, Matsuka Y, Minakuchi H. Four-year longitudinal course of TMD symptoms. *J Orofac Pain.* 2000;14:224-232.

62. Steed PA, Wexler GB. Temporomandibular disorders—traumatic etiology vs. nontraumatic etiology: a clinical and methodological inquiry into symptomatology and treatment outcomes. *Cranio.* 2001;19:188-194.

63. Stohler CS, Zarb GA. On the management of temporomandibular disorders: a plea for a low-tech, high-prudence therapeutic approach. *J Orofac Pain.* 1999;13:255-261.

64. Svensson P, Graven-Nielsen T. Craniofacial muscle pain: review of mechanisms and clinical manifestations. *J Orofac Pain.* 2001;15:17-145.

65. Rauhala K, Oikarinen KS, Raustia AM. Role of temporomandibular disorders (TMD) in facial pain: occlusion, muscle and TMJ pain. *Cranio.* 1999;17:254-261.

66. Satoh K, Yamaguchi T, Komatsu K, Inoue N, Minowa K, Kanayama T, et al. Analyses of muscular activity, energy metabolism, and muscle fiber type composition in a patient with bilateral masseteric hypertrophy. *Cranio.* 2001;19:294-301.

67. Kato T, Thie NM, Montplaisir JY, Lavigne GJ. Bruxism and orofacial movements during sleep. *Dent Clin North Am.* 2001;45:657-684.

68. Addante RR. Masseter muscle hypertrophy: report of case and literature review. *J Oral Maxillofac Surg.* 1994;52:1199-1202.

69. Mandel L, Kaynar A. Masseteric hypertrophy. *N Y State Dent J.* 1994;60:44-47.

70. Rosa RA, Kotkin HC. That acquired masseteric look. *ASDC J Dent Child.* 1996;63:105-107.

71. Rogers BA, Whear NM. Medical management of masseteric hypertrophy. *J Oral Maxillofac Surg.* 1995;53:492.

72. Roncevic R. Masseter muscle hypertrophy. Aetiology and therapy. *J Maxillofac Surg.* 1986;14:344-348.

73. Black MJ, Schloss MD. Masseteric muscle hypertrophy. *J Otolaryngol.* 1985;14:203-205.

74. Hui AC. Botulinum toxin for treatment of masseteric hypertrophy. *J Neurol.* 2002;249:345.

75. Ahn J, Horn C, Blitzer A. Botulinum toxin for masseter reduction in Asian patients. *Arch Facial Plast Surg.* 2004;6:188-191.

76. Dhanrajani PJ, Jonaidel O. Trismus: aetiology, differential diagnosis and treatment. *Dent Update.* 2002;29:88-9294.

77. Kadyan V, Clairmont AC, Engle M, Colachis SC. Severe trismus as a complication of cerebrovascular accident: a case report. *Arch Phys Med Rehabil.* 2005;86:594-595.

78. Warembourg H, Niquet G, Lekieffre J, Beaussart M, Goidin B. [Tirsmus in neurological disorders]. *Lille Med.* 1959;4:658-849.

79. Winterholler MG, Heckmann JG, Hecht M, Erbguth FJ. Recurrent trismus and stridor in an ALS patient: successful treatment with botulinum toxin. *Neurology.* 2002;58:502-503.

80. Zwart JA, Bovim G, Sand T, Sjaastad O. Tension headache: botulinum toxin paralysis of temporal muscles. *Headache.* 1994;34:458-462.

81. Mathew NT, Kaup AO. The use of botulinum toxin type A in headache treatment. *Curr Treat Options Neurol.* 2002;4:365-373.

82. Silberstein SD, Göbel H, Jensen R, Elkind AH, Degryse R, Walcott JM, et al. Botulinum toxin type A in a prophylactic treatment of chronic tension-type headache: a multicentre, double-blind, randomized placebo-controlled, parallel-group study. *Cephalalgia.* 2006;26:790-800.

83. Jensen R, Olesen J. Initiating mechanisms of experimentally induced tension-type headache. *Cephalalgia.* 1996;16:175-182.

84. Stohler CS. Muscle-related temporomandibular disorders. *J Orofac Pain.* 1999;13:273-284.

85. Freund BJ, Schwartz M. Relief of tension type headache symptoms in subjects with temporomandibular disorders treated with botulinum toxin-A. *Headache.* 2002;42:1033-1037.

86. Jankovic J, Schwartz K, Donovan DT. Botulinum toxin treatment of cranial-cervical dystonia, spasmodic dysphonia, other focal dystonias and hemifacial spasm. *J Neurol Neurosurg Psychiatry.* 1990;53:633-639.

87. Tan EK, Jankovic J. Botulinum toxin A in patients with oromandibular dystonia: Long-term follow-up. *Neurology.* 1999;53:2102-2105.

88. Tan EK, Jankovic J. Tardive and idiopathic oromandibular dystonia: A clinical comparison. *J Neurol Neurosurg Psychiatry.* 2000;68:186-190.

89. Tintner R, Jankovic J. Botulinum toxin type A in the management of oromandibular dystonia and bruxism. In Brin MF, Hallett M, Jankovic J, eds. *Scientific and Therapeutic Aspects of Botulinum Toxin*. Lippincott Williams & Wilkins; 2002:343-350.

90. Morris S, Benjamin S, Gray R, Bennett D. Physical, psychiatric and social characteristics of the temporomandibular disorder pain dysfunction syndrome: the relationship of mental disorders to presentation. *Br Dent J*. 1997;182:255-260.

Botulinum Toxin in **17** Headache Management

Stephen D. Silberstein

INTRODUCTION

Headache affects more than 45 million individuals in the United States, which makes it one of the most common nervous system disorders in existence.[1] The International Headache Society (IHS) diagnostic criteria for headache disorders have been revised[2] (International Classification of headache Disoders-2 [ICHD-2], 2004) and continue to classify primary headache disorders as those in which headache itself is the illness, with no other etiology diagnosed. Examples of a primary headache disorder include migraine and tension-type headache (TTH).[3] Headache disorders can be further classified as episodic (<15 headache days per month) or chronic (≥15 headache days per month for more than 3 months).[3]

Migraine is a primary episodic headache disorder characterized by various combinations of neurologic, gastrointestinal, and autonomic changes. "Migraine" is derived from the Greek word "hemicrania," (Galen ~200 AD).[4] The diagnosis of migraine is based on the retrospective reporting of headache characteristics and associated symptoms.[5] The physical and neurologic examinations, as well as laboratory studies, are usually normal and serve to exclude other, more ominous causes of headache.

The ICHD-2 (ICHD-2; 2004) provides criteria for a total of seven subtypes of migraine.[3]

The ICHD-2 diagnostic criteria for migraine include headache associated with at least two of the following: unilateral location, pulsating quality, moderate or severe pain intensity, and aggravation by or causing avoidance of routine physical activities; at least one of the following during headache: nausea or vomiting, photophobia and phonophobia; and headache not attributable to another disorder.[3]

Migraine prevalence is similar and stable in Western countries and the United States.[6] It is estimated that 28 million Americans, including 18% of women and 7% of men, are afflicted with severe, disabling migraines.[7] Migraine prevalence varies by age, gender, race, and income. Before puberty, migraine prevalence is approximately 4%[8]; after puberty, it increases more rapidly in girls than in boys. It increases until approximately age 40, then declines. Prevalence is lowest in Asian-Americans, intermediate in blacks, and highest in whites.[8] In the United States, migraine prevalence decreases as household income increases.[7-9]

The World Health Organization ranks migraine as one of the world's most disabling illnesses, profoundly impacting quality of life, causing functional impairment and disruption of household or social activities.[10] The economic burden of the disease to society is also considerable. In the United States, the yearly medical costs exceed one billion dollars, and costs to employers due to migraine-related absenteeism and reduced productivity is 13 billion dollars.[11]

Chronic daily headache (CDH) is a heterogeneous group of headache disorders that can include chronic migraine, chronic TTH (CTTH), and other headache types that occur 15 days or more a month in the absence of structural or systemic disease,[12] and affects 4% to 5% of the general population

The author is reporting that he is on the advisory panel, speaker's bureau, or serves as a consultant for Allergan, AstraZeneca, Endo Pharmaceuticals, GlaxoSmithKline, Medtronic, Merck, NuPathe, OrthoMcNeil, Pfizer, Pozen, and Valeant Pharmaceuticals. Also, he receives research support from Abbott, Advanced Bionics, AGA, Advanced NeuroModulation Systems, Allergan, AstraZeneca, Endo Pharmaceuticals, Lilly, GlaxoSmithKline, Medtronic, Merck, OrthoMcNeil, Pfizer, Pozen, ProEthic, Valeant Pharmaceuticals, and Vernalis.

worldwide.[13-15] Patients with CDH often over-use acute headache medications[2] and have greater disability and lower quality of life than patients with episodic headache.[15-17]

TTH is the most common of the primary headache disorders, with an annual prevalence as high as 38%.[15,18] TTH is associated with bilateral pain that is pressing or tightening in quality and mild to moderate in intensity. It is not associated with nausea/vomiting or routine physical activity but may be associated with photophobia or phonophobia.[3] Frequent episodic (at least 10 episodes occurring on ≥1 but <15 days per month) or chronic (≥15 days per month) TTH is associated with greatly decreased quality of life and high disability.[3,18]

PATHOPHYSIOLOGY OF HEADACHE DISORDERS

Migraine is believed to arise from activation of meningeal and blood vessel nociceptors, along with a change in central pain modulation mediated by the trigeminal system.[19] In response to stimulation of the trigeminal sensory neurons, perivascular nerve fibers that innervate blood vessels release peptide mediators, neurokinin A, substance P, and calcitonin gene–related peptide (CGRP), which transmit nociceptive activity to the brain stem autonomic nuclei via glutamate-mediated transduction. The trigeminovascular system can be activated by cortical spreading depression, a process characterized by shifts in cortical steady state potential; transient increases in potassium, nitric oxide, and glutamate; and transient increases followed by sustained decreases in cortical blood flow (Fig. 17-1).[19] Trigeminal activation results in release of vasoactive peptide–producing neurogenic inflammation, vasodilation, sensitization of nerve fibers, and, ultimately, pain and associated symptoms.[19] Migraine pain is likely a result of the combination of activation of pain-producing intracranial structures and reduction in endogenous pain control pathways.[19,20]

The pathophysiology underlying TTH is not well understood. The relative contributions of peripheral and central pain mechanisms to TTH remain unclear.[21]

TREATMENT OF HEADACHE

Acute (abortive) migraine treatments, which patients take at the time of occurrence in an

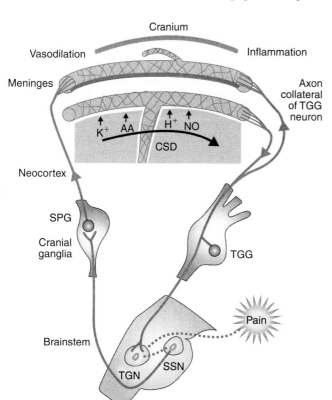

FIGURE 17-1. Cortical spreading depression. AA, arachidonic acid; CSD, cortical spreading depression; H+, hydrogen ions; K+, potassium ions; NO, nitric oxide; SPG, sphenopalatine ganglion; SSN, superior sagittal sinus; TGG, trigeminal ganglion; TGN, trigeminal nucleus. (Reproduced with permission from Silberstein SD. Migraine. *The Lancet.* 2004;363:381-391.)

attempt to relieve pain and disability and prevent progression, include migraine-specific medications, such as ergots or triptans, and non-specific agents, such as analgesics or opioids.[19] Prescription nonsteroidal anti-inflammatory drugs (NSAIDs) or combination analgesics may also be used. Patients with acute TTH typically self-medicate with over-the-counter analgesics, such as aspirin, acetaminophen, or NSAIDs, which could lead to drug overuse.

Preventive treatments are designed to reduce the frequency, severity, or duration of migraine attacks. These are indicated when acute medications are ineffective or overused, or headaches are very frequent or disabling.[19] Preventive agents include beta-adrenergic blockers, antidepressants, calcium channel and serotonin antagonists, anticonvulsants, and NSAIDs.[19]

Although daily, oral prophylactic treatments have proven effective, issues such as lack of compliance with daily dosing regimens and adverse effects have limited their usefulness[19,22] and resulted in a search for other modalities and agents, including botulinum neurotoxins (BoNTs), as potential preventive treatments.

BOTULINUM TOXIN IN HEADACHE DISORDERS

Botulinum Neurotoxin Formulations

The seven BoNT serotypes (A, B, C1, D, E, F, and G) produced by *Clostridium botulinum* are synthesized as single-chain polypeptides. All serotypes inhibit acetylcholine release, although their intracellular target proteins, physiochemical characteristics, and potencies are different.[23,24] Botulinum toxin type A (BoNT/A) has been the most widely studied serotype for therapeutic purposes.[23]

At present, BoNT is available for clinical use in the United States as BoNT/A products Botox (Allergan, Inc., Irvine, CA) and Dysport (Ipsen Ltd., Slough, UK), and the BoNTB product Myobloc/Neurobloc (Solstice Neurosciences, Inc., South San Francisco, CA, USA/Solstice Neurosciences Ltd., Dublin, Ireland). Botox is the only BoNT/A product approved by the US Food and Drug Administration and is indicated for the treatment of strabismus, blepharospasm, cervical dystonia, axillary hyperhidrosis, and glabellar lines.[25] It is also approved in other countries for the treatment of adult spasticity and juvenile cerebral palsy. Lyophilized Botox is available in vials containing 100 units (U) of BoNT/A and is diluted with 2 or 4 mL of preservative-free 0.9% saline to yield a concentration of 5.0 or 2.5 U per 0.1 mL, respectively.[25] Reconstituted solutions of Botox can be refrigerated but must be used within 4 hours.[25] Myobloc is available in 0.5-, 1-, and 2-mL vials containing 5000 U per mL.[24]

Mechanism of Action of Botulinum Toxin in Headache

BoNT inhibits the release of acetylcholine at the neuromuscular junction by binding to motor or sympathetic nerve terminals, then entering the nerve terminals and inhibiting the release of acetylcholine, thereby blocking neuromuscular transmission. This inhibition occurs as the BoNT cleaves one of several proteins integral to the successful docking and release of acetylcholine from vesicles situated within nerve endings. Following intramuscular injection, BoNT produces partial chemical denervation of the muscle, resulting in a localized reduction in muscle activity.[23,24]

The association between BoNT/A use and the alleviation of migraine headache symptoms was discovered during initial clinical trials of BoNT/A treatment for hyperfunctional lines of the face.[26] BoNT/A therapy has been used for a variety of disorders associated with painful muscle spasms. Because migraine attacks are frequently associated with muscle tenderness,[27] it was generally believed that intramuscular BoNT/A might prevent abnormal sensory signals in the affected muscle from traveling to the central nervous system (CNS). If abnormal muscle physiology can trigger migraine, one would predict that BoNT/A treatment would work prophylactically only in patients whose migraine attacks develop on the heels of episodic or chronic muscle tenderness.

Jakubowski et al[28] explored neurologic markers that might distinguish migraine patients who benefited from BoNT/A treatment from those who did not. The prevalence of neck tenderness, aura, photophobia, phonophobia, osmophobia, nausea, and throbbing was similar between responders and nonresponders. However, the two groups offered different accounts of their pain. Among nonresponders, 92% described a buildup of pressure inside their head (exploding headache).

Among responders, 74% perceived their head to be crushed, or clamped, or stubbed by external forces (imploding headache), and 13% attested to an eye-popping pain (ocular headache). The finding that exploding headache is not as responsive to extracranial BoNT/A injections is consistent with the view that migraine pain is mediated by intracranial innervation. The amenability of imploding and ocular headaches to BoNT/A treatment suggests that these types of migraine pain involve extracranial innervation as well.[29] The precise mechanisms by which BoNT/A alleviates headache pain are unclear. It inhibits the release of glutamate and the neuropeptides substance P and CGRP from nociceptive neurons, suggesting that its antinociceptive properties are distinct from its neuromuscular activity.[30]

BoNT/A may inhibit central sensitization of trigeminovascular neurons, which is believed to be key to migraine's development and maintenance.[30-33] Oshinsky et al[34] used a preclinical model of sensitizing dorsal horn neurons in the trigeminal nucleus caudalis (TNC) following chemical stimulation of the dura as a model for testing the effects of BoNT/A on central sensitization. They used single-neuron electrophysiology of second sensory neurons in the TNC with cutaneous receptive fields and microdialysis of the TNC to evaluate the effects of pretreatment of the periorbital region of the rat with BoNT/A. In saline-treated animals, extracellular glutamate increased steadily after 100 minutes following the application of inflammatory soup to the dura. The increase of glutamate reaches ~3 times the basal level at 3 hours after the inflammatory soup. Electrophysiologic recordings of neurons in the TNC before and after sensitization confirmed these data. Following the inflammatory soup, there was an increase in the magnitude of the response to sensory stimuli and an increase in the cutaneous receptive field of the second sensory neurons in the TNC.

Afferent-afferent communication happens in the nerve through axon-axon glutamate secretion, and at the level of the ganglion through nonsynaptic release of glutamate and peptides (CGRP and SP). Oshinsky's proposal is as follows: Following chemical stimulation of the dura during a migraine attack and in their rat model, the dural afferents may communicate with other trigeminal afferents on the ophthalmic division of the trigeminal nerve and recruit them to secrete glutamate and neuropeptides. This would recruit more afferents spreading activation and sensitization. The number of afferents activated on the dura is small compared with the total number of afferents in the whole trigeminal system, so activation of the dural afferents alone may not be sufficient to produce the large changes in the CNS that lead to central sensitization.

Oshinsky et al measured the extracellular level of glutamate following a 5-minute chemical stimulation of the dura and found that there is a 2- to 3-fold increase more than 1.5 hours following the stimulation. This increase was blocked by pretreating the face of the rat with BoNT/A. Producing the large changes in extracellular glutamate in the CNS requires a massive sensory activation. The afferents of the dura may recruit the afferents of the face and head, which leads to the sensitization of these areas seen in human and animal studies. Botulinum toxin may block the axon-to-axon and interganglionic communication of the afferents and thus prevent central and peripheral sensitization outside of rat dura. Electrophysiologic studies confirmed that there is no change in the magnitude of the sensory response in the TNC neurons or their receptive field in the rats with BoNT/A following the inflammatory soup. These data show that peripheral application of BoNT/A prevents central sensitization elicited by stimulation of the dura with inflammatory mediators.[34]

Treatment Guidelines

Selecting candidates for BoNT therapy begins with accurately diagnosing and classifying patients' headache type based on their medical history. BoNT/A therapy may be most appropriate for patients whose disabling headaches interfere with their daily routines despite acute therapy, or for patients who cannot tolerate other preventive strategies. Table 17-1 lists characteristics of headache patients who may be candidates for BoNT/A therapy. BoNT/A use is contraindicated for patients with sensitivity to toxins or with neuromuscular disorders, such as myasthenia gravis.[22]

Botulinum Neurotoxin Treatment Techniques

Sterile technique should be observed for the entire BoNT injection procedure. Injections do

TABLE 17-1 Candidates for Botulinum Toxin Type A (BoNT/A) Therapy For Headache[17]

- Patients with disabling primary headaches
- Patients who have failed to respond adequately to conventional treatments
- Patients with unacceptable side effects (from existing treatment)
- Patients in whom standard preventive treatments are contraindicated
- Patients in special populations or situations (the elderly, those at risk of unacceptable side effects from trial drugs or traditional treatments, airplane pilots, students studying and preparing for examinations)
- Patients misusing, abusing, or overusing acute headache medications
- Patients with coexistent jaw, head, or neck muscle spasm
- Patients who prefer this treatment
- Patients with imploding migraine headache

Used with permission from Blumenfeld AM, Binder W, Silberstein SD, Blitzer A. Procedures for administering botulinum toxin type A for migraine and tension-type headache. *Headache*. 2003;43:884-891.

not have to be intramuscular, but we use the muscles as reference sites for injections, which are most commonly administered in the glabellar and frontal regions, the temporalis muscle, the occipitalis muscle, and the cervical paraspinal region (Fig. 17-2).

The injection protocols commonly used are (1) the fixed-site approach, which uses fixed, symmetric injection sites and a range of predetermined doses; (2) the follow-the-pain approach, which adjusts the sites and doses depending on where the patient feels pain and where the examiner can elicit pain and tenderness on palpation of the muscle and often employs asymmetric injections; and (3) a combination approach, using injections

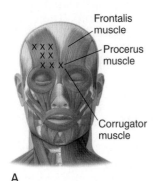

A

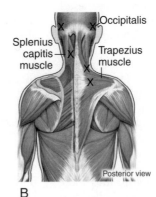

B

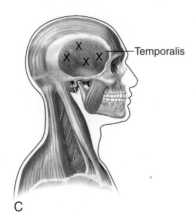

C

FIGURE 17-2. Injection site locations for headache treatment. **A,** Glabellar and frontal muscles. **B,** Occipital and suboccipital muscles, **C,** Temporalis muscle. (Reproduced with permission from Nucleus Medical Art. Copyright ©2003. All rights reserved. www.nucleusinc.com.)

TABLE 17-2 Anatomic Sites of Injection and Botulinum Toxin Type A (BoNT/A; Botox) Dose

Muscle	BoNT/A U/Site	Number of Injection Sites
Procerus*	2.5-5.0	1
Corrugator*	2.5	2 (1 per side)
Medial	2.5	2 (1 per side)
Lateral	2.5	2 (1 per side)
Frontalis*	2.5-5.0	2-4 per side
Temporalis*	2.5-5.0	8-10 (4-5 per side)
Occipitalis[†]	2.5-5.0	2 (1 per side)
Splenius capitis area* [†]	2.5-5.0	2 per side
Masseter[†]	2.5-5.0	1-2
Trapezius[†]	2.5-5.0	2–8 (1–4 per side)
Sternocleidomastoid[†]	2.5-5.0	2
Cervical paraspinal muscles[†]	2.5-5.0	1–3 per side

*For fixed-site or follow-the-trigeminal-nerve protocol, injections should be bilateral.
[†]For follow-the-pain protocol, injections may be unilateral or bilateral, depending on signs and symptoms.
Adapted from Blumenfeld AM, Binder W, Silberstein SD, Blitzer A. Procedures for administering botulinum toxin type A for migraine and tension-type headache. *Headache.* 2003;43:884-891.

at fixed frontal sites, supplemented with follow-the-pain injections (this approach typically uses higher doses of BoNT/A).[22] Table 17-2 lists recommended anatomic sites of injection for headache and the BoNT/A (Botox) dose per site.

Clinical Comparison of Efficacy of Botulinum Neurotoxin in Headache Disorders

Most studies on BoNT's efficacy and safety in headache treatment have used BOTOX®.[35] No large, well-controlled studies using other preparations have been published. Clinical trial results discussed in the next section are summarized in Table 17-3.[35]

Some studies support the efficacy of BoNT/A in migraine treatment. A double-blind, vehicle-controlled trial of 123 patients with moderate-to-severe migraine found that subjects treated with a single injection of 25 U BoNT/A (but not those treated with 75 U) showed significantly fewer migraine attacks per month, as well as reductions in migraine severity, number of days requiring acute medication, and incidence of migraine-induced vomiting.[36] The lack of significant effect in the higher dose group may be related to baseline group differences, for example, fewer migraines or a longer time since migraine onset in the higher-dose group.[36] Another double-blind, placebo-controlled, region-specific study found a significant

reduction in migraine pain among patients who received simultaneous injections of BoNT/A in the frontal and temporal regions, as well as an overall trend toward BoNT/A superiority to placebo in reducing migraine frequency and duration.[36] A randomized, double-blind, placebo-controlled study compared the efficacy of placebo, 16 U BoNT/A, and 100 U BoNT/A as migraine prophylaxis when injected into the frontal and neck muscles.[37] There were no statistically significant differences in reduction of migraine frequency among the groups, but the accompanying migraine symptoms were reduced in the 16 U BoNT/A group.[37]

New studies, however, have not demonstrated significant improvements over placebo. A recent study[38] of patients (N = 232) with moderate to severe episodic (four to eight episodes/month) migraine compared placebo with regional (frontal, temporal, or glabellar) or combined (frontal/temporal/glabellar) treatment with BoNT/A. Reductions from baseline in migraine frequency, maximum severity, and duration occurred with BoNT/A and placebo, but there were no significant between-group differences.[38] Elkind et al[39] conducted a series of three sequential studies of 418 patients with a history of four to eight moderate-to-severe migraines per month with re-randomization at each stage and BoNT/A doses ranging from 7.5 to 50 U. BoNT/A and placebo produced comparable decreases from baseline in migraine frequency at each time point examined, with no consistent,

TABLE 17-3 Summary of Randomized, Double-blind, Controlled Studies of the Efficacy of Botulinum Toxin Type A (BoNT/A) in the Treatment of Headache

Headache Type	Study Outcome
Migraine	
Silberstein et al 2000[36]	• Decreased migraine frequency and severity and acute medication use with BoNT/A 25 U but not with BoNT/A 75 U
Brin et al 2000[43]	• Decreased migraine pain compared with PBO with simultaneous frontal and temporal BoNT/A injections
Evers et al 2004[37]	• No difference from PBO in decreased frequency of migraine • Greater decrease in migraine-associated symptoms with BoNT/A 16 U
Saper et al 2007[38]	• Decreased frequency and severity of migraine in BoNT/A and PBO groups, with no between-group differences
Elkind et al 2006[39]	• Comparable decreases in migraine frequency in both BoNT/A and PBO groups, with no between-group differences
Chronic Daily Headache of Migraine Type	
Mathew et al 2005[40]	• No difference from PBO on primary efficacy end point change in headache-free days from baseline at day 180 • A significantly higher percentage of BoNT/A patients had a ≥50% decrease in headache days/month at day 180 compared with those taking PBO.
Dodick et al 2005[30]	• Greater decrease in headache frequency after two and three injections compared with PBO
Silberstein et al 2005[12]	• No difference from PBO on primary efficacy end point—change in headache frequency from baseline at day 180 • Greater decrease in headache frequency for BoNT/A 225 U and 150 U than PBO
Chronic Tension-Type Headache	
Silberstein et al 2006[21]	• No difference from PBO on primary efficacy endpoint mean change from baseline in CTTH headache days • Greater percentage of BoNT/A patients than PBO with ≥ 50% reduction in headache frequency at 90 and 120 days for several doses of BoNT/A

CTTH, chronic tension-type headache; PBO, placebo.

statistically significant, between-group differences observed.[39]

Several randomized, double-blind, placebo-controlled studies support the efficacy of BoNT for the treatment of CDH. In a large, placebo-controlled study (N = 355), Mathew et al[40] found that although BoNT/A did not differ from placebo in the primary efficacy measure (change from baseline in headache-free days at day 180), there were significant differences in several secondary end points, including a greater percentage of patients with a ≥50% decrease in headache frequency and a greater mean change from baseline in headache frequency at day 180.[40] A subgroup analysis of patients not taking concomitant preventive agents (n = 228) found that BoNT/A patients had a greater decrease in headache frequency compared with those taking placebo after two and three injections, and at most time points from day 180 to 270.[30] In a similar study (N = 702) by Silberstein et al,[12] which used several doses of BoNT/A (75, 150, and 225 U), the primary efficacy end point (mean improvement from baseline in headache frequency at day 180) was also not met.

However, all groups responded to treatment, and patients taking 150 and 225 U of BoNT/A had a greater decrease in headache frequency at Day 240 than those taking placebo.[12]

Studies evaluating the efficacy of BoNT/A in CTTH have been inconsistent. A double-blind, randomized, placebo-controlled study[21] of 300 patients found that although all treatment groups, including those taking placebo, improved in mean change from baseline in CTTH-free days per month (primary end point) at day 60, the group who received BoNT/A did not demonstrate improvement compared with the group taking placebo at any dose or regimen (50 to 150 U). However, a significantly greater percentage of patients in three BoNT/A groups at day 90 and two BoNT/A groups at day 120 had a ≥50% decrease in CTTH days than the placebo group.[21] Furthermore, a review evaluating clinical studies of TTH supports the benefit of BoNT/A in reducing frequency and severity of headaches, improving quality of life and disability scales, and reducing the need for acute medication,[41] while another review, which also included studies with both Botox and Dysport, concluded that randomized, double-blind, placebo-controlled trials present contradictory results attributable to variable doses, injection sites, and frequency of treatment.[42]

Adverse Events Associated With Use of Botulinum Neurotoxin

More than two decades of clinical use have established BoNT/A as a safe drug[24] with no systemic reactions in clinical trials for headache. Rash and flu-like symptoms can rarely occur as a result of an allergic reaction.[24] However, serious allergic reactions have never been reported. Injection of anterior neck muscles can cause dysphagia (swallowing difficulties) in some patients.[24] Dysphagia and dry mouth appear to be more common with injections of BoNT/B (Myobloc) because of its wider migration pattern.[24] The most common side effects when treating facial muscles are cosmetic and include ptosis or asymmetry of the position of the eyebrows.[24] Another possible, but rare, side effect is difficulty in holding the head erect because of neck muscle weakness.[24] Headache patients occasionally develop a headache following the injection procedure, although some have immediate relief of an acute attack. The latter is most likely due to the trigger point injection effect.[24] Worsening of headaches and neck pain can occur and last for several days or, rarely, weeks after the injections because of the irritating effect of the needling and delay in the muscle relaxing effect of BoNT.[24]

SUMMARY

Headache disorders, including migraine, CDH, and TTH, are common debilitating conditions that profoundly impact quality of life. Existing preventive and acute pharmacotherapies provide relief to some headache sufferers but vary in efficacy and may be associated with adverse events. Overuse and abuse of acute pharmacotherapies is an important problem in managing these conditions and should be avoided. Clinical studies suggest that BoNT is a safe treatment and may be efficacious for the prevention of some forms of episodic and chronic headache, including migraine and CDH. Further research is needed to understand the mechanism of action of BoNT in headache, further establish its safety and efficacy for these indications, and fully develop its therapeutic potential.

References

1. National Institute of Neurological Disorders and Stroke (NINDS). *Headache: Hope Through Research.* Bethesda, MD: US Department of Health and Human Services, National Institutes of Health. NIH publication 2002:02-158.
2. Headache Classification Committee of the International Headache Society. Classification and diagnostic criteria for headache disorders, cranial neuralgia, and facial pain. *Cephalalgia.* 1988;8(suppl 7):1-96.
3. Headache Classification Committee. The International Classification of Headache Disorders, 2nd ed. Cephalalgia 2004;24(suppl 1):1-160.
4. Critchley M. *Migraine: from Cappadocia to Queen Square.* London, UK: Heinemann; 1967.
5. Silberstein SD, Saper JR, Freitag F. Migraine: Diagnosis and treatment. In: Silberstein SD, Lipton RB, Dalessio DJ, eds. *Wolff's Headache and Other Head Pain.* 7th ed. New York: Oxford University Press; 2001:121-237.
6. Stewart WF, Shechter A, Rasmussen RK. Migraine prevalence. A review of population-based studies. *Neurology.* 1994;44:S17-S23.
7. Lipton RB, Stewart WF, Diamond S, Diamond ML, Reed M. Prevalence and burden of migraine in the United States: data from the American Migraine Study II. *Headache.* 2001;41:646-657.
8. Lipton RB, Hamelsky SW, Stewart WF. Epidemiology and impact of headache. In: Silberstein SD, Lipton RB, Dalessio DJ, eds. *Wolff's Headache and Other Head Pain.* 7th ed. New York: Oxford University Press; 2001:85-107.

9. Stewart WF, Lipton RB, Celentano DD, Reed ML. Prevalence of migraine headache in the United States. Relation to age, income, race and other sociodemographic factors. *JAMA*. 1992;267:64-69.

10. World Health Organization. *Headache disorders. Fact sheet No 277*. Available at: http://www.who.int/mediacentre/factsheets/fs277/en/print.html 2007

11. Hu XH, Markson LE, Lipton RB, Stewart WF, Berger ML. Burden of migraine in the United States: disability and economic costs. *Arch Intern Med*. 1999;159: 813-818.

12. Silberstein SD, Stark SR, Lucas SM, Christie SN, DeGryse RE, Turkel CC. Botulinum toxin type A for the prophylactic treatment of chronic daily headache: a randomized, double-blind, placebo-controlled trial. *Mayo Clin Proc*. 2005;80:1126-1137.

13. Scher AI, Stewart WF, Liberman J, Lipton RB. Prevalence of frequent headache in a population sample. *Headache*. 1998;38:497-506.

14. Castillo J, Munoz P, Guitera V, Pascual J. Epidemiology of chronic daily headache in the general population. *Headache*. 1999;39:190-196.

15. Wang SJ, Fuh JL, Lu SR, Liu CY, Hsu LC, Wang PN, et al. Chronic daily headache in Chinese elderly: prevalence, risk factors and biannual follow-up. *Neurology*. 2000;54:314-319.

16. Bigal ME, Rapoport AM, Lipton RB, Tepper SJ, Sheftell FD. Assessment of migraine disability using the Migraine Disabiilty Assessment (MIDAS) Questionnaire: a comparison of chronic migraine with episodic migraine. *Headache*. 2003;43:336-342.

17. Meletiche DM, Lofland JH, Young WB. Quality of life differences between patients with episodic and transformed migraine. *Headache*. 2001;41:573-578.

18. Schwartz BS, Stewart WF, Simon D, Lipton RB. Epidemiology of tension-type headache. *JAMA*. 1998;279:381-383.

19. Silberstein SD. Migraine. *Lancet*. 2004;363:381-391.

20. Goadsby PJ. Pathophysiology of headache. In: Silberstein SD, Lipton RB, Dalessio DJ, eds. *Wolff*. 7th ed. New York: Oxford University Press; 2001:57-72.

21. Silberstein SD, Gobel H, Jensen R, Elkind AH, deGryse R, Walcott JM, et al. Botulinum toxin type A in the prophylactic treatment of chronic tension-type headache: a multicentre, double-blind, randomized, placebo-controlled, parallel-group study. *Cephalalgia*. 2006;26:790-800.

22. Blumenfeld AM, Binder W, Silbrestein SD, Blizter A. Procedures for administering botulinum toxin type A for migraine and tension-type headache. *Headache*. 2003;43:884-891.

23. Aoki KR, Guyer B. Botulinum toxin type A and other botulinum toxin serotypes; a comparative review of biochemical and pharmacological actions. *Eur J Neurol*. 2001;8(suppl 5):21-29.

24. Mauskop A. The use of botulinum toxin in the treatment of headaches. *Pain Physician*. 2004;7:377-387.

25. BOTOX® package insert. Irvine, CA: Allergan, Inc. 2004.

26. Binder WJ, Brin MF, Blitzer A, Shoenrock LD, Pogoda JM. Botulinum toxin type A (Botox) for treatment of migraine headaches: an open-label study. *Otolaryngol Head Neck Surg*. 2000;123:669-676.

27. Jensen R, Bendtsen L, Olesen J. Muscular factors are of importance in tension-type headache. *Headache*. 1998;38:10-17.

28. Jakubowski M, Silberstein S, Ashkenazi A, Burstein R. Can allodynic migraine patients be identified interictally using a questionnaire? *Neurology*. 2005;65: 1419-1422.

29. Jakubowski M, McAllister PJ, Bajwa ZH, Ward TN, Smith P, Burstein R. Exploding vs. imploding headache in migraine prophylaxis with Botulinum Toxin A. *Pain*. 2006;125:286-295.

30. Dodick DW, Mauskop A, Elkind AH, deGryse R, Brin MF, Silberstein SD. Botulinum toxin type A for the prophylaxis of chronic daily headache: subgroup analysis of patients not receiving other prophylactic medications: a randomized double-blind, placebo-controlled study. *Headache*. 2005;45:315-324.

31. Aoki KR. Evidence for antinociceptive activity of botulinum toxin type A in pain management. *Headache*. 2003;43(suppl 3):S109-S115.

32. Cui M, Khanijou S, Rubino J, Aoki KR. Subcutaneous administration of botulinum toxin A reduces formalin-induced pain. *Pain*. 2004;107:125-133.

33. Oshinsky ML. Botulinum toxins and migraine: how does it work. *Practical Neurol*. 2004;Suppl:10-13.

34. Oshinsky M, Poso-Rosich P, Luo J, Hyman S, Silberstein SD. Botulinum toxin A blocks sensitization of neurons in the trigeminal nucleus caudalis [abstract]. *Cephalalgia*. 2004;24:781.

35. Schulte-Mattler WJ, Leinisch E. Evidence based medicine on the use of botulinum toxin for headache disorders. *J Neural Transm*. 2008;115:647-651.

36. Silberstein SD, Mathew N, Saper J, Jenkin S. Botulinum toxin type A as a migraine preventive treatment: for the Botox® Migraine Clinical Research Group. *Headache*. 2000;40:445-450.

37. Evers S, Vollmer-Haase J, Schwaag S, Rahmann A, Husstedt IW, Frese A. Botulinum toxin A in the prophylactic treatment of migraine - a randomized, double-blind, placebo-controlled study. *Cephalalgia*. 2004;24:838-843.

38. Saper JR, Mathew NT, Loder EW, deGryse R, VanDenburgh AM. A double-blind, randomized, placebo-controlled comparison of botulinum toxin type A injection sites and doses in the prevention of episodic migraine. *Pain Med*. 2007;8:478-485.

39. Elkind AH, O'Carroll P, Blumenfeld A, deGryse R, Dimitrova R. A series of three sequential, randomized, controlled studies of repeated treatments with botulinum toxin type A for migraine prophylaxis. *J Pain*. 2006;7:688-696.

40. Mathew NT, Frishberg BM, Gawel M, Dimitrova R, Gibson J, Turkel C. Botulinum toxin type A (BOTOX) for the prophylactic treatment of chronic daily headache: a randomized, double-blind, placebo-controlled trial. *Headache*. 2005;45:293-307.

41. Mathew NT, Kaup AO. The use of botulinum toxin type A in headache treatment. *Curr Treat Options Neurol*. 2002;4:365-373.

42. Rozen D, Sharma J. Treatment of tension-type headache with botox: a review of the literature. *Mt Sinai J Med*. 2006;73:493-4988.

43. Brin MF, Swope DM, O'Brien C, Abbasi S, Pogoda JM. Botox for migraine: double-blind, placebo-controlled, region-specific evaluation [abstract]. *Cephalalgia*. 2000;20:421-422.

Botulinum Toxin Therapy in Gastrointestinal Disorders

18

Rajasekhara Mummadi and Pankaj J. Pasricha

INTRODUCTION

Except at both extremities, the muscle of the gastrointestinal (GI) tract is dissimilar from skeletal muscle in terms of form (smooth versus striated), function, and control. Thus, its contractions and relaxations are under the immediate regulation of the intrinsic neurons of the enteric nervous system (ENS) contained within the wall of the GI tract itself, although significant modulation is provided by extrinsic autonomic nerves (both sympathetic and parasympathetic). ENS neurons can be both excitatory (predominantly cholinergic) and inhibitory (predominantly nitrinergic), and at any one time, the muscle tone in a given segment of the gut reflects a balance between these opposing influences.[1] In several disorders of motility, this system becomes imbalanced, often from partial or complete loss of inhibitory neurons. This provides the rationale for most of the GI use of botulinum neurotoxin (BoNT), which, by blocking excitatory neurotransmitter release, can reduce hypertonicity in the affected muscle. However, although many animal experiments have suggested that BoNT reduces muscle tone in the gut,[2] the underlying mechanisms remain to be clarified fully and there is some suggestion that it may also inhibit the responsiveness of smooth muscle to exogenous stimuli, an effect that is unique to the GI tract.[3]

After the pioneering work of Alan Scott, who used botulinum toxin A (BoNT/A) to treat strabismus in the 1970s,[4] another decade elapsed before the therapeutic potential of BoNT/A was applied to the smooth muscle. In 1993, Pasricha et al[5] demonstrated that BoNT/A can be of therapeutic value in treating GI smooth muscle disorders. Since then, BoNT/A has been used for a variety of indications in the gut with varying evidence of efficacy (Table 18-1). This chapter attempts to provide an overview of this emerging and exciting therapeutic area.

CRICOPHARYNGEAL DYSPHAGIA

Rationale

Unlike most of the other target muscles described in this chapter, the cricopharyngeus is a striated muscle. It is a major component of the upper esophageal sphincter (UES), and its dysfunction may be an important cause of oropharyngeal dysphagia. This condition, often called cricopharyngeal achalasia, is characterized by failure of timely and sufficient relaxation of the UES during the pharyngeal phase of swallowing. It can occur as an isolated abnormality or as part of a more generalized neuromuscular problem. Some but not all patients with this disorder may benefit from a surgical myotomy, and BoNT/A injections

Dr. Mummadi does not reported any conflicts of interest. Dr. Pasricha is reporting that he is a consultant on the advisory board of the following companies: Pentax, GI Supply, Proctor and Gamble, Amulet, Elixir, Transzyme, Dynogen, Altus, Apollo Endosurgery, Endopace, and Immersion.

TABLE 18-1 Applications of Botulinum Neurotoxin Type A in Gastrointestinal Disorders

Disorder	Site of Action	Level of Evidence*	Clinical Practice
UES disorders	Cricopharyngeus	Level II-2	Response predicts benefit by CPM. Used commonly in clinical practice.
Achalasia	LES	Level I	Used routinely in clinical practice. Alternative to myotomy in high risk patients. Short term response 70-90%
Diffuse esophageal spasm	Body of esophagus and LES	Level II-3	Reserved for patients who do not respond to medical therapy. Larger placebo controlled trials are needed to justify routine use.
Gastroparesis	Pylorus	Level I evidence for no efficacy	Not efficacious. Benefit only in uncontrolled trials. One randomized controlled trial (2007) showed no efficacy. Rarely used in routine practice.
Obesity	Antrum	Level I	One small RCT showing weight loss at 8 weeks. Clinical significance is not clear. Not used in clinical practice
Sphincter of Oddi dysfunction	Sphincter of Oddi	Level II-2	Can be used as a therapeutic trial to select patients who would benefit from ES
Anal fissure	Internal anal sphincter	Level I	Strong evidence for efficacy. Used routinely in clinical practice
Anismus	EAS or puborectalis	Level II-3	Evidence from small uncontrolled studies

CPM, cricopharyngeal myotomy; EAS, external anal sphincter; ES, endoscopic sphincterotomy; LES, lower esophageal sphincter; RCT, randomized controlled trial; UES, upper esophageal sphincter.

*Levels of evidence:
- Level I: Evidence obtained from at least one properly designed randomized controlled trial.
- Level II-1: Evidence obtained from well-designed controlled trials without randomization.
- Level II-2: Evidence obtained from well-designed cohort or case-control analytic studies, preferably from more than one center or research group.
- Level II-3: Evidence obtained from multiple time series with or without the intervention. Dramatic results in uncontrolled trials might also be regarded as this type of evidence.
- Level III: Opinions of respected authorities, based on clinical experience, descriptive studies, or reports of expert committees.

have been proposed both as a therapeutic trial to select patients for surgery as well as primary treatment for high-risk patients.

Technique

Because of its striated nature, the typical doses of BoNT/A used for cricopharyngeal injection are smaller than those for smooth muscle disorders. Multiple techniques[6-13] have been described, including percutaneous and endoscopic approaches (using rigid or flexible instruments), with guidance provided by electromyographic or radiologic techniques.

Efficacy

Multiple uncontrolled studies have been published to date[14-18] with mean short-term response rates varying from 70% to 100% and mean duration of around 7 months. Some authors have reported improvement in secondary cricopharyngeal dysfunction including Parkinson's disease[12] and post-stroke dysphagia.[19] Finally, there is a single report on the use of this drug for the poorly defined syndrome of globus.[20] Although generally safe, concerns regarding exacerbation of dysphagia and vocal cord paralysis exist.[21]

ACHALASIA

Achalasia ("failure to relax") is a motor disorder of the esophagus characterized by absent peristalsis and incomplete relaxation of the lower esophageal sphincter (LES). The latter appears to be functionally more significant, resulting in progressive dysphagia, chest discomfort, and regurgitation. There is no curative treatment for achalasia, and all the current treatment modalities aim to decrease the LES pressure, allowing gravity-aided emptying of esophagus. Conventional treatment options include pneumatic dilation (done endoscopically) of the LES or laparoscopic surgical myotomy. In 1993, Pasricha et al[5] described the first successful use of BoNT/A for the treatment of achalasia.

Rationale

LES tone, like that of other GI muscle, is under the influence of both excitatory and inhibitory nerves. Pathophysiologically, achalasia appears to result from a loss of the inhibitory (mainly nitrergic) nerves, leading to relatively unopposed excitatory cholinergic activity. BoNT/A acts by blocking acetylcholine release from these nerves and lowering resting LES tone. However, the precise effects of BoNT/A in this environment are incompletely understood and there are probably significant differences as compared with the skeletal muscle system.

Technique

Endoscopic injection of BoNT/A is a fairly simple and straightforward procedure. Although some variations have been described with minor differences in outcome, the technique used most often consists of 20 to 25 U being injected under direct vision with a sclerotherapy needle into each of the four quadrants in LES.[22]

Efficacy

BoNT/A therapy is comparable to surgical myotomy and pneumatic dilation in terms of immediate improvement, and considerable evidence exists to state that all three modalities report early benefit in 80% to 90% of patients. However, as expected, the effects of BoNT/A generally wane over the next few months. Overall, the remission rates drop to 67% at 6 months and 50% or less at 12 months according to a systematic review.[22] In a large randomized study by Vaezi et al[23] in Cleveland Clinic comparing BoNT/A and pneumatic dilation, 70% of patients treated with pneumatic dilation were in remission at the end of 12 months, whereas only 32% were

in remission in BoNT/A group. In general, older patients (age > 50 years) and those with vigorous achalasia do better with this modality.[24]

Safety and Other Concerns

In general, BoNT injections in the GI tract appear to be safe for most patients, with a small number of patients experiencing self-limited chest or epigastric pain.[25-27] Some studies have reported technical difficulties (in finding the submucosal plane) and a higher incidence of mucosal perforations in patients undergoing a myotomy after BoNT therapy, possibly due to induction of inflammation and fibrosis.[28,29] However, BoNT/A therapy does not appear to affect the outcome after either surgery or pneumatic dilation.[30,31]

Role of Botulinum Neurotoxin Type A Therapy in the Clinical Management Strategies for Achalasia

Because of its limited duration of action and its lack of efficacy in younger patients, BoNT/A therapy is not suitable for all patients. It is best used under the following circumstances:

1. Very elderly patients or those with extensive comorbidities in whom even the small risk of perforation with pneumatic dilation is unacceptable.
2. Patients with recurrence of symptoms after surgery and or pneumatic dilation, or in those whom the diagnosis of achalasia has not been unequivocally established. In such patients, BoNT may provide a useful way to assess the contribution of a dysfunctional LES to the reported symptoms.

DIFFUSE ESOPHAGEAL SPASM AND OTHER PUTATIVE DISORDERS OF ESOPHAGEAL MOTILITY

Diffuse esophageal spasm is a motor disorder of the esophagus that is considered by some to be part of the same spectrum as achalasia. In many cases, LES dysfunction is a notable feature and can be treated by the same approaches used for achalasia including BoNT/A. Generally, similar techniques are used with similar outcomes, although some investigators have not confined their injections to the LES but also targeted the body of the esophagus, where spasms is noticeable.[32] Other investigators have reported good outcomes from uncontrolled trials of BoNT/A injections in patients with noncardiac chest pain, presumably of esophageal origin.[33] However, these results need corroboration from randomized controlled trials.

GASTROPARESIS

Gastroparesis is a disorder of gastric motility characterized by delayed gastric emptying in absence of obstruction. Symptoms include early satiety, bloating, nausea, and vomiting. Etiologies include diabetes, previous gastric surgery, neurologic and rheumatologic disorders, or idiopathic causes.

Rationale

The pathologic and pathophysiologic basis of gastroparesis remains unclear. BoNT/A is injected into the pyloric muscle in these patients on the basis that "pylorospasm" has been reported in some patients, resulting in a functional obstruction that impedes gastric emptying.[34-36]

Technique

It can be difficult to localize the exact boundaries of the pyloric sphincter endoscopically, and consequently, intrapyloric injection is more difficult to perform. In the literature, this technique is less well standardized as compared with that used in achalasia. Furthermore, generally higher doses (200 IU) are used, distributed among four or more sites within the pyloric sphincter. Techniques reported are similar to the technique used for achalasia.

Efficacy

Several small case studies report improvement in gastric emptying and symptoms after BoNT/A therapy. However, the first placebo controlled randomized trial reported no benefit from BoNT/A injection,[37] and it is unlikely

that this treatment (using the current approaches, at least) will prove to be of significant value in this group of patients.

OBESITY

Rationale

Gastric contractions, mediated principally by acetylcholine are critical for normal gastric emptying. By blocking cholinergic contractions, BoNT/A is expected to induce a delay in gastric emptying and lead to premature satiety, limiting further food ingestion.

Technique

This is a technique that is still evolving, and investigators have variously targeted either just the antrum or the entire stomach, using 100 to 400 IU of BoNT/A.

Efficacy

Initial pilot studies have generally been disappointing.[38-40] However, more recently, in a placebo-controlled trial on 24 morbidly obese patients randomized to either BoNT/A injection or saline, Foschi et al[41] demonstrated significant reduction in weight (11 ± 1.09 vs 5.7 ± 1.1 kg, $P < 0.001$) associated with prolongation of gastric emptying and reduction in maximal gastric capacity for liquid at 8 weeks. These results need to be reproduced by other investigators but have provided considerable excitement about the use of endoscopic injection of gastric BoNT/A as a relatively simple method for producing mild to moderate weight loss on a temporary basis. Such an approach may have cosmetic appeal for consumers but may also be of value in the preoperative setting to reduce surgical risk.

SPHINCTER OF ODDI DYSFUNCTION

The sphincter of Oddi is a small muscular ring that surrounds the biliary and pancreatic ducts at their opening into the duodenum, and its dysfunction has been implicated in the pathogenesis of several syndrome including postcholecystectomy pain and recurrent pancreatitis.

However, the scientific evidence for this is weak at best. Furthermore, the usual treatment for this condition is endoscopic sphincterotomy, which may be associated with significant risk. Hence, there is a need for a technique that is both safer as well as more predictive of the role of sphincter spasm in the genesis of symptoms. Endoscopic injection of BoNT/A appears to satisfy these requirements in animal experiments,[42] and indeed, this technique has been used as a therapeutic trial with good effect in both uncontrolled as well as controlled studies.[42]

ANAL FISSURE

Rationale

Anal fissure is a tear in the mucosal lining of the anal canal extending from anal verge to dentate line that results in pain and bleeding. The internal anal sphincter (IAS) beneath the tear is often hypertonic, and this is postulated to further aggravate the lesion by producing vascular compression and ischemia. Treatment of chronic anal fissure involves reducing the tone of internal anal sphincter and increasing blood flow to promote healing of the mucosal defect. This can be accomplished by various modalities like topical nitroglycerin, BoNT/A therapy, and lateral sphincterotomy. Lateral sphincterotomy is the most frequently used surgical technique and has a high success rate[22] (71%–97%) but is associated with flatus (0%–36%) and fecal incontinence (0%–9%).[22] Topical nitrate therapy has a healing rate of 40% to 80%, but tachyphylaxis, need for frequent applications, and headache limit its widespread use. Some authors propose that BoNT/A therapy also helps in healing of the fissure owing to its antinociceptive properties.[43]

Technique

The dosages and sites of BoNT/A injection have widely varied among the studies. BoNT/A is usually injected without endoscopic guidance after palpating the lower round edge of the IAS, about 1 to 1.5 cm proximal to the dentate line. One report described retrograde endoscopic injection in 22 patients, and the authors believed that this technique may be less painful.[44] BoNT/A injected on either side of the anterior midline seems to yield better results than BoNT/A injected on either side of fissure.[45] The dosages ranged from 2.5 IU to 50 IU, and higher doses seem to result in better short- and long-term healing rates.[46] Injection into the external anal sphincter has also been shown to result in healing.[47] This effect most probably may be secondary to diffusion into the IAS, but generally, injection into the IAS is preferred due to lower incidence of side effects, such as incontinence.[47,48]

Evidence

Multiple studies have provided good (Level I) evidence in favor of the efficacy of BoNT/A injections for the treatment of anal fissure, with 2-month healing rates ranging from just higher than 40% to more than 90%.[49-66] The durability of the response has not been well characterized, but recurrence has been reported to occur in a significant proportion of patients in some series.[49] However, these patients may benefit from repeat injections with or without higher doses.

Adverse Effects

Transient flatus incontinence and mild fecal incontinence occur in less than 10% of patients.[47] However, two cases of long-term fecal incontinence following BoNT/A injection have also been reported.[67,68]

OTHER ANORECTAL DISORDERS

Animus

Animus (also known as pelvic floor dyssenergia) is defined as inappropriate (paradoxical) contraction or failed relaxation of the puborectalis and external anal sphincter (EAS), resulting in chronic constipation. This is usually considered to be secondary to maladaptive learning but sometimes could be the result of systemic diseases like parkinsonism. Uncontrolled trials of BoNT injections suggest that 75% or more patients with this condition may respond.[69-71] However, technical aspects like dose of BoNT/A, site of injection (puborectalis versus EAS) and the use of guidance with electromyography or ultrasonography, need to be standardized, and placebo-controlled trials are necessary. Anecdotally, BoNT/A injection has also been found to be helpful in reducing symptoms in various other conditions such as posthemorrhoidectomy,[72,73] proctalgia fugax,[74,75] and radiation proctitis.[76]

CONCLUSIONS

It is clear that BoNT can significantly affect GI motility, a property that can be exploited for therapeutic benefit in those conditions in which a discrete region of muscle can be confidently implicated in the pathophysiology. Taking this a step further, one can make the case that the clinical response to local injection of BoNT (the "toxin test") reliably predicts the need for more invasive treatments such as surgical or endoscopic ablation of the target muscle. Failure to respond is then either because dysfunction of the muscle is not a major contributor to the clinical symptoms, or the targeted muscle is completely denervated and its tone is generated by purely myogenic mechanisms, which are not expected to respond to BoNT.

Ongoing clinical trials are clarifying the utility of BoNT in GI syndromes. It is unlikely, for instance, that intrapyloric injections will be of significant value in the management of gastroparesis. On the other hand, its use in obesity may represent an exciting new application. There is much that also needs to be learned about the biologic mechanisms underlying the observed effects on GI muscle, and such research may provide the opportunity for novel discoveries in the ENS.

References

1. Hansen M. The enteric nervous system I: organisation and classification. *Pharmacol Toxicol.* 2003;92:105-113.
2. Pasricha P, Ravich W, Kalloo A. Effects of intrasphincteric botulinum toxin on the lower esophageal sphincter in piglets. *Gastroenterology.* 1993;105:1045-1049.
3. James A, Ryan J, Parkman H. Inhibitory effects of botulinum toxin on pyloric and antral smooth muscle. *Am J Physiol Gastrointest Liver Physiol.* 2003;285:G291-G297.
4. Scott A. Botulinum toxin injection into extraocular muscles as an alternative to strabismus surgery. *Ophthalmology.* 1980;87:1044-1049.
5. Pasricha P, Ravich W, Kalloo A. Botulinum toxin for achalasia. *Lancet.* 1993;341:244-245.
6. Atkinson S, Rees J. Botulinum toxin for cricopharyngeal dysphagia: case reports of CT-guided injection. *J Otolaryngol.* 1997;26:273-276.
7. Blitzer A, Brin M. Use of botulinum toxin for diagnosis and management of cricopharyngeal achalasia. *Otolaryngol Head Neck Surg.* 1997;116:328-330.

8. Brant C, Siqueira E, Ferrari AJ. Botulinum toxin for oropharyngeal dysphagia: case report of flexible endoscope-guided injection. *Dis Esophagus.* 1999;12:68-73.
9. Alberty J, Oelerich M, Ludwig K, Hartmann S, Stoll W. Efficacy of botulinum toxin A for treatment of upper esophageal sphincter dysfunction. *Laryngoscope.* 2000;110:1151-1156.
10. Restivo D, Marchese Ragona R, Staffieri A, de Grandis D. Successful botulinum toxin treatment of dysphagia in oculopharyngeal muscular dystrophy. *Gastroenterology.* 2000;119:1416.
11. Haapaniemi J, Laurikainen E, Pulkkinen J, Marttila R. Botulinum toxin in the treatment of cricopharyngeal dysphagia. *Dysphagia.* 2001;16:171-175.
12. Restivo D, Palmeri A, Marchese-Ragona R. Botulinum toxin for cricopharyngeal dysfunction in Parkinson's disease. *N Engl J Med.* 2002;346:1174-1175.
13. Restivo D, Maimone D, Patti F, Marchese-Ragona R, Marino G, Pavone A. Trismus after stroke/TBI: botulinum toxin benefit and use pre-PEG placement. *Neurology.* 2005;64:2152-2153.
14. Schneider I, Thumfart W, Pototschnig C, Eckel H. Treatment of dysfunction of the cricopharyngeal muscle with botulinum A toxin: introduction of a new, noninvasive method. *Ann Otol Rhinol Laryngol.* 1994;103:31-35.
15. Murry T, Wasserman T, Carrau R, Castillo B. Injection of botulinum toxin A for the treatment of dysfunction of the upper esophageal sphincter. *Am J Otolaryngol.* 2005;26:157-162.
16. Chiu M, Chang Y, Hsiao T. Prolonged effect of botulinum toxin injection in the treatment of cricopharyngeal dysphagia: case report and literature review. *Dysphagia.* 2004;19:52-57.
17. Liu L, Tarnopolsky M, Armstrong D. Injection of botulinum toxin A to the upper esophageal sphincter for oropharyngeal dysphagia in two patients with inclusion body myositis. *Can J Gastroenterol.* 2004;18: 397-399.
18. Zaninotto G, Marchese Ragona R, Briani C, Costantini M, Rizzetto C, Portale G, et al. The role of botulinum toxin injection and upper esophageal sphincter myotomy in treating oropharyngeal dysphagia. *J Gastrointest Surg.* 2004;8:997-1006.
19. Masiero S, Briani C, Marchese-Ragona R, Giacometti P, Costantini M, Zaninotto G. Successful treatment of long-standing post-stroke dysphagia with botulinum toxin and rehabilitation. *J Rehabil Med.* 2006;38: 201-203.
20. Halum S, Butler S, Koufman J, Postma G. Treatment of globus by upper esophageal sphincter injection with botulinum A toxin. *Ear Nose Throat J.* 2005;84:74.
21. Ravich W. Toxin for UES dysfunction: therapy or poison? *Dysphagia.* 2001;16:168-170.
22. Gui D, Rossi S, Runfola M, Magalini S. Review article: botulinum toxin in the therapy of gastrointestinal motility disorders. *Aliment Pharmacol Ther.* 2003;18: 1-16.
23. Vaezi M, Richter J, Wilcox C, Schroeder P, Birgisson S, Slaughter R, et al. Botulinum toxin versus pneumatic dilatation in the treatment of achalasia: a randomised trial. *Gut.* 1999;44:231-239.
24. Neubrand M, Scheurlen C, Schepke M, Sauerbruch T. Long-term results and prognostic factors in the treatment of achalasia with botulinum toxin. *Endoscopy.* 2002;34:519-523.
25. Khoshoo V, LaGarde D, Udall JJ. Intrasphincteric injection of Botulinum toxin for treating achalasia in children. *J Pediatr Gastroenterol Nutr.* 1997;24:439-441.

26. Dughera L, Battaglia E, Maggio D, Cassolino P, Mioli P, Morelli A, et al. Botulinum toxin treatment of oesophageal achalasia in the old old and oldest old: a 1-year follow-up study. *Drugs Aging.* 2005;22: 779-783.

27. Bassotti G, D'Onofrio V, Battaglia E, Fiorella S, Dughera L, Iaquinto G, et al. Treatment with botulinum toxin of octo-nonagerians with oesophageal achalasia: a two-year follow-up study. *Aliment Pharmacol Ther.* 2006;23:1615-1619.

28. Woltman T, Pellegrini C, Oelschlager B. Achalasia. *Surg Clin North Am.* 2005;85:483-493.

29. Horgan S, Hudda K, Eubanks T, McAllister J, Pellegrini C. Does botulinum toxin injection make esophagomyotomy a more difficult operation? *Surg Endosc.* 1999;13:576-579.

30. Mikaeli J, Yaghoobi M, Montazeri G, Ansari R, Bishehsari F, Malekzadeh R. Efficacy of botulinum toxin injection before pneumatic dilatation in patients with idiopathic achalasia. *Dis Esophagus.* 2004;17: 213-217.

31. Mikaeli J, Bishehsari F, Montazeri G, Mahdavinia M, Yaghoobi M, Darvish-Moghadam S, et al. Injection of botulinum toxin before pneumatic dilatation in achalasia treatment: a randomized-controlled trial. *Aliment Pharmacol Ther.* 2006;24:983-989.

32. Storr M, Allescher H, Rösch T, Born P, Weigert N, Classen M. Treatment of symptomatic diffuse esophageal spasm by endoscopic injection of botulinum toxin: a prospective study with long term follow-up. *Gastrointest Endosc.* 2001;54:18A.

33. Miller L, Pullela S, Parkman H, Schiano T, Cassidy M, Cohen S, et al. Treatment of chest pain in patients with noncardiac, nonreflux, nonachalasia spastic esophageal motor disorders using botulinum toxin injection into the gastroesophageal junction. *Am J Gastroenterol.* 2002;97:1640-1646.

34. Zárate N, Mearin F, Wang X, Hewlett B, Huizinga J, Malagelada J. Severe idiopathic gastroparesis due to neuronal and interstitial cells of Cajal degeneration: pathologic findings and management. *Gut.* 2003;52:966-970.

35. Lacy B, Zayat E, Crowell M, Schuster M. Botulinum toxin for the treatment of gastroparesis: a preliminary report. *Am J Gastroenterol.* 2002;97:1548-1552.

36. Lacy B, Crowell M, Schettler-Duncan A, Mathis C, Pasricha P. The treatment of diabetic gastroparesis with botulinum toxin injection of the pylorus. *Diabetes Care.* 2004;27:2341-2347.

37. Arts J, Holvoet L, Caenepeel P, Bisschops R, Sifrim D, Verbeke K, et al. A randomized controlled cross-over study of intra-pyloric injection of botulinum toxin in gastroparesis. *Aliment Pharmacol Ther.* 2007;21: 1251-1258.

38. Júnior A, Savassi-Rocha P, Coelho L, Spósito M, Albuquerque W, Diniz M, et al. Botulinum A toxin injected into the gastric wall for the treatment of class III obesity: a pilot study. *Obes Surg.* 2006;16:335-343.

39. Gui D, Mingrone G, Valenza V, Spada P, Mutignani M, Runfola M, et al. Effect of botulinum toxin antral injection on gastric emptying and weight reduction in obese patients: a pilot study. *Aliment Pharmacol Ther.* 2006;23:675-680.

40. García-Compean D, Mendoza-Fuerte E, Martínez J, Villarreal I, Maldonado H. Endoscopic injection of botulinum toxin in the gastric antrum for the treatment of obesity. Results of a pilot study. *Gastroenterol Clin Biol.* 2005;29:789-791.

41. Foschi D, Corsi F, Lazzaroni M, Sangaletti O, Riva P, La Tartara G, et al. Treatment of morbid obesity by intraparietogastric administration of botulinum toxin: a randomized, double-blind, controlled study. *Int J Obes (Lond).* 2007;31:707-712.

42. Pasricha P, Miskovsky E, Kalloo A. Intrasphincteric injection of botulinum toxin for suspected sphincter of Oddi dysfunction. *Gut.* 1994;35:1319-1321.

43. Runfola M, Di Mugno M, Balletta A, Magalini S, Gui D. Antinociceptive effect of botulinum toxin: an added value to chemical sphincterotomy in anal fissure? *Dis Colon Rectum.* 2006;49:1078-1079.

44. Kinney T, Shah A, Rogers B, Ehrenpreis E. Retrograde endoscopic delivery of botulinum toxin for anal fissures. *Endoscopy.* 2006;38:654.

45. Maria G, Brisinda G, Bentivoglio A, Cassetta E, Gui D, Albanese A. Influence of botulinum toxin site of injections on healing rate in patients with chronic anal fissure. *Am J Surg.* 2000;179:46-50.

46. Brisinda G, Maria G, Sganga G, Bentivoglio A, Albanese A, Castagneto M. Effectiveness of higher doses of botulinum toxin to induce healing in patients with chronic anal fissures. *Surgery.* 2002;131:179-184.

47. Jost W. One hundred cases of anal fissure treated with botulin toxin: early and long-term results. *Dis Colon Rectum.* 1997;40:1029-1032.

48. Maria G, Sganga G, Civello I, Brisinda G. Botulinum neurotoxin and other treatments for fissure-in-ano and pelvic floor disorders. *Br J Surg.* 2002;89:950-961.

49. Minguez M, Herreros B, Espi A, Garcia-Granero E, Sanchiz V, Mora F, et al. Long-term follow-up (42 months) of chronic anal fissure after healing with botulinum toxin. *Gastroenterology.* 2002;123:112-117.

50. Lindsey I, Jones O, Cunningham C, George B, Mortensen N. Botulinum toxin as second-line therapy for chronic anal fissure failing 0.2 percent glyceryl trinitrate. *Dis Colon Rectum.* 2003;46:361-366.

51. Mentes B, Irkörücü O, Akin M, Leventoglu S, Tatlicioglu E. Comparison of botulinum toxin injection and lateral internal sphincterotomy for the treatment of chronic anal fissure. *Dis Colon Rectum.* 2003;46:232-237.

52. Arroyo SA, Pérez VF, Miranda TE, Sánchez RA, Serrano PP, Calpena RR. Surgical (close lateral internal sphincterotomy) versus chemical (botulinum toxin) sphincterotomy as treatment of chronic anal fissure. *Med Clin (Barc).* 2005;124:573-575.

53. Arroyo A, Perez F, Serrano P, Candela F, Calpena R. Long-term results of botulinum toxin for the treatment of chronic anal fissure: prospective clinical and manometric study. *Int J Colorectal Dis.* 2005;20:267.

54. Arroyo A, Pérez F, Serrano P, Candela F, Lacueva J, Calpena R. Surgical versus chemical (botulinum toxin) sphincterotomy for chronic anal fissure: long-term results of a prospective randomized clinical and manometric study. *Am J Surg.* 2005;189:429-434.

55. Iswariah H, Stephens J, Rieger N, Rodda D, Hewett P. Randomized prospective controlled trial of lateral internal sphincterotomy versus injection of botulinum toxin for the treatment of idiopathic fissure in ano. *ANZ J Surg.* 2005;75:553-555.

56. Massoud B, Mehrdad V, Baharak T, Alireza Z. Botulinum toxin injection versus internal anal sphincterotomy for the treatment of chronic anal fissure. *Ann Saudi Med.* 2005;25:140-142.

57. De Nardi P, Ortolano E, Radaelli G, Staudacher C. Comparison of glycerine trinitrate and botulinum toxin-a for the treatment of chronic anal fissure: long-term results. *Dis Colon Rectum.* 2006;49:427-432.

58. Fruehauf H, Fried M, Wegmueller B, Bauerfeind P, Thumshirn M. Efficacy and safety of botulinum toxin a injection compared with topical nitroglycerin ointment for the treatment of chronic anal fissure: a prospective randomized study. *Am J Gastroenterol.* 2006;101:2107-2112.

59. Jones O, Ramalingam T, Merrie A, Cunningham C, George B, Mortensen N, et al. Randomized clinical trial of botulinum toxin plus glyceryl trinitrate vs. botulinum toxin alone for medically resistant chronic anal fissure: overall poor healing rates. *Dis Colon Rectum.* 2006;49:1574-1580.

60. Lysy J, Israeli E, Levy S, Rozentzweig G, Strauss-Liviatan N, Goldin E. Long-term results of "chemical sphincterotomy" for chronic anal fissure: a prospective study. *Dis Colon Rectum.* 2006;49: 858-864.

61. Tranqui P, Trottier D, Victor C, Freeman J. Nonsurgical treatment of chronic anal fissure: nitroglycerin and dilatation versus nifedipine and botulinum toxin. *Can J Surg.* 2006;49:41-45.

62. Witte M, Klaase J. [Favourable results with local injections of botulinum-A toxin in patients with chronic isosorbide dinitrate ointment-resistant anal fissures]. *Ned Tijdschr Geneeskd.* 2006;150: 1513-1517.

63. Brisinda G, Cadeddu F, Brandara F, Marniga G, Maria G. Randomized clinical trial comparing botulinum toxin injections with 0.2 per cent nitroglycerin ointment for chronic anal fissure. *Br J Surg.* 2007;94:162-167.

64. Kelly T, Ballal M, Khera G. Randomized clinical trial comparing botulinum toxin injections with 0.2 per cent nitroglycerin ointment for chronic anal fissure (Br J Surg 2007;94:162-167). *Br J Surg.* 2007; 94:646; author reply -7.

65. Sileri P, Mele A, Stolfi V, Grande M, Sica G, Gentileschi P, et al. Medical and surgical treatment of chronic anal fissure: a prospective study. *J Gastrointest Surg.* 2007;11:1541-1548.

66. Witte M, Klaase J. Botulinum toxin A injection in ISDN ointment-resistant chronic anal fissures. *Dig Surg.* 2007;24:197-201.

67. Smith M, Frizelle F. Long-term faecal incontinence following the use of botulinum toxin. *Colorectal Dis.* 2004;6:526-527.

68. Brown S, Matabudul Y, Shorthouse A. A second case of long-term incontinence following botulinum injection for anal fissure. *Colorectal Dis.* 2006;8:452-453.

69. Joo J, Agachan F, Wolff B, Nogueras J, Wexner S. Initial North American experience with botulinum toxin type A for treatment of anismus. *Dis Colon Rectum.* 1996;39:1107-1111.

70. Shafik A, El-Sibai O. Botulin toxin in the treatment of nonrelaxing puborectalis syndrome. *Dig Surg.* 1998;15:347-351.

71. Ron Y, Avni Y, Lukovetski A, Wardi J, Geva D, Birkenfeld S, et al. Botulinum toxin type-A in therapy of patients with anismus. *Dis Colon Rectum.* 2001;44:1821-1826.

72. Patti R, Angileri M, Migliore G, Sammartano S, Termine S, Crivello F, et al. [Effectiveness of contemporary injection of botulinum toxin and topical application of glyceryl trinitrate against postoperative pain after Milligan-Morgan haemorrhoidectomy]. *Ann Ital Chir.* 2006;77:503-508.

73. Patti R, Almasio P, Luigi A, Arcara M, Matteo A, Sammartano S, et al. Botulinum toxin vs. topical glyceryl trinitrate ointment for pain control in patients undergoing hemorrhoidectomy: a randomized trial. *Dis Colon Rectum.* 2006;49:1741-1748.

74. Katsinelos P, Kalomenopoulou M, Christodoulou K, Katsiba D, Tsolkas P, Pilpilidis I, et al. Treatment of proctalgia fugax with botulinum A toxin. *Eur J Gastroenterol Hepatol.* 2001;13:1371-1373.

75. Sánchez RA, Arroyo SA, Pérez VF, Serrano PP, Candela PF, Calpena RR. [Treatment of proctalgia fugax with botulinum toxin: results in 5 patients]. *Rev Clin Esp.* 2006;206:137-140.

76. De Micheli C, Fornengo P, Bosio A, Epifani G, Pascale C. Severe radiation-induced proctitis treated with botulinum anatoxin type A. *J Clin Oncol.* 2003;21:2627.

77. Eckardt V, Gockel I, Bernhard G. Pneumatic dilation for achalasia: late results of a prospective follow up investigation. *Gut.* 2004;53:629-633.

Mechanism of Action 19 of Botulinum Neurotoxin in the Lower Urinary Tract

Michael B. Chancellor, George T. Somogyi, and Christopher P. Smith

INTRODUCTION

Botulinum neurotoxins (BoNTs) are well known for their ability to potently and selectively disrupt and modulate neurotransmission. Only recently have urologists become interested in the potential use of BoNT in patients with detrusor overactivity and other urologic disorders. We will review mechanisms by which BoNT modulates acetylcholine (ACh) and other biochemical messengers at presynaptic nerve terminals in the detrusor smooth muscle and possibly the urothelium. We will also review what is known about potentially important noncholinergic mechanisms modulating the function of detrusor smooth muscle and bladder afferent sensory processing.

BoNT has received regulatory approval for a number of conditions characterized by excessive and unwanted muscle contractility or tonus in striated muscle (e.g., cervical dystonia, blepharospasm, hemifacial spasm, and limb spasticity secondary to central nervous system injury) or overactive secretion (e.g., hyperhidrosis). More recently, researchers have discovered that BoNT is effective in the treatment of conditions such as overactive bladder and esophageal spasm, suggesting that BoNT's effects on neurotransmission in smooth muscle appear to be similar to those in striated muscle.[1] BoNT is currently undergoing regulatory evaluation for urologic disorders in the United States and the European Union. However, as the uses of BoNT continue to expand, it is important to be familiar with the mechanism by which the toxin works and to investigate any differences that may exist when it is applied to different tissue types.

A stepwise mechanism of action for the botulinum toxins was first suggested by Simpson[2] and involves toxin binding to, and internalization within, the presynaptic membrane of cholinergic neurons, followed by translocation into the neuronal cytosol and then inhibition of ACh release. his review explores these processes with regard to BoNT, its structure and its effects on the function of the lower urinary tract.

ACTION OF BOTULINUM NEUROTOXIN ON URINARY TRACT STRIATED VERSUS SMOOTH MUSCLE

None of the clinically available clostridial neurotoxins cause death of neurons or myocytes, or alteration of other cellular constituents. Thus, these neurotoxins are not toxic to tissue. Rather, in muscle, they act as biochemical neuromodulators, temporarily inactivating cholinergic transmission at the neuromuscular junction. Historically, the molecular mechanisms of BoNT have mostly been elucidated in studies of striated muscle. More recently, as a result of recognizing new clinical applications of BoNT, there have been studies conducted on

The authors of this chapter are disclosing that they have been research investigators and consultants for Allergan, Inc., the manufacturer of Botox.

the biological effects of BoNT on smooth muscle.[3-5]

In striated muscle, BoNT administration interferes with signaling between alpha motor neurons and extrafusal muscle fibers, as well as signaling between gamma motor neurons and the intrafusal fibers of muscle spindles.[6-9] In the initial weeks after injection, BoNT-treated muscles show some variability in muscle fiber size and intracellular changes consistent with denervation (i.e., central mitochondria dispersed toward the periphery).[10-12] However, these effects are temporary and BoNT appears to produce no persistent changes in muscle fiber internal architecture after recovery from paralysis. BoNT may even produce beneficial gross muscular changes, such as reversing hypertrophy in dystonic muscle groups.[13]

Physiologic changes induced by BoNT include a fall of resting membrane potential, fibrillation potentials, and the elimination of extrajunctional acetylcholinesterase activity.[14] Morphologically, there is evidence for subsequent compensatory nerve sprouting and the creation of functional synapses extrajunctionally.[15-18] When exocytosis at the parent terminal eventually recovers, the sprouts are retracted and endplate functioning returns to normal.[15,19]

EFFECT OF BOTULINUM NEUROTOXIN ON THE DETRUSOR MUSCLE

Despite some apparent differences at the cellular level, BoNT administration has the same clinical effect on both smooth and striated muscle. In the case of BoNT administration to the bladder wall, there is an increase in bladder capacity, with a reduction in incontinence episodes and symptoms of urgency. A more complete neuromuscular blockade of the detrusor results in impaired voiding andr urinary retention if relatively larger doses of BoNT are used.[1,20-23]

FROM CELLULAR ACTION TO CLINICAL EFFECT

In normal bladders, the smooth muscle bundles of the detrusor are not well coupled electrically and thus the detrusor's smooth muscle requires dense innervation. During filling of the normal bladder, parasympathetic excitatory neurons are silent and the detrusor is relatively quiescent, allowing storage of urine at a low pressure. Micturition is induced by activation of the parasympathetic nerves and release of ACh, which stimulates postjunctional M3 receptors to induce a large amplitude detrusor contraction. ACh also stimulates prejunctional M1 muscarinic receptors on post-ganglionic parasympathetic nerve terminals to facilitate its own release and thereby amplify excitatory input to the detrusor.[24] The overactive bladder meanwhile exhibits a number of histologic and neurologic changes that disrupt these processes and contribute to the disorder's symptoms.[25]

In overactive bladders, there is increased coupling of the smooth muscle bundles of the detrusor, which leads to greater excitability in response to low-grade efferent stimuli.[25] Experimentally, in bladder strips from spinal cord–injured animals, there is upregulation of presynaptic muscarinic facilitatory mechanisms in cholinergic nerve terminals.[26] This would also contribute to a greater contractile response to low-grade stimulation and suggests that such increased synaptic activity would render the neurons associated with the smooth muscle of the detrusor highly susceptible to BoNT binding and internalization.

Recent studies show that BoNT injected in the overactive human bladder appears to exert a complex inhibitory effect on vesicular release of excitatory neurotransmitters as well as on axonal expression of other SNARE-complex–dependent proteins in the urothelium and suburothelium.[27]

MECHANISM OF ACTION

Efferent Effect

Smith and colleagues found significant decreases in the release of labeled ACh in BoNT injected in normal rat bladders, suggesting that BoNT could reduce cholinergic nerve–induced bladder activity (Fig. 19-1).[23] Although BoNT is known to exhibit cholinergic specificity, release of other transmitters can be inhibited, particularly if adequate concentrations are used.[28-31] For example, contractile data suggest that BoNT may impair atropine triphosphate (ATP) release in addition to ACh release from isolated bladder tissue (Fig. 19-2).[32] These results have clinical

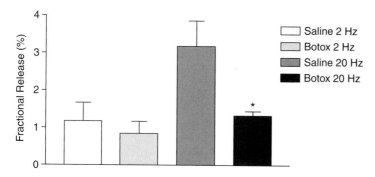

FIGURE 19-1. Release of ^{13}C-choline from rat bladder strips 5 days following injection with saline (sham) or 50 units botulinum neurotoxin type A (BoNT/A). Each value is the mean + SEM from three to four experiments. Note the significant decrease in release of acetylcholine from BoNT/A-treated rats at the higher frequency (20 Hz), $P < 0.05$ using the unpaired t test and following log rhythmic transformation of the data.

significance in lieu of recent investigations demonstrating alterations in P2X receptor expression and increased purinergic bladder response in patients with idiopathic detrusor instability. In fact, O'Reilly and colleagues[33] found that approximately 50% of the nerve-mediated contractions in bladder tissues extracted from patients with idiopathic detrusor overactivity were purinergic in origin.

Afferent Effect

BoNT's efficacy in conditions of detrusor overactivity may result not only from an inhibitory effect on detrusor muscle, but some effects of the drug may be mediated by altering afferent (sensory) input. Urothelium possesses muscarinic receptor populations with a density two times as high as detrusor smooth muscle, and dorsal root ganglionectomy experiments demonstrating the persistence of acetylcholinesterase staining nerves near the urothelium suggest that parasympathetic nerves supply some innervation to urothelium.[34,35] Besides receiving cholinergic innervation, human urothelium has also been shown to release the neurotransmitter ACh at rest.[36] Thus, ACh, released from urothelium and acting on nearby muscarinic receptor populations (i.e., urothelium or afferent nerves) or neuronal sources of ACh binding to muscarinic receptors within urothelium or afferent nerves, could have a significant impact on bladder sensory input to the central nervous system and may be affected by BoNT treatment.

In addition, recent basic and clinical evidence suggests that BoNT may have sensory inhibitory effects unrelated to its actions on ACh release. For example, an in vitro model of mechanoreceptor-stimulated urothelial ATP release was tested in spinal cord–injured rat bladders to determine whether intravesical botulinum neurotoxin A (BoNT/A) administration would inhibit urothelial ATP release, a measure of sensory nerve activation.[37] The results demonstrated that hypoosmotic stimulation of bladder urothelium evoked a significant release of ATP that was markedly inhibited by BoNT/A (e.g., 53%, Fig. 19-3), suggesting that impairment of urothelial ATP release may be one mechanism by which BoNT reduces detrusor overactivity. BoNT has also been shown to inhibit release of

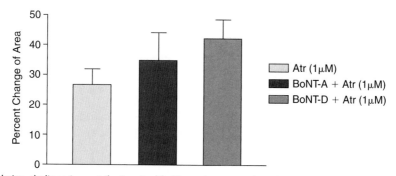

FIGURE 19-2. Relative cholinergic contribution to bladder strip contractions in untreated (n = 4), botulinum neurotoxin (BoNT/A) (n = 5) and BoNT/D (n = 5) preparations. No significant difference in percent change of contractile area was observed following atropine administration (1 μM) between untreated or BoNT-treated bladder strips. These results suggest that BoNT/A and BoNT/D impaired both purinergic and cholinergic transmitter release from bladder nerve terminals.

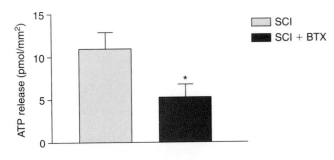

FIGURE 19-3. Bar graph representing hypoosmotic evoked release of atropine triphosphate from urothelium in bladders from spinal cord–injured rats both pretreated and untreated with intravesical botulinum neurotoxin type A (BoNT/A, 20 U/mL).

neuropeptides such as calcitonin gene–related peptide (CGRP), substances thought to play a role in overactive bladder conditions such as sensory urgency or chronic bladder inflammation (i.e., interstitial cystitis).[38,39]

Effects on Acetylcholine and Atropine Triphosphatase Release

In animal bladder models, BoNT inhibited the release of ACh in response to high-grade stimulation but not low-grade stimulation (see Fig. 19-1),[23] suggesting that it may act on the muscarinic facilitatory mechanism mediated by protein kinase C.

ATP has also been implicated as a neurotransmitter in the generation of unstable contractions in idiopathic detrusor overactivity (IDO).[33,40] Studies on guinea pig[28] and rat[23] bladder strips have shown that BoNT is capable of inhibiting the release of both ACh and ATP, providing a rationale for its possible use in treating patients with IDO (see Fig. 19-2).

Although ATP release has been widely demonstrated from efferent cholinergic and adrenergic terminals,[41-43] ATP release from bladder urothelial cells has only recently been confirmed.[44-47]

Bladder urothelium may play an important role in the sensory transduction mechanisms modulating micturition, particularly in conditions of increased sensory nerve transmission following chronic inflammation and spinal cord injury (SCI).[37] Urothelial cells can release ATP,[45,47] and the increased release of ATP from the urothelium of SCI bladders could activate P2X3 receptors in epithelial and subepithelial layers to increase afferent nerve activity, accounting for the higher frequency of bladder contractions seen in both human and animal models of SCI.

Recently BoNT was shown to inhibit ATP release from the urothelial but not the serosal side of the bladder, suggesting that BoNT treatment inhibits transmitter release not only from efferent nerve endings but from sensory nerve terminals and urothelium as well (see Fig. 19-3).[37] That BoNT significantly impairs urothelial ATP release following SCI presents a plausible explanation for its clinical efficacy in the treatment of human neurogenic bladder dysfunction.

Effect on P2X3 and Capsaicin-Sensitive TRPV1 Sensory Receptors

Extracellular ATP is implicated in a large number of sensory processes that range from pain response to regulation of organ motility. The ATP receptor P2X3 is almost exclusively expressed in sensory neurons. There is accumulating evidence that this receptor has a specific role in nociception. For example, activation of P2X3 by ATP leads to a much stronger nociceptive effect in inflamed compared with normal tissue.[48,49]

Originally described as a capsaicin receptor related to natural irritants (called vanilloids), the Transient Receptor Potential channel, Vanilloid family member 1 (TRPV1) receptor is believed to function as an integrator of noxious stimuli, such as acids, heat, pollutants with a negative electronic charge, and endogenous proinflammatory substances.[50] Specifically, TRPV1 plays a key role in the perception of peripheral thermal and inflammatory pain.[51]

Recent findings indicate that BoNT blocks TRPV1 membrane translocation induced by protein kinase C, suggesting that activity-dependent delivery of channels to the neuronal surface may contribute to the buildup and maintenance of thermal inflammatory hyperalgesia in peripheral nociceptor terminals.[51]

Successful BoNT treatment for overactive bladder is associated with a significant decrease of TRPV1 and/or P2X3 in suburothelial nerve fibers.[52] These changes may reflect a direct effect of BoNT on the afferent innervation of the bladder or may occur as a secondary effect to the action of BoNT on the efferent innervation of the detrusor.[52a]

Clinical Effects on Calcitonin Gene-Related Peptide and Substance P Release

Sensory axons in the bladder contain both CGRP and substance P. These neuropeptides, which are released from nociceptive sensory endings in response to noxious stimuli, function as inflammatory response mediators.[53] Substance P acts on mast cells to produce degranulation, resulting in release of histamine and cytokines, which directly sensitize or excite nociceptors. In addition, both substance P and CGRP produce edema (substance P through plasma extravasation, and CGRP through dilation of peripheral blood vessels), causing liberation of bradykinin, all of which can lead to further activation of primary afferent fibers.[53] Together with bradykinin and prostaglandins, substance P and CGRP also cause migration of leukocytes to the site of injury and clotting responses.[54,55]

BoNT has been shown in several preclinical models to block the release of CGRP, SP, and glutamate from afferent nerve terminals.[39,54] The effect of BoNT on sensory pathways is supported by results reported in preclinical models of bladder pain, in which intravesical application of BoNT significantly reduced pain responses and inhibited CGRP release from afferent nerve terminals, suggesting that BoNT may have clinical applications for the treatment of disorders such as interstitial cystitis and sensory urgency.[38,39]

Inhibition of Nerve Growth Factor Release and Receptor Transport

In both animals and humans, the bladder increases production of nerve growth factor (NGF) in response to conditions such as SCI, denervation, inflammation, distension, or hypertrophy.[56] NGF is a signaling protein that interacts with specific receptors along autocrine, paracrine, and endocrine pathways. It is produced in the smooth muscle of the urinary tract and urothelium of the bladder, and elevated NGF levels have been reported to trigger bladder overactivity, such as that seen

in men with benign prostatic hyperplasia, women with interstitial cystitis, and in patients with IDO.

Intravesical BoNT injection reduces NGF content in the bladder tissue of patients with neurogenic detrusor overactivity, but it is unknown whether reduced bladder NGF results from decreased production, decreased uptake or a combination of both.[56] The result of this action of BoNT is to decrease the hyperexcitability of C-fiber bladder afferents, thereby reducing neurogenic detrusor overactivity.[57]

Sensory Effects of Botulinum Neurotoxin: Evidence from Nonurologic Medical Specialties

Neurologists have long recognized the relief of pain induced by intramuscular injection of BoNT; the benefit can be seen before evidence of muscle relaxation, and pain relief often outlasts reduction in spasm, suggesting a direct analgesic effect.[58-60] In patients receiving BoNT for cervical dystonia, pain relief often exceeds motor benefit; thus pain relief by BoNT cannot be entirely due to its effects on muscle contraction.[61,62]

Changes in afferent activity may influence pain through both direct sensory effects and via central reorganization due to prolonged reduced muscle spindle feedback into the CNS; that is, reduced Ia afferent input from muscle spindle fibers to the spinal cord due to inhibition of ACh release from γ-motor neurons.[59]

Histologic Impact of Botulinum Neurotoxin Type A Injection

Only one study has looked at ultrastructural changes in overactive human detrusor tissue following BoNT injection. Haferkamp et al[63] collected 30 biopsies from 24 patients with a diagnosis of neurogenic overactive bladder. Biopsies were taken before and 3 months after BoNT injection and during the wearing-off phase of the toxin's efficacy. They observed no significant changes in muscle cell fascicles, intercellular collagen content, or muscle cell degeneration when comparing biopsies taken before and after BoNT administration, although these results cannot be extrapolated to the possible structural effects of repeat injections. Unlike striated muscle, axonal sprouting in detrusor smooth muscle was limited following BoNT administration, and further research is required to determine if prolonged toxin dosing will elicit such a response. The results of an immunohistochemical study also suggested no significant axonal sprouting in the suburothelium of successfully treated patients.[52]

A single published study to date has retrospectively investigated histopathologic changes in excised human neurogenic overactive bladders that could be associated with intradetrusor BoNT injections. Full-thickness specimens from bladders previously treated with one or more injections of BoNT showed significantly less fibrosis, but no differences in inflammation and edema compared with untreated ones; degrees of inflammation, edema, and fibrosis were comparable in the two groups. Treated bladders had been injected with a mean number of 1.5 ± 0.8 injections, and the mean time between the last injection and surgery was 6.8 ± 2.8 months.[64]

Because the action of BoNT is reversible over time and does not appear to induce any enduring pathologic changes, it has theoretical longevity in terms of its clinical usefulness in urologic dysfunction. Indeed, regular BoNT blockade of striated muscle activity over a 12-year period was shown to be clinically safe and effective.[65] However, because biopsies were not performed, the long-term effects at a cellular level cannot be determined.

Although the majority of long-term results are positive, more data are needed from both smooth and striated muscle. A case study by Coletti Moja and colleagues has described acute neuromuscular failure in a patient who had a 2-year history of regular BoNT treatment (Dysport [Ipsen, Milford, MA] 800–1000 U every 3 months for limb spasticity).[66] Biopsy investigations showed subacute denervation and inflammation of the deltoid muscle with unspecified diffuse abnormalities of group II afferent fibers at a site distal to the area of drug administration, with clinical features resembling an acute myasthenic-like syndrome. Such findings indicate that there is still much to learn about the effects of long-term exposure to BoNT.

Repeat Botulinum Neurotoxin Type A Injections

Grosse and colleagues[67] evaluated the effectiveness of repeated detrusor injections of BoNT/A. A total of 49 patients with refractory neurogenic detrusor overactivity received between two and five injections of BoNT/A. The authors found significant and similar reductions in detrusor overactivity and in the use of anticholinergic medication, in addition to significant increases in bladder capacity and compliance after both the first and second injection with BoNT/A. The average interval between injections was 11 months. As more patients are repeatedly treated with BoNT/A injections into the lower urinary tract, urologists will gain better insight into patients' risk of developing antibodies and becoming clinically nonresponsive. Similar to studies in adults, investigators have also found that children respond favorably to repeated injections with BoNT/A.[68-70]

ADVERSE LOCAL EFFECTS

Most patients would refuse to choose BoNT/A treatment if there was a significant risk of long-term catheterization. Surprisingly, Popat and colleagues[21] described de novo self-catheterization rates of as high as 69% in neurogenic and 19% in idiopathic patients after injection of 300 units and 200 units of BoNT/A, respectively. In addition, Kessler et al[71] described de novo catheterization rates of 45% in idiopathic and neurogenic overactive bladder patients following detrusor injection of 300 units of BoNT/A. The high rates of self-catheterization observed in some series might be explained by differences in what each study defines as a clinically relevant post-void residual (PVR); e.g., >100 mL in the study by Popat et al[21] versus >150 mL in the study by Kessler et al.[71] However, two other series reported low postinjection PVRs of 15 mL[69,70] and 42 mL[22] after injection of 300 units and 100 to 300 units of BoNT/A, respectively. Although the efficacy of BoNT/A treatment has been demonstrated in all the studies to date, the impact of toxin dosage and delivery (i.e., toxin dose and dilution, and the site and depth of injections) on the development of adverse events remains to be established.

CONCLUSION

BoNT is efficacious across a wide variety of disorders that involve pathologic neuromuscular activity. Advances have been made in our understanding of how BoNT works at a molecular level, yet questions remain.

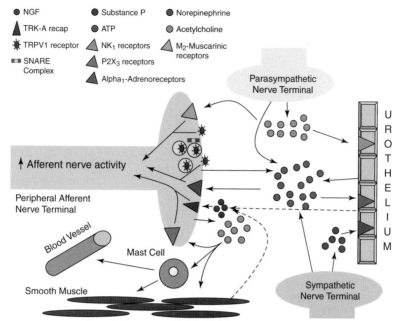

FIGURE 19-4. Potential sites of botulinum neurotoxin type A (BoNT/A) modulation within bladder sensory pathways. By decreasing local pools of transmitters, growth factors, and sensory receptors, BoNT/A could thereby inhibit bladder afferent nerve activity, particularly in conditions of increased excitability (e.g., detrusor overactivity). *See Color Plate*

Further research is needed to characterize the protein receptors to which BoNT binds, to expand our understanding of light chain translocation within the motor neuron, to establish the process by which the light chain interacts with SNAP-25, and to explore the toxin's long-term effects on smooth muscle cells. Although there has been speculation that diffusion or proteolysis of the toxin's light chain eventually occurs, the mechanism that accounts for the durability as well as the loss of toxin action remains to be determined.

Commonly occurring urologic conditions like detrusor overactivity are often characterized by involuntary contractions of the detrusor muscle. BoNT acts by binding to the nerve endings within muscles, blocking the release of ACh, and probably other neurotransmitters, to modulate muscle contraction and reduce the sensitization of sensory nerve endings (Fig. 19-4). Selective injection permits specific paralysis of the detrusor muscle while leaving surrounding tissues and distant muscles unaffected. Therapy with BoNT would appear to not only help alleviate muscle spasticity but, in view of its proposed anti-nociceptive properties and impact on sensory feedback loops, could provide substantial relief of hyperalgesia associated with a variety of lower urinary tract disorders.

References

1. Schurch B, de Sèze M, Denys P, Chartier-Kastler E, Haab F, Everaert K, et al. Botulinum toxin type a is a safe and effective treatment for neurogenic urinary incontinence: results of a single treatment, randomized, placebo controlled 6-month study. *J Urol.* 2005;174:196-200.
2. Simpson LL. The action of botulinal toxin. *Rev Infect Dis.* 1979;1:656-662.
3. Atiemo H, Wynes J, Chuo J, Nipkow L, Sklar GN, Chai TC. Effect of botulinum toxin on detrusor overactivity induced by intravesical adenosine triphosphate and capsaicin in a rat model. *Urology.* 2005;65:622-626.
4. Holman ME, Spitzer NC. Action of botulinum toxin on transmission from sympathetic nerves to the vas deferens. *Br J Pharmacol.* 1973;47:431-433.
5. Pasricha PJ, Ravich WJ, Kalloo AN. Effects of intrasphincteric botulinum toxin on the lower esophageal sphincter in piglets. *Gastroenterology.* 1993;105:1045-1049.
6. Filippi GM, Errico P, Santarelli R, Bagolini B, Manni E. Botulinum A toxin effects on rat jaw muscle spindles. *Acta Otolaryngol.* 1993;113:400-404.
7. Rosales RL, Arimura K, Takenaga S, Osame M. Extrafusal and intrafusal muscle effects in experimental botulinum toxin-A injection. *Muscle Nerve.* 1996;19:488-496.
8. Modugno N, Priori A, Berardelli A, Vacca L, Mercuri B, Manfredi M. Botulinum toxin restores presynaptic inhibition of group Ia afferents in patients with essential tremor. *Muscle Nerve.* 1998;21:1701-1705.

9. Giannantoni A, Di Stasi SM, Nardicchi V, Zucchi A, Macchioni L, Bini V, et al. Botulinum-A toxin injections into the detrusor muscle decrease nerve growth factor bladder tissue levels in patients with neurogenic detrusor overactivity. *J Urol.* 2006;175:2341-2344.

10. Borodic GE, Ferrante R. Effects of repeated botulinum toxin injections on orbicularis oculi muscle. *J Clin Neuroophthalmol.* 1992;12:121-127.

11. Spencer RF, McNeer KW. Botulinum toxin paralysis of adult monkey extraocular muscle. Structural alterations in orbital, singly innervated muscle fibers. *Arch Ophthalmol.* 1987;105:1703-1711.

12. Harris CP, Alderson K, Nebeker J, Holds JB, Anderson RL. Histologic features of human orbicularis oculi treated with botulinum A toxin. *Arch Ophthalmol.* 1991;109:393-395.

13. Borodic GE, Mills L, Joseph M. Botulinum A toxin for the treatment of adult-onset spasmodic torticollis. *Plast Reconstr Surg.* 1991;87:285-289.

14. Thesleff S, Molgo J, Tagerud S. Trophic interrelations at the neuromuscular junction as revealed by the use of botulinal neurotoxins. *J Physiol (Paris).* 1990;84:167-173.

15. de Paiva A, Meunier FA, Molgo J, Aoki KR, Dolly JO. Functional repair of motor endplates after botulinum neurotoxin type A poisoning: biphasic switch of synaptic activity between nerve sprouts and their parent terminals. *Proc Natl Acad Sci U S A.* 1999;96: 3200-3205.

16. Alderson K, Holds JB, Anderson RL. Botulinum-induced alteration of nerve-muscle interactions in the human orbicularis oculi following treatment for blepharospasm. *Neurology.* 1991;41:1800-1805.

17. Juzans P, Comella JX, Molgo J, Faille L, Angaut-Petit D. Nerve terminal sprouting in botulinum type-A treated mouse levator auris longus muscle. *Neuromuscul Disord.* 1996;6:177-185.

18. Angaut-Petit D, Molgo J, Comella JX, Faille L, Tabti N. Terminal sprouting in mouse neuromuscular junctions poisoned with botulinum type A toxin: morphological and electrophysiological features. *Neuroscience.* 1990;37:799-808.

19. Van Putten MJ, Padberg M, Tavy DL. In vivo analysis of end-plate noise of human extensor digitorum brevis muscle after intramuscularly injected botulinum toxin type A. *Muscle Nerve.* 2002;26:784-790.

20. Chancellor MB, O'Leary M, Erickson J, Cannon TW, Chermansky C, Leng WW, et al. Successful use of bladder botulinum toxin injection to treat refractory overactive bladder [abstract DP50]. 98th Annual Meeting of the American Urological Association 2003, Chicago, IL, USA.

21. Popat R, Apostolidis A, Kalsi V, Gonzales G, Fowler CJ, Dasgupta P. A comparison between the response of patients with idiopathic detrusor overactivity and neurogenic detrusor overactivity to the first intradetrusor injection of botulinum-A toxin. *J Urol.* 2005; 174:984-989.

22. Smith CP, Nishiguchi J, O'Leary M, Yoshimura N, Chancellor MB. Single-institution experience in 110 patients with botulinum toxin A injection into bladder or urethra. *Urology.* 2005;65:37-41.

23. Smith CP, Franks ME, McNeil BK, Ghosh R, de Groat WC, Chancellor MB. Effect of botulinum toxin A on the autonomic nervous system of the rat lower urinary tract. *J Urol.* 2003;169:1896.

24. Somogyi GT, Tanowitz M, Zernova G, de Groat WC. M1 muscarinic receptor-induced facilitation of ACh and noradrenaline release in the rat bladder is mediated by protein kinase C. *J Physiol.* 1996;496(Pt 1):245-254.

25. Chu FM, Dmochowski R. Pathophysiology of overactive bladder. *Am J Med.* 2006;119(3 suppl 1):3-8.

26. Somogyi GT, Zernova GV, Yoshiyama M, Yamamoto T, de Groat WC. Frequency dependence of muscarinic facilitation of transmitter release in urinary bladder strips from neurally intact or chronic spinal cord transected rats. *Br J Pharmacol.* 1998;125:241-246.

27. Apostolidis A, Dasgupta P, Fowler CJ. Proposed mechanism for the efficacy of injected botulinum toxin in the treatment of human detrusor overactivity. *Eur Urol.* 2006;49:644-650.

28. MacKenzie I, Burnstock G, Dolly JO. The effects of purified botulinum neurotoxin type A on cholinergic, adrenergic and non-adrenergic, atropine-resistant autonomic neuromuscular transmission. *Neuroscience.* 1982;7:997-1006.

29. Kim HJ, Seo K, Yum KW, Oh YS, Yoon TG, Yoon SM. Effects of botulinum toxin type A on the superior cervical ganglia in rabbits. *Auton Neurosci.* 2002;102:8.

30. Morris JL, Jobling P, Gibbins IL. Differential inhibition by botulinum neurotoxin A of cotransmitters released from autonomic vasodilator neurons. *Am J Physiol Heart Circ Physiol.* 2001;281:H2124.

31. Ishikawa H, Mitsui Y, Yoshitomi T, Mashimo K, Aoki S, Mukono K, et al. Presynaptic effects of botulinum toxin type A on the neuronally evoked response of albino and pigmented rabbit iris sphincter and dilator muscles. *Nippon Ganka Gakkai Zasshi.* 2001;105:218.

32. Smith CP, Boone TB, de Groat WC, Chancellor MB, Somogyi GT. Effect of stimulation intensity and botulinum toxin isoform on rat bladder strip contractions. *Brain Res Bull.* 2003;61:165.

33. O'Reilly BA, Kosaka AH, Knight GF, Chang TK, Ford AP, Rymer JM, et al. P2X receptors and their role in female idiopathic detrusor instability. *J Urol.* 2002;167:157-164.

34. Hawthorn MH, Chapple CR, Cock M, Chess-Williams R. Urothelium-derived inhibitory factor(s) influence detrusor muscle contractility in vitro. *Br J Pharmacol.* 2000;129:416-419.

35. Wakabayashi Y, Kojima Y, Makiura Y, Tomoyoshi T, Maeda T. Acetylcholinesterase positive axons in the mucosa of urinary bladder of adult cats: retrograde tracing and degeneration studies. *Histol Histopathol.* 1995;10:523-530.

36. Andersson KE, Yoshida M. Antimuscarinics and the overactive detrusor—which is the main mechanism of action. *Eur Urol.* 2003;43:1-5.

37. Khera M, Somogyi GT, Kiss S, Boone TB, Smith CP. Botulinum toxin A inhibits ATP release from bladder urothelium after chronic spinal cord injury. *Neurochem Int.* 2004;45:987-993.

38. Rapp DE, Turk KW, Bales GT, Cook SP. Botulinum toxin type A inhibits calcitonin gene-related peptide release from isolated rat bladder. *J Urol.* 2006;175(3 Pt 1):1138-1142.

39. Chuang YC, Yoshimura N, Huang CC, Chiang PH, Chancellor MB. Intravesical botulinum toxin A administration produces analgesia against acetic acid induced bladder pain responses in rats. *J Urol.* 2004; 172(4 Pt 1):1529-1532.

40. Bayliss M, Wu C, Newgreen D, Mundy AR, Fry CH. A quantitative study of atropine-resistant contractile responses in human detrusor smooth muscle, from stable, unstable and obstructed bladders. *J Urol.* 1999;162:1833-1839.

41. Sperlagh B, Vizi ES. Is the neuronal ATP release from guinea-pig vas deferens subject to alpha 2-adrenoceptor-mediated modulation? *Neuroscience.* 1992;51: 203-209.

42. Todorov LD, Mihaylova-Todorova S, Craviso GL, Bjur RA, Westfall DP. Evidence for the differential release of the cotransmitters ATP and noradrenaline from sympathetic nerves of the guinea-pig vas deferens. *J Physiol.* 1996;496(Pt 3):731-748.

43. Tong YC, Hung YC, Shinozuka K, Kunitomo M, Cheng JT. Evidence of adenosine 5'-triphosphate release from nerve and P2x-purinoceptor mediated contraction during electrical stimulation of rat urinary bladder smooth muscle. *J Urol.* 1997;158:1973-1977.

44. Ferguson DR, Kennedy I, Burton TJ. ATP is released from rabbit urinary bladder epithelial cells by hydrostatic pressure changes—a possible sensory mechanism? *J Physiol.* 1997;505(Pt 2):503-511.

45. Birder LA, Nakamura Y, Kiss S, Nealen ML, Barrick S, Kanai AJ, et al. Altered urinary bladder function in mice lacking the vanilloid receptor TRPV1. *Nat Neurosci.* 2002;5:856-860.

46. Ferguson DR. Urothelial function. *BJU Int.* 1999;84:235-242.

47. Sun Y, Keay S, De Deyne PG, Chai TC. Augmented stretch activated adenosine triphosphate release from bladder uroepithelial cells in patients with interstitial cystitis. *J Urol.* 2001;166:1951-1956.

48. Ford AP, Gever JR, Nunn PA, Zhong Y, Cefalu JS, Dillon MP, et al. Purinoceptors as therapeutic targets for lower urinary tract dysfunction. *Br J Pharmacol.* 2006;147(Suppl 2):S132-S143.

49. Paukert M, Osteroth R, Geisler HS, Brandle U, Glowatzki E, Ruppersberg JP, et al. Inflammatory mediators potentiate ATP-gated channels through the P2X(3) subunit. *J Biol Chem.* 2001;276:21077-21082.

50. Cortright DN, Szallasi A. Biochemical pharmacology of the vanilloid receptor TRPV1. *An update.* 2004;271:1814-1819.

51. Morenilla-Palao C, Planells-Cases R, Garcia-Sanz N, Ferrer-Montiel A. Regulated exocytosis contributes to protein kinase C potentiation of vanilloid receptor activity. *J Biol Chem.* 2004;279:25665-25672.

52. Apostolidis A, Popat R, Yiangou Y, Cockayne D, Ford AP, Davis JB, et al. Decreased sensory receptors P2X3 and TRPV1 in suburothelial nerve fibers following intradetrusor injections of botulinum toxin for human detrusor overactivity. *J Urol.* 2005;174: 977-982.

52a. Apostolidis A, Dasgupta P, Fowler CJ. Proposed mechanism for the efficacy of injected botulinum toxin in the treatment of human detrusor overactivity. *Eur Urol.* 2006;49:644-650.

53. Basbaum AI, Jessell TM. The perception of pain. In: Kandel ER, Schwartz JH, Jessell TM, eds. *Principles of Neural Science.* 4th ed. New York: McGraw Hill; 2000:472-491.

54. Aoki KR. Review of a proposed mechanism for the antinociceptive action of botulinum toxin type A. *Neurotoxicology.* 2005;26:785-793.

55. Zubrzycka M, Janecka A. Substance P: transmitter of nociception (Minireview). *Endocr Regul.* 2000;34: 195-201.

56. Steers WD, Tuttle JB. Mechanisms of disease: the role of nerve growth factor in the pathophysiology of bladder disorders. *Nat Clin Pract Urol.* 2006;3:101-110.

57. Giannantoni A, Di Stasi SM, Nardicchi V, Zucchi A, Macchioni L, Bini V, et al. Botulinum-A toxin injections into the detrusor muscle decrease nerve growth factor bladder tissue levels in patients with neurogenic detrusor overactivity. *J Urol.* 2006;175: 2341-2344.

58. Relja M, Telarovic S. Botulinum toxin type-A and pain responsiveness in cervical dystonia: A dose response study. *Mov Disord.* 2005;20:S10.

59. Foster KA. The analgesic potential of clostridial neurotoxin derivatives. *Expert Opin Investig Drugs.* 2004;13:1437-1443.

60. Tarsy D, First ER. Painful cervical dystonia: clinical features and response to treatment with botulinum toxin. *Mov Disord.* 1999;14:1043-1045.

61. Brin MF, Fahn S, Moskowitz C, Friedman A, Shale HM, Greene PE, et al. Localized injections of botulinum toxin for the treatment of focal dystonia and hemifacial spasm. *Adv Neurol.* 1988;50:599-608.

62. Tsui JK, Fross RD, Calne S, Calne DB. Local treatment of spasmodic torticollis with botulinum toxin. *Can J Neurol Sci.* 1987;14(3 suppl):533-535.

63. Haferkamp A, Schurch B, Reitz A, Krengel U, Grosse J, Kramer G, et al. Lack of ultrastructural detrusor changes following endoscopic injection of botulinum toxin type A in overactive neurogenic bladder. *Eur Urol.* 2004;46:784-791.

64. Comperat E, Reitz A, Delcourt A, Capron F, Denys P, Chartier-Kastler E. Histologic features in the urinary bladder wall affected from neurogenic overactivity—a comparison of inflammation, oedema and fibrosis with and without injection of botulinum toxin type A. *Eur Urol.* 2006;50:1058-1064.

65. Mejia NI, Vuong KD, Jankovic J. Long-term botulinum toxin efficacy, safety, and immunogenicity. *Mov Disord.* 2005;20:592-597.

66. Coletti Moja M, Dimanico U, Mongini T, Cavaciocchi V, Gerbino Promis PC, Grasso E. Acute neuromuscular failure related to long-term botulinum toxin therapy. *Eur Neurol.* 2004;51:181-183.

67. Grosse J, Kramer G, Stohrer M. Success of repeat detrusor injections of botulinum a toxin in patients with severe neurogenic detrusor overactivity and incontinence. *Eur Urol.* 2005;47:653-659.

68. Altaweel W, Jednack R, Bilodeau C, Corcos J. Repeated intradetrusor botulinum toxin type A in children with neurogenic bladder due to myelomeningocele. *J Urol.* 2006;175(3 Pt 1):1102-1105.

69. Schulte-Baukloh H, Weiss C, Stolze T, Sturzebecher B, Knispel HH. Botulinum-A toxin for treatment of overactive bladder without detrusor overactivity: urodynamic outcome and patient satisfaction. *Urology.* 2005;66:82-87.

70. Schulte-Baukloh H, Knispel HH, Stolze T, Weiss C, Michael T, Miller K. Repeated botulinum-A toxin injections in treatment of children with neurogenic detrusor overactivity. *Urology.* 2005;66:865-870; discussion 870.

71. Kessler TM, Danuser H, Schumacher M, Studer UE, Burkhard FC. Botulinum A toxin injections into the detrusor: an effective treatment in idiopathic and neurogenic detrusor overactivity? *Neurourol Urodyn.* 2005;24:231-236.

72. Kuo HC. Clinical effects of suburothelial injection of botulinum A toxin on patients with nonneurogenic detrusor overactivity refractory to anticholinergics. *Urology.* 2005;66:94-98.

73. Meunier FA, Schiavo G, Molgo J. Botulinum neurotoxins: from paralysis to recovery of functional neuromuscular transmission. *J Physiol (Paris).* 2002;96:105-113.

Botulinum Toxin in 20 Overactive Bladder

Brigitte Schurch and Dennis Dykstra

SUMMARY

Anticholinergics are usually the gold standard used to treat overactive bladder (OAB). Side effects and lack of efficacy are the two main causes for considering alternative treatments. Until recently, invasive surgery (mainly bladder augmentation) was the only available treatment option for these intractable bladders. This chapter considers botulinum neurotoxin (BoNT) injection as an alternative treatment to surgery in patients with detrusor overactivity (DO) in whom anticholinergic therapy has failed.

There is convincing evidence that BoNT injection into the detrusor is a very effective method to treat urinary incontinence secondary to neurogenic detrusor overactivity (NDO) as well as to idiopathic detrusor overactivity (IDO). In both conditions, the duration of effect is at least 6 months. The overall success rate seems to be similar in both patient populations. For NDO, two evidence-based medicine level 1 studies are available; for IDO only evidence-based medicine level 3 or 4 studies have been published. Injection technique and outcome parameters vary from study to study, and standardization is required. Outcome following repeated injections has been the object of several publications: the efficacy remains as good as after the first injection, and there is no evidence of change in bladder compliance or detrusor fibrosis. However, long-term observation studies remain necessary to assess these last points. To date, there is no proposed clear ratio for Botox or Dysport for treatment of NDO or IDO. However, clinical experience using 200-300 units Botox or 500-750 units Dysport are comparable. The current BoNT/A (Botox versus Dysport) reported dose appears to be safe, and few side effects have been reported by using these toxins.

INTRODUCTION

The report of the International Continence Society (ICS) of 2002 has defined the overactive bladder syndrome as urgency, with or without urge incontinence, usually with frequency and nocturia, in the absence of local pathologic or hormonal factors.[1] DO is defined as urodynamic observation characterized by involuntary detrusor contractions during the filling phase that may be spontaneous or provoked. Detrusor overactivity is subdivided into NDO when there is an established neurologic cause, or IDO when no known cause for the overactivity is present. Anticholinergic medication has been the primary treatment for patients with OAB in recent years. These drugs act on muscarinic receptors as competitive inhibitors of acetylcholine (Ach) and inhibit involuntary bladder contractions. Unfortunately, they are also associated with troublesome side effects, including dry mouth, constipation, blurred vision, drowsiness, and tachycardia. Newer, slow-release or long-acting preparations of tolterodine and oxybutynin, the two most common drugs prescribed in OAB, have fewer side effects.[2,3] However, some patients cannot tolerate even these side effects and suffer from a poor quality of life (QoL).

Alternative pharmacologic agents are being investigated and include potassium channel openers,[4] beta-3 adrenoreceptor agonists,[5] alpha-1 adrenoreceptor antagonists,[6] and neurokinin receptor antagonists.[7] Alternative methods of drug delivery for traditional anticholinergics have also been tried and include

Dr. Schurch is disclosing that she is a consultant for Allergan, Inc., Irvine, CA; Astellas, Switzerland; Pfizer, Switzerland; Pfizer, England; and receives lecture fees from Allergan, Irvine, CA and Allergan, Switzerland and Astellas International. Dr. Dykstra is disclosing that he has been a lecturer and consultant for Allergan and Solstice.

intravesical preparations[8] and transdermal application of oxybutynin.[9] Intravesical application of vanilloid substances has been tried as an alternative treatment for patients with severe DO who did not tolerate side effects from anticholinergic drugs.[10,11] However, results have been disappointing or not yet fully evaluated. BoNT is another highly effective second-line treatment for patients who have urodynamically proven DO. After systemic absorption, BoNT binds irreversibly to the presynaptic nerve endings, where it inhibits the release of Ach and blocks the signal transduction to the target organ: muscle or gland. In the initial report of botulism, an often deadly poisoning, a complete urinary retention and bowel paralysis were mentioned.[12] After weeks or even months of recovery, the symptoms of the intoxication disappear in inverse order and a restoration of all disturbed body functions can be observed. The action of the toxin is reversed by the synthesis of new SNARE proteins; therefore, for medical purposes, BoNT treatment must be repeated to guarantee a constant therapeutic effect.

MECHANISM OF ACTION

The mechanism of action of BoNT in the detrusor has been described in detail in Chapter 19 and will be only summarized here.

Most of the effects of BoNT are thought to result from the inhibition of Ach release from the presynaptic nerve terminal. When this occurs, Ach receptors in the muscle are not stimulated. Specifically with intradetrusor injections, affected muscarinic receptors in the detrusor muscle cannot be stimulated and detrusor in voluntary contractions are suppressed. Review of the clinical data shows a profound effect of BoNT on involuntary detrusor contractions and elevated detrusor pressures. However, it is clear that neurotransmitters other than Ach are also affected by BoNT, including sensory/afferent neurotransmitters. It is likely that these also play a role in the therapeutic effects of BoNT in OAB. Botulinum toxin type A (BoNT/A) has been found to inhibit Ach and adenosine triphosphate release from urothelium in rats and guinea pigs.[13,14] BoNT/A has been shown to inhibit stimulated (but not basal) release of calcitonin gene–related peptide (CGRP) from trigeminal ganglia neurons[15] and sensory neurons in the isolated rat bladder.[16] BoNT/A has also been shown to inhibit the release of glutamate[17] and substance P[18]

from sensory neurons. Apostolidis and colleagues[19] studied human bladder biopsy specimens from patients with NDO and IDO. They found that BoNT/A-treated bladders had decreased levels of TRPV1 (vanilloids) and P2X3 (purinergic), two sensory receptors found in the suburothelium.

Two recent publications addressed the effects of acute BoNT/A treatment on the detrusor muscle. Comperat et al[20] studied cystectomy specimens from patients with NDO who received or did not receive BoNT/A injections. The investigators found no difference in inflammation or edema between the groups, but there was significantly less fibrosis in the BoNT/A-treated bladders. Giannantoni et al[21] found that BoNT/A decreased bladder tissue content of nerve growth factor (NGF) at 1 and 3 months after treatment. They theorized that this occurred either as a result of decreased Ach or other neurotransmitter release at the presynaptic level. NGF has a key role in the survival of sensory neurons maintaining the normal properties of C afferent fibers. All of these data help support the belief that BoNT/A works to treat DO and OAB by both sensory and motor pathways and may have a positive effect on bladder wall structure and fibrosis. Confirmatory studies regarding the latter are necessary to make definitive conclusions.

BOTULINUM NEUROTOXIN: INTRADETRUSOR INJECTION TECHNIQUE

A number of variables must be considered for BoNT administration, including type and amount of toxin; dilution volume; location, number, and depth of injections; instrumentation; and anesthesia technique. A number of protocols have been proven to work well; however, the optimal amount and dilution of toxin and injection site protocol have not been established. Tables 20-1 and 20-2 summarize these variables for the trials discussed in this chapter. As one can imagine, with so many variables involved, establishing an "optimal protocol" is very challenging. Most of the work on IDO and NDO has been done with BoNT/A, with few studies on BoNT type B. The Botox formulation of BoNT/A has been studied the most; however, there are a number of studies on Dysport as well. At this time, Botox is the only formulation of BoNT/A available in

TABLE 20-1 NDO and BoNT Injection

Author	Year	Number of Patients NDO	Dose (U)	Vol/Inj (mL)	Number of Injections	Duration (Months)	Success Rate*	Reported Side Effects: (Number of Patients)
Adults								
Schurch et al[25]	2000	21	Botox 300	1.0	30 sparing trigone	9	89%	
Del Popolo et al[37]	2003	93	Dysport 500, 750, 1000	Not reported	20–30 sparing trigone	At least 4 months	100%	Hypoastenia (5)
Harper et al[76]	2003	39 (mixed cohort NDO and IDO)	Botox 300 Botox 200	1.0 1.0	20–30 sparing trigone	4	100%	
Loch et al[54]	2003	30 (mixed cohort NDO and IDO)	Botox 200	Not reported	20 sparing trigone	8	67%	Acute retention (1)
Kennely et al[39]	2003	10	Botox 300	1.0	30 sparing trigone	Up to 6	73%	
Reitz et al[33]	2004	200	Botox 300	1.0	30 sparing trigone	9	96%	
Giannantoni et al[34]	2004	40	Botox 300	1.0	30 sparing trigone	6–8	73%	Mild asthenia (1)
Giannantoni et al[39]	2004	12	Botox 300	1.0	30 sparing trigone		75%	
Kuo[40]	2004	12	Botox 200	0.2	40 sparing trigone	5.3 (3–9)	73.3%	Not reported
Bagi and Petersen[87]	2004	15	Dysport 500, 750, 1000	1.0	30 sparing trigone	7	87%	
Patki et al[35]	2006	37	Dysport 1000	Not reported	30 trigone not stated	9	82%	Transient general weakness (2)

Grosse et al[77]	2005	66	Botox 300 Dysport 750	0.5 0.2	30 sparing trigone 25 sparing trigone	>9	86.3%	Muscle weakness (4) (Dysport group)
Kessler et al[58]	2005	11	Botox 300	1.0	30 sparing trigone	5	72%	CISC (5)
Smith et al[24]	2005	21	Botox 100–300	1.0	10–30 sparing trigone	6	80%	
Klaphajone et al[42]	2005	10	Botox 300	1.0	30 sparing trigone	At least 4	70%	
Hajebrahimi et al[41]	2005	10	Botox 300–400	1.0	30–40 sparing trigone	At least 3	33%	
Popat et al[57]	2005	44	Botox 300	1.0	30 sparing trigone	4	97.4% 64.1% continent	CISC (30)
Schurch et al[32]	2005	59	Botox 200/ 300/ Placebo	1.0	30 sparing trigone	At least 6	83%	
Children								
Schulte-Baukloh et al[44]	2002	17 children with NDO	Botox Max 300 (12 U/kg)	Not reported	30–40 sparing trigone	6	100%	
Schulte-Baukloh et al[45]	2003	20 children with NDO	Botox Max 300 (12 U/kg)	0.3–0.5	30–50 sparing trigone	6	54%	
Riccabona et al[46]	2004	15 children with NDO	Botox Max 300 (10 U/kg)	1.0	25–40 sparing trigone	10.5	100% 86.6% continent	
Corcos et al[47]	2004	20 children with NDO	Botox Max 300 (5/kg)	Not reported	10–30 sparing trigone	8.1	81% 68% continent	

CISC, clean intermittent self-catheterization; IDO, idiopathic detrusor overactivity; NDO, neurogenic detrusor overactivity.
*Based on reduced incontinence episode.

TABLE 20-2 IDO and BoNT injection

Authors	Year	Number of Patients IDO	Dose (U)	Vol/Inj	Number of Injections	Duration (months)	Success Rate*	Reported Side Effects: (Number of Patients)
Radziszweski et al[55]	2002	12	Dysport 300	0.1-0.2	10–15 sparing trigone	1 (follow-up)	100%	
Loch et al[54] See Table 20-1	2003							
Flynn et al[56]	2004	7	Botox 150	0.2	10-12 sparing trigone	3-6	100%	
Kuo[40]	2004	30	Botox 200	0.2	40 sparing trigone	5.3 (3-9)	73.3%	
Harper et al[76] See Table 20-1	2003							
Rapp et al[16]	2004	29	Botox 300	0.1	30 including trigone	6	60%	0
Sahai et al[51]	2005	18	Botox 200 vs placebo			3 (follow-up)		Retention (3)
Kessler et al[58]	2005	11	Botox 300	1.0	30 sparing trigone	5	91%	Retention (4 plus 1 SPC)
Rajkumar et al[52]	2005	15	Botox 300	1.0	30 sparing trigone	6	96%	
Dykstra et al[53]	2005	15	Myobloc BTXB 2500, 3750, 5000, 10000, 15000	0.4	10 sparing trigone	mean 6 weeks (range 10-52)	93%	General malaise and dry mouth (2 receiving 15000 units)
Schulte-Baukloh et al[44]	2005	7	Botox 300 including trigone 50–100 into sphincter if evidence of PVR	<0.5	40	>6	86%	

Schulte-Baukloh et al[44]	2005	44	Botox 200–300 including trigone 50–100 into sphincter if evidence of PVR	<0.5	40–50	6	86%	
Ghei et al[65]	2005	20 (3 NOB)	BoNT/B—5000 or placebo	0.2	20 sparing trigone	>6 weeks	Decrease frequency and incontinence episode	Retention (2) Dry mouth and malaise (2)
Kuo[22]	2005	20	Botox 200	0.4	10 suburothelial, sparing trigone	>6	85% 45% continent	Retention (6) Difficulty in voiding (15)
Popat et al[57]	2005	31	Botox 200	1.0	20 sparing trigone	4	92% 54.2% continent	Retention (6)
Werner et al[49]	2005	26	Botox 100	1.0	30 sparing trigone	>9	100%	
Schmid et al[60]	2006	100	Botox 100	1.0	30 sparing trigone	9 (7–11)	88%	Retention (4)

BoNT/B, botulinum neurotoxin type B; IDO, idiopathic detrusor overactivity; PVR, postvoid residual volume; SPC, suprapubic catheter.
*Based on reduced incontinence episode. Reduction of number of incontinence has not been analyzed here because most of the papers differ, some authors using the percentage of patients who improved and others using the percentage improvement in the number of urinary incontinence episodes. Also assessment of frequency and urgency differs from author to author.

the United States. BoNT has been injected directly into the detrusor in almost all studies. One investigator has reported on submucosal injections, perhaps to take advantage of the presumed effect on afferent sensory nerves.[22] In the initial studies, toxin was injected into the lateral and posterior bladder wall, sparing the dome (to avoid intraperitoneal injection) and the trigone. The trigone was avoided because of the fear of reflux, but this has not turned out to be a problem in series in which the trigone was injected.[23] Nevertheless, because initial protocols spared the trigone, many subsequent studies did as well (see Tables 20-1 and 20-2).

Some investigators have proposed injecting the bladder base and trigone only, but the usefulness of this technique needs to be confirmed.[24] The dilution of toxin and the amount of liquid injected into the bladder have also varied. Initial studies diluted 100 U of Botox in 10 mL of preservative-free normal saline.[25] Although more concentrated dilutions have been used, most experts agree that a higher volume (e.g., at least 5 mL per 100 U Botox) provides better coverage of the bladder.[26] Thus, based on the current literature, 10 to 30 mL of total volume injected (the same would apply for Botox, Dysport, or type B toxin) seems a reasonable estimate. The number of injection sites has varied from 10 to 50, with most studies doing 20 to 30 injections (see Tables 20-1 and 20-2). To see how much of the bladder was covered by injections, Boy and colleagues[27] injected six patients who had NDO with BoNT/A (Botox) plus a magnetic tracer and then studied the patients with magnetic resonance imaging to determine the dispersion of the injected liquid. Two common volumes were used: three patients received 300 U in 30 mL normal saline at 30 sites (10 U/site), and three patients received 300 U in 10 mL normal saline at 10 sites (30 U/site). Both protocols achieved good coverage, with the larger volume covering 33% of bladder versus 25% for the smaller volume. Overall, 12.9% of the liquid was found in the perivesical fat.

BoNT can be delivered with a rigid or flexible cystoscope, depending on patient or surgeon preference. Rigid systems allow for quicker, more controllable injections, whereas flexible scopes are generally more comfortable for patients, especially men. Both local and general anesthesia has been used for BoNT injection. We have found local anesthesia to work well, with excellent patient tolerability,

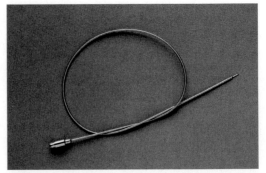

FIGURE 20-1. Flexible injection needle for detrusor muscle injection (Storz, Charr. 8, length: 50 cm).

and to be ideal for the office setting. Conscious sedation may also be used for more anxious or sensitive patients, although we rarely find it necessary. General anesthesia may be considered for extremely anxious or sensitive patients and for neurogenic patients who are at high risk for autonomic dysreflexia. General anesthesia is required for most pediatric applications.

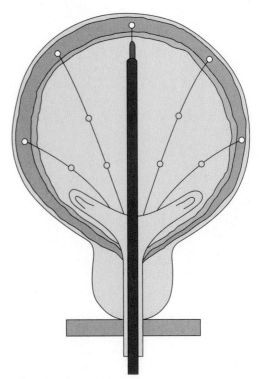

FIGURE 20-2. Detrusor mapping.

NEUROGENIC DETRUSOR OVERACTIVITY

Especially in neurogenic patients, side effects of oral anticholinergic medication like dry mouth, constipation, dyspepsia, changes in visual accommodation, dizziness, and somnolence are troublesome and reduce patient compliance.[28-31] The effect of injecting BoNT/A into the human detrusor muscle in spinal cord–injured patients was first reported by our group in a nonrandomized prospective study.[25] The patients with spinal cord injury selected for this first clinical study had severe NDO and suffered from incontinence resistant to anticholinergic drugs. One of the main inclusion criteria was that patients had to be able to perform intermittent self-catheterization. Patients with low bladder compliance due to organic detrusor muscle changes or fibrosis were excluded. Using a rigid cystoscope, 200 to 400 U Botox were injected into the detrusor muscle, sparing the trigone (Figs. 20-1 and 20-2). The reason for sparing the trigone was to avoid vesicorenal reflux (see earlier) and the lack of knowledge about the effect of BoNT/A on the adrenergic nerves and on the release of nociceptive neuropeptides. In total, 19 of the 21 treated patients could be regularly observed over a period of 9 months by clinical and urodynamic checks. Six-week follow-up showed a significant increase in the reflex volume (RV) and in the maximum cystometric bladder capacity. There was also a significant decrease in the maximum detrusor voiding pressure. At the 36-week follow-up, ongoing improvement occurred. The amount of oral anticholinergics could be reduced or even completely abolished. Continence was restored in all but two patients, and patients' satisfaction was high. The further experience of the European group increased to 200 patients with the same result profile.[33]

The first controlled study of BoNT/A in NDO was reported by Giannantoni et al[34] in 2004. They randomized patients with NDO to receive either 300 U BoNT/A (Botox) (diluted in 30 mL, 30 injection sites) or 0.6 umol/L of intravesical resiniferotoxin (RTX) in 50 mL of sodium chloride (NaCl) 0.9%. Repeat injections or instillations were allowed. Both treatments resulted in improvement in continence and urodynamic parameters at 6, 12, and 18 months; however, the improvements were significantly better with BoNT/A for all variables at all time points. In addition, patients administered RTX received a mean of 8.6 instillations, whereas patients administered BoNT/A received a mean of 2.1 injections over an 18-month period.

A recent multicenter, randomized, placebo-controlled, 24-week study, examining the effect of two different doses of BoNT/A (200 and 300 Botox U) injected into the detrusor to treat NDO has confirmed the efficacy and safety of this treatment.[32] Out of the recruited 59 patients, 57 completed the study. The mean reduction of urinary incontinence (UI) was about 50% at all posttreatment time points in the BoNT/A groups and none in the placebo group ($P < 0.05$). Overall, 29 patients (49.2%) reported no UI episodes for at least 1 week post-treatment period, of whom 24 (82.8%) were in the BoNT/A treatment group. Significant changes in key urodynamic parameters versus baseline were observed in each BoNT/A group at all time points after treatment, which was not the case for the placebo group ($P < 0.05$). There were robust improvements in the mean change from baseline in incontinence quality of life (QoL) questionnaire (I-QOL) total scores in patients treated with BoNT/A at all post-treatment time points ($P < 0.002$), which were maintained throughout the 24 study weeks. Two hundred units appeared to work as well as 300 units regarding all outcome parameters (clinic and urodynamic). However, no definitive conclusion can be drawn regarding the best dose to be used for NDO because the study was not powered to compare 200 and 300 units. Moreover, differences between 200 and 300 units might have been seen if the study would have been prolonged into a 36-week study.

Recently, Patki et al[35] reported on the first prospective assessment of intradetrusor injections of Dysport as treatment for drug-resistant NDO in spinal cord–injured patients. One thousand units were cystoscopically injected (30 injection sites) into the detrusor, in 37 patients with drug-resistant NDO. Maximum cystometric capacity (MCC), maximum detrusor pressure (MDP), NDO, continence and oral anticholinergic requirement were used as outcome parameters. The International Consultation on Incontinence questionnaire (ICIQ) was used to assess QoL pre- and post-injection. Mean follow-up was 7 months. Maximum cystometric capacity increased from a mean 259 mL to 521.5 mL. Maximum detrusor pressure decreased from a mean 54.3 cmH_2O to 24.4 cmH_2O. Incontinence and NDO were abolished in 82% and 76% patients, respectively. Eighty-six percent of the patients were able to stop or reduce anticholinergics, with a similar number of patients scoring favorably on ICIQ. The mean period of improvement was 9 months. Acceptable failure rates with 24% persistence of NDO and 18% persistence of incontinence were observed. An even more recently published study compared a single injection of BoNT/A (500 units Dysport, diluted in 25 mL saline and injected into 25 injection sites) with placebo in 31 patients with NDO and urinary incontinence. Time of follow-up was 26 weeks. Patients in the BoNT/A group had a significant change regarding intake of anticholinergic drugs, cystometric bladder capacitiy, maximum detrusor pressure, frequency of urinary leakage, and QoL parameters.[36]

Other groups have also reported positive effects of BoNT/A injected into the detrusor to treat NDO.[22,34,37-42] Their results are summarized in Table 20-1.

Myelomeningocele

About 10% of the children with myelomeningocele (MMC) and NDO are nonresponders to anticholinergic medication or suffer of side effects from anticholinergic drugs, even if administered intravesically.[43] There is increasing evidence that BoNT is a highly effective second-line treatment for children with MMC and NDO. Only four prospective studies have evaluated the efficacy of BoNT/A injection in the pediatric neurogenic population and NDO. Schulte-Baukloh injected 20 children with NDO and MMC with 12 U/kg (maximum 300 U) Botox. Urodynamic follow-up at 2 and 4 weeks revealed significant increases in mean MCC (35% increase) as well as significant decreases in MDP (41% decrease).[44,45] However, while significant increases in MCC were demonstrated up to 6 months after treatment, no significant difference in MDP was seen at 3- to 6-month follow-up.

A more recent pediatric study with longer follow-up in 15 patients (mean age 5.8 years) supports earlier studies by demonstrating 118% increase in MCC ($P < 0.001$) and a 46% decrease in MDP ($P < 0.001$) following BoNT/A injection.[46]

Corcos et al[47] evaluated 20 children with MMC and NDO. Their results were less positive

than those of Schulte-Baukloh and Ricabonna. The lower dose they used might be a reason for this lower efficacy. The clinical effects of BoNT/A in MMC children with NDO lasted on average 6 to 10.5 months and were similar after repeated injection.[46-48] None of these studies reported side effects related to the toxin or the injection procedure.

The results of BoNT injection into the detrusor in children are summarized in Table 20-1.

In Summary

The preliminary results of these prospective studies on NDO are overwhelming, especially considering the fact, that in all these studies the included patients were difficult cases for conservative treatment. This treatment option seems to establish its indication in cases in which anticholinergic medication fails or is intolerable and self-intermittent catheterization can be performed by the patient. This new therapeutic approach also appears to be a valuable alternative to surgery.

IDIOPATHIC OVERACTIVE BLADDER WITH OR WITHOUT DETRUSOR OVERACTIVITY

Experience of BoNT application for IDO differs in dosage, dilution, injection sites, number of injections and injection rate. Most of the published studies deal with low patient numbers and there is often a mixture of both IDO and NDO (see Table 20-2).[22,40,45,49-53]

In 2003, Loch et al[54] reported on the effect of injections of 200 U Botox into the detrusor muscle in 30 patients with severe DO. Twenty of the 30 patients reported improved continence, the effect lasting 8 months. Therapy-resistant patients were all patients with interstitial cystitis. These authors noted high residual volume and one acute retention, that might be explained by the high amount of toxin used for this indication. On the other hand, Radzieszweski and Borkowski observed marked improvement of DO in 12 patients at 1 month follow up without change in the residual volume by using 300 Dysport U.[55]

Flynn et al[56] reported on their open-label uncontrolled clinical trial on seven patients who received 150 U Botox (50 U/mL) at

12 sites for severe urge urinary incontinence. They saw a decrease of more than 50% of symptoms at all visits up to 3 months, with signs of recurrence by 6 months in all subjects.

In a prospective, open-label study, Popat et al[57] injected patients (44 NDO, 31 IDO) who had urgency or urgency incontinence due to urodynamically proven intractable DO with 300 units NDO or 200 Botox U (IDO). All patients improved after BoNT/A treatment, and complete continence was achieved in 60.3%. The continence rate appeared better in patients with NDO at 4 weeks, whereas no difference was noted between the 2 groups at 16 weeks. Of patients with NDO, 69.2% had to perform de novo clean intermittent self-catheterization (CISC) after BoNT/A. Despite using a lower dose, post-treatment incomplete emptying associated with lower urinary tract symptoms (LUTS) that necessitated the use of CISC developed in 19.3% of patients with IDO.

In their prospective study, Kessler et al[58] injected 300 Botox U into the detrusor in 11 patients with IDO and 11 with NDO resistant to anticholinergic treatment. BoNT/A injections into the detrusor had a significant and comparable therapeutic effects in both groups. However, owing to postvoid residuals (PVR) > 150 ml following BoNT/A injections, de novo CISC was necessary in nine patients (four with IDO [36%] and five [45%] with NDO), and in one patient with IDO, a suprapubic catheter was placed.

In their prospective nonrandomized ongoing study, Schmid et al[59,60] evaluated the efficacy and safety of BoNT/A injections into the detrusor muscle to treat patients suffering from IDO resistant to conventional treatment such as anticholinergic drugs. One hundred patients suffering from IDO (including urgency-frequency syndrome) and incontinence despite administration of maximal doses of anticholinergics were consecutively treated by injections of 100 Botox U into the detrusor muscle at 30 different sites under cystoscopic control. Micturition diary, full urodynamics, neurologic status, and urine probes were performed in all participants before treatment. Special attention was given to RV, MCC, detrusor compliance (DC), PVR, urgency, and frequency/nocturia. Clinical and urodynamic checks and QoL assessment (King's Health Questionnaire) were performed at baseline and 4, 12, and 36 weeks after BoNT/A treatment. Overall, after 4 and 12 weeks, 88% of the patients showed a significant ($P < 0.001$) improvement of their

bladder function in regard to subjective symptoms, QoL as well as to urodynamic parameters. Urgency disappeared in 82% and incontinence in 86% within 1 to 2 weeks after BoNT/A injections. Frequency decreased from mean 14 to 7 micturitions/day (-50%) and nocturia from mean 4 to 1.5, respectively. Maximum cystometric bladder capacity increased from mean 246 to 381 mL (+56%), DC rose from mean 24 to 41 mL/cmH$_2$O and pretreatment DO (RV mean 169 mL) improved in 74% of patients. Volume at first desire to void increased from mean 126 to 212 mL, and urge volume increased from mean 214 to 309 mL. There were no severe side effects except four patients had temporary urine retention. In only eight patients, clinical benefit was poor and analysis revealed preoperative very low DC. Efficacy duration lasted 9 (± 2) months.

Only one study showed benefit of BoNT/A in treating children with IDO.[61] Twenty-one children, with a mean age of 10 years, with IDO and daytime incontinence, in whom medical therapy had failed, were injected with 100 U of BoNT (Botox). The authors reported an increase in functional bladder capacity, with a reduction in DO and urgency symptoms.

One of the downsides of using the BoNT/A for IDO is the risk of CISC, which can occur according to the literature in 5% to 45% of patients. This is particularly important in this patient group because they do not usually need any auxiliary means for emptying their bladder. According to the above-mentioned studies, it appears that the risk of needing CISC in IDO increases with the injected dose. However, because only few escalation dose studies have yet been performed, it remains difficult to decide which dose is the best for IDO.[62] Moreover, it is well known that the duration of the effect of the toxin depends on the injected amount.

Thinking in another way, Schulte-Baukloh[50,63] investigated the effect of BoNT/A injections into the detrusor and external sphincter in patients with IDO. They were interested in the benefit of additional sphincter injection in these patients. When small amounts of preoperative residual urine (≥15 mL) were detected, the patients were believed to be at risk for symptomatic residual volume after BoNT/A detrusor injection alone. Twenty-two patients received 200 to 300 Botox U into the detrusor (group D) and 22 "at-risk" patients 200 to 300 Botox U distributed between the detrusor and the external sphincter (group D + S), by which 50 to 100 units of the 200 to 300 units were separately applied into the sphincter. There was no significant difference between the groups after either treatment concerning the primary outcomes (continence, improvement of QoL, and urodynamic parameters). The only difference was that the post-treatment residual volume was higher in the D group than in the D + S group. The authors concluded that for patients who might be expected to have residual urine after injection only into the detrusor, additional injection of a low dose of BoNT/A into the external sphincter muscle could be one option to reduce that risk. However, the definition of "at-risk" patients and especially the volume at which the residual volume has to be considered as problematic. In the Schulte-Baukloh paper,[63] this volume has a mean of 20 mL, which might be entirely physiologic. Moreover, residual volume of the group D patients was on average 80 mL after treatment, indicating that they may not have needed CISC unless symptomatic. Indeed, there is no mention of the need of CISC in the author's report. Different doses between groups were employed, and it is difficult to make a firm judgment on the dose needed in any particular clinical situation. Finally using an additional injection into the external urethral sphincter, one has to carefully counsel these patients about the possible risk of de novo stress incontinence after combined injections because this is a symptom they did not previously have. The authors themselves agreed with the fact that according to the answers given by the patients to the urogenital-distress-distress inventory (UDI-6) questionnaire, a slightly higher incidence of urinary stress incontinence after additional injection into the sphincter muscle could not be excluded. In our opinion, additional sphincter injection might be of value to minimize the risk of retention in IDO at the price of a possible de novo stress incontinence.

In Summary

BoNT injections into the detrusor muscle might represent an alternative treatment for patients with severe IDO resistant to conservative treatment. Before reasonable randomized control studies aiming at comparing different techniques and different dosages are done, it remains difficult to decide what is the best technique to treat patients who suffer from IDO who are not willing to perform CISC. Such studies remain necessary to compare different dosages with the risk of needing CISC in regard to the duration of the effect.

BOTULINUM TOXIN TYPE B AND OVERACTIVE BLADDER

There are only three reports on the primary use of botulinum toxin type B (BoNT/B) in urology. The first is a case report in a female patient with multiple sclerosis, NDO, and reflex incontinence, who was injected with 5000, 7500, and 10000 U Myobloc diluted in 3 mL saline (500 units/injection site in 0.3 mL).[64] After each injection, she was dry without having to catheterize herself. The effect lasted for 4 months. In an open-label dose-escalation study, the same authors aimed at testing the efficacy of BoNT/B in the treatment of 15 patients with non-neurogenic OAB (see Table 20-2).[53] The doses used in this study were 2500, 5000, 7500, 10000, and 15000 U Myobloc diluted in 4 mL normal saline (0.4 mL at 250 units per injection site). A paired t-test of the pre and post frequency difference indicates that these 15 patients experienced an average of 5.27 fewer frequency episodes per day after treatment ($P < 0.001$). The longest duration effect was 3 months using 10000 to 15000 units ($P < 0.001$). Recently, Ghei et al[65] tested the efficacy and safety of BoNT/B for the treatment of the OAB in a randomized, double-blind, placebo-controlled crossover trial. A total of 20 patients, 18 to 80 years old, with DO unresponsive to oral antimuscarinic agents participated in the study. They were injected with either placebo (20 mL normal saline, 10 injection sites) or BoNT/B (5000 units diluted up to 20 mL, 10 injection sites) intravesically in an outpatient setting. After 6 weeks, the treatments were crossed over without washout period. The primary outcome was the paired difference in change in average voided volumes. Frequency, incontinence episodes and paired differences in QoL measured by the King's Health Questionnaire were the secondary outcome measures. The Wilcoxon signed ranks test was used to test the paired difference in change between treatment phases. Little carryover effect was noted in the second-arm placebo, and the placebo data from both arms were included in the analysis. There were statistically significant paired differences in the change in average voided volume, urinary frequency and episodes of incontinence between active treatment and placebo (respectively, $P = 0.012$, $P = 0.033$, $P = 0.001$). There were similarly significant paired differences in the change in QoL affecting five domains of the King's Health Questionnaire (see Table 20-2). The strength of this article is that it is a prospective randomized placebo-controlled study of BoNT/B injection for bladder overactivity. However, one undesirable feature of the study is that the hypothesis was tested on a mixed population of patients (patients with mixed etiologies of DO, three neurogenic and 17 non-neurogenic with detrusor overactivity). This limits the generalizability of the findings. The authors made a strong argument why a crossover design was appropriate, and their data were valid. However, because some studies have shown that BoNT/B might have duration of efficacy of approximately 3 to 4 months, most experts in the field would still question the merit of a crossover at 6 weeks because not all the patients returned to preinjection clinical and urodynamic values assessed at 6 weeks. Most experts would submit that a washout period after the crossover might have been appropriate. Moreover, because there are limited experiences with BoNT/B in the bladder, assessment of duration of response would have been of value.

In two case reports BoNT/B injections (5000 to 7500 U diluted in 20 mL normal saline and 20 injection sites) into the detrusor were used in patients with neurogenic incontinence showing acquired resistance to BoNT/A.[66,67] Resistance to BoNT/A was confirmed by measuring the extensor digitorum brevis compound muscle action potential (CMAP) amplitude elicited by electrical stimulation of the peroneal nerve.[68] Results on bladder dysfunction observed after BoNT/B injections were comparable to those obtained after BoNT/A. However, duration of effect was only 4 to 6 weeks. There is no study published on the use BoNT/B to treat OAB in children.

In Summary

According to these reports, it appears that BoNT/B may be an option for patients with DO who became secondarily resistant to the BoNT/A after repeated injections. However, it must be pointed out that in animal models and in human experiments, the injection of type B toxin in striated muscles has been shown to have a shorter duration of action than the type A toxin.[69,70] This was also observed in the few urologic reports on injection of BoNT/B into the detrusor. When using the type B toxin, this needs to be considered, especially if the intention is to treat the patient primarily with BoNT/B. It should be clear that antibody production against the type A toxin does not necessarily interfere with the type B toxin. Therefore, we think that in patients with a primary resistance to the type A toxin, which we define as the absence of a clinical and urodynamic effect after injection of an adequate dose of the type A toxin in the detrusor smooth muscle, an attempt with the type B toxin may be justified. Both toxins interact with different target proteins, and a primary lack of response to the type A toxin does not necessarily imply a lack of response to the type B toxin.

DURATION OF EFFECT AND REPEATED INJECTION

The recovery of the paralyzed functions has been understood as a nerve sprouting from the nerve terminal, which establishes new neuromuscular junctions.[71,72] However, de Paiva et al[73] observed in a study in mice that the blocked original nerve ending may regain its function after several weeks and that with the return of synaptic function of the original nerve endings the so-called functional nerve sprouts lose their exocytotic activity and disappear. When injected into the smooth detrusor muscle, the effect of BoNT/A lasts usually 6 to 9 months (occasionally up to 12 months), as opposed to BoNT/B, which lasts only a few weeks, as mentioned before.[25,33,74] The reason for the prolonged efficacy in the smooth muscle is unknown, the lack of axonal sprouting observed in detrusor biopsies after toxin injection has been recently discussed.[75] As BoNT injections into the detrusor gain more and more clinical significance in the treatment of DO, a constant efficacy even after repeated injections needs to be ensured. The purpose of one of our recent studies was to assess the effect of repeated BoNT/A injections (300 U Botox) into the detrusor in patients with NDO and incontinence. We evaluated the safety of repeated injections, persistence of the clinical and urodynamic treatment efficacy, and potential changes in bladder compliance. Seventeen patients with NDO who had three or more BoNT/A injections into the detrusor were studied. Clinical and urodynamic data were analysed before the first injection, after the first injection, and after the last repeated injection. No systemic side effects were observed for the total number of 91 injections. Mean number of injections per patient was 5.4, with a range of three to nine. The mean number of incontinence episodes per day decreased from 2.6 per day at baseline to 0 after the first injection, and remained 0 after the last injection. Maximum cystometric bladder capacity and RV increased significantly after the first and last reinjection compared with baseline. Maximum detrusor pressure decreased significantly after the first and last reinjection compared with baseline. No difference in compliance was found among examination 1, 2, and 3.

From the clinical point of view, repeated injections in our patients were as efficient as the first injection. From the urodynamic point of view, repeated injections of BoNT/A remained effective on maximum cystometric bladder capacity and maximum detrusor pressure, and did not have a negative effect on bladder compliance. In particular, the unchanged bladder compliance even after repeated injections suggest that repeated injections into the detrusor muscle do not induce fibrosis of the bladder wall. There was neither evidence of drug tolerance nor exacerbation of regional symptoms, which could have occurred from enhancement of pathological innervation.[76] Our findings are in line with those reported by other teams.

Grosse et al[77] evaluated the effect of two to seven repeated injections of BONT/A to treat NDO due to acquired spinal cord lesions in adults. A sustained clinical improvement was observed at all follow-up examinations. Persistent urodynamic improvement as well as absence of change in the DC was also documented, although only after two reinjections. No increase in drug tolerance after multiple treatments was observed. Recently, in a paediatric population Schulte-Baukloh et al[48] reported on the outcome of repeated BoNT/A injections in children with NDO who had received at least three injections. Although without statistical analysis, there was no evidence for drug tolerance or lack of efficacy as

measured by RV, maximum detrusor pressure, MCBC, and bladder compliance.

Corcos et al[47] reported on repeated injections in a population of 20 patients with MMC (average age 13 years); they showed that the MCC increased from 197.7 mL to 285.3 mL ($P < 0.01$) after the first injection, the maximum detrusor pressure decreased from 44.7 to 29.9 cmH_2O ($P < 0.01$), and the compliance increased from 4.95 to 12.75 mL/cmH_2O ($P < 0.01$). After a second and subsequent treatments (up to four), the same range of improvement was observed in these three parameters.

SIDE EFFECTS OF BOTULINUM TOXIN-A INJECTIONS

In more than 6 years of clinical use of BoNT/A (Botox) in more than 300 patients, including multiple repeated injections in some patients, we have not observed any systemic side effects.[32,33] However, occasionally, systemic side effects have been reported, including a case of fatal heart block after BoNT injection for achalasia, although no direct causal link was established.[78] In general, weakness is an uncommon event following BoNT therapy, although it has been reported as an adverse event in nine patients with NDO following bladder injection with 1000 U Dysport as well as in three patients with NDO following bladder injection with 300 U Botox.[74,79,80] In Patki's study,[35] two cases (5.4%) reported transient self-limiting (4–6 weeks) generalized muscle weakness after injection of 1000 U Dysport into the detrusor. It could be argued that the reduction of total dose to 750 U would avoid this side effect.[74,79] Dykstra and Sidi also noted mild generalized upper extremity weakness in three patients with spinal cord injury following injection of 140 to 240 U Botox into the urethral sphincter.[81] In contrast to the patients treated by Dykstra and Sidi[81] and Del Popolo,[79] who recovered upper extremity function within 2 to 4 weeks, Wyndaele and Van Dromme[80] noted that in their patients with bladder injection, muscle weakness lasted 3 months.

When considering the dose equivalence between the different commercially available BoNTs like Dysport and Botox, it is important to note the different range of ratios mentioned in the literature.[82,83] However, the weight of information from the studies in skeletal muscle diseases would suggest an approximate ratio of 1:3 Botox to Dysport units.[83] As reported by Leippold et al,[84] this ratio has not been established for smooth muscle. Also the technique being the same as for Botox,[32] it is likely that the higher diffusion of Dysport in smooth muscle may be the reason for the systemic side effects.[85] A prior dose-escalation study or randomization to different dosage arms is necessary for deciding optimum Dysport dosage for DO.

COST OF BOTULINUM NEUROTOXIN THERAPY

By using BoNT in urology, one has to be aware that it is a "off-label use" indication. Therefore, treatment is not reimbursed by health insurance. When deciding on long-term or, in case of spinal cord-injured patients, lifetime treatment, the cost factor becomes prohibitive. This issue was assessed by Kalsi et al[86] proposing a cost-effectiveness model for BoNT/A in the treatment of DO. The average cost per patient per injection was 826 pounds. Studies aiming at comparing BoNT costs over years with costs related to enterocystoplasty would be of relevance to evaluate long-term cost-efficiency of each treatment. Also, it is anticipated that the number of patients requiring repeated injections will continually increase. This may have a significant impact on the procedure time required by the urologist.

CONCLUSION

BoNT injections have an increasing place in the urologic therapeutic arsenal. However, it should be pointed out that most of the indications for using BoNT are for diseases refractory to usual conservative treatment and before irreversible surgery. Moreover, large randomized controlled studies are still lacking. They are necessary to prove the efficacy of BoNT injections on an evidence-based medicine level.

References

1. Abrams P, Cardozo L, Fall M, Griffiths D, Rosier P, Ulmsten U, et al. The standardisation of terminology of lower urinary tract function: report from the Standardisation Sub-committee of the International Continence Society. *Neurourol Urodyn.* 2002;21: 167-178.

2. Anderson RU, Mobley D, Blank B, Saltzstein D, Susset J, Brown JS. Once daily controlled versus immediate release oxybutynin chloride for urge urinary incontinence. OROS Oxybutynin Study Group. *J Urol.* 1999;161:1809-1812.

3. Van Kerrebroeck P, Kreder K, Jonas U, Zinner N, Wein A. Tolterodine once-daily: superior efficacy and tolerability in the treatment of the overactive bladder. *Urology.* 2001;57:414-421.

4. Wojdan A, Freeden C, Woods M, Oshiro G, Spinelli W, Colatsky TJ, et al. Comparison of the potassium channel openers, WAY-133537, ZD6169, and celikalim on isolated bladder tissue and in vivo bladder instability in rat. *J Pharmacol Exp Ther.* 1999;289:1410-1418.

5. Igawa Y, Yamazaki Y, Takeda H, Kaidoh K, Akahane M, Ajisawa Y, et al. Relaxant effects of isoproterenol and selective beta3-adrenoceptor agonists on normal, low compliant and hyperreflexic human bladders. *J Urol.* 2001;165:240-244.

6. Noble AJ, Chess-Williams R, Couldwell C, Furukawa K, Uchiyuma T, Korstanje C, et al. The effects of tamsulosin, a high affinity antagonist at functional alpha 1A- and alpha 1D-adrenoceptor subtypes. *Br J Pharmacol.* 1997;120:231-238.

7. Kamo I, Imai S, Okanishi S, Doi T. Possible site of action of TAK-637, a tachykinin NK(1) receptor antagonist, on the micturition reflex in guinea pigs. *Eur J Pharmacol.* 2000;401:235-240.

8. Enzelsberger H, Helmer H, Kurz C. Intravesical instillation of oxybutynin in women with idiopathic detrusor instability: a randomised trial. *Br J Obstet Gynaecol.* 1995;102:929-930.

9. Dmochowski RR, Nitti V, Staskin D, Luber K, Appell R, Davila GW. Transdermal oxybutynin in the treatment of adults with overactive bladder: combined results of two randomized clinical trials. *World J Urol.* 2005;23:263-270.

10. Fowler CJ, Jewkes D, McDonald WI, Lynn B, de Groat WC. Intravesical capsaicin for neurogenic bladder dysfunction. *Lancet.* 1992;339:1239.

11. Cruz F, Guimaraes M, Silva C, Reis M. Suppression of bladder hyperreflexia by intravesical resiniferatoxin. *Lancet.* 1997;350:640-641.

12. Kerner J. *Das Fettgift oder die Fettsäure und ihre Wirkungen auf den tierischen Orgismus; ein Beytrag zur Untersuchung des in Verdorbenen Würsten giftig wirkenden Stoffes,* Stuttgart, Cotta. 1822.

13. Smith CP, Franks ME, McNeil BK, Ghosh R, de Groat WC, Chancellor MB, et al. Effect of botulinum toxin A on the autonomic nervous system of the rat lower urinary tract. *J Urol.* 2003;169:1896-1900.

14. MacKenzie I, Burnstock G, Dolly JO. The effects of purified botulinum neurotoxin type A on cholinergic, adrenergic and non-adrenergic, atropine-resistant autonomic neuromuscular transmission. *Neuroscience.* 1982;7:997-1006.

15. Durham PL, Cady R. Regulation of calcitonin gene-related peptide secretion from trigeminal nerve cells by botulinum toxin type A: implications for migraine therapy. *Headache.* 2004;44:35-42; discussion 43.

16. Rapp DE, Turk KW, Bales GT, Cook SP. Botulinum toxin type a inhibits calcitonin gene-related peptide release from isolated rat bladder. *J Urol.* 2006;175(3 Pt 1):1138-1142.

17. Cui M, Khanijou S, Rubino J, Aoki KR. Subcutaneous administration of botulinum toxin A reduces formalin-induced pain. *Pain.* 2004;107(1-2):125-133.

18. Lucioni A, Bales GT, Turk KW, Lotan T, Cook SP, Rapp DE. Botulinum toxin type A inhibits substance P

release in inflammatory rat bladder model. *J Urol.* 2006;175(4 suppl):91-93.

19. Apostolidis A, Popat R, Yiangou Y, Cockayne D, Ford AP, Davis JB, et al. Decreased sensory receptors P2X3 and TRPV1 in suburothelial nerve fibers following intradetrusor injections of botulinum toxin for human detrusor overactivity. *J Urol.* 2005;174:977-982; discussion 82-83.

20. Comperat E, Reitz A, Delcourt A, Capron F, Denys P, Chartier-Kastler E. Histologic features in the urinary bladder wall affected from neurogenic overactivity—a comparison of inflammation, oedema and fibrosis with and without injection of botulinum toxin type A. *Eur Urol.* 2006;50:1058-1064.

21. Giannantoni A, Di Stasi SM, Nardicchi V, Zucchi A, Macchioni L, Bini V, et al. Botulinum-A toxin injections into the detrusor muscle decrease nerve growth factor bladder tissue levels in patients with neurogenic detrusor overactivity. *J Urol.* 2006;175:2341-2344.

22. Kuo HC. Clinical effects of suburothelial injection of botulinum A toxin on patients with nonneurogenic detrusor overactivity refractory to anticholinergics. *Urology.* 2005;66:94-98.

23. Karsenty G, Elzayat E, Delapparent T, St-Denis B, Lemieux MC, Corcos J. Botulinum toxin type A injections into the trigone to treat idiopathic overactive bladder do not induce vesicoureteral reflux. *J Urol.* 2007;177:1011-1014.

24. Smith CP, Nishiguchi J, O'Leary M, Yoshimura N, Chancellor MB. Single-institution experience in 110 patients with botulinum toxin A injection into bladder or urethra. *Urology.* 2005;65:37-41.

25. Schurch B, Stohrer M, Kramer G, Schmid DM, Gaul G, Hauri D. Botulinum-A toxin for treating detrusor hyperreflexia in spinal cord injured patients: a new alternative to anticholinergic drugs? Preliminary results. *J Urol.* 2000;164(3 Pt 1):692-697.

26. Karsenty G, Carsenac A, Boy S, Reitz A, Tournebise H, Bladou F, et al. Botulinum toxin-A (BTA) in the treatment of neurogenic detrudor overcativity (NDOI)—A prospective randomized study to compare 30 vs. 10 injection sites. *Eur Urol.* 2007;2:245.

27. Boy S, Schmid M, Reitz A, Von Hessling A, Hodler J, Schurch B. Botulinum toxin injections into the bladder wall—A morphological evaluation of the injection technique using magnetic resonance imaging. *J Urol.* 2006;175(4 suppl):415.

28. Abrams P, Freeman R, Anderstrom C, Mattiasson A. Tolterodine, a new antimuscarinic agent: as effective but better tolerated than oxybutynin in patients with an overactive bladder. *Br J Urol.* 1998;81:801-810.

29. Drutz HP, Appell RA, Gleason D, Klimberg I, Radomski S. Clinical efficacy and safety of tolterodine compared to oxybutynin and placebo in patients with overactive bladder. *Int Urogynecol J Pelvic Floor Dysfunct.* 1999;10:283-289.

30. Appell RA. Clinical efficacy and safety of tolterodine in the treatment of overactive bladder: a pooled analysis. *Urology.* 1997;50(6A suppl):90-96; discussion 7-9.

31. Kreder K, Mayne C, Jonas U. Long-term safety, tolerability and efficacy of extended-release tolterodine in the treatment of overactive bladder. *Eur Urol.* 2002;41:588-595.

32. Schurch B, de Seze M, Denys P, Chartier-Kastler E, Haab F, Everaert K, et al. Botulinum toxin type A is a safe and effective treatment for neurogenic urinary incontinence: results of a single treatment, randomized, placebo controlled 6-month study. *J Urol.* 2005;174:196-200.

33. Reitz A, Stohrer M, Kramer G, Del Popolo G, Chartier-Kastler E, Pannek J, et al. European experience of 200 cases treated with botulinum-A toxin injections into the detrusor muscle for urinary incontinence due to neurogenic detrusor overactivity. *Eur Urol.* 2004;45:510-515.

34. Giannantoni A, Di Stasi SM, Stephen RL, Bini V, Costantini E, Porena M. Intravesical resiniferatoxin versus botulinum-A toxin injections for neurogenic detrusor overactivity: a prospective randomized study. *J Urol.* 2004;172:240-243.

35. Patki P, Hamid R, Arumugam K, Shah J, Craggs M. Botulinum-A txoin (Dysport) in the treatment of drug resistant neurogenic detrusor overactivity following traumatic spinal cord injury. *BJU Int.* 2006;98:77-82.

36. Ehren I, Volz D, Farrelly E, Berglund L, Brundin L, Hultling C, et al. Efficacy and impact of botulinum toxin A on quality of life in patients with neurogenic detrusor overactivity: a randomised, placebo-controlled, double-blind study. *Scand J Urol Nephrol.* 2007;41:335-340.

37. Del Popolo G, Li Marzi V, Panariello G, Lombardi G. English Botulinum toxin-A in the treatment of neurogenic detruos overactivity. *Neurourol Urodyn.* 2003;22:498.

38. Giannantoni A, Merini E, Di Stasi SM, Constantini E, Zuchhi A, Mearini L, et al. New therapeutic option for refractory neurogenic detrusor overactivity. *Minerva Urol Nephrol.* 2004;56:78-87.

39. Kennely M, Kang J. Botulinum-A toxin injection into the detrusor as treatment for refractory detrusor hyperreflexia. *Top Spinal Cord Inj Rehabil.* 2003;8:46-53.

40. Kuo HC. Urodynamic evidence of effectiveness of botulinum A toxin injection in treatment of detrusor overactivity refractory to anticholinergic agents. *Urology.* 2004;63:868-872.

41. Hajebrahimi S, Altaweel W, Cadoret J, Cohen E, Corcos J. Efficacy of botulinum-A toxin in adults with neurogenic overactive bladder: initial results. *Can J Urol.* 2005;12:2543-2546.

42. Klaphajone J, Kitisomprayoonkul W, Sriplakit S. Botulinum toxin type A injections for treating neurogenic detrusor overactivity combined with low-compliance bladder in patients with spinal cord lesions. *Arch Phys Med Rehabil.* 2005;86:2114-2118.

43. Hernandez RD, Hurwitz RS, Foote JE, Zimmern PE, Leach GE. Nonsurgical management of threatened upper urinary tracts and incontinence in children with myelomeningocele. *J Urol.* 1994;152(5 Pt 1):1582-1585.

44. Schulte-Baukloh H, Michael T, Schobert J, Stolze T, Knispel HH. Efficacy of botulinum-A toxin in children with detrusor hyperreflexia due to myelomeningocele: preliminary results. *Urology.* 2002;59:325-327; discussion 7-8.

45. Schulte-Baukloh H, Michael T, Sturzebecher B, Knispel HH. Botulinum-A toxin detrusor injection as a novel approach in the treatment of bladder spasticity in children with neurogenic bladder. *Eur Urol.* 2003;44:139-143.

46. Riccabona M, Koen M, Schindler M, Goedele B, Pycha A, Lusuardi L, et al. Botulinum-A toxin injection into the detrusor: a safe alternative in the treatment of children with myelomeningocele with detrusor hyperreflexia. *J Urol.* 2004;171(2 Pt 1):845-848; discussion 8.

47. Corcos J, Al-Taweed W, Robichaud C. Botulinum toxin as an alternative treatment to bladder augmentation in children with neurogenic bladder due to myelomeningocele [abstract]. *J Urol.* 2004;171:181.

48. Schulte-Baukloh H, Knispel HH, Stolze T, Weiss C, Michael T, Miller K. Repeated botulinum-A toxin injections in treatment of children with neurogenic detrusor overactivity. *Urology.* 2005;66:865-870; discussion 70.

49. Werner M, Schmid DM, Schussler B. Efficacy of botulinum-A toxin in the treatment of detrusor overactivity incontinence: a prospective nonrandomized study. *Am J Obstet Gynecol.* 2005;192:1735-1740.

50. Schulte-Baukloh H, Weiss C, Schobert J, Stolze T, Sturzebecher B, Knispel HH. [Subjective patient satisfaction after injection of botulinum-A toxin in detrusor overactivity]. *Aktuelle Urol.* 2005;36:230-233.

51. Sahai A, Khan M, Smith K, Dasgupta P. Botulinum toxin for patients with detrusor overactivity: Early results from a randomised, double blind placebo-controlled trial. *International Continence Society Annual Meeting, Montreal.* 2005;Abstract 468(5).

52. Rajkumar GN, Small DR, Mustafa AW, Conn G. A prospective study to evaluate the safety, tolerability, efficacy and durability of response of intravesical injection of botulinum toxin type A into detrusor muscle in patients with refractory idiopathic detrusor overactivity. *BJU Int.* 2005;96:848-852.

53. Dykstra D, Enriquez A, Valley M. Treatment of overactive bladder with botulinum toxin type B: a pilot study. *Int Urogynecol J Pelvic Floor Dysfunct.* 2003;14:424-426.

54. Loch A, Loch T, Osterhage J, Alloussi S, Stöckle M. Botulinum-A toxin detrusor injections in the treatment of non-neurologic and neurologic cases of urge incontinence [abstract]. *Eur Urol.* 2003;2:172.

55. Radziszewski P, Borkowski A. Botulinum toxin type A intravesical injections for instable bladder overactivity. *Eur Urol.* 2002;1:134.

56. Flynn MK, Webster GD, Amundsen CL. The effect of botulinum-A toxin on patients with severe urge urinary incontinence. *J Urol.* 2004;172(6 Pt 1):2316-2320.

57. Popat R, Apostolidis A, Kalsi V, Gonzales G, Fowler CJ, Dasgupta P. A comparison between the response of patients with idiopathic detrusor overactivity and neurogenic detrusor overactivity to the first intradetrusor injection of botulinum-A toxin. *J Urol.* 2005;174:984-989.

58. Kessler TM, Danuser H, Schumacher M, Studer UE, Burkhard FC. Botulinum A toxin injections into the detrusor: an effective treatment in idiopathic and neurogenic detrusor overactivity? *Neurourol Urodyn.* 2005;24:231-236.

59. Schmid DM, Schurch B, John H, Hauri D. Botulinum toxin injection to treat overactive bladder. *Eur Urol.* 2004;(Suppl 3):131.

60. Schmid DM, Sauermann P, Werner M, Schuessler B, Blick N, Muentener M, et al. Experience of 100 cases treated with botulinum-A toxin injections into the detrusor muscle for idiopathic overactive bladder refractory to anticholinergics. *J Urol.* 2006;176:177-185.

61. Hoebeke P, De Caestecker K, Vande Walle J, Dehoorne J, Raes A, Verleyen P, et al. The effect of botulinum-A toxin in incontinent children with therapy resistant overactive bladder. *J Urol.* 2006;176:328-330.

62. Kuo HC. Will suburothelial injection of small dose of botulinum A toxin have similar therapeutic effects and less adverse events for refractory detrusor overactivity? *Urology.* 2006;68:993-997; discussion 7-8.

63. Schulte-Baukloh H, Weiss C, Stolze T, Herholz J, Sturzebecher B, Miller K, et al. Botulinum-A toxin detrusor and sphincter injection in treatment of overactive bladder syndrome: objective outcome and patient satisfaction. *Eur Urol.* 2005;48:984-990; discussion 90.

64. Dykstra DD, Pryor J, Goldish G. Use of botulinum toxin type B for the treatment of detrusor hyperreflexia in a patient with multiple sclerosis: a case report. *Arch Phys Med Rehabil.* 2003;84:1399-1400.

65. Ghei M, Maraj BH, Miller R, Nathan S, O'Sullivan C, Fowler CJ, et al. Effects of botulinum toxin B on refractory detrusor overactivity: a randomized, double-blind, placebo controlled, crossover trial. *J Urol.* 2005;174:1873-1877; discussion 7.

66. Reitz A, Schurch B. Botulinum toxin type B injection for management of type A resistant neurogenic detrusor overactivity. *J Urol.* 2004;171(2 Pt 1):804-805 discussion.

67. Pistolesi D, Selli C, Rossi B, Stampacchia G. Botulinum toxin type B for type A resistant bladder spasticity. *J Urol.* 2004;171(2 Pt 1):802-803.

68. Kessler KR, Benecke R. The EBD test—a clinical test for the detection of antibodies to botulinum type A. *Mov Disord.* 1997;12:95-99.

69. Aoki KR. Pharmacology and immunology of botulinum toxin serotypes. *J Neurol.* 2001;248 (Suppl 1):3-10.

70. Matarasso SL. Comparison of botulinum toxin types A and B: a bilateral and double-blind randomized evaluation in the treatment of canthal rhytides. *Dermatol Surg.* 2003;29:7-13; discussion.

71. Alderson K, Holds JB, Anderson RL. Botulinum-induced alteration of nerve-muscle interactions in the human orbicularis oculi following treatment for blepharospasm. *Neurology.* 1991;41:1800-1805.

72. Printer MJ, Vanden Noven S, Muccio D, Wallace N. Axotomy-like changes in cat motor neuron electrical properties elicited by botulinum toxin depend on the complete elimination of neuromuscular transmission. *J Neurosci.* 1991;11:657-666.

73. de Paiva A, Meunier FA, Molgo J, Aoki KR, Dolly JO. Functional repair of motor endplates after botulinum neurotoxin type A poisoning: biphasic switch of synaptic activity between nerve sprouts and their parent terminals. *Proc Natl Acad Sci U S A.* 1999;96:3200-3205.

74. Grosse J, Kramer G, Schurch B, Stöhrer M. Repeat injections of botulinum-A toxin in patients with neurogenic lower urinary tract dysfunction do not cause increased drug tolearnce. *Neurourol Urodyn.* 2002;21:287-386.

75. Haferkamp A, Schurch B, Reitz A, Krengel U, Grosse J, Kramer G, et al. Lack of ultrastructural detrusor changes following endoscopic injection of botulinum toxin type A in overactive neurogenic bladder. *Eur Urol.* 2004;46:784-791.

76. Karsenty G, Reitz A, Lindemann G, Boy S, Schurch B. Persistence of therapeutic effect after repeated injections of botulinum A to treat incontinence due to neurogenic detrusor overactivity. *Urology.* 2006;68:1193-1197.

77. Grosse J, Kramer G, Stohrer M. Success of repeat detrusor injections of botulinum a toxin in patients with severe neurogenic detrusor overactivity and incontinence. *Eur Urol.* 2005;47:653-659.

78. Malnick SD, Metchnik L, Somin M, Bergman N, Attali M. Fatal heart block following treatment with botulinum toxin for achalasia. *Am J Gastroenterol.* 2000;95:3333-3334.

79. Del Popolo G. Botulinum-A toxin in the treatment of detrusor hyperreflexia. *Neurourol Urodyn*. 2001;20:522.

80. Wyndaele JJ, Van Dromme SA. Muscular weakness as side effect of botulinum toxin injection for neurogenic detrusor overactivity. *Spinal Cord*. 2002;40:599-600.

81. Dykstra DD, Sidi AA. Treatment of detrusor-sphincter dyssynergia with botulinum A toxin: a double-blind study. *Arch Phys Med Rehabil*. 1990;71:24-26.

82. Ranoux D, Gury C, Fondarai J, Mas JL, Zuber M. Respective potencies of Botox and Dysport: a double blind, randomised, crossover study in cervical dystonia. *J Neurol Neurosurg Psychiatry*. 2002;72:459-462.

83. Van den Bergh PY, Lison DF. Dose standardization of botulinum toxin. *Adv Neurol*. 1998;78:231-235.

Botulinum Toxin in **21** the Treatment of Chronic Pelvic Pain Syndromes

Phillip P. Smith and Christopher P. Smith

INTRODUCTION AND THERAPEUTIC RATIONALE

In the absence of an identified cause of acute pain, chronic pelvic pain is nonmalignant pain perceived as arising from the pelvic organs. There is no ideal classification system for chronic pelvic pain because its etiology is often obscure, which contributes to the difficulty of characterization and formulation of rational therapy. The European Association of Urology has proposed a classification scheme dividing chronic pelvic pain into prostatic, bladder, urethral, scrotal, gynecologic, and pelvic floor pain syndromes.[1] More recently, it has been suggested that the nomenclature of pelvic pain should avoid statements of etiology and preferably refer to the apparent organ or region. For example, the term interstitial cystitis (IC) is replaced by painful bladder syndrome (PBS). The terms inflammatory prostatitis and prostatism are replaced by male chronic pelvic pain syndrome or prostatic pain syndrome. Because these syndromes are of unknown etiology, assigning etiologic names implies knowledge that may not be present.[2] Despite the superficially clear classification, these syndromes may have etiologic overlaps[3] and thus are amenable to common therapeutic goals and agents.

Botulinum neurotoxin (BoNT) is elaborated by *Clostridium botulinum* and is among the most potent naturally occuring toxins. Its primary mode of action, such as in botulinum toxin poisoning, is chemodenervation of muscle via blockade of presynaptic acetylcholine release at the neuromuscular junction, with subsequent flaccid paralysis. In therapeutic use, BoNT has demonstrated effectiveness in the treatment of several pain disorders including focal dystonia, cervical dystonia/spastic torticollis, spasmodic dysphonia, oromandibular dystonia, temporomandibular disorder, refractory myofascial pain syndrome, and tension- and migraine-type headache.[4] Several modes of action appear to be important to its effectiveness in this regard.[5] The flaccid paralysis induced by BoNT eliminates abnormal muscle tone and spasm, and thus prevents ischemia-induced release of inflammatory mediators.[6-10] Inflammation-induced pain appears to be most susceptible to modulation with BoNT.[11,12] More direct suppression of afferent activity and related reflexive responses has also been described.[11,13,14] Other suggested antinociceptive actions include direct and secondary autonomic effects, induced CNS plasticity, and central effects.[7,15-18]

Pelvic pain disorders are marked by functional abnormalities of muscle tensioning and relaxation (e.g., vaginismus) and inflammation (e.g., chronic prostatitis), thus making them prime potential targets for the therapeutic use of botulinum toxin. The first report of the use of botulinum toxin for disorders of the lower urogenital tract was a case series of its use for the treatment of detrusor-sphincter dyssynergia in spinal cord injury in 1988.[19] Almost 10 years later, the first use of botulinum toxin for the treatment of a chronic pelvic pain syndrome was reported. In a case report of the use of

Dr. Phillip Smith does not report any conflicts of interest. Dr. Christopher Smith is disclosing that he was a consultant and research investigator for Allergan, Inc., Irvine, CA.

BoNT/A in the treatment of severe vaginismus associated with interstitial cystitis, 10 U were injected into two anterior vaginal wall sites, with reported effectiveness 24 months post injection. The results were attributed to relieving inappropriate spasm of vaginal wall muscles.[20]

GENITOURINARY PAIN SYNDROMES TREATED WITH BOTULISM NEUROTOXIN TYPE A

Botulinum neurotoxin type A (BoNT/A) has been investigated for use in three general categories of chronic genitourinary pelvic pain syndromes, chronic female pelvic pain syndromes, chronic prostatitis/male chronic pelvic pain syndrome, and painful bladder syndrome/interstitial cystitis. Its antinociceptive effects, as well as its effect as a paralyzing agent, are thought to be central to its effectiveness in these pain syndromes. A summary of published trials of the use of BoNT/A in genitourinary pain syndromes is presented in Table 21-1.

Chronic Female Pelvic Pain Syndromes

Chronic female pelvic pain syndromes are frequently encountered, result in significant detriments of quality of life (QoL) for their sufferers, and are frustrating for both the patient and the treating physician. The incidence has been estimated at 21.5/1000 women, and the costs (1996) estimated at $880 million.[21] The etiologies of chronic female pain include conditions affecting the reproductive viscera such as endometriosis and the sequela of pelvic inflammatory disease, and conditions of nonreproductive origin such as irritable bowel syndrome and painful bladder syndrome. Often, despite thorough investigation including pelvic imaging and diagnostic laparoscopy, there is no readily identified etiology. Many of these cases may be related to pelvic floor hypertonus[22]; thus, therapies aimed at diminishing nociceptive reflex activity may be of value. Related treatment modalities that have potential benefit include pelvic floor relaxation and biofeedback.[1] Preliminary work suggests that sacral neuromodulation may be effective in female chronic pelvic pain.[23,24]

The use of botulinum toxin for the treatment of chronic female pelvic pain has focused on three potentially related pain syndromes: vulvodynia, vaginismus, and levator ani spasm/pain.

Vulvodynia

Vulvodynia is a complex syndrome of unexplained vulvar pain or burning and sexual dysfunction. The condition is estimated to affect 200,000 American women each year.[25] It is regarded as a complex regional pain syndrome resulting from inappropriate activity in nonmyelinated pain fibers, although there is minimal evidence to suggest an infectious or inflammatory etiology.[26] Commonly used treatment modalities include tricyclic antidepressants, gabapentin, estrogens, a variety of injections including steroids and interferon, postural and pelvic floor exercises, soft tissue mobilization/myofascial release, bowel and bladder retraining, contact avoidance, dietary changes, and psychiatric referral.[25,27] Traditional conservative and surgical therapies are often suboptimally effective, frequently have significant side effects and risks, and lack prospective study on their efficacy. Treatment with sacral nerve neuromodulation for voiding-associated pelvic and perineal pain (including vulvodynia) associated with voiding dysfunction was associated with a reduction in pain Visual Analog Score from 5.8 to 3.7 at up to 24 months follow-up, but the complication rate was 18.7%.[28] This study primarily evaluated the effect of neuromodulation on voiding function, however, and the primary use of this modality for vulvodynia remains to be defined.

In 2004, an initial case report describing the successful management of refractory vulvodynia with BoNT/A and surgery was published.[29] Later, in an open-label pilot study, 19 patients with provoked vestibulodynia were treated with BoNT/A, seven received 35 U, and 12 received 50 U. Reductions in a standard pain scale (0–10) were observed with both doses (8.1 to 2.9 and 7.4 to 1.8, respectively) 30 days following treatment. Improvements in QoL scores and decreased medication use were reported. The duration of response averaged 14 weeks. No side effects were reported.[30]

The only other published report of the use of BoNT/A for the treatment of vulvodynia is a recent case series of seven women, both pre- and postmenopausal, with vulvodynia that was unresponsive to standard treatments. Pain interrupted sexual activities in all patients,

Table 21-1 Botulinum Toxin and Genitourinary Pain Syndromes

Authors	Year	Symptoms	Type	n	Total dose	Method	Followup (mo)	Results	Adverse Events
Female Pelvic Pain Syndromes									
Brin and Vapnick[26]	1997	Vaginismus	CR	1	20	Anterior vaginal wall injection	24	Relief of pain and spasm	None
Shafik et al[32]	2000	Vaginismus	CT	13	25 U	Bulbospongiosus injection	10	Eight patients with BTX able to achieve intercourse, five injected with saline unsuccessful	None
Gunter et al[29]	2004	Vulvodynia	CR	1				Successful treatment of refractory case	
Jarvis et al[38]	2004	Chronic pelvic pain	CS	12	40	Intramuscular injection	3	Improvements in dyspareunia, dysmenorrhea, sexual activity scores. No change in vaginal manometry, uroflow	None
Romito et al[37]	2004	Chronic pelvic pain	CR	2		Intramuscular injection	Several	Relief of pain and spasm	
Ghazizadeh and Nikzad[33]	2004	Vaginismus	CS	24	150–400 U	Puborectalis injections, 3 sites each side	12.3	96% resolution, 75% achieved intercourse, no recurrences	None
Thomson et al[39]	2005	Chronic pelvic pain, pelvic floor tenderness	CR	1	40–80	Repeated intramuscular injection	18	Improvement of QoL scores, pain VAS scores, pelvic floor resting tone (manometry)	None

Continued

Table 21-1 Botulinum Toxin and Genitourinary Pain Syndromes—Cont'd

Authors	Year	Symptoms	Type	n	Total dose	Method	Followup (mo)	Results	Adverse Events
Brown et al.	2006	Vestibulodynia	CS	2	20–40		3	Reduced coital pain in one, reduced levator hypertonicity, no change in vestibular hyperalgesia	None
Abbott et al[40]	2006	Pelvic pain, pelvic floor myalgia	RCT	60	80	Transvaginal puborectal and pubococcygeal injection, two sites	6	Less nonmenstrual pain, improved QoL scores, improved resting manometry. No changes in bladder/bowel questionaires or uroflow.	Transient SUI
Dykstra et al[30]	2006	Vestibulodynia	CS	19	35 (7) 50 (12)	Intramuscular injection	3	Improvements in pain scores, QoL, less medication use	None
Yoon et al[31]	2007	Vulvodynia	CS	7	20–40 U	Vestibule, LA, perineal injection, repeated q 2 wks	11.6	Pain score improved, no recurrences	None

Chronic Prostatitis/Male Chronic Pelvic Pain Syndrome (CP/CPPS)

Maria et al[62]	1968	CS	4	30	Transperineal injection	2	Improved symptoms in three or four, improved duration of maximum flow, no change in flow parameters	None
Zermann et al[69]	2000	CS	11	200	Transurethral perisphincteric injection	<1	Tenderness and pain improved in all patients. Decreased FUL, PVR, improved flow rates	None

Interstitial Cystitis/Painful Bladder Syndrome (IC/PBS)

Smith et al[40]	2004	CS	13	100–200	Submucosal trigone	6	Frequency, nocturia reduced 45%, pain reduced 79%, first desire to void and cystometric capacity improved 58/59%	None
Kuo[66]	2005	CS	10	100–200	Submucosal trigone	3	Symptomatic and cystometric improvements in only two patients.	Seven patients with voiding difficulty
Smith et al[101]	2005	CR	1	100	Intravesical	6	Improvement in irritative symptoms, bother and pain, lasting 3–6 months.	None

BTX, Botox; PVR, post-void residual; QoL, quality-of-life; RCT, randomized controlled trial; SUI, stress urinary incontinence.

and none had gross abnormalities or lesions. Two of the seven had elevated levator ani tone without vaginismus. Questionnaires using a Visual Analog Scale (VAS) were completed before and at 2 weeks after treatment. Injections were at tender points of the vestibule, levator ani, or perineal body, as determined by gentle digital palpation and touching with cotton-tip swab. Initial injections were 20 U in 0.2 to 0.3 mL per site, no closer to each other than 1 cm. Injections were repeated 2 weeks later with 40 U, if pain persisted. Follow-up ranged from 2 to 24 months and averaged 11.6 months. There was no comment on durability of treatment.[31]

Vaginismus

Vaginismus is the persistent involuntary contraction of striated muscle surrounding the lower third of the vagina that occurrs upon attempted penetration. It may be primary, meaning successful vaginal intercourse has not been achieved despite voluntary attempts, or acquired, often due to dyspareunia resulting from organic or functional pathology. Anxiolytics, local anesthetics, and lubricants have been the standard therapies, but a significant proportion of patients do not respond to these measures. Therefore, treatment directed toward inhibition of involuntary muscle contraction, analogous to the BoNT chemodenervation treatment of torticollis or blepharospasm, may benefit these women.

Despite evidence for success of BoNT/A in other disorders of chronic muscle spasm, only three reports directly address its use for vaginismus. The first is the aforementioned case report; this patient was able to achieve vaginal intercourse for the first time in 8 years, following BoNT/A injection into the anterior vaginal wall.[20] A nonrandomized, nonblinded control trial was then reported, in which eight women were injected with BoNT/A and five controls were injected with saline.[32] The bulbospongiosus muscles were injected with either 25 U of BoNT/A in 1 mL saline, or 1 mL saline alone, and patients were followed for a mean of 10 months. All patients injected with BoNT/A were subsequently able to achieve satisfactory vaginal intercourse, whereas none of the patients injected with saline were successful. No reinjections, recurrences, or complications were reported.[32] The most recent report is a case series of 24 women with significant vaginismus for whom standard therapies had failed.[33] The mean age in this study was 25 years, and all were premenopausal. Under local anesthetic with sedation, 150 to 400 U of BoNT/A were injected into the puborectalis muscle in three sites on each side. Patients were evaluated with subjective assessment of vaginal muscle resistance and their ability to achieve vaginal intercourse following the injections. At a mean follow-up of 12.4 months, 96% were found to have little or no muscular resistance at examination, and 75% had achieved successful intercourse. There were no recurrences, nor were any significant side effects noted.[33]

Levator ani pain

Spasm of the levator ani muscles are commonly linked to chronic pelvic pain.[34] Conversely, female chronic pelvic pain in the absence of other detectable pathology is associated with altered levator ani electromyographic (EMG) activity consistent with abnormal levator function.[35] A study of levator trigger point injection with a mixture of local anesthetics produced improvements in Visual Analog Score, perceived cure, and global satisfaction scores, suggesting the value of local antinociceptive therapy.[36] Owing to the direct neuromuscular and antinociceptive effects of botulinum toxin, injection of the levator muscles with BoNT/A has been proposed as a treatment modality for female chronic pelvic pain and vulvodynia. Certainly the subset of women with this problem overlaps the subset of women with vaginismus, although in the studies available, the focus of the treatment of levator pain and spasm is on women with chronic pelvic pain rather than sexual dysfunction.

Two published abstracts mark the first appearances of the use of BoNT/A for the treatment of chronic female pelvic pain in the literature. A review of 167 patients with chronic pelvic pain demonstrated that all had chronic urethral and levator tenderness, inefficient voluntary control of the pelvic striated muscle, voiding dysfunction, and elevated urethral pressures. This may be the result of poorly coordinated pelvic floor muscle action with subsequent impaired overall motor function despite normal or heightened localized contractile activity. The result is, in essence, a form of repetitive motion stress injury that could be an etiologic factor in chronic pelvic pain.[22] Botulinum toxin injected into the levator ani with the intent of relieving muscle spasm in two patients produced symptomatic relief within a few days that lasted for several months.[37]

A pilot study of BoNT/A injection of the pubococcygeus and puborectalis muscles for the treatment of chronic pelvic pain in women with chronic pelvic pain and pelvic floor muscle hypertonicity by digital and manometric assessment demonstrated improvements in both objective and subjective measures.[38] Twelve nonpregnant premenopausal women with pelvic pain (dysmenorrhea, dyspareunia, dyschesia and/or nonmenstrual pelvic pain) of at least 2 years' duration and pelvic floor hypetonicity as defined by a resting vaginal pressure of >40 cm/w were assessed by VAS pain scores, SF12, EuroQoL-5D, pelvic floor manometry and uroflow. 10 U of BoNT/A were injected transvaginally in each of four sites for the puborectalis and for the pubococcygeus bilaterally, using three different concentrations of BoNT/A (10, 20, and 100 U/mL). At 12 weeks' follow-up, significant pain reduction scores for dyspareunia and dysmenorrhea, improvements in sexual activity scores and improvements in bladder function scores were observed. No significant improvements in QoL scores, vaginal manometry, or uroflow were detected. No differences were found with respect to different concentrations of BoNT/A. One woman who had prior stress urinary incontinence (SUI) had mild incontinence following injection, but there was no de novo SUI. The authors inferred that a reduction in dyspareunia might be the result of a direct sensory effect of BoNT/A.[38]

The use of BoNT/A in the presence of known endometriosis was described in a case report of a 34-year-old woman with dysmenorrhea, dyspareunia, and intermenstrual pain. Laparoscopy-proven endometriosis had been previously resected with partial relief of her symptoms. The puborectalis and pubococcygeus muscles were tender on examination, and pelvic floor manometry demonstrated elevated resting tone (48 cm/w vs normal <30 cm/w). Local anesthetic injection into levator muscles relieved pain and reduced manometric resting pressure for less than 2 weeks. BoNT/A 10 U/0.5 mL normal saline (NS) was injected into right and left puborectalis and right and left pubococcygeus. Significant improvements in QoL questionnaire (SF-12, EuroQoL-5D scores), pain VAS and resting manometry were observed, with maximal improvement at 8 weeks. Symptoms and findings returned by 18 to 20 weeks after injection. Treatment was repeated twice at 20 U/injection with similar findings. No major or minor side effects were described.[39]

In a double-blind, randomized controlled trial of BoNT/A versus saline, 60 patients with 2 years or more of chronic pelvic pain disruptive to daily activities were studied. In this group, the painful levator muscles (pelvic floor myalgia) were accompanied by elevated vaginal pressures per manometry. The patients were randomized to receive either 80 U (20 U/mL) of BoNT/A or NS injections into the puborectalis and pubococcygeus muscles.[40] Most of these patients (92% overall) had undergone surgery, with 55% having histologically confirmed endometriosis. Only 11% had negative laparoscopic findings; thus, possibly as many as 80% of the patients in this study had identifiable disease associated with their pelvic pain. After 26 weeks of follow-up, QoL measures (EuroQOL-5D, SF-12 mental component, and VAS for sexual pleasure, frequency of intercourse, and dyspareunia) were improved in both BoNT/A and placebo groups, with the difference between BoNT/A and placebo improvements not reaching statistical significance. Resting pelvic floor pressure in the BoNT/A group was significantly reduced. No significant changes were found in uroflow and bowel and bladder function questionnaire responses. Two women in the BoNT/A group had transient SUI, with one of these women also having intermittent incontinence of flatus and stool for four months. The investigators concluded that while their QoL measurements did not demonstrate greater improvements following BoNT/A compared with placebo, the objective measurement of pelvic floor pressure was reduced. Therefore, a lack of significant superiority of BoNT/A in QoL improvements might have been related to the relatively small study size and imperfect QoL assessment tools.[40]

Chronic Prostatitis/Male Chronic Pelvic Pain Syndrome

The syndrome of chronic prostatitis/male chronic pelvic pain (CP/CPPS) corresponds to Category III of the NIH prostatitis categorization.[41] It is characterized by perineal, lower abdominal, testicular, penile, and scrotal/testicular pain.[42] It is the most common form of prostatitis, constituting 90% to 95% of prostatitis cases. It has a reported incidence of 2 million men in the United States, and is estimated to generate 5% of urologic office visits.[43] CP/CPPS has a significant negative impact on patient QoL.[44] Compared with controls, men with CP/CPPS reported a significantly greater lifetime prevalence of non-specific urethritis, cardiovascular disease, neurologic disease, psychiatric conditions, and hematopoietic, lymphatic, or infectious disease.[45]

Pain is the prerequisite symptom for CP/CPPS/Category III prostatitis. In addition to pain, irritative urinary symptoms and ejaculatory pain may accompany CP/CPPS.[46] Because the syndrome is multifaceted and of uncertain etiology, the diagnostic evaluation is poorly defined. A history and physical, including digital rectal examination (DRE), urinalysis, and urologic referral have been recommended.[46] The value of Stamey-Meares four-glass test in the evaluation of men with CP/CPPS is unclear. Although men with CP/CPPS are more likely than controls to have higher leukocyte counts (but not semen) in urine samples with and without prostatic massage, the predictive value of the test is small. The presence of pathogenic and nonpathogenic bacteria in segmented urine specimens of men with prostatitis has a similar incidence to controls.[47] Prostate-specific antigen (PSA), percent-free PSA and free PSA isoforms are slightly elevated in men with CP/CPPS but have low sensitivity and specificity for the condition.[48] The potassium sensitivity test does not have good predictive value for CP/CPPS, although men with CP/CPPS frequently have a positive test.[49] However, administration of the NIH Chronic Prostatitis Symptom Index (NIH-CPSI) may be useful both for diagnosis and treatment assessment. This questionnaire has been shown to be valid, reliable, and responsive to prostatitis symptoms in primary and secondary care patients and should be used as a research outcome in clinical studies.[50-52] The Giessen Prostatitis Symptom score (GPSS) and International Prostate Symptom Score (IPSS) likewise are valid assessment tools.[53]

Standard therapy for CP/CPPS includes symptomatic treatment with a variety of anti-inflammatory drugs, anesthetics, muscle relaxants, and analgesics, as well as therapies aimed at treating presumed etiologies such as infection (i.e., antibiotics) or obstruction (i.e., alpha-adrenergic blockade).[44] Pentosan polysulfate has demonstrated mixed results, reducing pain scores in an open-label multicenter pilot study.[54] A subsequent randomized controlled trial[55] demonstrated only modest improvements in QoL scores but no significant improvements of urinary symptoms or pain.

Neither antibiotic therapy nor alpha-adrenergic blockade have been shown to be superior or effective in a majority of patients.[56-58] The natural history of the condition in a treated population is marked by wide variability in symptom severity over time, with significant improvement observed in one third of men with CP/CPPS, suggesting available treatments are not adequate.[59]

Botulinum toxin holds promise as a treatment for CP/CPPS by relieving voiding dysfunction and by reducing pain sensation. Men with CP/CPPS report a greater intensity of heat or burning sensation in response to perineal application of capsaicin than do controls,[60] suggesting that altered sensory processing is involved in the syndrome. As discussed earlier, BoNT/A inhibits responses to inflammatory pain, which suggests that CP/CPPS may be responsive to BoNT/A. In a rat model of capsaicin-induced nonbacterial inflammatory prostatitis, inflammatory and pain responses were assessed by behavioral analysis, COX-2 protein concentration, and plasma protein extravasation by Evans blue injection. In animals injected with up to 20 U BoNT/A into the prostate 1 week before capsaicin injection, BoNT/A reversed pain and inflammatory changes in a dose-dependent manner.[61] CP/CPPS has also been viewed as a result or complication of voiding dysfunction; therefore, improving urodynamic parameters may improve CP/CPPS symptoms. Intraprostatic BoNT/A injection improved subjective voiding symptoms, America Urological Association (AUA) symptom scores, and flow patterns in two series.[62,63]

Several studies have demonstrated the utility of BoNT/A in the treatment of male voiding dysfunction due to BPH.[64-68] Only one clinical study is found specifically addressing the use of BoNT/A for the treatment of CP/CPPS.[69] Eleven men with chronic prostatic pain of greater than 12 months' duration, ages 32 to 66 years, were studied. Patients were assessed by physical examination, VAS pain assessment, and urodynamics. All patients were neurologically normal, and had a normal bladder and urethra by cystoscopy. Patients studied had hypersensitive/hyperalgesic urethral sphincter and bladder neck, pathologic pelvic muscle tenderness, poor voluntary control of the pelvic floor muscles, resting urethral sphincter pressure greater than 80 cm/w and/or maximum uroflow less than 15 mL/s. A dose of 200 U of BoNT/A was administered by transurethral perisphincteric injection under direct vision using a 22-gauge Bard needle at three to four injection sites. At 2- to 4-week follow-up, nine of 11 patients reported subjective improvement. VAS pain scores decreased from 7.2 to 1.6. Significant decreases in pelvic floor tenderness, functional urethral length, urethral closure pressure, post-void residual (PVR), and increases in average and maximal uroflow were observed. One patient had SUI; no other problems were noted.[69]

Interstitial Cystitis/Painful Bladder Syndrome

Interstitial cystitis/Bladder Pain Syndrome (IC/PBS) is a syndrome of chronic lower urinary tract irritative symptoms and pelvic pain in the absence of other pathology. IC and painful bladder syndrome may be descriptions of the same entity, distinct from other pelvic/genitourinary pain syndromes.[70,71] Although traditionally viewed to be more common in women, the syndrome affects both men and women; the incidence in men may be underestimated because some men with IC may be misclassified as having CP/CPPS.[72] Pain and

urinary frequency in the absence of other identifiable cause are consistent characteristics of the syndrome.[70,73] The pain typically increases with bladder filling, is usually suprapubic but may localize elsewhere in the pelvis and perineum, and is often extreme in intensity (i.e., during flare-ups). Requirements for the clinical diagnosis of IC/PBS have recently been reviewed.[74] Diagnostic criteria were proposed by the National Institute of Diabetes and Digestive and Kidney Diseases (NIDDK) in 1988 (Table 21-2), intended for research purposes rather than clinical practice. These criteria have been criticized for underestimating the clinical incidence of IC/PBS.[73] In practical clinical terms, the diagnosis is made by a combination of a history of urgency/frequency, bladder pain in the absence of infection or malignancy, and typical examination findings of tenderness. A symptom questionnaire may be helpful, such as the University of Wisconsin IC Scale, the O'Leary-Sant Symptom Index or the Pelvic Pain and Urinary Frequency (PUF) Score.[74] The cystoscopic presence of glomerulations after

---

TABLE 21-2 NIDDK Diagnostic Criteria for Interstitial Cystitis

To be diagnosed with interstitial cystitis, patients must have either glomerulations on cystoscopic examination or classic Hunner's ulcer, and they must have either pain associated with the bladder or urinary urgency. An examination for glomerulations should be undertaken after distention of the bladder with the patient under anesthesia to 80 to 100 cm/water pressure for 1 to 2 minutes. The bladder may be distended up to two times before evaluation. The glomerulations must be diffuse, present in at least three quadrants of the bladder, and there must be at least 10 glomerulations per quadrant. The glomerulations must not be along the path of the cystoscope (to eliminate artifact from contact instrumentation). The presence of any of the following criteria excludes the diagnosis of interstitial cystitis:
1. Bladder capacity greater than 350 mL on awake cystometry using either a gas or liquid filling medium
2. Absence of an intense urge to void with the bladder filled to 100 mL gas or 150 mL water during cystometry, using an infusion rate of 30 to 100 mL/min
3. The demonstration of phasic involuntary bladder contractions on cystometry using the fill rate described previously
4. Duration of symptoms less than 9 months
5. Absence of nocturia
6. Symptoms relieved by antimicrobials, urinary antiseptics, anticholinergics or antispasmodics
7. A frequency of urination, while awake, of less than eight times a day
8. A diagnosis of bacterial cystitis or prostatitis within a 3-month period
9. Bladder or ureteral calculi
10. Active genital herpes
11. Uterine, cervical, vaginal or urethral cancer
12. Urethral diverticulum
13. Cyclophosphamide or any type of chemical cystitis
14. Tuberculous cystitis
15. Radiation cystitis
16. Benign or malignant bladder tumors
17. Vaginitis
18. Age less than 18 years

NIDDK, National Institute of Diabetes and Digestive and Kidney Diseases.
From Hanno PM, Landis JR, Matthews-Cook Y, Kusek J, Nyberg L Jr. The diagnosis of interstitial cystitis revisited: lessons learned from the National Institutes of Health Interstitial Cystitis Database study. *J Urol.* 1999;161:553-557.

hydrodistension, long-accepted as diagnostic of IC, has not been proven.[1] However, cystoscopy is not without potential benefit. The presence or absence of ulceration (Hunner's ulcers) at cystoscopy may denote two subtypes of IC/PBS, representing separate entities, based upon demographic, endoscopic, cystometric, and histologic responses, as well as response to therapy.[75]

IC/PBS occurs in the absence of identifiable bacterial or viral infectious agents, and thus, not surprisingly, antibiotics are not helpful.[1] Ulcerative IC/PBS is associated with a pancystitis, but this feature is absent in nonulcerative disease. Mast cell activation with release of inflammatory mediators such as histamine, leukotrienes, cytokines, and serotonin is increased 10-fold in ulcerative IC/PBS.[76] Disruption of the protective glycosaminoglycan (GAG) layer at the urothelial apex may expose nerve endings to noxious urine components.[77,78] Urothelial release of adenosine triphosphate (ATP) in response to stretch is enhanced in IC/PBS patients, and P2X3 receptors in cultured urothelial cells are upregulated by stretch to a greater degree in urothelial tissue from IC/PBS patients.[79,80] Neuroplasticity due to enhanced activation of nociceptive afferent pathways results in prolonged pain responses, spread of the pain response to previously uninvolved neurons, and enhanced responsiveness of select neurons.[5] Sensory nerve dysfunction may underlie IC. The function of capsaicin-sensitive primary sensory neurons from the bladder and urethra includes regulation of the micturition threshold, activation of viscerovascular reflexes, and perception of bladder pain. In the presence of chronic inflammation, transmitters (ATP, NO) released by efferent nerve endings sensitize afferent terminals.[81] Enhanced sensory signaling resulting in central changes may or may not originate in the bladder. Significant bidirectional neural cross-talk and cross-sensitization between the colon and lower urinary tract due to convergence of pelvic afferents result in overlap of clinical pain syndromes. These cross-organ reflexes are likely important for normal integration of sexual, bowel, and bladder function. Sensitization of afferent pathways of one viscera by irritation in another viscera may play a role in pelvic pain syndromes.[82] Possible mechanisms for visceral cross-sensitization include prespinal convergence, afferent interactions by means of spinal interneurons, sympathetic reflexes or cross-sphincteric reflexes.[83]

Available treatments for IC/PBS are often of limited benefit, and realistic expectations by the physician and patient are an important component of the therapeutic plan.[1] At present, a therapeutic approach aimed at multiple "pathologic targets" is recommended.[84] This typically includes efforts at reinforcement of GAG layer function with oral pentosan polysulfate sodium (PPS),[85,86] hyaluronic acid instillations,[87,88] and intravesical heparin.[89] Hydroxyzine may be used for suppression of mast cell histamine release, with or without concurrent PPS.[90,91] The H2 histamine blocker cimetidine has also demonstrated some therapeutic benefit,[92] although its effect may not be histamine mediated.[93] The third arm of multimodal therapy is suppression or modulation of neurosensory activity. This may be accomplished with oral therapy such as amitriptyline,[94] duloxetine,[95] nortriptyline, gabapentin or topiramate,[83] or by means of bladder instillations with dimethyl sulfoxise,[96] bacille Calmette-Guérin vaccine,[97] the novel synthetic peptide RDP58,[98] and C-fiber desensitization with resiniferatoxin instillation.[99] A variety of other intravesical cocktails have been demonstrated to produce at least short-term relief of symptoms.[84]

Owing to its various antinociceptive effects, BoNT/A has been investigated as a treatment for PBS/IC.[76] BoNT/A inhibits urothelial acetylcholine and norepinephrine (NE) release in response to electrical stimulation, as well as release of ATP in response to hypo-osmotic stress[100-102] in an animal cystitis model. Depletion of neurotransmitters from sensory afferents diminishes urothelial mast cell release and bladder afferent sensitization in response to colorectal irritation,[103] suggesting BoNT/A-induced inhibition of neurotransmitter release may diminish the release of inflammatory agents (Fig. 21-1). Because calcitonin gene–related peptide (CGRP) is contained primarily in unmyelinated afferent fibers in the bladder, CGRP release from nerve terminals has been used to assess bladder nociceptive responses.[104,105] When compared with rats treated with protamine only, intravesical treatment with BoNT/A following protamine sulfate disruption of the uroethelial barrier was found to diminish CGRP release from afferent nerve terminals as well as irritative cystometric responses to acetic acid seven days after treatment.[106] In a whole rat bladder in vitro model, CGRP release in response to ATP/capsaicin (10 μM/30 nM bath) was studied. ATP/capsaicin increased the release of CGRP by 75% over

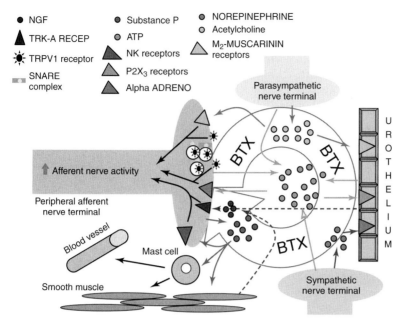

● NGF
▲ TRK-A RECEP
☀ TRPV1 receptor
▭ SNARE complex

● Substance P
○ ATP
△ NK receptors
△ P2X$_3$ receptors
▲ Alpha ADRENO

◐ NOREPINEPHRINE
○ Acetylcholine
△ M$_2$-MUSCARININ receptors

Parasympathetic nerve terminal

BTX

BTX

BTX

U R O T H E L I U M

↑ Afferent nerve activity

Peripheral afferent nerve terminal

Blood vessel

Mast cell

Smooth muscle

Sympathetic nerve terminal

FIGURE 21-1. Representation of neuronal (autonomic) and non-neuronal (urothelial) sources of neurotransmitters modulating bladder afferent nerve activity and the effect of botulinum neurotoxin (BoNT) in the treatment of interstitial cystitis/painful bladder syndrome. BoNT inhibits neurotransmitter release, reducing sensory afferent excitability, thus diminishing or eliminating symptoms. *See Color Plate*

baseline, although neither ATP nor capsaicin individually promoted CGRP release. Pretreatment in a BoNT/A organ bath (50 mM) did not significantly reduce baseline CGRP levels, but ATP/capsaicin-induced CGRP release was significantly reduced by 62%,[107] indicating that BoNT/A suppresses the inflammatory response to noxious stimuli.

Human data on the use of BoNT/A for IC/PBS are limited. The first report was a case series of 13 women with NIDDK-defined IC. The patients underwent submucosal transurethral injections of 100 to 200 U of Dysport (Ipsen, Milford, MA) (seven patients) or BoNT/A (six patients) into 20 to 30 sites in trigone and bladder base. Validated questionnaire (Interstitial Cystitis Symptom Index, Interstitial Cystitis Problem Index) or voiding charts and a VAS were evaluated at baseline, 1 month, and subsequently, at 3-month intervals. Statistically significant improvements in frequency, nocturia, and pain were observed 1 month following treatment, with improvements in first desire to void and cystometric capacity in those patients so evaluated. Onset of symptom relief occurred 5 to 7 days following treatment, and the mean duration of symptom relief was 3.7 months.[108]

In a case series investigating the broader use of BoNT/A injection for the treatment of voiding dysfunction, four patients with IC were included in the cohort of 68 treated patients.[109] For the entire group of patients, frequency and pad use decreased, cystometric capacity increased, no change in maximum voiding detrusor pressure nor in post-void residual bladder volume, with no patient having retention or pyelonephritis despite targeting the bladder base and trigone. Trigone injection was used to maximize C-fiber exposure to the drug. The maximal effect was observed 7 to 30 days following injection. However, interpretation of these results with regard to IC/PBS is difficult because the IC data were not segregated from other voiding dysfunctions in this report and the number of IC/PBS patients was small in comparison to the total cohort.[109]

Somewhat less encouraging is a case series of eight women and two men with chronic IC unresponsive to other therapy. Five were injected with suburothelial 100 U BoNT/A (20 sites), the other five also had 100 U injected into trigone. Functional and cystometric bladder capacity increased, and frequency and pain scores improved mildly. Significant improvements were noted in only two patients. No patient was symptom free following treatment with BoNT/A. There were no therapeutic or adverse differences between the nontrigone and trigone injection groups.[66]

Bladder instillation of BoNT/A rather than injection has also been used. In a case report of a 42-year-old woman with recalcitrant IC, the bladder was instilled with 100 U BoNT/A/100 mL NS following hydrodistension. Decreased irritative symptoms, reduced pain with a 50% decrease in pain medication use, and a 50% decrease in VAS scores for bother were reported 1 week following treatment. Maximum benefit lasted 3 months, with some improvement remaining at six months. Repeating BoNT/A treatment with protamine instillation to disrupt the urothelial barrier instead of hydrodistension had similar clinical benefits.[109]

INJECTION TECHNIQUES

This section presents a summary of our techniques for injection of botulinum toxin into the bladder, prostate and sphincteric tissues.

For the treatment of levator ani spasm, direct transvaginal injection into the levator muscles is made using a standard obstetric pudendal nerve block kit. A solution of BoNT/A is prepared in preservative-free saline, 100 U in 4 mL. The plastic spacer is removed from the needle hub, allowing a 1 cm injection depth. Using the trumpet to protect the operator's index finger, the needle is guided to the levator muscle and the vaginal wall is pierced, the tip of the needle entering the muscle. One milliliter is injected into each of four sites, typically posterolateral, following aspiration to ensure avoidance of intravascular injection. Proximal injections target the pubococcygeus muscles, at the 4 o'clock and 8 o'clock positions, just distal to the ischial spine. Distal injection sites target the puborectalis muscle, at the 4 o'clock and 8 o'clock positions just inside the hymenal ring. Four milliliters of 25 U/mL BoNT/A are used. Superficial perineal muscle injection for vulvodynia is accomplished under direct vision using a small-gauge needle. Injection sites are placed posterolaterally within the posterior fourchette and vulva.

Male CP/CPPS is treated with ultrasound-guided transrectal intraprostatic injection following a periprostatic lidocaine nerve block. BoNT/A 100 to 200 U is diluted in 4 mL saline, and two injections are given bilaterally into the transition zone. Concurrent injections into the external urethral sphincter are given. This is accomplished by means of a rigid cystoscope and a 25-gauge Williams needle (Cook Urologic, Spencer, IN). One injection into each side, 50 U BoNT/A in 1 ml saline, is administered.

Bladder injection for the treatment of IC/PBS is accomplished under brief general anesthesia to allow adequate bladder distension. BoNT/A is prepared by diluting one to three vials (100-300 U) in 10- to 30-mL preservative-free NS for an injectable concentration of 10 U/mL. A rigid cystoscope and a 25-gauge Williams needle are used to inject 20 to 30 0.5- to 1-ml aliquots into the bladder base and trigone. The needle is positioned sufficiently superficial in the bladder wall so that injection is seen to raise a bleb, but not so shallow as to create a blister. The dome of the bladder is avoided to minimize risk to the bowel. Figure 21-2 illustrates typical injection patterns.

SUMMARY

The use of BoNT/A in the treatment of chronic genitourinary pain syndromes holds promise. The toxin likely provides relief by means of a combination of chemical denervation of striated muscle, thereby relieving muscle tension and its induced pain, as well as direct antinociceptive effects. The latter may be the prominent mechanism of relief in PBS/IC. Inconsistencies in the definition and characterization of these syndromes complicate study

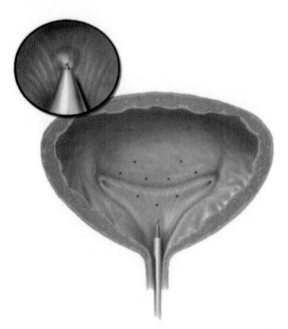

FIGURE 21-2. Suggested urothelial injection technique for botulinum neurotoxin type A in the treatment of interstitial cystitis/painful bladder syndrome. Note multiple small blebs raised by injection of 0.5 to 1 mL (5–10 U) per site on bladder base and trigone, because the intent of therapy is to reduce afferent/sensory activity rather than neuromuscular blockade. An extended injection pattern is avoided to minimize risk of bladder hypotonia and secondary voiding difficulties.

design, although a standard research definition for PBS/IC has been promulgated. Studies of chronic pelvic pain syndromes have used a variety of outcome measures, although syndrome-specific validated tools are available, such as the NIH-CPSI for CP/CPPS. Acceptance of a descriptive taxonomy of pelvic pain syndromes should precede prospective randomized trials with standardized outcome measures in order to fully evaluate the clinical effectiveness of this treatment modality. Continuing efforts toward understanding the antinociceptive actions of BoNT/A will more clearly define its role in specific pain syndromes.

References

1. Fall M, Baranowski AP, Fowler CJ, Lepinard V, Malone-Lee JG, Messelink EJ, et al. EAU guidelines on chronic pelvic pain. *Eur Urol.* 2004;46:681-689.
2. Abrams P, Baranowski A, Berger RE, Fall M, Hanno P, Wesselmann U. A new classification is needed for pelvic pain syndromes—are existing terminologies of spurious diagnostic authority bad for patients? *J Urol.* 2006;175:1989-1990.
3. Moldwin RM. Similarities between interstitial cystitis and male chronic pelvic pain syndrome. *Curr Urol Rep.* 2002;3:313-318.
4. Smith HS, Audette J, Royal MA. Botulinum toxin in pain management of soft tissue syndromes. *Clin J Pain.* 2002;18(6 suppl):S147-S154.
5. Arezzo JC. Possible mechanisms for the effects of botulinum toxin on pain. *Clin J Pain.* 2002;18(6 Suppl):S125-S132.
6. Brin MF, Fahn S, Moskowitz C, Friedman A, Shale HM, Greene PE, et al. Localized injections of botulinum toxin for the treatment of focal dystonia and hemifacial spasm. *Mov Disord.* 1987;2:237-254.
7. Giladi N. The mechanism of action of botulinum toxin type A in focal dystonia is most probably through its dual effect on efferent (motor) and afferent pathways at the injected site. *J Neurol Sci.* 1997;152:132-135.
8. Kessler KR, Benecke R. Botulinum toxin: from poison to remedy. *Neurotoxicology.* 1997;18:761-770.
9. Cui M, Khanijou S, Rubino J, Aoki KR. Subcutaneous administration of botulinum toxin A reduces formalin-induced pain. *Pain.* 2004;107:125-133.11.
10. Aoki KR. Review of a proposed mechanism for the antinociceptive action of botulinum toxin type A. *Neurotoxicology.* 2005;26:785.
11. Mense S. Neurobiological basis for the use of botulinum toxin in pain therapy. *J Neurol.* 2004;251(suppl 1):I1-I7.
12. Park HJ, Lee Y, Lee J, Park C, Moon DE. The effects of botulinum toxin A on mechanical and cold allodynia in a rat model of neuropathic pain. *Can J Anaesth.* 2006;53:470-477.
13. Filippi GM, Errico P, Santarelli R, Bagolini B, Manni E. Botulinum A toxin effects on rat jaw muscle spindles. *Acta Otolaryngol.* 1993;113:400-404.
14. Rosales RL, Arimura K, Takenaga S, Osame M. Extrafusal and intrafusal muscle effects in experimental botulinum toxin-A injection. *Muscle Nerve.* 1996;19:488-496.
15. Rand MJ, Whaler BC. Impairment of sympathetic transmission by botulinum toxin. *Nature.* 1965;206:588-591.
16. Nix WA, Butler IJ, Roontga S, Gutmann L, Hopf HC. Persistent unilateral tibialis anterior muscle hypertrophy with complex repetitive discharges and myalgia: report of two unique cases and response to botulinum toxin. *Neurology.* 1992;42(3 Pt 1):602-606.
17. Davis D, Jabbari B. Significant improvement of stiff-person syndrome after paraspinal injection of botulinum toxin A. *Mov Disord.* 1993;8:371-373.
18. Cosgrove AP, Corry IS, Graham HK. Botulinum toxin in the management of the lower limb in cerebral palsy. *Dev Med Child Neurol.* 1994;36:386-396.
19. Dykstra DD, Sidi AA, Scott AB, Pagel JM, Goldish GD. Effects of botulinum A toxin on detrusor-sphincter dyssynergia in spinal cord injury patients. *J Urol.* 1988;139:919-922.
20. Brin MF, Vapnek JM. Treatment of vaginismus with botulinum toxin injections. *Lancet.* 1997;349:252-253.
21. Stones W, Cheong Y, et al. Interventions for treating chronic pelvic pain in women. *Cochrane Database of Systematic Reviews.* 2005;2:CD000387.
22. Doggweiler R, Zerman D, et al. *Chronic Spasm of Pelvic Floor Muscles in Patients with Chronic Pelvic Pain.* ICS 29th Annual Scientific Meeting, Denver CO, 1999.
23. Brookoff D, Bennett DS. Neuromodulation in intractable interstitial cystitis and related pelvic pain syndromes. *Pain Med.* 2006;7(Suppl 1):S166-S184.
24. Kapural L, Narouze SN, Janicki TI, Mekhail N. Spinal cord stimulation is an effective treatment for the chronic intractable visceral pelvic pain. *Pain Med.* 2006;7:440-443.
25. Updike GM, Wiesenfeld HC. Insight into the treatment of vulvar pain: a survey of clinicians. *Am J Obstet Gynecol.* 2005;193:1404-1409.
26. Smart OC, MacLean AB. Vulvodynia. *Curr Opin Obstet Gynecol.* 2003;15:497-500.
27. Hartmann D, Strauhal MJ, Nelson CA. Treatment of women in the United States with localized, provoked vulvodynia: practice survey of women's health physical therapists. *J Reprod Med.* 2007;52:48-52.
28. Aboseif S, Tamaddon K, Chalfin S, Freedman S, Kaptein J. Sacral neuromodulation as an effective treatment for refractory pelvic floor dysfunction. *Urology.* 2002;60:52-56.
29. Gunter J, Brewer A, Tawfik O. Botulinum toxin a for vulvodynia: a case report. *J Pain.* 2004;5:238-240.
30. Dykstra DD, Presthus J. Botulinum toxin type A for the treatment of provoked vestibulodynia: an open-label, pilot study. *J Reprod Med.* 2006;51:467-470.
31. Yoon H, Chung WS, Shim BS. Botulinum toxin A for the management of vulvodynia. *Int J Impot Res.* 2007;19:84-87.
32. Shafik A, El-Sibai O. Vaginismus: results of treatment with botulin toxin. *J Obstet Gynaecol.* 2000;20:300-302.
33. Ghazizadeh S, Nikzad M. Botulinum toxin in the treatment of refractory vaginismus. *Obstet Gynecol.* 2004;104(5 Pt 1):922-925.
34. Everaert K, Devulder J, et al: The Pain Cycle, Implications for the Diagnosis and Treatment of Pelvic Pain Syndromes. ICS 29th Annual Scientific Meeting, Denver CO, 1999.
35. Glazer HI, Jantos M, Hartmann EH, Swencionis C. Electromyographic comparisons of the pelvic floor in women with dysesthetic vulvodynia and asymptomatic women. *J Reprod Med.* 1998;43:959-962.

36. Langford CF, Udvari Nagy S, Ghoniem GM. Levator ani trigger point injections: An underutilized treatment for chronic pelvic pain. *Neurourol Urodyn.* 2007;26:59-62.

37. Romito S, Bottanelli M, Pellegrini M, Vicentini S, Rizzuto N, Bertolasi L. Botulinum toxin for the treatment of genital pain syndromes. *Gynecol Obstet Invest.* 2004;58:164-167.

38. Jarvis SK, Abbott JA, Lenart MB, Steensma A, Vancaillie TG. Pilot study of botulinum toxin type A in the treatment of chronic pelvic pain associated with spasm of the levator ani muscles. *Aust N Z J Obstet Gynaecol.* 2004;44:46-50.

39. Thomson AJ, Jarvis SK, Lenart M, Abbott JA, Vancaillie TG. The use of botulinum toxin type A (BOTOX) as treatment for intractable chronic pelvic pain associated with spasm of the levator ani muscles. *BJOG.* 2005;112:247-249.

40. Abbott JA, Jarvis SK, Lyons SD, Thomson A, Vancaille TG. Botulinum toxin type A for chronic pain and pelvic floor spasm in women: a randomized controlled trial. *Obstet Gynecol.* 2006;108:915-923.

41. Nickel JC, Nyberg LM, Hennenfent M. Research guidelines for chronic prostatitis: consensus report from the first National Institutes of Health International Prostatitis Collaborative Network. *Urology.* 1999;54: 229-233.

42. Krieger JN, Egan KJ, Ross SO, Jacobs R, Berger RE. Chronic pelvic pains represent the most prominent urogenital symptoms of chronic prostatitis. *Urology.* 1996;48:715-721; discussion 721-722.

43. Collins MM, Stafford RS, O'Leary MP, Barry MJ. How common is prostatitis? A national survey of physician visits. *J Urol.* 1998;159:1224-1228.

44. Zermann DH, Ishigooka M, Doggweiler-Wiygul R, Schubert J, Schmidt RA. The male chronic pelvic pain syndrome. *World J Urol.* 2001;19:173-179.

45. Pontari MA, McNaughton-Collins M, O'Leary MP, Calhoun EA, Jang T, Kusek JW, et al. A case-control study of risk factors in men with chronic pelvic pain syndrome. *BJU Int.* 2005;96:559-565.

46. Habermacher GM, Chason JT, Schaeffer AJ. Prostatitis/chronic pelvic pain syndrome. *Annu Rev Med.* 2006;57:195-206.

47. Nickel JC, Alexander RB, Schaeffer AJ, Landis JR, Knauss JS, Propert KJ; Chronic Prostatitis Collaborative Research Network Study Group. Leukocytes and bacteria in men with chronic prostatitis/chronic pelvic pain syndrome compared to asymptomatic controls. *J Urol.* 2003;170:818-822.

48. Nadler RB, Collins MM, Propert KJ, Mikolajczyk SD, Knauss JS, Landis JR, et al. Prostate-specific antigen test in diagnostic evaluation of chronic prostatitis/chronic pelvic pain syndrome. *Urology.* 2006;67: 337-342.

49. Yilmaz U, Liu YW, Rothman I, Lee JC, Yang CC, Berger RE. Intravesical potassium chloride sensitivity test in men with chronic pelvic pain syndrome. *J Urol.* 2004;172:548-550.

50. Litwin MS. A review of the development and validation of the National Institutes of Health Chronic Prostatitis Symptom Index. *Urology.* 2002;60(6 suppl):14-18; discussion 18-19.

51. Turner JA, Ciol MA, Von Korff M, Berger R. Validity and responsiveness of the national institutes of health chronic prostatitis symptom index. *J Urol.* 2003;169:580-583.

52. Propert KJ, Litwin MS, Wang Y, Alexander RB, Calhoun E, Nickel JC, et al. Responsiveness of the National Institutes of Health Chronic Prostatitis Symptom Index (NIH-CPSI). *Qual Life Res.* 2006;15:299-305.

53. Schneider H, Ludwig M, Weidner W, Brähler E. Experience with different questionnaires in the management of patients with CP/CPPS: GPSS, IPSS and NIH-CPSI. *World J Urol.* 2003;21:116-118; discussion 115.

54. Nickel JC, Johnston B, Downey J, Barkin J, Pommerville P, Gregoire M, et al. Pentosan polysulfate therapy for chronic nonbacterial prostatitis (chronic pelvic pain syndrome category IIIA): a prospective multicenter clinical trial. *Urology.* 2000;56:413-417.

55. Nickel JC, Forrest JB, Tomera K, Hernandez-Graulau J, Moon TD, Schaeffer AJ, et al. Pentosan polysulfate sodium therapy for men with chronic pelvic pain syndrome: a multicenter, randomized, placebo controlled study. *J Urol.* 2005;173:1252-1255.

56. Mehik A, Alas P, Nickel JC, Sarpola A, Helström PJ. Alfuzosin treatment for chronic prostatitis/chronic pelvic pain syndrome: a prospective, randomized, double-blind, placebo-controlled, pilot study. *Urology.* 2003;62:425-429.

57. Alexander RB, Propert KJ, Schaeffer AJ, Landis JR, Nickel JC, O'Leary MP, et al. Ciprofloxacin or tamsulosin in men with chronic prostatitis/chronic pelvic pain syndrome. *Ann Intern Med.* 2004;141:581.

58. Nickel JC, Narayan P, McKay J, Doyle C. Treatment of chronic prostatitis/chronic pelvic pain syndrome with tamsulosin: a randomized double-blind trial. *J Urol.* 2004;171:1594.

59. Chuang YC, Yoshimura N, Wu M, Huang CC, Chiang PH, Tyagi P, et al. Intraprostatic capsaicin injection as a novel model for nonbacterial prostatitis and effects of botulinum toxin A. *Eur Urol.* 2007;51:1119-1127.

60. Propert KJ, McNaughton-Collins M, Leiby BE, O'Leary MP, Kusek JW, Litwin MS, et al. A prospective study of symptoms and quality of life in men with chronic prostatitis/chronic pelvic pain syndrome: the National Institutes of Health Chronic Prostatitis Cohort study. *J Urol.* 2006;175:619-623; discussion 623.

61. Turini D, Beneforti P, Spinelli M, Malagutti S, Lazzeri M. Heat/burning sensation induced by topical application of capsaicin on perineal cutaneous area: new approach in diagnosis and treatment of chronic prostatitis/chronic pelvic pain syndrome? *Urology.* 2006;67:910-913.

62. Maria G, Destito A, Lacquaniti S, Bentivoglio AR, Brisinda G, Albanese A. Relief by botulinum toxin of voiding dysfunction due to prostatitis. *Lancet.* 1998;352:625.

63. Maria G, Cadeddu F, Brisinda D, Brandara F, Brisinda G. Management of bladder, prostatic and pelvic floor disorders with botulinum neurotoxin. *Curr Med Chem.* 2005;12:247-265.

64. Maria G, Brisinda G, Civello IM, Bentivoglio AR, Sganga G, Albanese A. Relief by botulinum toxin of voiding dysfunction due to benign prostatic hyperplasia: results of a randomized, placebo-controlled study. *Urology.* 2003;62:259-264; discussion 264-265.

65. Chuang YC, Chiang PH, Huang CC, Yoshimura N, Chancellor MB. Botulinum toxin type A improves benign prostatic hyperplasia symptoms in patients with small prostates. *Urology.* 2005;66:775-779.

66. Kuo HC. Preliminary results of suburothelial injection of botulinum a toxin in the treatment of chronic interstitial cystitis. *Urol Int.* 2005;75:170-174.

67. Chuang YC, Chiang PH, Yoshimura N, De Miguel F, Chancellor MB. Sustained beneficial effects of

intraprostatic botulinum toxin type A on lower urinary tract symptoms and quality of life in men with benign prostatic hyperplasia. *BJU Int.* 2006;98:1033-1037; discussion 1337.

68. Park DS, Cho TW, Lee YK, Lee YT, Hong YK, Jang WK. Evaluation of short term clinical effects and presumptive mechanism of botulinum toxin type A as a treatment modality of benign prostatic hyperplasia. *Yonsei Med J.* 2006;47:706-714.

69. Zermann D, Ishigooka M, Schubert J, Schmidt RA. Perisphincteric injection of botulinum toxin type A. A treatment option for patients with chronic prostatic pain? *Eur Urol.* 2000;38:393-399.

70. Nickel JC. Interstitial cystitis: the paradigm shifts: international consultations on interstitial cystitis. *Rev Urol.* 2004;6:200-202.

71. Bogart LM, Berry SH, Clemens JQ. Symptoms of interstitial cystitis, painful bladder syndrome and similar diseases in women: a systematic review. *J Urol.* 2007;177:450-456.

72. Forrest JB, Nickel JC, Moldwin RM. Chronic prostatitis/chronic pelvic pain syndrome and male interstitial cystitis: enigmas and opportunities. *Urology.* 2007;69 (4 suppl):S60-S63.

73. Hanno PM, Landis JR, Matthews-Cook Y, Kusek J, Nyberg L Jr. The diagnosis of interstitial cystitis revisited: lessons learned from the National Institutes of Health Interstitial Cystitis Database study. *J Urol.* 1999;161:553-557.

74. Evans RJ, Sant GR. Current diagnosis of interstitial cystitis: an evolving paradigm. *Urology.* 2007; 69(4 Suppl):S64-S72.

75. Peeker R, Fall M. Toward a precise definition of interstitial cystitis: further evidence of differences in classic and nonulcer disease. *J Urol.* 2002;167:2470-2472.

76. Toft BR, Nordling J. Recent developments of intravesical therapy of painful bladder syndrome/interstitial cystitis: a review. *Curr Opin Urol.* 2006;16:268-272.

77. Parsons CL, Stauffer C, Schmidt JD. Bladder-surface glycosaminoglycans: an efficient mechanism of environmental adaptation. *Science.* 1980;208:605-607.

78. Parsons CL, Boychuk D, Jones S, Hurst R, Callahan H. Bladder surface glycosaminoglycans: an epithelial permeability barrier. *J Urol.* 1990;143:139-142.

79. Sun Y, Keay S, De Deyne PG, Chai TC. Augmented stretch activated adenosine triphosphate release from bladder uroepithelial cells in patients with interstitial cystitis. *J Urol.* 2001;166:1951-1956.

80. Sun Y, Chai TC. Up-regulation of P2X3 receptor during stretch of bladder urothelial cells from patients with interstitial cystitis. *J Urol.* 2004;171:448-452.

81. Maggi CA. The dual function of capsaicin-sensitive sensory nerves in the bladder and urethra. *Ciba Found Symp.* 1990;151:77-83; discussion 83-90.

82. Pezzone MA, Liang R, Fraser MO. A model of neural cross-talk and irritation in the pelvis: implications for the overlap of chronic pelvic pain disorders. *Gastroenterology.* 2005;128:1953-1964.

83. Wesselmann U. Neurogenic inflammation and chronic pelvic pain. *World J Urol.* 2001;19:180-185.

84. Moldwin RM, Evans RJ, Stanford EJ, Rosenberg MT. Rational approaches to the treatment of patients with interstitial cystitis. *Urology.* 2007;69(4 suppl):S73-S81.

85. Mulholland SG, Hanno P, Parsons CL, Sant GR, Staskin DR. Pentosan polysulfate sodium for therapy of interstitial cystitis. A double-blind placebo-controlled clinical study. *Urology.* 1990;35:552-558.

86. Hanno PM. Analysis of long-term Elmiron therapy for interstitial cystitis. *Urology.* 1997;49(5A suppl):93-99.

87. Daha LK, Riedl CR, Lazar D, Hohlbrugger G, Pflüger H. Do cystometric findings predict the results of intravesical hyaluronic acid in women with interstitial cystitis? *Eur Urol.* 2005;47:393-397; discussion 397.

88. Kallestrup EB, Jorgensen SS, Nordling J, Hald T. Treatment of interstitial cystitis with Cystistat: a hyaluronic acid product. *Scand J Urol Nephrol.* 2005;39:143-147.

89. Parsons CL. Successful downregulation of bladder sensory nerves with combination of heparin and alkalinized lidocaine in patients with interstitial cystitis. *Urology.* 2005;65:45-48.

90. Theoharides TC, Sant GR. Hydroxyzine therapy for interstitial cystitis. *Urology.* 1997;49(5A suppl): 108-110.

91. Sant GR, Propert KJ, Hanno PM, Burks D, Culkin D, Diokno AC, et al. A pilot clinical trial of oral pentosan polysulfate and oral hydroxyzine in patients with interstitial cystitis. *J Urol.* 2003;170:810-815.

92. Seshadri P, Emerson L, Morales A. Cimetidine in the treatment of interstitial cystitis. *Urology.* 1994;44: 614-616.

93. Dasgupta P, Sharma SD, Womack C, Blackford HN, Dennis P. Cimetidine in painful bladder syndrome: a histopathological study. *BJU Int.* 2001;88:183-186.

94. van Ophoven A, Hertle L. Long-term results of amitriptyline treatment for interstitial cystitis. *J Urol.* 2005;174:1837-1840.

95. van Ophoven A, Hertle L. The dual serotonin and noradrenaline reuptake inhibitor duloxetine for the treatment of interstitial cystitis: results of an observational study. *J Urol.* 2007;177:552-555.

96. Rossberger J, Fall M, Peeker R. Critical appraisal of dimethyl sulfoxide treatment for interstitial cystitis: discomfort, side-effects and treatment outcome. *Scand J Urol Nephrol.* 2005;39:73-77.

97. Mayer R, Propert KJ, Peters KM, Payne CK, Zhang Y, Burks D, et al. A randomized controlled trial of intravesical Bacillus Calmette-Guerin for treatment refractory interstitial cystitis. *J Urol.* 2005;173: 1186-1191.

98. Luo Y. A potential modality for interstitial cystitis: intravesical use of anti-inflammatory peptide RDP58. *J Urol.* 2005;173:340.

99. Payne CK, Mosbaugh PG, Forrest JB, Evans RJ, Whitmore KE, Antoci JP, et al. Intravesical resiniferatoxin for the treatment of interstitial cystitis: a randomized, double-blind, placebo controlled trial. *J Urol.* 2005;173:1590-1594.

100. Smith CP, Franks ME, McNeil BK, Ghosh R, de Groat WC, Chancellor MB, et al. Effect of botulinum toxin A on the autonomic nervous system of the rat lower urinary tract. *J Urol.* 2003;169:1896-1900.

101. Smith CP, Vemulakonda VM, Kiss S, Boone TB, Somogyi GT. Enhanced ATP release from rat bladder urothelium during chronic bladder inflammation: effect of botulinum toxin A. *Neurochem Int.* 2005;47:291-297.

102. Vemulakonda VM, Somogyi GT, Kiss S, Salas NA, Boone TB, Smith CP. Inhibitory effect of intravesically applied botulinum toxin A in chronic bladder inflammation. *J Urol.* 2005;173:621-624.

103. Ustinova EE, Gutkin DW, Pezzone MA. Sensitization of pelvic nerve afferents and mast cell infiltration in the urinary bladder following chronic colonic irritation is mediated by neuropeptides. *Am J Physiol Renal Physiol.* 2007;292:F123-F130.

104. Gabella G, Davis C. Distribution of afferent axons in the bladder of rats. *J Neurocytol.* 1998;27:141-155.

105. Huang H, Wu X, Nicol GD, Meller S, Vasko MR. ATP augments peptide release from rat sensory neurons in culture through activation of P2Y receptors. *J Pharmacol Exp Ther*. 2003;306:1137-1144.

106. Chuang YC, Yoshimura N, Huang CC, Chiang PH, Chancellor MB. Intravesical botulinum toxin A administration produces analgesia against acetic acid induced bladder pain responses in rats. *J Urol*. 2004;172(4 Pt 1):1529-1532.

107. Rapp DE, Turk KW, Bales GT, Cook SP. Botulinum toxin type a inhibits calcitonin gene-related peptide release from isolated rat bladder. *J Urol*. 2006;175(3 Pt 1):1138-1142.

108. Smith CP, Radziszewski P, Borkowski A, Somogyi GT, Boone TB, Chancellor MB. Botulinum toxin a has antinociceptive effects in treating interstitial cystitis. *Urology*. 2004;64:871-875; discussion 875.

109. Smith CP, Nishiguchi J, O'Leary M, Yoshimura N, Chancellor MB. Single-institution experience in 110 patients with botulinum toxin A injection into bladder or urethra. *Urology*. 2005;65:37-41.

110. Kuo HC. Prostate botulinum A toxin injection—an alternative treatment for benign prostatic obstruction in poor surgical candidates. *Urology*. 2005;65: 670-674.

Application of 22 Botulinum Toxin in the Prostate

Yao-Chi Chuang and Michael B. Chancellor

INTRODUCTION

Benign prostatic hyperplasia (BPH) is a non-malignant enlargement of the prostate in aging men. Although there is debate regarding the exact definition, the fundamental aspects of the disease include the interaction between the prostatic hyperplasia, bladder outlet obstruction, and lower urinary tract symptoms (LUTS).[1] The LUTS associated with BPH can be categorized into voiding symptoms and storage symptoms. The degree to which the symptoms bother the patient and impair quality of life is the key factor for seeking medical treatment with an urologist.

Although the etiology of BPH remains unknown, it has been suggested that excessive growth (static component) and contraction (dynamic component) are the two main components. The static component is under parasympathetic control and regulated by androgen, whereas the stromal smooth muscle is sympathetically influenced. Alpha-1 adrenoceptor antagonists and 5 alpha reductase inhibitors are the most common medical therapies used today to treat BPH.[2,3] However, both types of drugs require daily administration, and some patients discontinue treatment due to intolerable side effects, such as postural hypotension, retrograde ejaculation, and impotence. Transurethral resection of the prostate (TURP) is used when there is no response to medical treatment or when BPH-related complications occur. Nevertheless, concerns have been raised about the safety of TURP.[3] Minimally invasive therapies for BPH have been developed for those who have a poor response to medical treatment and are unwilling or too high risk to take TURP.[3]

The human prostate is innervated by sympathetic and parasympathetic efferents, as well as by sensory afferents. The prostatic epithelium receives a cholinergic innervation, whereas the stroma receives a predominantly noradrenergic innervation.[4-6] Cholinergic innervation of the prostate gland has an important role in regulation of the functions of the prostate epithelium, with effects on growth and secretion, whereas the noradrenergic innervation has been implicated in the contraction of smooth muscle and etiology of outflow obstruction accompanying BPH.[4-6] In addition, excessive sympathetic activity stimulates epidermal growth factor in the prostate, which results in trophic function in prostate growth.[7,8]

Botulinum neurotoxin type A (BoNT/A), an agent known to inhibit acetylcholine release at the presynaptic cholinergic junction, has been injected into the bladder and urethra to treat various types of voiding dysfunction.[9] Recently, more studies have demonstrated that BoNT/A could also inhibit other neurotransmitters, including norepinephrine and sensory neurotransmitters.[10-12] Therefore, the application of BoNT/A has been expanded to treat symptomatic BPH patients with exciting primary results. The purpose of this chapter is to review the mechanisms of action and results of BoNT/A treatment for BPH, and to provide perspectives on potential therapy for prostatic diseases.[13]

Dr. Chuang is disclosing that he is a consultant for Allergan, Inc. Dr. Chancellor is disclosing that he is both a consultant and investigator for Allergan, Inc.

EXPERIMENTAL EVIDENCE

In the rat prostate, it has been reported that the stromal and glandular components account for 48.3% and 51.8% of the entire prostate, respectively.[14] Doggweiler and colleagues used single or serial injections of BoNT/A into the rat prostate and observed a generalized atrophy and apoptosis of glandular elements.[15] BoNT/A, inhibiting the release of acetylcholine at the nerve terminal, can suppress the secretomotor function of acetylcholine on the prostate and result in a decrease of the prostate weight. We know that the prostate is under the influence of not only acetylcholine but also norepinephrine and testosterone.[4-6] Therefore, additional mechanisms might be involved, but this remains to be explored. In a male rat prostate model, we have demonstrated a significant increase in apoptotic cells after BoNT/A injection (12-fold, 16-fold, and 22-fold increase for 5 U, 10 U, and 20 U Botox [Allergan, Irvine, CA], respectively). Although there was no change in the androgen receptor, there were decreases in alpha-1A adrenergic receptor of 13%, 80%, and 81% for 5 U, 10 U, and 20 U Botox, respectively. We also observed a decrease in proliferative cells of 38%, 77%, and 80% for 5 U, 10 U, and 20 U Botox, respectively.[16]

These studies suggest that BoNT/A may have an effect on both the dynamic and static components of BPH. We must keep in mind that there are differences among species in the make up of the prostate gland. The rat prostate is primarily epithelium, whereas the human prostate is primarily stroma, and the results of BoNT-A effects on the rat prostate cannot be generalized to the human therapeutic arena without due caution.

The dog is one of a few animals that can develop BPH spontaneously and is frequently used as an animal model for the study of human prostatic hyperplasia.[17] Chuang et al[18] investigated morphologic and apoptotic changes in the canine prostate after BoNT/A injection. Results demonstrated that injection of BoNT/A induced marked atrophy and diffuse apoptosis of prostate glands associated with decreased cell proliferation (Figs. 22-1 and 22-2). The effect persisted for at least 3 months without any notable side effects.

Doggweiler et al[15] suggested that denervation can alter growth factor expression in the rat prostate and resulted in programmed cell death. Thus apoptotic changes in the prostate after BoNT/A treatment are likely to be related

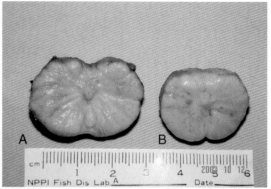

FIGURE 22-1. Coronal section of canine prostate one month after botulinum neurotoxin type A (BoNT/A) or saline injection. Smaller in size and less indurations after BoNT/A injection (**B**) than the control (**A**). (With permission from BMC Urology.)

with reduced neurotrophic influence on the gland. Expression of specific prostate apoptosis-related genes, such as bcl2 and transforming growth factor-β has been implicated in the pathogenesis of BPH.[19] Thus, induction of apoptosis may emerge as an attractive target for the management of BPH.

The dynamic component of BPH comes from contraction of smooth muscle cells in the stroma, which are adrenergically innervated. Lin et al[20] reported that injection of 200 U BoNT/A into the canine prostate significantly reduced the prostate urethral pressure response to intravenous norepinephrine and electrostimulation, and induced pronounced atrophic changes in prostate gland and vacuoles formation in smooth muscle cells of the stromal tissue. However, these effects were less significant in the group injected with 100 U. They concluded that BoNT/A reduces contractile function while maintaining relaxation response of the prostate, enabling BoNT/A a viable option to manage prostate-related symptoms.

PROSTATE APPLICATIONS

BoNT-A BPH Clinical Results

In 2003, Maria and colleagues[21] first reported on BoNT/A injection into the prostate in men with voiding dysfunction due to BPH. A total of 30 men were treated with either Botox (200 units in 4 mL saline) or saline by transperineal injection into bilateral lobes of prostate. Thirteen of 15 patients (86.6%) in

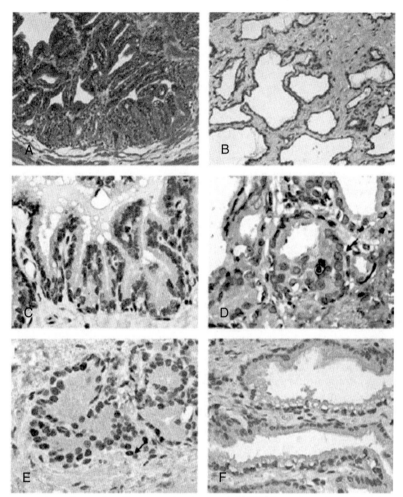

FIGURE 22-2. Representative saline or botulinum neurotoxin type A (BoNT/A) treatment in canine prostate at 3 months for H & E, terminal deoxynucleotidyl-mediated deoxyuridine triphosphate nick end labeling (TUNEL) and proliferative cell nuclear antigen (PCNA) staining. Significant glandular proliferation with papillary infolding in the lumen was seen in the control canine (**A**). Atrophy change of glandular component with flattening of the lining epithelium was seen in the BoNT/A-treated canine (**B**). More TUNEL-stained cells are recognized in the BoNT/A-treated animal (**D**) than the saline-treated animal (**C**). More PCNA-stained cells are recognized in the control animal (**E**) than the BoNT/A-treated animal (**F**). (With permission from BJU International.) *See Color Plate*

the treated group versus three of the 15 patients (20%) in the control group had symptomatic improvement at the 2-month follow-up examination. In BoNT/A-treated patients, significant increases in maximum flow rates from 8.1 to 16.8 mL/sec (52%), as well as significant decreases in post void residual (PVR) from 126.3 to 21.0 mL (83%), were seen. Prostate volumes decreased from 52.6 to 16.8 mL (68%), prostate specific antigen (PSA) levels dropped from 3.7 to 1.8 ng/mL (51%), and American Urological Association (AUA) symptom scores improved from 23.2 to 8.0 (65%). Signs and symptoms were stable through 6 and 12 months in the BoNT/A-treated patients.

There are no local complications or systemic side effects observed in an average of 19.6 months follow-up. None of these parameters improved in the patients who received saline injection.

Recently, Kuo reported on 10 patients with video urodynamically proved benign prostatic obstruction and chronic urinary retention or large residual urine who received Botox (200 U in 20 mL saline) injection into 10 sites of transitional zone of prostate via cystoscopy.[22] All patients had an improvement in spontaneous voiding, with significant increases in maximum flow rates from 7.6 to 9.9 mL/sec (30.3%) as well as significant decreases in

PVR from 243.0 to 53.9 mL (77.8%), prostate volumes from 65.6 to 49.5 mL (29.9%), voiding detrusor pressure from 65.0 to 54.1 cm H_2O (16.8%) and quality of life index from 4.5 to 2.3 (48.9%) at 3 months follow-up. The maximal effects of BoNT/A appeared at 1 week and were maintained at the end of study, with a mean of 9 months follow-up. No local or systemic side effects were reported in any patients. Interestingly, there is no significant change in the transition zone index. This study suggested that BoNT/A might be effective throughout the prostate gland in addition to the transition zone.

Chuang et al[18] have reported on eight BPH patients refractory to alpha blockers treated with transperineal injection of 200 U of BoNT/A into the prostate. Two injections of equal volume (2 mL) were given in each lobe. All patients had a prostate volume of greater than 40 mL and a peak urine flow rate less than 12 mL/sec. No local or systemic side effects were observed. Most patients reported improvement starting from 3 to 7 days after BoNT-A treatment, reaching maximal effect in about 1 month, and maintaining effects for as long as 8 months. At 1-month follow-up, the prostate volume, mean symptom score and quality of life index were significantly reduced by 18.8% (from 61.6 ± 8.7 to 50.0 ± 5.9 mL, $P < 0.05$), 73.1% (from 19.0 ± 1.8 to 5.1 ± 2.0, $P < 0.05$) and 61.5% (from 3.9 ± 0.3 to 1.5 ± 0.2, $P < 0.05$), respectively. The maximal flow rate was increased by 72.0% (from 7.5 ± 1.8 to 12.9 ± 0.5 mL/sec, $P < 0.05$). The residual urine was decreased by 86.2% (from 177.6 ± 71.7 to 24.5 ± 4.5 mL, $P = 0.064$). Two patients with chronic urinary retention can void spontaneously 1 week after BoNT/A injection. One patient did not have decrease of prostate volume but had improvement in symptom score and flow rate. It raised the possibility that BoNT/A has effects on the dynamic component of BPH.

In a report from Italy, Guercini et al[23] treated 16 men with prostate gland size of more than 80 mL and low flow rate (maximal flow rate < 10 mL/sec) with prostatic BoNT/A injection. The authors used intraprostatic injection of 150 U of BoNT/A dissolved in saline solution into each lobe. Improvement was seen at 1 month follow-up and sustained for 6 months. The prostate volume and mean symptom score were significantly reduced by 38.7% (from 106 to 65 mL) and 45.8% (from 24 to 13) at 1 month, respectively.

Most interestingly PSA and residual urine were significantly reduced by 28.4% (from 9.5 to 6.8 ng/dL), and 64.1% (295 to 106 mL), respectively.

The prostate size has an impact on the therapeutic effect of one treatment for BPH. Chuang et al[24] expanded the clinical use of BoNT/A in treating patients with a small prostate and symptomatic BPH. A total of 16 patients with small prostate size (less than 30 mL), symptomatic BPH, and a peak urine flow rate less than 12 mL/sec received intraprostatic injection of BoNT/A (100 U/4 mL). One injection of equal volume (2 mL) into each lobe of the gland was performed.[24] No significant local or systemic side effects were observed in any of the patients. All patients reported subjective improvement starting approximately 1 week, achieving maximal effect after 1 month, and maintaining at a mean follow-up of 10 months. The mean prostate volume, symptom score, and quality of life index were significantly reduced by 13.3% (from 19.6 ± 1.2 mL to 17.0 ± 1.1 mL), 52.6% (from 18.8 ± 1.6 to 8.9 ± 1.9), and 44.7% (from 3.8 ± 0.3 to 2.1 ± 0.3), respectively. The maximal flow rate was significantly increased by 39.8% (7.3 ± 0.7 mL/sec to 11.8 ± 0.8 mL/sec). In two patients who received biopsy 1 month after BoNT/A injection, the TUNEL staining demonstrated increase in apoptotic activity not only in the glandular component but also in the stromal component of the prostate tissue. This study suggests that BoNT-A disrupted the trophic effect of autonomic systemic on the prostate gland and induced cellular apoptosis. However, four of 16 patients had an increased peak flow rate and improved symptoms without shrinkage of the prostate volume.

In an open-label study, Larson et al[25] reported symptomatic improvement in International Prostate Symptom Score (IPSS), bother score, and peak flow rate in 10 patients with BPH who were transrectally injected with 100 U Botox 3 months after injection. In contrast to the positive response report of BoNT on the prostate gland summarized earlier, another study did not find any therapeutic benefit from intraprostatic BoNT injection. There was no change in prostate volume as measured by pelvic magnetic resonance imaging in a sham double-blind study using 200 U BoNT/A or saline in 30 patients.

Park et al[26] reported that 39 out of 52 patients with symptomatic improvement:

decreased IPSS by 30.3%, QOL by 34.4%, prostate volume by 13.1%, residual urine by 34.3%, and increased peak flow rate by 15.5% after transperineal injection of various doses of BoNT/A from 100 U to 300 U in a 3-month follow-up study. The authors reported that voiding symptoms improved but not to the same extent as storage symptoms.

In our series,[27] a total of 41 men (mean age 69.1 ± 7.1 years) with an IPSS ≧8, peak flow rate less than 12 mL/sec, and refractory to medical treatment were injected with 100 U (N = 21, for prostate volume less then 30 mL) or 200 U (N = 20, for prostate volume greater than 30 mL) of BoNT/A into the prostate transperineally under transrectal ultrasound guidance. No significant local or systemic side effects were observed in any of the patients. Thirty-one of 41 patients (75.6%) had more than 30% improvement on LUTS and QOL indices. Four of 5 patients (80%) with urinary retention for more than 1 month can void spontaneously from 1 week to 1 month after BoNT/A injection. Twelve of 41 patients (29.2%) did not have a change in prostate volume; however, seven of the 12 patients (58.3%) still have more than 30% improvement in the maximal flow rate, LUTS, and QOL. Current studies suggest that the mechanisms on relief of LUTS through intraprostatic BoNT/A injection may not totally depend on the volume of shrinkage. The inhibitory effect on the smooth muscle tone and sensory nerve function may play an important role. A summary of published reports on prostate BoNT injection is listed in Table 22-1. It appears that intraprostatic BoNT/A injection improved LUTS associated with various degrees of reduction of prostate volume and increase of flow rate. The duration of effect is reported to last 6 months or longer. Because the use of botulinum toxin for therapy of disorders of the prostate is currently off label, caution should be applied until larger randomized clinical studies are completed that will guide physicians in making decisions about the use of botulinum toxin for this indication.

Prostate Botulinum Toxin Type A Injection Technique and Dosage

Intraprostatic injection therapy for BPH has been explored to reduce prostate volume since early 1900s.[28] The indication for treatment was shifting to LUTS associated with various sizes of prostate. Chalfin and Bradley's work on injecting local anesthetic into the prostate demonstrated the disappearance of detrusor overactivity in patients with benign prostatic obstruction.[29] The study lends to support the concept that ablation of sensory stimuli from the prostate would be of therapeutic benefit. Therefore, BoNT may produce its effects not by apoptosis leading to gland shrinkage, but by denervation causing storage symptoms to improve.

As demonstrated in Table 22-1, successful BoNT/A injections can be performed using transperineal, transurethral, or transrectal approaches. The transperineal and transrectal route eliminates the need for cystoscopy and can be performed even without local anesthesia and temporary urethral catheter drainage. Therapeutic doses have been reported from 100 U to 300 U of Botox in different volumes from 4 to 20 mL. Unlike alcohol-induced tissue necrosis and inflammation, there has been no report of local or systemic complications with injection of the prostate with BoNT.

We perform BoNT prostate injections by mixing one vial (100 U) of BoNT/A with 4 mL of saline just before injection. The total units of Botox used in our group were from 100 to 200 U, depending on the size of the prostate. In patients with a smaller prostate (i.e., <30 mL), we selected 100 U, and for those with a larger prostate (>30 mL), we selected 200 U. However, for those with a prostate larger than 60 mL, more than 200 U may be necessary. The patients were placed in a lithotomy position and treated using transperineal injection under ultrasound-guided transrectal control. A 21-gauge, 20-cm long needle (Chiba, Denmark) was placed in the adapter of the transrectal linear 7.5-MHz endosonic multiplane transducer (BK, type 8551, B-K medical, Denmark) and was inserted 1 cm to the left and 1 cm to the right of the median raphe and 1 to 3 cm above the anal sphincter (Fig. 22-3).[18,24] The transverse view was used to ensure proper placement of the needle, which appeared as a bright spot in the center of the transitional zone. The scanning plane was changed to longitudinal, and the needle was further advanced until 0.5 to 1.0 cm from the bladder neck. BoNT was injected at the cranial, middle, and caudal aspect of lateral lobe. Diffusion of hyperechoic BoNT over the lateral lobe of the prostate was noted by transrectal ultrasound (TRUS) monitoring.

TABLE 22-1 Benign Prostatic Hyperplasia Patients' Response to Intraprostatic Injection of Botulinum Neurotoxin Type A

Reference	Study Design	Patient Criteria and Number	BoNT Dose	Method	% of Improvement at First and Last Follow-Up	Mean Follow-Up
Smith et al[10] (paper)	Double blind, placebo controlled 1:1 ratio	IPSS > 8 Qmax < 15 mL/sec N = 30	200 U 50 U/mL	Transperineal, 22-gauge needle	IPSS: 54%, 62% QOL: NA Qmax: 46%, 46% RU: 60%, 81% Prostate size: 54%, 61% PSA: 42%, 38% At 1 and 12 months	19.6 months
Chuang et al[11] (paper)	Prospective	BPO poor surgical candidates; prostate > 30 mL N = 10	200 U 10 U/mL	Transurethral, 23-gauge needle	QOL: 49%, 51% Qmax: 30%, 53% RU: 78%, 85% Prostate size: 30%, 24% PSA: NA At 3 and 6 months	9 months
Welch et al[12] (paper)	Prospective	Symptomatic BPH prostate < 30 mL Qmax < 12 mL/sec N = 16	100 U 25 U/mL	Transperineal, 21-gauge needle	IPSS: 53%, 53% QOL: 45%, 45% Qmax: 62%, 73% RU: 63%, 60% Prostate size: 13%, 16% PSA: NA At 1 and 10 months	10 months
Chuang et al[13] (paper)	Prospective	Symptomatic BPH prostate > 40 mL Qmax <12 mL/sec N = 8	200 U 25 U/mL	Transperineal, 21-gauge needle	IPSS: 73%, 79% QOL: 62%, 59% Qmax: 72%, 73% RU: 86%, 88% Prostate size: 19%, 20% PSA: NA At 1 and 3 months	4.8 months

Study	Design	Indication	Dose	Technique	Outcomes	Follow-up
Guercini et al[23] (abstract)	Prospective	Severe BPH prostate >80 mL Qmax < 10 mL/sec N = 16	300 U 50 U/mL	Transperineal	IPSS: 46%, 63% QOL: NA Qmax: 89%, 121% RU: 64%, 71% Prostate size: 39%, 50% PSA: 28%, 74% At 1 and 6 months	6 months
Larson et al[25] (abstract)	Open label	BPH with LUTS N = 10	100 U 25 U/mL	Transrectal 22-gauge needle	IPSS: 16%, 46% QOL: 44%, 59% Qmax: NS, 34% RU: NA Prostate size: NA PSA: NA At 1 and 3 months	3 months
Larson et al[25] (abstract)	2:1 treated to sham double blind	BPH with LUTS N = 30	200 U 50 U/mL	Transrectal 22-gauge needle	QOL: NA Qmax: NA RU: NA Prostate size: NA PSA: NA NA	NA
Park et al[26] (paper)	Prospective	Symptomatic BPH N = 52	100 U to 300 U 4 to 9 mL saline	Transperineal	IPSS: 30%, NA QOL: 34%, NA Qmax: 16%, NA RU: 34%, NA Prostate size: 13%, NA% PSA: NA At 3 months	3 months

BPH, benign prostatic hyperplasia; IPSS, International Prostate Symptom Score; LUTS, lower urinary tract symptoms; NA, not available; PSA, prostate specific antigen; QOL, quality of life. With permission from BIU International. *J Urol.* 2006;98:28-32.

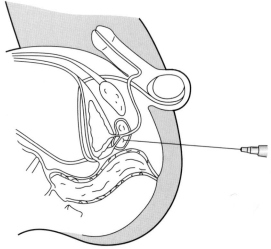

FIGURE 22-3. Transperineal injection position. (With permission from BJU International.)

POSSIBLE ADDITIONAL USES OF BOTULINUM NEUROTOXIN TYPE A FOR THE TREATMENT OF PROSTATIC DISEASES

Botulinum Neurotoxin Effects on the Rat Model of Prostatitis

Chronic nonbacterial prostatitis, or chronic pelvic pain syndrome, is a common but frustrating clinical entity characterized by prostate pain or pelvic pain in the absence of identifiable infection. Abnormal sensory function of the prostate has been claimed for the symptoms of chronic prostatitis or protatodynia.[30] The prostatic afferent neurons that contain calcitonin gene–related peptide and substance P convey nociceptive information from the prostate and may contribute to the symptoms of prostatitis and prostatodynia. The non-nociceptive afferent neurons might be responsible for baroreceptors that sense build-up of prostate secretions.[4,31] Does sensory C-fibers play a role in prostate pain? A recent study demonstrated the existence of a rich TRPV1 sensory innervation in the human prostate, which might explain the pain and burning sensation reported by patients with chronic prostatitis or irritative voiding symptoms.[32]

Using a capsaicin-induced prostatitis model in rats, we demonstrated the analgesic and anti-inflammatory properties of BoNT/A in the prostate.[33] The painful behavioral changes,

accumulation of polymorphonuclear cells (PMNs), and cyclooxygenase 2 (COX-2) expression induced by capsaicin injection were inhibited in a dose-dependent fashion by BoNT/A 1 week pretreatment. BoNT/A 1 week pretreatment resulted in an eightfold reduction of PMN accumulation and decrease of COX-2 expression from 21.5-fold to 1.6-fold. The effects were decreased at 2 weeks pretreatment with BoNT/A. In addition to decreased COX-2 expression in the prostate gland, intraprostatic BoNT/A injection also suppressed COX-2 expression in the L6 ventral horn and dorsal horn.[34] BoNT/A pretreatment could inhibit the capsaicin-induced COX-2 expression from the peripheral organ to L6 spinal cord and inhibit prostatic pain and inflammation. This finding suggests a potential clinical benefit of BoNT/A for the treatment of nonbacterial prostatitis.

Effects of Botulinum Neurotoxin Type A on Human Nonbacterial Prostatitis or Chronic Prostatic Pain

Maria et al[35] first reported that four men with chronic nonbacterial prostatitis and poor bladder emptying associated with nonrelaxing external urethral sphincter received bilateral injections of 30 U BoNT/A. All patients had a striking improvement in voiding symptoms lasting from 1 week to 12 months. Zermann et al. performed transurethral perisphincteric injection of 200 U BoNT/A in 11 patients with chronic prostatic pain. In nine patients, the severity of paing was reduced from 7.2 to 1.6.[36] Shin et al[37] reported that multi-regional injections of BoNT/A (including four intraprostatic injection) improved symptoms in 59% of patients with chronic pelvic pain syndrome (CPPS). Therefore, urethral injection, perisphincteric, or intraprostatic BoNT/A injection might have therapeutic benefits for patients with human nonbacteria prostatitis or chronic prostatic pain.

Effects of Botulinum Neurotoxin Type A on Prostate Cancer

Although there are currently no published reports of BoNT/A being used as therapy for prostate cancer, in the clinical papers published that included PSA, there has been a reduction of PSA level with BoNT injection.[21,23] In the rat, dog, and human prostate tissue that has been assessed histologically, apoptosis has been noted.[15,16,18,24] Inflammatory change and COX-2 elevation have been reported to play a role in the pathogenesis of prostate cancer.[38] Thus, the fact that BoNT/A inhibits inflammatory change and downregulates COX-2 expression may affect prostate cancer. We acknowledge that using BoNT/A in prostate cancer is conjectural and it is not clear whether a therapy would involve a single or multiple injections. However, we believe that a new agent and new mechanisms of action for the treatment of prostate cancer is exciting and should be studied.

CONCLUSIONS

Prostate diseases are central to the practice of urology, and a new drug or substance such as botulinum toxin that can affect the prostate gland has has had a profound impact in our field. Translational research suggests that the novel mechanism of action of botulinum toxin could be useful in the prostate as therapy for BPH or chronic nonbacterial prostatitis, or even as an adjuvant therapy for prostate cancer.[13] Clinical series have demonstrated sustained efficacy of 6 months or longer after prostate BoNT/A injection. Because the use of BoNT/A in the prostate is currently off label and, in support of evidence-based medicine practices, caution should be applied until larger randomized clinical studies are completed. More basic research is needed to identify the mechanisms in which botulinum toxin may affect the prostate.

ACKNOWLEDGMENT

We would like to thank Dr. Catherine Thomas and Ms. Leica Sciulli for their excellent review of this manuscript.

References

1. Lepor H. The pathophysiology of lower urinary tract symptoms in the ageing male population. *Br J Urol.* 1998;81:29-33.
2. Walsh PC. Treatment of benign prostatic hyperplasia. *N Engl J Med.* 1996;335:557-563.
3. Roehrborn C, McConnell J, Barry M, Benaim E, Bruskewitz R, Blute M, et al. AUA guideline on management of benign prostatic hyperplasia (2003). Chapter 1: diagnosis and treatment recommendations. *J Urol.* 2003;170:530-547.
4. Pennefather JN, Lau WAK, Mitchelson F, Ventura S. The autonomic and sensory innervation of the smooth muscle of the prostate gland: a review of pharmacological and histological studies. *J Auton Pharmacol.* 2000;20:193-206.
5. Ventura S, Pennefather JN, Mitchelson F. Cholinergic innervation and function in the prostate gland. *Pharmacol Ther.* 2002;94:93-112.
6. Coffey DS, Walsh PC. Clinical and experimental studies of benign prostatic hyperplasia. *Urol Clin North Am.* 1990;17:461.
7. Ravindranath N, Wion D, Brachet P, Djakiew D. Epidermal growth factor modulates the expression of vascular endothelial growth factor in the human prostate. *J Androl.* 2001;22:432.
8. Mariness D, Patel R, Walden PD. Mechanistic investigation of the adrenergic induction of ventral prostate hyperplasia in mice. *Prostate.* 2003;54:230.
9. Smith CP, Chancellor MB. Emerging role of botulinum toxin in the treatment of voiding dysfunction. *J Urol.* 2004;171:2128-2137.
10. Smith CP, Franks ME, McNeil BK, Ghosh R, de Groat WC, Chancellor MB, et al. Effect of botulinum toxin A on the autonomic nervous system of the rat lower urinary tract. *J Urol.* 2003;169:1896-1900.
11. Chuang YC, Yoshimura N, Huang CC, Chiang PH, Chancellor MB. Intravesical botulinum toxin A administration produces analgesia against acetic acid induced bladder pain responses in rats. *J Urol.* 2004;172:1529-1532.
12. Welch MJ, Purkiss JR, Foster KA. Sensitivity of embryonic rat dorsal root ganglia neurons to Clostridium botulinum neurotoxins. *Toxicon.* 2000;38:245-258.
13. Chuang YC, Chancellor MB. The application of Botulinum toxin in the prostate. *J Urol.* 2006;176:2376-2386.
14. Lujan M, Paez A, Llanes L, Angulo J, Berenguer A. Role of autonomic innervation in rat prostatic structure maintenance: a morphometric analysis. *J Urol.* 1998;160:1919-1923.
15. Doggweiler R, Zermann DH, Ishigooka M, Schmidt RA. Botox induced prostatic involution. *Prostate.* 1998;37:44.
16. Chuang YC, Huang CC, Kang HY, Chiang PH, DeMiguel F, Yoshimura N, et al. Novel action of Botulinum toxin on the stromal and epithelial components of prostate gland. *J Urol.* 2006;173:1158-1163.
17. Lin ATL, Chen MT, Chiang H, Yang CH, Chang LS. Effect of orchiectomy on the alpha adrenergic contractile response of dog prostate. *J Urol.* 1995;154:1930.
18. Chuang YC, Tu CH, Huang CC, Lin HJ, Chiang PH, Yoshimura N, Chancellor MB. Intraprostatic Botulinum toxin type A injection relieves bladder outlet obstruction and induces prostate apoptosis. *BMC Urol.* 2006;6:12.
19. Kyprianou N. Doxazosin and terazosin suppress prostate growth by inducing apoptosis: clinical significance. *J Urol.* 2003;169:1520-1525.
20. Lin ATL, Yang AH, Chen KK. Effect of Botulinum toxin A on the contractile function of dog prostate. *Eur Urol.* 2007;52:539-582.
21. Maria G, Brisinda G, Civello IM, Bentivoglio AR, Sganga G, Albanese A. Relief by botulinum toxin of voiding dysfunction due to benign prostatic hyperplasia: Results of a randomized, placebo-controlled study. *Urology.* 2003;62:259.
22. Kuo HC. Prostate Botulinum toxin A injection- an alternative treatment for benign prostatic obstruction in poor surgical candidates. *Urology.* 2005;65:670.

23. Guercini F, Giannantoni A, Bard RL, Brisinda G, Cadeddu F, Maria G, et al: Intraprostatic botulin toxin injection in patients with severe benign prostatic hyperplasia a multicenter feasibility study [abstract]. *J Urol.* 2005;173:376-377.

24. Chuang YC, Chiang PH, Huang CC, Yoshimura N, Chancellor MB. Botulinum toxin type A improves benign prostatic hyperplasia symptoms in patients with small prostates. *Urology.* 2005;66:775.

25. Larson TR, Scottsdale AZ, Huidobro C, Acevedo C. Intraprostatic injection of botulinum toxin in the treatment of symptomatic LUTS, including sequential MRIS for accurate changes in size of the prostate [abstract]. *J Urol.* 2005;173:376-377.

26. Park DS, Cho TW, Lee YK, Lee JH, Hong YK, Lee YT. Evaluation of short term clinical effects and presumptive mechanism of Botulinum toxin type A as a treatment modality of benign prostatic hyperplasia. *Yonsei Med J.* 2006;31:706-714.

27. Chuang YC, Chiang PH, Yoshimura N, DeMigue F, Chancellor M. Sustained beneficial effects of intraprostatic Botulinum toxin type A injection on lower urinary tract symptoms and quality of life in men with benign prostatic hyperplasia. *BJU Int.* 2006;98:1033-1037.

28. Plante MK, Folsom JB, Zvara P. Prostatic tissue ablation by injection: a literature review. *J Urol.* 2004;172:20.

29. Chalfin SA, Bradley WE. The etiology of detrusor hyperreflexia in patients with infravesical obstruction. *J Urol.* 1982;127:938-942.

30. Pontari MA, Ruggiori MR. Mechanisms in prostatitis/chronic pelvic pain syndrome. *J Urol.* 2004;172:839.

31. Danuser H, Springer JP, Katofiasc MA, Thor KB. Extrinsic innervaiton of the cat prostate gland: a combined tracing and immunohistochemical study. *J Urol.* 1997;157:1018.

32. Dinis P, Charrua A, Avelino A, Nagy I, Quintas J, Ribau U, Cruz F. The distribution of sensory fibers immunoreactive for the TRPV1 (capsaicin) receptor in the human prostate. *Eur Urol.* 2005;48:162.

33. Chuang YC, Yoshimura N, Huang CC, Chiang PH, Wu M, Chancellor MB. Intraprostatic capsaicin injection as a novel model for non-bacteria prostatitis. *Eur Urol.* 2007;51:1119-1127.

34. Chuang YC, Yoshimura N, Huang CC, Chiang PH, Wu M, Chancellor MB. Intraprostatic botulinum toxin a injection inhibits COX-2 expression and suppresses prostatic pain on capsaicin induced prostatitis model in rat. *J Urol.* 2008;180:742-748.

35. Maria G, Destitio A, Lacquaniti S, Bentivoglio AR, Albanese A. Relief by Botulinum toxin of voiding dysfunction due to prostatitis. *Lancet.* 1998;352:625.

36. Zermann D, Ishigooka M, Schubert J, Schmidt RA. Perisphincteric injection of botulinum toxin type A. A treatment option for patients with chronic prostatic pain? *Eur Urol.* 2000;38:393-399.

37. Shin SM, Park DS. Multi-regional injections of low dose Botulinum toxin A for men with chronic pelvic pain syndrome. *J Urol.* 2006;175(suppl):34.

38. Nelson WG, De Marzo AM, De Weese TL, Isaacs WB. The role of inflammation in the pathogenesis of prostate cancer. *J Urol.* 2004;172:S6.

Clinical Application of 23 Botulinum Neurotoxin in the Treatment of Myofascial Pain Syndromes

Martin K. Childers

INTRODUCTION

Myofascial pain syndrome (MPS) is a disorder characterized by the presence of myofascial trigger points (MTrPs), distinct sensitive spots in a palpable taut band of skeletal muscle fibers[1,2] that produce local and referred pain. Synonyms for MPS include myogelosis,[3,4] fibrositis,[5-7] and fibromyalgia.[7-12] MPS is characterized by both a motor abnormality (a taut or hard band within the muscle) and also by a sensory abnormality (tenderness and referred pain).[13] In addition to pain, the disorder is accompanied by referred autonomic phenomena as well as anxiety and depression.[14] The pathophysiology of MPS is not clearly understood due, in part, to the scarcity of reliable valid studies.[15] Moreover, concomitant disorders, and frequent behavioral and psychosocial contributing factors[16] in patients with MPS contribute to the complexity of human studies. Symptoms of MPS are generally associated with physical activities thought to contribute to "muscle overload," either acutely by sudden overload, or gradually with prolonged repetitive activity.[17] MPS can be classified as regional or generalized. Some authors broaden the definition of myofascial pain to include a regional pain syndrome of any soft-tissue origin. Thus, MPS may be considered either a primary disorder causing local or regional pain syndromes, or a secondary disorder that occurs as a consequence of some other condition.[1,13,16,18-20]

PHYSICAL EXAMINATION

Finding and localizing MTrPs is generally considered the most important part of the physical examination to provide an accurate diagnosis of MPS.[1,17,21] Simons and Travell's *Myofascial Pain and Dysfunction The Trigger Point Manual*[22] is considered the criterion standard reference on locating and treating MTrPs. Active MTrPs, which are believed to cause pain, exhibit marked localized tenderness, and may refer pain to distant sites, disturb motor function, or produce autonomic changes. Specific clinical training is required to become adept at identifying MTrPs, because evidence suggests that nontrained clinicians do not reliably detect the taut band and local twitch response.[23] As Simons and Mense point out, "The diagnostic skill required depends on considerable innate palpation ability, authoritative training, and extensive clinical experience."[17] To clinically identify MTrPs, the clinician palpates a localized tender spot in a nodular portion of a taut ropelike band of muscle fibers. Manual pressure over a trigger point should elicit pain at that area and may also elicit pain at a distant site (referred pain) from the point under the fingertip. MTrPs when palpated, should also elicit pain that mirrors the patient's experience. Applied pressure often earns the response "That's my pain!" Insertion of a needle, abrupt palpation, or even a brisk tap with the fingertip directly over the trigger point may induce a brief

Dr. Childers is reporting that he has consulted for McNeil, Allergan, and Ipsen.

muscle contraction detectable by the examiner. This rapid contraction of muscle fibers of the ropy taut band is termed a local twitch response.[17] In muscles that move a relatively small mass or are large and superficial (like the finger extensors or the gluteus maximus), the response is easily seen and may cause the limb to visibly move when the examiner introduces a needle into the trigger point. Localized abnormal response from the autonomic nervous system may cause piloerection, localized sweating, or even regional temperature changes in the skin attributed to altered blood flow.[24-26]

Features of Myofascial Trigger Points

Characteristic features of MTrPs have been described in both human and animal studies. Animal studies reported myofascial trigger spots (MTrSs) in taut bands of rabbit muscle fibers similar to that observed in human MTrP in several respects.[27] Equine MTrPs have also been identified with similar features to those documented in humans and rabbits with the exception that referred pain patterns cannot be determined in animals.[28] One such feature of the MTrP is the so-called twitch response. This local response is considered a characteristic finding of the MTrP. Mechanical stimulation ("snapping" palpation, pressure, or needle insertion) can elicit a local twitch response frequently accompanied by referred pain.[29] The twitch response accompanied by a burst of electrical activity (e.g., endplate noise) within the muscle band contains the activated trigger point, whereas no activity is seen at other muscle bands. Endplate noise is significantly more prevalent in MTrPs than in sites that lie outside of an MTrP but still within the endplate zone.[30] This observation has been attributed to a spinal reflex,[27,29] becaue the response is abolished by motor nerve ablation or infusion of local anesthetic. Moreover, spinal cord transection above the neurologic level of the MTrP fails to permanently alter the characteristic response.

Several hypotheses[21,26] propose to explain the findings observed in MTrPs. One theory is related to excessive release of acetylcholine in abnormal endplates,[27] as the EMG activity recorded at trigger points resembles findings described at the endplate region.[30] This idea has led to studies of botulinum neurotoxin injection (BoNT) into MTrPs in an attempt to reduce release of excessive acetylcholine. To date, results of small cohort studies[31-37] examining effects of BoNT on MTrPs have yielded inconsistent findings. Another theory proposes that MTps are found only at the muscle spindle in an attempt to explain beneficial effects of alpha-adrenergic antagonists. However, this idea does not fully explain the electromyographic (EMG) findings recorded at the MTrP. Furthermore, there appears to be little evidence that painful muscle areas, such as MTrPs, are associated with any structural changes in the appearance of the muscle spindle.

Botulinum Toxin Use in Myofascial Pain Syndrome—Evidence in Peer-Reviewed Literature

A literature search of the PubMed database from September 2007 to the earliest available year using the terms BoNT and myofascial pain yielded 61 publications. Limiting the publications to prospective, randomized, placebo-controlled studies in humans or animals yielded less than six publications. The following section briefly describes the primary results from selected prospective studies.[42-50]

In an attempt to address the question of whether or not BoNT might be superior to injection with local anesthetic in patients with MPS, Graboskie et al compared effects of botulinum neurotoxin type A (BoNT/A) to bupivacaine injections in a single-center randomized crossover superiority trial.[51] As an enrollment criterion, only subjects who responded favorably to bupivacaine injections into MTrPs were included in the trial. In this study, 18 patients with MPS received MTrP injections with either 25 units BoNT/A or 0.5 ml of 0.5% bupivacaine per trigger point. A maximum of eight trigger points were injected per subject. Subjects were followed until their pain returned to 75% or more of their preinjection pain for 2 consecutive weeks, after which there was a 2-week wash-out period. The subjects then crossed over and had the same trigger points injected with the other agent. All subjects participated in a home exercise program involving static stretches of the affected muscles. Both treatments were effective in reducing pain when compared with baseline ($P = 0.0067$). There were no significant differences detected between either study groups with respect to duration or magnitude of pain relief, function, satisfaction or cost of care (cost of injectate excluded). The authors concluded that bupivacaine is more a cost-effective treatment for MPS compared with BoNT/A.

Querama et al[52] investigated effects of BoNT/A on pain and EMG activity in 30 subjects with infraspinatus MTrPs. Perhaps based on the finding that BoNT reduces endplate noise in rabbit MTrPs,[53] Querama et al carried out a double-blind, randomized, placebo-controlled, parallel clinical trial on the effects of BoNT/A on pain from MTrPs and on EMG activity. Thirty patients with MTrPs in the infraspinatus muscles received either 50 units of BoNT/A or 0.25 mL of isotonic saline. Results indicated that BoNT/A reduced motor endplate activity and the interference pattern of EMG but had no effect either on pain (spontaneous or referred) or pain thresholds compared with isotonic saline. The authors concluded that their results do not support an analgesic effect of BoNT/A in MPS.

Ojala et al[54] studied effects of small doses of BoNT/A in neck and shoulder MPS. Their rationale for studying small doses was due to the fact that injections of large amounts of BoNT may cause muscle weakness and other adverse events. Therefore, they studied the effects of small doses (5 U) of BoNT/A injected directly into active MTrPs using a double-blind crossover technique. Thirty-one patients were studied. Patients received either BoNT/A or physiologic saline injections on two occasions 4 weeks apart. The total dose of BoNT/A varied from 15 to 35 U. The follow-up measurements were carried out at 4 weeks after each treatment. Neck pain and result of treatment were assessed with questionnaires. Pressure pain thresholds were measured using a dolorimeter. Their results indicated that no statistically significant changes in the neck pain and pressure pain threshold values occurred between the experimental groups, nor were there significant differences detected in side effects between groups. The authors concluded that there were no significant differences in analgesic effects following small doses of BoNT/A or physiologic saline in the treatment of MPS.

Ferrente and colleagues[42] studied the effects of BoNT/A in patients with cervicothoracic MPS. One hundred thirty-two patients with cervical or shoulder MPS or both and active MTrPs were enrolled in a 12-week, randomized, double-blind, placebo-controlled trial. Patients were given one of three doses (10, 25, or 50 U) of BoNT/A into up to five active MTrPs, with the maximum doses in each experimental group of 0, 50, 125, and 250 U. Patients also received myofascial release physical therapy, amitriptyline, ibuprofen, and propoxyphene-acetaminophen napsylate. Results failed to demonstrate significant differences between the placebo and BoNT/A groups with respect to Visual Analog Pain scores, pressure algometry, or rescue medication. Thus, the authors concluded that BoNT/A injections into MTrP points did not improve cervicothoracic MPS.

Kamanli et al[35] compared MTrP injection with BoNT-A with dry needling and lidocaine injection in a single-blind study of 29 patients with MPS. Patients were randomly assigned to three groups: lidocaine injection (n = 10, 32 MTrPs), dry needling (n = 10, 33 MTrPs), and BoNT/A injections (n = 9, 22 MTrP). Results indicated that pain pressure thresholds improved in all three groups. Of interest, Visual Analog Scores significantly decreased in the lidocaine and BoNT/A groups but not in the dry needle group. Similarly, quality of life scores significantly improved only in the lidocaine and BoNT/A groups, but not in the dry needle group. Depression and anxiety scores significantly improved only in the BoNT/A group. The authors concluded that lidocaine injection is more practical and rapid than dry needling and is more cost effective than BoNT-A injection. Therefore, lidocaine seems to be the treatment of choice in MPS. On the other hand, the authors speculated that BoNT/A could be selectively used in MPS patients who are resistant to conventional treatments.

One pivotal trial has reported efficacy of BoNT in MPS. In a large multicenter study[55] in Europe, the efficacy and tolerability of BoNT/A was evaluated in 145 patients with MPS of the upper back. In this prospective, randomized, double-blind, placebo-controlled, 12-week study, patients with chronic moderate-to-severe MPS affecting cervical or shoulder muscles, or both, were randomized to receive either BoNT/A or saline injections into the 10 most tender MTrPs (40 U per site). The primary outcome was in the proportion of patients with mild or no pain at Week 5. Secondary outcomes included changes in pain intensity and the number of pain-free days per week. Tolerability and safety were also assessed. Results demonstrated that at Week 5, significantly more patients in the BoNT/A group reported mild or no pain (51%), compared with the patients in the placebo group (26%; $P = 0.002$). Furthermore, compared with patients who received placebo, patients who received BoNT/A reported significantly greater improvement from baseline in pain intensity during Weeks 5 to 8 ($P < 0.05$), and significantly fewer days per week without pain between Weeks 5 and 12 ($P = 0.036$). Treatment was well tolerated, with most side effects resolving within 8 weeks. This study was the first large multicenter evaluation of BoNT/A in patients with chronic MPS to support the hypothesis that BoNT can safely and effectively reduce pain attributed to MTrPs in the upper back.

Botulinum Toxin in Regional Myofascial Pain Syndrome

To test the idea that BoNT might work to relieve regional MPS, the author conducted a pilot study[56] on the use of BoNT/A in a cohort of subjects with regional MPS of the lower limb, in a condition termed piriformis syndrome. Blunt trauma, such as a fall onto the buttocks, has been reported to result in this painful chronic musculoskeletal disorder, which is thought to involve the piriformis muscle because of its close proximity to the sciatic nerve. Piriformis syndrome is associated with buttock, hip, and lower limb pain and occurs predominantly in women. It has been suggested that hip, buttock, and leg pain results as a consequence of prolonged or excessive contraction of the piriformis muscle.[57,58] Subsequent to the location of this muscle and its close association with the sciatic nerve, excessive or sustained muscular force might also compress the sciatic nerve and result in lower limb pain. Thus, agents such as BoNT known to locally decrease muscle force[59-61] might bring about pain relief by decreasing muscle tension and also by presumably decreasing tension on nerve axons. Accordingly, it was hypothesized that injection into this muscle with the potent paralytic agent BoNT/A would diminish buttock, hip, and lower limb pain.

Ten women with piriformis syndrome participated in a double-blind crossover pilot to test effects of local intramuscular BoNT/A (100 U) directly injected into the piriformis muscle. Pain scores and nerve conduction studies were measured in each participant over several weeks. Results of the main outcome measures (pain scores) suggested a clinical benefit—probably as a result of a modest analgesic response from toxin injection. Others[47,62] have similarly reported afavorable response to BoNT in piriformis syndrome.

If clinical benefit was due, at least in part, to local decrease in muscular force and subsequent decrease in motor axon compression as a result of BoNT injection, then it was anticipated that associated changes would be observed in nerve conduction (H reflex) studies.[63] However, no changes in H reflexes were detected either before or after experimental interventions. Thus, the idea that sciatic nerve compression resulted from local increase in piriformis muscle tension was not supported by the findings. This line of evidence pointed to an alternative mechanism of action[64] of BoNT in pain syndromes and also raised questions about the very nature of MPS. There are no clear biochemical markers that distinguish patients with MPS. However, although the pathogenesis is still unknown, there has been evidence of increased corticotropin-releasing hormone and substance P (SP) in the cerebrospinal fluid (CSF) of fibromyalgia patients, as well as increased SP, interleukin-6 (IL-6), and interleukin-8 (IL-8) in their serum.[65] One hypothesis supports the idea that MPS is an immunoendocrine disorder in which the increased release of CRH and SP from neurons triggers local mast cells to release proinflammatory and neurosensitizing molecules. This hypothesis fits well with recent discoveries of neuropeptides found in the muscles of patients with active MTrPs.[66,67]

Regional Examination of the Lower Extremity for Piriformis Syndrome

To evaluate individuals for piriformis syndrome,[68,69] their usual buttock, hip and lower limb pain may be reproduced during the following maneuvers: palpation over a point midway between the sacrum and greater trochanter of the femur, active hip abduction in the lateral recumbent position, and rectal palpation of the ipsilateral side of the involved limb.[56] A number of similar maneuvers have been described. Freiberg's maneuver of forceful internal rotation of the extended thigh elicits buttock pain by stretching the piriformis muscle, and Pace's maneuver elicits pain by having the patient abduct the legs in the seated position, which causes contraction of the piriformis muscle.[70] Beatty described a maneuver[71,72] performed by the patient lying with the painful side up, the painful leg flexed, and the knee resting on the table. Buttock pain is produced when the patient lifts and holds the knee several inches off the table. Beatty reported that the maneuver he described produced deep buttock pain in three patients with piriformis syndrome. In 100 consecutive patients with surgically documented herniated lumbar discs, the maneuver often produced lumbar and leg pain but not deep buttock pain. Also, in 27 patients with primary hip abnormalities, pain was often produced in the trochanteric area but not in the buttock. The maneuver described by Beatty presumably relies on contraction of the muscle rather than stretching, which might reproduce pain due to an actively contracting piriformis muscle. A positive finding in at least two of the preceding maneuvers is sufficient to confirm a diagnosis of piriformis syndrome, provided that other potential causes have been eliminated from the differential diagnosis (described later). For example, patients with trochanteric bursitis generally present with chronic intermittent aching pain over the lateral aspect of the affected hip. Pain is worsened by sitting in a deep chair or car seat, or by climbing stairs. In contrast, patients with regional MPS of the lower limb (piriformis syndrome) report pain primarily in the buttocks, with occasional radiation into the lateral thigh. Clinical criteria for trochanteric bursitis should include the first and second and at least one of the remaining findings: (1) history of lateral aching hip pain; (2) localized tenderness over the greater trochanter; (3) radiation of pain over the lateral thigh; (4) pain of resisted hip abduction; (5) pain at extreme ends of rotation, particularly a positive Patrick (Fabere) test.

Diagnostic Studies

No definitive laboratory test or imaging method is diagnostic of MPS. Thus, diagnosis is made primarily on history and physical examination. Although no specific laboratory tests confirm (or refute) a diagnosis of MPS,[2,14,73] some tests can be helpful in the search for predisposing conditions, such as hypothyroidism, hypoglycemia, and vitamin deficiencies. Specific tests that may be helpful include complete blood count, chemistry profile, erythrocyte sedimentation rate (ESR), and levels of vitamins C, B_1, B_6, B_{12}, and folic

acid. If clinical features of thyroid disease are present, an assay for thyrotropin may be indicated.[74,75] A presumptive diagnosis of piriformis syndrome is based principally on clinical evidence because well-established laboratory or imaging studies to confirm such a diagnosis are not available. Therefore, other sources of buttock, hip, and lower limb pain must be excluded before such a diagnosis can be made. Although laboratory or imaging studies are not diagnostic for this condition, delayed H-reflex latencies have been reported in at least one case series,[76] presumably because of sciatic nerve compression by the piriformis muscle.

Procedures used in the treatment of piriformis muscle syndrome include therapeutic stretch, ultrasound, massage, manipulation, and oral analgesic agents. Caudal epidural steroid injections, local intramuscular steroid injections, and surgical resection of the muscle have also been reported as effective. The rationale for use of botulinum toxins in MPS may involve presynaptic blockade of nociceptive peptides in affected muscles, reduction in force of contracting muscles, or some combination of both mechanisms.[40,41,64,80,81]

GENERAL TREATMENT APPROACH TO MYOFASCIAL PAIN SYNDROME

A wide variety of therapy is available to patients with MPS. Much of the variation in forms of treatment (and diagnoses) of this disorder probably results from differences in culture, training and recognition of an often undiagnosed syndrome of pain, dysfunction, and autonomic dysregulation. The following section discusses treatment strategies for patients with MPS, including those individuals who develop chronic pain.

Early use of therapeutic modalities such as, biofeedback, ultrasound, lasers, and massage may be useful adjuncts in relieving initial pain to allow participation in an active exercise program. Although therapeutic modalities are commonly used for MPS, most of these modalities have not been rigorously investigated. Appropriate controls, sample sizes, and blinding measures are often lacking. Despite these issues, results from published reports generally indicate therapeutic efficacy.[82] For example, Hou et al[83] investigated the immediate effect of physical therapeutic modalities on myofascial pain in the upper trapezius muscle in 119 subjects with active MTrPs. Their findings suggested that therapeutic combinations such as hot pack plus active range of motion and stretch with vapocoolant spray are effective adjuncts for pain relief in patients with MPS. To investigate the immediate effectiveness of electrotherapy on MTrPs of the upper trapezius muscle, Hsueh et al[84] studied 60 patients with MTrPs in one side of the upper trapezius muscle. The involved upper trapezius muscles were treated with three different methods according to a random assignment. One group received a placebo treatment, another group was given electrical nerve stimulation (ENS) therapy; and a third group given electrical muscle stimulation (EMS) therapy. The effectiveness of each treatment was assessed by conducting three measurements on each muscle before and immediately after treatment: subjective pain intensity, pressure pain threshold, and range of motion. Results indicated that electrical nerve stimulation is more effective for immediate pain relief than electrical muscle stimulation, whereas muscle stimulation appeared to have a greater benefit on immediate release of muscle tightness compared with nerve stimulation. Together, the results of these and other studies suggest that addition of therapeutic physical modalities[1,7,16,85,88] such as heat and various forms of muscle and nerve stimulation are beneficial in the initial treatment of MPS.

The use of physical therapy techniques that focus on correction of muscle shortening by targeted stretching, strengthening of affected muscles, and correction of aggravating postural and biomechanical factors are generally considered to be the most effective treatment for MPS.[87-89] This idea is supported by a line of evidence examining the relationship between muscle overload and MTrPs. For example, Itoh et al[90] developed an experimental model of MTrPs in which healthy volunteers underwent repetitive eccentric exercise of the third finger of one hand. Pain thresholds of the skin, fascia, and muscle were measured immediately afterward and for 7 days. Following exercise, pressure pain thresholds decreased, then gradually returned to baseline values. A ropy band was palpated in the exercised forearm muscle, and the electrical pain threshold of the fascia at the palpable band was the lowest among the measured loci and tissues. Needle EMG activity accompanied with dull pain sensation was recorded only when the electrode was located on or near the fascia of the palpable band.

As another example of exercise as a treatment for MPS, a study was conducted in 20 patients with MPS localized to the temporomandibular region.[1,88] The exercise treatment consisted of jaw movements and correction of body posture. After treatment, six patients reported no pain at all and seven patients reported improvement in the ability to chew. Together findings from these and other studies suggest a direct relationship between exercise and MPS, although definitive large multicenter trials appear to be lacking.

The goal for the treatment of MPS is to engage patients in active therapy to prevent the development of chronic pain syndrome, or if it has developed, to rehabilitate patients from its disabling interacting symptoms. Chronic MPS is not a diagnosis but a descriptive term for individuals who not only report persistent pain, but who demonstrate poor coping, self-limitations in functional activities, significant life disruption, and dysfunctional pain behavior.[91] Other common symptoms of chronic pain syndrome related to an accompanying disuse syndrome include the multiple physical systems effects of deconditioning, as well as insomnia, fatigue, anxiety, and depression.[92] A central feature of chronic MPS is avoidance of activity based on the fear that engaging in functional activity will increase pain (fear/avoidance).[92] The critical importance of addressing such a belief is underscored by prior studies that indicated that patients' beliefs about their pain were the best predictors of task performance,[93] medical utilization,[94] and long-term rehabilitation.[95]

Oral Medications

Nonsteroidal anti-inflammatory drugs (NSAIDs) may be a useful adjunct to active exercise-based treatment of MPS, but NSAIDs are generally considered beneficial when used in conjunction with an active treatment program. However, no randomized placebo-controlled clinical trials exist to support efficacy of NSAIDs use in this condition. Interestingly, when injected into the MTrP, the NSAID diclofenac was shown to be superior to lidocaine in one small clinical trial.[96] Low-dose amitriptyline is widely used in patients with fibromyalgia, and is thought to help improve the patient's sleep cycle.[65,97-99] Muscle relaxants may provide benefit to patients with

MPS. For example, cyclobenzaprine hydrochloride, a commonly prescribed muscle relaxant, is indicated as an adjunct to rest and physical therapy for the relief of muscle spasm associated with acute, painful musculoskeletal conditions. In contrast to low-dose (5 mg TID) cyclobenzaprine, a higher dose (10 mg TID) is associated with more somnolence and dry mouth. Importantly, there does not appear to be a relationship between somnolence and pain relief. A large, multicenter, community-based trial of patients with acute pain and muscle spasm evaluated low-dose cyclobenzaprine (5 mg TID) alone compared with combination therapy using two doses of ibuprofen. It is possible that low-dose cyclobenzaprine or high-dose ibuprofen alone may be sufficient to relieve acute musculoskeletal pain, and that no additional benefit is incurred by adding another medication. Future trials comparing various doses of muscle relaxants and NSAIDs, alone or in combination, will be required to address these questions in the treatment of patients with MPS.

Procedures

When combined with other therapies, interventional techniques can be an effective adjunct in the multidisciplinary management of patients with MPS.[100] In treating MPS, other than trigger point injections, interventional procedures (e.g., epidural steroid injections, sacroiliac joint injections, and blocks of medial branch nerves feeding out from facet joints of the spine) are usually not employed. However, at times myofascial pain is associated with or caused by other underlying conditions. For instance, lumbar myofascial pain may also have some component of lumbar facet arthropathy. Lumbar medial branch blocks and radiofrequency denervation, alone or in combination with the other therapies (e.g., muscle relaxants), may work together to relieve myofascial pain. Similarly, epidural steroid injection may provide lumbar pain relief in a patient with spondylosis. It has been suggested by Romanoff et al[1] that cervical epidural steroid injections may be used to treat cervical myofascial pain syndrome if conservative treatments fail. Therefore, underlying pathology may respond to more aggressive interventional methods, and in turn, synergistically provide pain relief to the patient with MPS.

MTrP injections should be individualized for both the patient and clinician. Alcohol, if used to clean skin, should be allowed to dry completely to prevent additional pain. Use of operating rooms or special procedure (sterile) rooms equipped with monitoring devices for the purpose of intramuscular injections using small caliber needles is not necessary. Most patients can be treated safely in an office setting by experienced clinicians. The diagnostic skill required to find active MTrPs depends on considerable innate palpation ability, authoritative training, and extensive clinical experience.[17] Application of trigger point injection begins by first determining the equipment needs according to the needs of the patient, the clinician's training, and the anatomic target for injection. Typically, a 1.0-mL tuberculin-type syringe with 5/8-inch 25-gauge needle is adequate for superficial muscles. For small muscles (e.g., facial muscles), a 1-inch 30-gauge needle is sufficient. For larger muscles, a 1-inch or 1.5-inch 25-gauge needle is adequate. After placing the patient in a position that facilitates relaxation of the desired muscle, the MTrP is located. In the prone position, the MTrP is ascertained using gentle pressure from the end of a fingertip or a ballpoint pen applied at regular 1-cm intervals. The patient is observed closely during palpation because pressure on the markedly tender MTrP usually causes the patient to jump, wince, or cry out. Each muscle has a characteristic pattern of referred pain that, for active MTrPs, is familiar to the patient. Thus, the patient will respond that this pressure reproduces their usual pain and, when questioned, will describe painful sensations at a site slightly distant to the point under the examiner's finger. Once the MTrP has been located, the skin is marked, and the site is injected with saline, anesthetic agent, or corticosteroid solution.

Piriformis Muscle Injection

To inject the piriformis muscle (Fig. 23-1), the patient is placed in the prone position, the skin over the largest bulk of the buttocks is swabbed with iodine, and sterile drapes are applied. Under pulsed fluoroscopy, the greater trochanter of the femur, the body of the sacrum, and the sciatic notch can easily be identified (Fig. 23-2). The skin is marked corresponding to a location midway between a line that bisected the middle of the sciatic notch and the greater trochanter of the hip. A sterile 5 1/2-inch 20-guage dual-purpose injection/EMG needle is inserted through the overlying

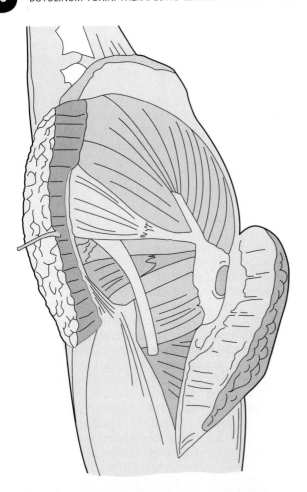

FIGURE 23-1. Posterior view of the piriformis muscle *(arrow)*. The gluteus maximus has been cut. Note the relationship between the piriformis muscle and the sciatic nerve, which lies directly caudal to the muscle belly. The piriformis muscle originates along the anterior lateral portion of the sacrum and inserts onto the greater trochanter of the femur. (Reproduced with permission from S. Kargo AE, Basel.)

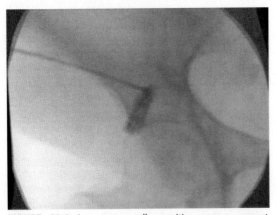

FIGURE 23-2. Incorrect needle position versus correct needle position for piriformis injection using fluoroscopic guidance. A 6-inch spinal needle was used to inject contrast dye into the piriformis muscle to confirm needle placement before injection with BoNT/A. In the image shown, the outline of the piriformis muscle *(darkly outlined by the contrast dye)* is shown to enhance outside of the predicted pattern of the piriformis muscle. Note that the outline of the injected muscle does not run from the greater trochanter to the sciatic notch, but appears to be slightly cephalad to this position.

skin marking. The needle should be angled slightly lateral to medial. Once the iliacus encountered, the needle is withdrawn slightly and the injection site is visualized by fluoroscopy (Fig. 23-3).

To further verify that the needle tip is placed accurately within the piriformis muscle, before injection and subsequent to fluoroscopic localization of needle placement, an electromyograph can be connected to the hub of the needle. A ground and a reference electrode are secured to the skin overlying the lateral upper thigh. The patient is instructed to externally rotate the thigh to activate the piriformis muscle. If brisk motor unit action potentials are not observed, the needle should be repositioned slightly, and the procedure repeated. Three milliliters of an iodine-based radiotracer dye is subsequently injected. The pattern of radiotracer spread is subsequently examined under pulsed fluoroscopy. If the radiotracer pattern does not correspond with the parallel alignment of piriformis muscle fibers, the needle

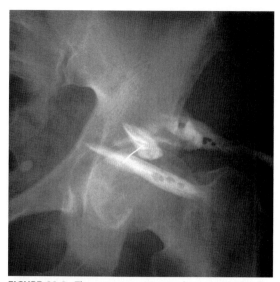

FIGURE 23-3. The correct position is shown, with the dye pattern clearly entering fibers that insert along the greater trochanter and extend directly toward the sciatic notch. In piriformis syndrome, needle entry into the piriformis muscle typically elicits a twitch response with marked external rotation of the femur. Patients also report that the injected material reproduces their usual pain, including radiation of pain at a site distant to the injected muscle.

should be repositioned and the procedure (including electromyography) repeated. If the needle tip is too shallow, radiotracer dye patterns will appear to correlate with those of the gluteus maximus. Similarly, if the needle tip is too proximal or distal, dye patterns will appear to correlate with fibers of the obturator internus or gemelli muscles. After needle tip placement is verified by both fluoroscopic and electromyographic techniques, syringes are changed, and medication is injected.

POTENTIAL DISEASE COMPLICATIONS

Patients with MPS may go on to develop a chronic pain syndrome. Treatment of individuals with chronic MPS is described earlier. Perhaps the biggest complication of untreated and progressive MPS is the development of a syndrome of physical inactivity that may lead to cardiovascular disease.[101-104] Evidence of a dose-response relation between physical activity and cardiovascular disease end points has been proposed,[102] although a majority of the literature in this area has relied on prospective observational studies, and few randomized

trials of physical activity and cardiovascular disease as a clinical outcome have been reported. This notwithstanding, evidence indicates that cardiovascular disease incidence and mortality are causally related to physical activity in an inverse, dose-response fashion. Thus, left untreated, patients with MPS who go on to develop chronic pain and lack physical activity are at high risk for cardiovascular disease and early death.

Potential Complications of Injections for Myofascial Pain Syndrome

The greatest risk of treatment of the patent with MPS is related to MTrP injections in the thoracic area. Because of the anatomic proximity of the apex of the lung to the upper trapezius and scalene muscles, the clinician must be aware of the potential for pneumothorax as a result of MTrP injection involving these muscles. The use of long (>1 inch) small gauge needles should be avoided because long, thin needles can easily bend once inserted into the muscle, and the tip can inadvertently puncture the pleura. Rather, use of short (< 1 inch) needles should be used for MTrP injections anywhere near the apex of the lung. In addition, the needle should be directed away from structures at risk of inadvertent puncture. To provide additional proprioceptive feedback during injection, grasping the muscle between the thumb and forefinger will allow the clinician to palpate the thickness of the tissue to be injected. Thin patients or those with reduced lung capacity from underlying diseases are particularly at risk, and thus, the clinician should use extra precautions when performing MTrP injections in these individuals.

SUMMARY

MPS is a disorder characterized by distinct sensitive spots in a palpable taut band of skeletal muscle fibers (MTrPs) that produce local and referred pain. In addition to pain, MPS is accompanied by referred autonomic phenomena as well as anxiety and depression and is poorly understood owing to the scarcity of reliable studies. BoNT has been reported to be an effective treatment for MPS, but only one multicenter European trial has published data in a randomized clinical trial setting (as of September 2007). More studies are necessary to fully understand the role of BoNT in MPS.

References

1. Borg-Stein J, Simons DG. Focused review: myofascial pain. *Arch Phys Med Rehabil.* 2002;83(3 suppl 1): S40-S49.
2. Auleciems LM. Myofascial pain syndrome: a multidisciplinary approach. *Nurse Pract.* 1995;20(18):21-28, passim.
3. Windisch A, Reitinger A, Traxler H, Radner H, Neumayer C, Feigl W, et al. Morphology and histochemistry of myogelosis. *Clin Anat.* 1999;12: 266-271.
4. Wallraff J. [Histology of myogelosis.]. *Munch Med Wochenschr.* 1951;93:913-916.
5. Inanici F, Yunus MB. History of fibromyalgia: past to present. *Curr Pain Headache Rep.* 2004;8:369-378.
6. Bengtsson A. The muscle in fibromyalgia. *Rheumatology.* 2002;41:721-724(Oxford).
7. Schneider MJ. Tender points/fibromyalgia vs. trigger points/myofascial pain syndrome: a need for clarity in terminology and differential diagnosis. *J Manipulative Physiol Ther.* 1995;18:398-406.
8. Buskila D. Fibromyalgia, chronic fatigue syndrome, and myofascial pain syndrome. *Curr Opin Rheumatol.* 2001;13:117-127.
9. Gerwin RD. A review of myofascial pain and fibromyalgia—factors that promote their persistence. *Acupunct Med.* 2005;23:121-134.
10. Goldenberg DL. Fibromyalgia, chronic fatigue syndrome, and myofascial pain syndrome. *Curr Opin Rheumatol.* 1991;3:247-258.
11. Henriksson KG. Is fibromyalgia a distinct clinical entity? Pain mechanisms in fibromyalgia syndrome. A myologist's view. *Baillieres Best Pract Res Clin Rheumatol.* 1999;13:455-461.
12. Pongratz DE, Sievers M. Fibromyalgia-symptom or diagnosis: a definition of the position. *Scand J Rheumatol Suppl.* 2000;113:3-7.
13. Gerwin RD. Classification, epidemiology, and natural history of myofascial pain syndrome. *Curr Pain Headache Rep.* 2001;5:412-420.
14. Escobar PL, Ballesteros J. Myofascial pain syndrome. *Orthop Rev.* 1987;16:708-713.
15. Bohr TW. Fibromyalgia syndrome and myofascial pain syndrome. Do they exist? *Neurol Clin.* 1995;13:365-384.
16. Fricton JR. Myofascial pain syndrome. *Neurol Clin.* 1989;7:413-427.
17. Simons DG, Mense S. [Diagnosis and therapy of myofascial trigger points]. *Schmerz.* 2003;17:419-424.
18. Aronoff GM. Myofascial pain syndrome and fibromyalgia: a critical assessment and alternate view. *Clin J Pain.* 1998;14:74-85.
19. Buskila D. Fibromyalgia, chronic fatigue syndrome, and myofascial pain syndrome. *Curr Opin Rheumatol.* 1999;11:119-126.
20. Mikhail M, Rosen H. History and etiology of myofascial pain-dysfunction syndrome. *J Prosthet Dent.* 1980;44:438-444.
21. Simons DG. Myofascial pain syndromes: where are we? Where are we going? *Arch Phys Med Rehabil.* 1988;69(3 Pt 1):207-212.
22. Simons DG, Travell JG, Simons LS: *Myofascial Pain and Dysfunction the Trigger Point Manual.* 2nd ed. Baltimore: Williams & Wilkins; 1999.
23. Hsieh CY, Hong CZ, Adams AH, Platt KJ, Danielson CD, Hoehler FK, et al. Interexaminer reliability of the palpation of trigger points in the trunk and lower limb muscles. *Arch Phys Med Rehabil.* 2000;81:258-264.
24. McPartland JM. Travell trigger points—molecular and osteopathic perspectives. *J Am Osteopath Assoc.* 2004;104:244-249.
25. Mense S, Simons DG, Hoheisel U, Quenzer B. Lesions of rat skeletal muscle after local block of acetylcholinesterase and neuromuscular stimulation. *J Appl Physiol.* 2003;94:2494-2501.
26. Rivner MH. The neurophysiology of myofascial pain syndrome. *Curr Pain Headache Rep.* 2001;5: 432-440.
27. Hong CZ, Simons DG. Pathophysiologic and electrophysiologic mechanisms of myofascial trigger points. *Arch Phys Med Rehabil.* 1998;79:863-872.
28. Macgregor J, Graf von SD. Needle electromyographic activity of myofascial trigger points and control sites in equine cleidobrachialis muscle—an observational study. *Acupunct Med.* 2006;24:61-70.
29. Hong CZ. Pathophysiology of myofascial trigger point. *J Formos Med Assoc.* 1996;95:93-104.
30. Simons DG, Hong CZ, Simons LS. Endplate potentials are common to midfiber myofacial trigger points. *Am J Phys Med Rehabil.* 2002;81:212-222.
31. Ho KY, Tan KH. Botulinum toxin A for myofascial trigger point injection: A qualitative systematic review. *Eur J Pain.* 2007;11:519-527.
32. Qerama E, Fuglsang-Frederiksen A, Kasch H, Bach FW, Jensen TS. A double-blind, controlled study of botulinum toxin A in chronic myofascial pain. *Neurology.* 2006;67:241-245.
33. Ojala T, Arokoski JP, Partanen J. The effect of small doses of botulinum toxin a on neck-shoulder myofascial pain syndrome: a double-blind, randomized, and controlled crossover trial. *Clin J Pain.* 2006;22:90-96.
34. Graboski CL, Gray DS, Burnham RS. Botulinum toxin A versus bupivacaine trigger point injections for the treatment of myofascial pain syndrome: a randomised double blind crossover study. *Pain.* 2005;118: 170-175.
35. Kamanli A, Kaya A, Ardicoglu O, Ozgocmen S, Zengin FO, Bayik Y. Comparison of lidocaine injection, botulinum toxin injection, and dry needling to trigger points in myofascial pain syndrome. *Rheumatol Int.* 2005;25:604-611.
36. Kuan TS, Chen JT, Chen SM, Chien CH, Hong CZ. Effect of botulinum toxin on endplate noise in myofascial trigger spots of rabbit skeletal muscle. *Am J Phys Med Rehabil.* 2002;81:512-520.
37. Wheeler AH, Goolkasian P, Gretz SS. A randomized, double-blind, prospective pilot study of botulinum toxin injection for refractory, unilateral, cervicothoracic, paraspinal, myofascial pain syndrome. *Spine.* 1998;23:1662-1666.
38. Schalow G, Zach GA. Reorganization of the human central nervous system. *Gen Physiol Biophys.* 2000;19(Suppl 1):11-240.
39. Bishop B. Spasticity: its physiology and management. Part II. Neurophysiology of spasticity: current concepts. *Phys Ther.* 1977;57:377-384.
40. Mense S. Neurobiological basis for the use of botulinum toxin in pain therapy. *J Neurol.* 2004;251(suppl 1):I1-I7.
41. Sycha T, Kranz G, Auff E, Schnider P. Botulinum toxin in the treatment of rare head and neck pain syndromes: a systematic review of the literature. *J Neurol.* 2004;251(Suppl 1):I19-I30.
42. Ferrante FM, Bearn L, Rothrock R, King L. Evidence against trigger point injection technique for the

treatment of cervicothoracic myofascial pain with botulinum toxin type A. *Anesthesiology.* 2005;103:377-383.

43. Graboski CL, Gray DS, Burnham RS. Botulinum toxin A versus bupivacaine trigger point injections for the treatment of myofascial pain syndrome: a randomised double blind crossover study. *Pain.* 2005;118: 170-175.

44. Kamanli A, Kaya A, Ardicoglu O, Ozgocmen S, Zengin FO, Bayik Y. Comparison of lidocaine injection, botulinum toxin injection, and dry needling to trigger points in myofascial pain syndrome. *Rheumatol Int.* 2005;25:604-611.

45. Lang AM. A preliminary comparison of the efficacy and tolerability of botulinum toxin serotypes A and B in the treatment of myofascial pain syndrome: a retrospective, open-label chart review. *Clin Ther.* 2003;25:2268-2278.

46. Ojala T, Arokoski JP, Partanen J. The effect of small doses of botulinum toxin a on neck-shoulder myofascial pain syndrome: a double-blind, randomized, and controlled crossover trial. *Clin J Pain.* 2006;22:90-96.

47. Porta M. A comparative trial of botulinum toxin type A and methylprednisolone for the treatment of myofascial pain syndrome and pain from chronic muscle spasm. *Pain.* 2000;85:101-105.

48. Qerama E, Fuglsang-Frederiksen A, Kasch H, Bach FW, Jensen TS. A double-blind, controlled study of botulinum toxin A in chronic myofascial pain. *Neurology.* 2006;67:241-245.

49. Richards BA, Jensen TS. A double-blind, controlled study of botulinum toxin A in chronic myofascial pain. *Neurology.* 2007;68:963-964.

50. Wheeler AH, Goolkasian P, Gretz SS. A randomized, double-blind, prospective pilot study of botulinum toxin injection for refractory, unilateral, cervicothoracic, paraspinal, myofascial pain syndrome. *Spine.* 1998;23:1662-1666.

51. Graboski CL, Gray DS, Burnham RS. Botulinum toxin A versus bupivacaine trigger point injections for the treatment of myofascial pain syndrome: a randomised double blind crossover study. *Pain.* 2005;118:170-275.

52. Qerama E, Fuglsang-Frederiksen A, Kasch H, Bach FW, Jensen TS. A double-blind, controlled study of botulinum toxin A in chronic myofascial pain. *Neurology.* 2006;67:241-245.

53. Kuan TS, Chen JT, Chen SM, Chien CH, Hong CZ. Effect of botulinum toxin on endplate noise in myofascial trigger spots of rabbit skeletal muscle. *Am J Phys Med Rehabil.* 2002;81:512-520.

54. Ojala T, Arokoski JP, Partanen J. The effect of small doses of botulinum toxin a on neck-shoulder myofascial pain syndrome: a double-blind, randomized, and controlled crossover trial. *Clin J Pain.* 2006;22:90-96.

55. Gobel H, Heinze A, Reichel G, Hefter H, Benecke R. Efficacy and safety of a single botulinum type A toxin complex treatment (Dysport) for the relief of upper back myofascial pain syndrome: results from a randomized double-blind placebo-controlled multicentre study. *Pain.* 2006;125:82-88.

56. Childers MK, Wilson DJ, Gnatz SM, Conway RR, Sherman AK. Botulinum toxin type A use in piriformis muscle syndrome: a pilot study. *Am J Phys Med Rehabil.* 2002;81:751-759.

57. Papadopoulos EC, Khan SN. Piriformis syndrome and low back pain: a new classification and review of the literature. *Orthop Clin North Am.* 2004;35:65-71.

58. Parziale JR, Hudgins TH, Fishman LM. The piriformis syndrome. *Am J Orthop.* 1996;25:819-823.

59. Dressler D, Saberi FA, Barbosa ER. Botulinum toxin: mechanisms of action. *Arq Neuropsiquiatr.* 2005;63:180-185.

60. Dolly O. Synaptic transmission: inhibition of neurotransmitter release by botulinum toxins. *Headache.* 2003;43(suppl 1):S16-S24.

61. Simpson LL. Studies on the mechanism of action of botulinum toxin. *Adv Cytopharmacol.* 1979;3:27-34.

62. Lang AM. Botulinum toxin type B in piriformis syndrome. *Am J Phys Med Rehabil.* 2004;83:198-202.

63. Fishman LM, Zybert PA. Electrophysiologic evidence of piriformis syndrome. *Arch Phys Med Rehabil.* 1992;73:359-364.

64. Aoki KR. Review of a proposed mechanism for the antinociceptive action of botulinum toxin type A. *Neurotoxicology.* 2005;26:785-793.

65. Lucas HJ, Brauch CM, Settas L, Theoharides TC. Fibromyalgia—new concepts of pathogenesis and treatment. *Int J Immunopathol Pharmacol.* 2006;19:5-10.

66. Gerwin RD, Dommerholt J, Shah JP. An expansion of Simons' integrated hypothesis of trigger point formation. *Curr Pain Headache Rep.* 2004;8:468-475.

67. Shah JP, Phillips TM, Danoff JV, Gerber LH. An in vivo microanalytical technique for measuring the local biochemical milieu of human skeletal muscle. *J Appl Physiol.* 2005;99:1977-1984.

68. Burton DJ, Enion D, Shaw DL. Pyomyositis of the piriformis muscle in a juvenile. *Ann R Coll Surg Engl.* 2005;87:W9-W12.

69. Jankiewicz JJ, Hennrikus WL, Houkom JA. The appearance of the piriformis muscle syndrome in computed tomography and magnetic resonance imaging. A case report and review of the literature. *Clin Orthop Relat Res.* 1991;262:205-209.

70. Nakamura H, Seki M, Konishi S, Yamano Y, Takaoka K. Piriformis syndrome diagnosed by cauda equina action potentials: report of two cases. *Spine.* 2003;28:E37-E40.

71. Beatty RA. Piriformis syndrome. *J Neurosurg Spine.* 2006;5:101-102.

72. Beatty RA. The piriformis muscle syndrome: a simple diagnostic maneuver. *Neurosurgery.* 1994;34:512-514.

73. Graff-Radford SB. Myofascial pain: diagnosis and management. *Curr Pain Headache Rep.* 2004;8: 463-467.

74. Saravanan P, Dayan CM. Thyroid autoantibodies. *Endocrinol Metab Clin North Am.* 2001;30:315-337, viii.

75. Schussler GC. Diagnostic tests and physiological relationships in thyroid disease. *Mod Treat.* 1969;6:443-464.

76. Fishman LM, Zybert PA. Electrophysiologic evidence of piriformis syndrome. *Arch Phys Med Rehabil.* 1992;73:359-364.

77. Fanucci E, Masala S, Sodani G, Varrucciu V, Romagnoli A, Squillaci E, et al. CT-guided injection of botulinic toxin for percutaneous therapy of piriformis muscle syndrome with preliminary MRI results about denervative process. *Eur Radiol.* 2001;11:2543-2548.

78. Fishman LM, Konnoth C, Rozner B. Botulinum neurotoxin type B and physical therapy in the treatment of piriformis syndrome: a dose-finding study. *Am J Phys Med Rehabil.* 2004;83:42-50.

79. Monnier G, Tatu L, Michel F. New indications for botulinum toxin in rheumatology. *Joint Bone Spine.* 2006;73:667-671.

80. Raj PP. Botulinum toxin therapy in pain management. *Anesthesiol Clin N Am.* 2003;21:715-731.

81. Reilich P, Fheodoroff K, Kern U, Mense S, Seddigh S, Wissel J, et al. Consensus statement: botulinum toxin

in myofascial [corrected] pain. *J Neurol.* 2004;251(suppl 1):I36-I38.

82. Harris RE, Clauw DJ. The use of complementary medical therapies in the management of myofascial pain disorders. *Curr Pain Headache Rep.* 2002;6:370-374.

83. Hou CR, Tsai LC, Cheng KF, Chung KC, Hong CZ. Immediate effects of various physical therapeutic modalities on cervical myofascial pain and trigger-point sensitivity. *Arch Phys Med Rehabil.* 2002;83:1406-1414.

84. Hsueh TC, Cheng PT, Kuan TS, Hong CZ. The immediate effectiveness of electrical nerve stimulation and electrical muscle stimulation on myofascial trigger points. *Am J Phys Med Rehabil.* 1997;76:471-476.

85. Graff-Radford SB. Regional myofascial pain syndrome and headache: principles of diagnosis and management. *Curr Pain Headache Rep.* 2001;5:376-381.

86. Wheeler AH. Myofascial pain disorders: theory to therapy. *Drugs.* 2004;64:45-62.

87. McClaflin RR. Myofascial pain syndrome. Primary care strategies for early intervention. *Postgrad Med.* 1994;96:56-59.

88. Nicolakis P, Erdogmus B, Kopf A, Nicolakis M, Piehslinger E, Fialka-Moser V. Effectiveness of exercise therapy in patients with myofascial pain dysfunction syndrome. *J Oral Rehabil.* 2002;29:362-368.

89. Rosen NB. Physical medicine and rehabilitation approaches to the management of myofascial pain and fibromyalgia syndromes. *Baillieres Clin Rheumatol.* 1994;8:881-916.

90. Itoh K, Okada K, Kawakita K. A proposed experimental model of myofascial trigger points in human muscle after slow eccentric exercise. *Acupunct Med.* 2004;22:2-12.

91. Feldman JB. The neurobiology of pain, affect and hypnosis. *Am J Clin Hypn.* 2004;46:187-200.

92. Aronoff GM, Feldman JB, Campion TS. Management of chronic pain and control of long-term disability. *Occup Med.* 2000;15:755-770, iv.

93. Lackner JM, Carosella AM. The relative influence of perceived pain control, anxiety, and functional self efficacy on spinal function among patients with chronic low back pain. *Spine.* 1999;24:2254-2260.

94. Reitsma B, Meijler WJ. Pain and patienthood. *Clin J Pain.* 1997;13:9-21.

95. Jensen MP, Turner JA, Romano JM. Changes in beliefs, catastrophizing, and coping are associated with improvement in multidisciplinary pain treatment. *J Consult Clin Psychol.* 2001;69:655-662.

96. Frost A. Diclofenac versus lidocaine as injection therapy in myofascial pain. *Scand J Rheumatol.* 1986;15:153-156.

97. Arnold LM. Biology and therapy of fibromyalgia. New therapies in fibromyalgia. *Arthritis Res Ther.* 2006;8:212.

98. Borg-Stein J. Treatment of fibromyalgia, myofascial pain, and related disorders. *Phys Med Rehabil Clin N Am.* 2006;17:491-510, viii.

99. Rudin NJ. Evaluation of treatments for myofascial pain syndrome and fibromyalgia. *Curr Pain Headache Rep.* 2003;7:433-442.

100. Criscuolo CM. Interventional approaches to the management of myofascial pain syndrome. *Curr Pain Headache Rep.* 2001;5:407-411.

101. Dubbert PM, Carithers T, Sumner AE, Barbour KA, Clark BL, Hall JE, et al. Obesity, physical inactivity, and risk for cardiovascular disease. *Am J Med Sci.* 2002;324:116-126.

102. Kohl HW, III. Physical activity and cardiovascular disease: evidence for a dose response. *Med Sci Sports Exerc.* 2001;33(6 suppl):S472-S483.

103. Vitale C, Marazzi G, Volterrani M, Aloisio A, Rosano G, Fini M. Metabolic syndrome. *Minerva Med.* 2006;97:219-929.

104. Warburton DE, Nicol CW, Bredin SS. Health benefits of physical activity: the evidence. *CMAJ.* 2006;14(174):801-809.

Botulinum Toxin for **24**
Osteoarticular Pain

Maren Lawson Mahowald, Hollis E. Krug, Jasvinder A. Singh, and Dennis Dykstra

INTRODUCTION

Osteoarticular pain that is refractory to oral and intra-articular (IA) therapies in patients too young or too old and frail for arthroplasty represents a growing unmet need for new joint pain treatments.

Medical management of chronic refractory joint pain is difficult because of the high rate of potentially serious side effects from nonsteroidal anti-inflammatory drugs and systemic analgesics. Joint replacement surgery has been a major advance in the treatment of end-stage joint destruction; however, many patients are too young or too old and frail to undergo arthroplasty. Selective chemodenervation of articular pain fibers offers a novel approach to local treatment of joint pain with IA injection of neurotoxins. We describe herein our clinical experience with IA botulinum neurotoxin (IA-BoNT) injections and the animal models of joint pain with a menu of murine pain behavior measure that will facilitate screening of neurotoxins for use as joint analgesics.

NEUROBIOLOGY OF OSTEOARTICULAR PAIN

Polymodal C- and A-delta fibers in the joint serve analogous functions to cutaneous nociceptors.[1] The C fiber nociceptors form a diffuse lattice throughout the articular capsule. A-delta fiber free nerve endings are found in IA and periarticular ligaments.[2] Mechanical joint pain may also be produced by nociceptors in ligaments, joint capsules, entheses, and blood vessels that are activated by stretch, increased IA pressure with effusions, and abnormal forces and torque due to joint deformities, independent of inflammation in the joint.

In the synovium, nerve fibers positive for substance P (SP) and calcitonin gene–related peptide (CGRP) are associated with blood vessels and also form a network of free endings up to the intima layer. Sympathetic fibers are localized to blood vessels. Articular nerves transmit afferent nociceptive and proprioceptive signals to the central nervous system and antidromic efferent signals to stimulate perivascular peripheral fibers and tissue mast cells. This antidromic stimulation produces neurogenic inflammation, vasodilatation and plasma extravasations in the joint.[2] The dorsal root ganglion cells of C fibers and A-delta fibers synthesize neuropeptides that are transported centrally to the dorsal horn as neurotransmitters and also distally to interact with resident articular cells, inflammatory cells, blood vessels, and lymphatics (i.e., neurogenic inflammation). Efferent sympathetic fibers may also contribute to neurogenic inflammation. In the setting of joint inflammation, articular primary afferent neurons are sensitized to mechanical, thermal, and chemical stimuli (peripheral sensitization) producing articular allodynia (joint pain with normal movement) and hyperalgesia (exaggerated pain with synovial palpation). With sustained nociceptive afferent input, spinal cord neurons become increasingly sensitized to the afferent input from the painful joint

Dr. Mahowald is disclosing she has received research support from NIH, Minnesota Veterans Research Institute, Minnesota Medical Foundation, Genentech, Allergan, Amgen, Pfizer, and Merck. Dr. Krug is disclosing that she has received research support from Allergan, Inc., Irvine, CA. Dr. Singh is disclosing he has received speaker fees from Abbott Laboratories, IL; Investigator-initiated research and travel grants from Allergan Pharmaceuticals, CA; and Investigator-initiated grant from TAP Pharmaceuticals, Lake Forest, IL. Dr. Dykstra is disclosing that he has been a lecturer for Allergan and Solstice. Additionally, he has attended consultant meetings for both companies.

(i.e., central sensitization). The peripheral and central sensitization amplifies nociceptive processing. The severity of adjuvant arthritis in rats is attenuated by sectioning the nerve to the joint or applying capsaicin, which depletes articular SP to the limb.[3] Levels of SP, CGRP, and nerve growth factor in arthritic joints and dorsal root ganglia were reduced after subcutaneous injection of capsaicin in rats. The inflammatory response was also reduced in this model.[4] The density of nerve fibers in synovium and periarticular bone that release SP and CGRP are reduced later in the course of adjuvant arthritis (autodenervation), followed by a regenerative phase and altered morphology.[2] Similar reductions in free nerve endings and sympathetic fibers on blood vessels in the superficial layer are also seen in the rheumatoid synovium. Immunocytochemical localization studies done in murine antigen-induced arthritis showed that an apparent reduction in SP and CGRP nerves in arthritic synovium was likely due to failure of synovial reinnervation because neural fiber sprouting was unable to keep up with intense synovial tissue proliferation rather than actual destruction of nerve tissue.[5] Sensitization of articular nociceptors causes normally inactive primary afferents to become spontaneously active at rest and responsive to non-noxious movements and touch.[6] SP contributes to the inflammatory response by stimulating the resident synovial cells to produce inflammatory mediators and cytokines, and appears to be the principal neurotransmitter of pain in arthritis.[7] SP can activate mast cells, synoviocytes, neutrophils, T cells, B cells, and macrophages, thereby amplifying the inflammatory response. Neurokinin receptors that bind SP are coupled to regulatory G proteins and activate hydrolysis of inositol-containing phospholipids for the second response in cell activation.[7] Opioid receptors are upregulated on peripheral sensory nerves during inflammation, and resident immune cells express endogenous opioids; thus, IA opioids reduce pain and possibly inflammation.[8]

The spinal cord is the integrative site for afferent sensory information and reflex antidromic efferent functions.[1] Noxious stimulation of peripheral tissues causes expression of C-fos, presumably for synthesis of neuropeptides. Levels of transmitters and receptors in dorsal root ganglia and the spinal cord change when there is acute or chronic inflammation in a peripheral joint. Glutamate and N-methyl-D-aspartate (NMDA) receptors transmit nociceptive information from an inflamed joint to the spinal cord. Serotonin and norepinephrine, transmitters in descending inhibition of spinal neurons, are increased under inflammatory conditions. Neuro-peptides synthesis (SP, CGRP, dynorphin, enkephalin) in dorsal ganglia and the spinal cord is also increased during joint inflammation.[2] The full functional consequences of the changes in neuropeptides, transmitters, and receptors remain to be elucidated, and the role of the spinal cord in regulation of peripheral joint inflammation is just beginning to be defined.[9] Investigators have started to delineate neuromolecular signatures of the three different pain states using mouse models of bone cancer pain, neuropathic pain, and inflammatory pain. The characteristic neuromolecular signature for bone cancer pain was an increase in a spinal cord astrocyte marker (reflecting hypertrophy of astrocytes), increased dynorphin in deep spinal laminae, no changes in SP or CGRP, but increased internalization of SP receptors and increased C-fos expression in lamina I of the dorsal horn, demonstrating sensitization of primary afferent neurons.[10] In the setting of pain due to paw inflammation, there was upregulation of SP and CGRP in laminae I and II of the dorsal horn and increased protein kinase C and SP receptor. In contrast, downregulation of SP and CGRP and upregulation of galanin, neuropeptide Y, and GAP-43 in both primary afferent neurons and the spinal cord was found with peripheral nerve injury.[11] Interestingly, one group of investigators demonstrated that osteoprotegerin prevented cancer-induced bone destruction by osteoclasts, reduced pain, and blocked sensitization in the spinal cord.[10] Such advances in our understanding of the neuromolecular signatures for different pain states will provide a new framework for the mechanism-based development of new analgesics.

RATIONALE FOR SELECTING BOTULINUM TOXIN TO TREAT OSTEOARTICULAR PAIN

The phenomenon of neurogenic inflammation that involves the release of neurotransmitters such as SP and CGRP in the periphery may be involved in the explanation of our recent observation of reduced pain following IA injection of botulinum toxin type A (see discussion below of references 13 to 17). Clinically

IA-BoNT/A (Botox, Allergan, Irvine, CA) injections into joints made painful by both inflammatory and noninflammatory joint disorders produced significant pain relief, suggesting that persistent pain in and of itself may produce neurogenic inflammation and augmented joint pain. BoNT/A can bind to nociceptor C-fibers, undergo endocytosis, and block vesicle release of substance P, CGRP, and glutamate, agents involved in joint pain generation, transmission, and nociceptor sensitization by neurogenic inflammation.[12] Thereby, BoNT/A could disrupt nociceptor function and decrease pain generation, transmission, and neurogenic inflammation. This data suggests that IA therapies directed against efferent nerve function (i.e., sensory nerve release of neurotransmitters in the periphery) may be a new approach to IA therapy of refractory joint pain.[13-17]

MEASURING PAIN BEHAVIORS IN ANIMAL MODELS OF ARTHRITIS PAIN

While studying IA neurotoxin for human arthritis pain, we identified a need for an animal model to screen additional neurotoxins and carry out dose-ranging studies in preparation for further human studies. Although major advances in the neurobiology of bone pain have been made,[10] analysis of pain in animal models of arthritis pain has been limited by the lack of behavioral measures of animal pain. The purpose of these studies was to develop functional measures of articular pain in murine models of arthritis in order to demonstrate the effectiveness of IA neurotoxins as analgesics. We examined published measures used in animal pain models and measures analogous to those used in human clinical studies and adapted them to murine models of arthritis pain. We developed protocols for measuring pain behaviors to test neurotoxin effects on arthritis joint pain in order to do drug screening, dose-ranging studies, and safety assessment for rapid translation into human clinical trials.

Measures of Pain Behavior in Murine Models of Acute and Chronic Arthritis Pain

Three models of arthritis pain were produced in C57B16 adult female mice. Acute inflammatory arthritis pain was produced by the injection of 10 lambda of 3% carrageenan intra-articularly into the left knee. Acute inflammatory arthritis was evident within 1 hour, peaked at 3 to 4 hours, then declined substantially by 8 hours, and was completely resolved by 24 hours. Chronic noninflammatory arthritis pain was produced by injection of 10 lambda containing 10 international units of collagenase type IV intra-articularly into the left knee. IA collagenase injection produced severe joint laxity and degenerative arthritis by 4 weeks. Chronic inflammatory arthritis pain was produced by injection of 30 lambda of 1 mg/mL Complete Freund's adjuvant (CFA) intra-articularly into the left knee. CFA arthritis was maximal within 3 weeks. IA injection was performed through the patellar tendon just superior to the tibial plateau. Accuracy was ensured by using a sheathed needle to limit insertion depth (Fig. 24-1).

Both inflammatory (acute and chronic) and chronic noninflammatory arthritis pain was quantified using a menu of pain behavior measures including clinical examination for inflammation, tenderness and joint deformities, evoked pain responses, and electronically measured nocturnal activity. Clinical joint examination measured erythema on a 0 to 3 scale and swelling on a 0 to 3 scale. (Fig. 24-2). Evoked pain behavior (fights, bites, and vocalizations) was elicited by applying firm pressure to the knee using the thumb and index finger. All examiners were trained by using a Palpometer® (Palpometer Systems, Inc., Victoria, BC) (see Fig. 24-1) to develop consistency and precision of palpation pressure. A standardized and reproducible stimulus was found to be very important for reliable and accurate evoked pain measures. Joint tenderness was quantitated as the number of fights and vocalizations in 1 minute during firm palpation of the knee. Spontaneous pain behavior was identified by measuring nocturnal spontaneous activity with Mini-Mitter infrared motion detectors, Nalgene running wheels, and VitalView Data Acquisition software (Mini Mitter, Bend, OR) (see Fig. 24-1). Evoked pain measures and spontaneous nocturnal activity were both sensitive and specific measures of arthritis pain behavior in all three models of arthritis pain. Diurnal variations in activity in the mouse, a nocturnal animal, significantly affected pain behavior measurements (see Fig. 24-2). Daytime spontaneous activity was minimal and insensitive to change due to arthritis pain. Visual gait analysis

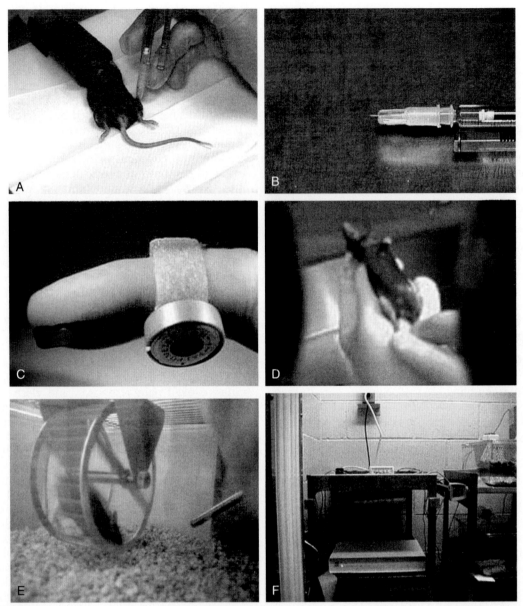

FIGURE 24-1. A, Mice are anesthetized with isofluorane, and the left knee is injected through an infrapatellar approach. **B,** The needle for injection is sheathed, allowing only 2 to 3 mm of the needle to protrude from the sheath, ensuring accurate needle depth. **C,** The Palpometer allows examiners to be trained to produce exactly 1100 gf/cm^2 with each knee palpation, ensuring accurate and consistent examination technique. **D,** Mice are restrained to reduce mobility during examination, minimizing spontaneous movement to ensure adequate sensitivity and specificity for evoked pain behaviors (fights and vocalization). **E,** Spontaneous nocturnal activity is measured using running wheels *(shown)* designed to electronically count the number of revolutions per time period, as well as motion detectors *(not shown)* designed to count periods of spontaneous activity. **F,** Data is captured using the Mini-Mitter system with Vital View data acquisition software (Mini Mitter, Bend, OR).

(limp, 1-4 scale) and manually counting the number of rearings and ambulation distance in 2 minutes pre- and postpalpation were not sufficiently sensitive to change due to arthritis pain (not shown).

Acute Inflammatory Arthritis Pain Model Induced by Carrageenan

Mice were pretreated with 0.3 to 0.5 U BoNT/A in 10 lambda sterile normal saline injected

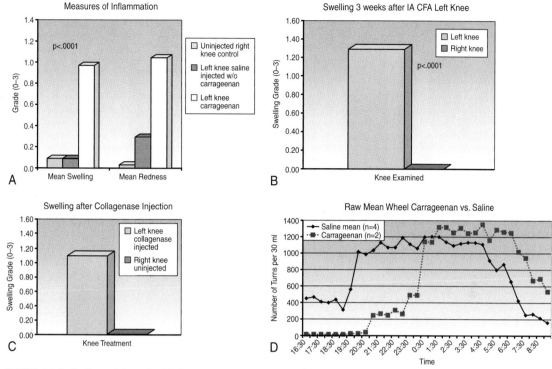

FIGURE 24-2. A, Knees injected with 3% carrageenan were significantly more swollen and erythematous at the time of examination, confirming the presence of inflammation. **B,** Three weeks following Complete Freund's adjuvant injection, the injected knees demonstrated significant soft tissue swelling. **C,** Four weeks following injection of 10 IU type IV collagenase into the left knee, there was significant bony swelling, demonstrating the presence of chronic degenerative noninflammatory arthritis. **D,** Mice exhibited significant diurnal variations in spontaneous activity. They were very inactive during daytime hours, but spontaneous activity increased significantly between 8 PM and 6 AM. During this time, changes in spontaneous activity could easily be detected, such as a decrease in wheel running in mice injected with carrageenan seen here. During daytime hours when mice were inactive, changes in activity due to arthritis pain could not be seen.

intra-articularly into the left knee 3 days before IA injection of carrageenan and pain behavior testing. Treatment controls were injected with an equal volume (10 lambda) of normal saline. Evoked pain behavior measures were performed followed by nocturnal spontaneous activity. Acute inflammatory arthritis pain produced significant changes in evoked joint pain behaviors and spontaneous nocturnal activity (Fig. 24-3). Systemic morphine (an analgesic control) improved evoked pain responses but produced paradoxical hyperactivity measured by spontaneous nocturnal activity, which confounded measurement of potential analgesic effects (data not shown). IA-BoNT/A pretreatment 3 days before production of acute inflammatory arthritis decreased clinical measures of inflammation and reduced evoked pain behaviors to nonarthritic levels (see Fig. 24-3). However, at this dose, pretreatment also produced transient limping due to mild reversible limb weakness. Pretreatment with IA-BoNT/A

had no effect on spontaneous nocturnal wheel running in mice with acute inflammatory arthritis but did reduce spontaneous nocturnal wheel running in normal mice likely due to limb weakness (see Fig. 24-3).

Chronic Noninflammatory Arthritis Pain Model Induced by Intra-Articular Collagenase

There was palpable bony enlargement (swelling) and tenderness of the joint 4 weeks after IA collagenase (see Fig. 24-2). Spontaneous nocturnal activity was reduced compared with nonarthritic controls. Mean spontaneous nocturnal wheel running was also decreased in arthritic mice as compared with nonarthritic mice; however, the results were highly variable and not statistically significant (Fig. 24-4). IA-BoNT/A 3 days before pain behavior testing reduced evoked pain behaviors to near

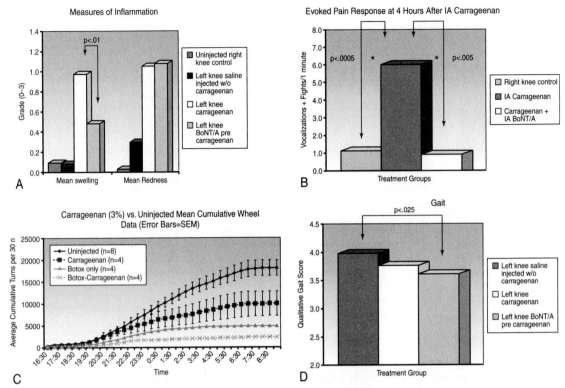

FIGURE 24-3. A, IA injection of carrageenan produced significant swelling and erythema that peaked 4 hours after injection. Pretreatment with IA botulinum toxin type A significantly reduced swelling but not erythema. **B,** IA injection of carrageenan produced significantly increased evoked pain responses to palpation of the arthritic left knee as compared with the uninjected normal right knee. Pretreatment with IA botulinum toxin normalized these evoked pain responses. **C,** Spontaneous nocturnal wheel running was significantly reduced by production of carrageenan-induced acute arthritis. Pretreatment with botulinum toxin type A did not normalize spontaneous wheel running; however, injection of botulinum toxin alone, without production of arthritis with carrageenan, produced similar reductions in spontaneous nocturnal wheel running. **D,** Qualitative gait analysis showed only slightly abnormal gait in the carrageenan-injected animals as compared with saline-injected controls, which was not statistically significant. However, mice injected with botulinum toxin A had a statistically significant alteration in gait, probably due to mild left lower extremity weakness.

nonarthritic levels but, due to high variability, the change was not statistically significant (see Fig. 24-4). IA-BoNT/A again produced weakness in the injected lower extremity and did not restore spontaneous nocturnal activity and wheel running to normal levels (see Fig. 24-4). There was no weakness of forepaw muscles after IA-BoNT/A into the knee (data not shown), indicating no systemic effect of botulinum toxin on motor function. There are several possible explanations for the high degree of variability seen in these studies. Some mice were more avid wheel runners. First-generation running wheels were subject to intermittent obstruction by cage bedding. Importantly, our early IA injections may not have been as accurate as assumed, producing variable degrees of arthritis pain.

Weakness due to botulinum toxin was also variable. All of these factors likely added to the variability of the results seen.

Chronic Inflammatory Arthritis Pain Model Induced by Complete Freund's Adjuvant

Significantly increased evoked pain responses to joint palpation (Fig. 24-5) and significant soft tissue swelling (see Fig. 24-2) was noted 3 weeks after IA CFA. Spontaneous nocturnal activity and wheel running were decreased in arthritis mice compared with that of nonarthritic controls. This decrease in spontaneous activity was statistically significant for wheel running (see Fig. 24-5). Preliminary results of

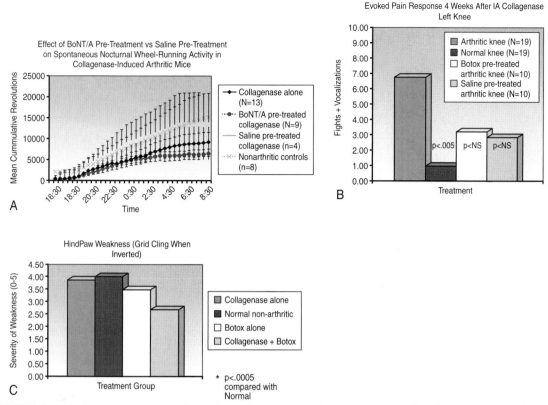

FIGURE 24-4. A, Spontaneous nocturnal wheel running was reduced on average by both collagenase-induced chronic noninflammatory arthritis and by botulinum toxin A injection. However, results were highly variable and not statistically significant. Interestingly, treatment with saline as a control appeared to improve spontaneous nocturnal wheel running, but these results were again highly variable and not significant. **B,** Evoked pain response 4 weeks after collagenase injection in the left knee was significantly increased as compared with the uninjected right knee. Both botulinum toxin A treatment and saline treatment appeared to reduce this evoked pain response, but results were variable and not statistically significant. **C,** Injection of botulinum toxin A into the left knee produced measurable mild weakness of the left hind limb that was significant when compared with the same limb of uninjected animals. This was true in both arthritic and nonarthritic animals.

treatment studies of chronic inflammatory arthritis suggest that evoked pain responses were reduced and spontaneous nocturnal wheel running improved after treatment with IA-BoNT/A (data not shown).

Our preliminary work described earlier indicates that murine models of acute and chronic arthritis joint pain caused by inflammatory and noninflammatory pathologies can be quantified with pain behavior protocols. The sensitivity and specificity of the measures permits quantitative screening of neurotoxins as IA analgesics. Measured evoked pain responses and quantitative spontaneous activity measures are necessary to maximize sensitivity to change. Treatment with IA-BoNT toxin reduces pain behavior in murine models of arthritis pain when quantified by evoked measures. The high doses of botulinum toxin used in these studies was associated with

significant temporary local weakness but not with systemic weakness or other observed toxicity. This weakness confounded measures of spontaneous nocturnal activity. Dose-ranging studies will be important for determining the optimum analgesic dose without significant limb weakness or other toxicity.

EFFECTS OF INTRA-ARTICULAR BOTULINUM TOXIN TYPE A IN HUMAN ARTHRITIS PAIN

In an open-label pilot study of IA-BONT/A,[17] we studied the effects of 25 to 100 U of BONT/A with 2 mL of 2% bupivacaine in nine shoulder joints, three knee joints, and three ankle joints. Pain decrease began

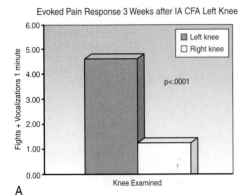

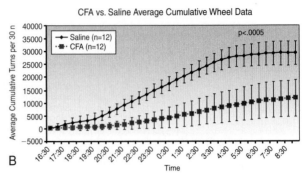

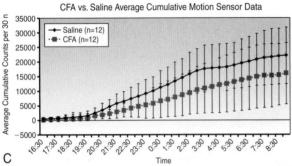

FIGURE 24-5. A, Injection of Complete Freund's adjuvant into the left knee produced significantly increased evoked pain responses as compared with the uninjected right knee. **B,** Spontaneous nocturnal wheel running was significantly decreased in animals with chronic inflammatory arthritis as compared with saline-injected nonarthritic control mice ($P < .0005$). **C,** Spontaneous nocturnal activity appeared to be decreased in mice with chronic inflammatory arthritis but was highly variable and not statistically different from that of saline-injected nonarthritic control mice.

within 2 to 14 days. Mean maximum decrease in pain severity 4 to 12 weeks after joint injection was 55% (from 6.8 to 2.9 on the Numeric Rating Scale [NRS], $P = .018$) in lower extremity joints and 71% (from 8.2 to 2.41, $P = <.001$) in the shoulders. Fourteen of 15 joints had more than 30% pain reduction, and 10/15 joints had more than 50% pain reduction. Pain relief lasted 3 to 10 months, and repeat injections produced 42% to 100% pain reduction that lasted up to 12 months in some patients. Based on this open-label observational study, we found that IA-BoNT/A injection for sustained analgesia is a promising new treatment approach to persistent joint pain. Safety concerns requiring further study included the possible development of increased joint pain and inflammation, weakness of limb muscles, effects on other sensory nerves, and potential neuropathic joint degeneration.

In another open-label pilot study, we evaluated the effects and safety of injecting BoNT/A and BoNT/B (Myobloc, Solstice Neurosciences, Malvern, PA) into sacroiliac joints, cervical/lumbar facet joints, C-2 roots, sternoclavicular joint, and lumbar disc in 11 patients with refractory pain. Eight of 11 patients had a decrease in their pain score. All patients who responded to the injections noted improved function in activities of daily living and range of motion when pain was reduced. No side effects were noted. The mean duration of pain relief for the first BoNT treatments was 2.0 months. The median difference of duration of pain relief between BoNT and previous steroid injection was 1.6 months, with BoNT being superior. The median change in pain score (0 to 10) after BoNT injection was a three-point decrease (see reference 14 for additional study data). We concluded that BoNT injections lasted longer than steroid injections and gave excellent pain relief. Based on these positive findings, randomized controlled trials for the use of BoNT/A and BoNT/B in root and joint pain are warranted.[14]

We have extended these observations in the pilot studies and obtained approval from the US Food and Drug Administration (FDA) for our investigational new drug application to conduct prospective, randomized, placebo-controlled studies of IA-BONT/A and saline placebo in patients with refractory knee pain due to advanced rheumatoid arthritis and osteoarthritis, refractory shoulder pain, and painful prosthetic knee joints.

Interim analysis of 1-month data on 37 patients with moderate to severe refractory knee pain due to osteoarthritis were randomized to receive 100 U IA-BoNT/A + lidocaine or IA saline + lidocaine (placebo). Double-blind assessments were made for baseline and follow-up at 1 month, 3 months, and 6 months from the time of withdrawal from the study. The primary outcome measure at 1 month was the McGill Pain Inventory and the Western Ontario McMaster OA index (WOMAC) (Pain score, Function score, WOMAC question 1 [walking pain], and WOMAC Total score). Secondary outcome measures included the $10\times$ Timed Stands Test of lower extremity function,[36] severity of Day Pain and Night Pain on 0-10 Numerical Rating Scale (NRS) and passive arc of motion

Patients in the severe pain group had baseline NRS pain greater than 7, whereas the moderate pain group had baseline NRS pain 4.5 to less than 7. The protocol was approved by the Investigational Review Board and participants gave signed, informed consent.

We studied 37 patients with osteoarthritis (36 men, 1 woman); 19 had severe pain, and 18 had moderate pain. Seventeen patients were randomized to IA-BONT/A, and 20 were randomized to IA placebo. In this interim 1-month study analysis, there was no significant change in the means of the outcome measures of pain or function in the whole group because of large standard deviations. Examination of the scatter plots revealed groups with dichotomous responses (i.e., no or minimal change versus those with greater than 30% decrease in pain) based on baseline pain severity indicating multiple models analysis adjusting for baseline pain will be necessary for analysis of the completed study dataset. Exploratory analysis of subgroups based on moderate or severe baseline pain severity rating (on NRS) was carried out after examination of the scatter plots. Of the 17 patients with moderate pain, eight had been randomized to IA-BONT/A and 10 to

IA placebo. Two patients dropped out before the 1-month follow-up examination due to lack of efficacy (both placebo). In the severe knee pain group, significant changes were observed in the IA-BONT/A group but not the placebo group 1 month after the IA injections (Fig. 24-6). There was a significant decrease in the WOMAC Pain score—12.4 (standard error [s.e.] 1.5) to 8.9 (s.e. 3.1), $P = .006$; improvement in WOMAC Physical Function score—42.4 (4.2) to 31.8 (10.3), $P = .033$; decrease in Q1-walking pain from 2.6 (0.7) to 1.7 (1.0), $P = .035$. The WOMAC Total Score decreased 27% in the IA-BONT/A group ($P = .018$ and only 14% in the IA placebo group ($P = .19$). The Short Form McGill Pain Inventory (SF-M) yields three scores: a sensory score, an affective score, and a total pain score. IA-BONT/A produced a 47% decrease in the sensory score from 17 (s.d. 1.9) to 9 (s.d. 1.9), $P = .04$; a 51% decrease in the affective score from 6.3 (s.d. 1.2) to 3.1 (s.d. 1.1) $P = .02$; and a 48% decrease in the total pain score from 23 (s.d. 2.6) to 12 (s.d. 2.9), $P = .03$). The IA placebo injections produced no significant changes in this group. In patients with severe pain, the IA-BONT/A injection produced a 38% decrease in daytime pain from 7.6 (s.d. 0.3) to 4.7 (s.d. 0.7), $P = .003$ and a 25% decrease in nighttime pain from 5.4 (s.d. 0.9) to 4.1 (s.d. 0.7), $P = .015$. The IA placebo injections produced a 24% decrease in daytime pain from 7.7 (s.d. 0.3) to 5.8 (s.d. 0.9), a 19% decrease in nighttime pain from 4.8 (s.d. 0.8) to 3.9 (s.d. 0.8), both non significant changes.

In the moderate pain group, IA-BoNT/A and placebo injections produced little change.

However, there was a strong placebo response in those with moderate pain who had a 25% decrease in pain from 6.11 (s.d. 0.1) to 4.6 (s.d. 0.6), $P = .018$ (a statistically significant decrease that is not clinically significant). Calculation of the percentage of patients who had 30% and 50% reduction in pain adds to the interpretability of the study results. In the severe pain group, IA-BoNT/A produced a 30% pain reduction (a clinically important pain decrease) in 55% of patients and a 50% reduction (an excellent pain decrease) in 44% of the patients. Interestingly, IA placebo produced 30% pain reduction and 50% reduction in 33% of injected patients at this interim time point of the study. This strong placebo response was surprising because these patients had all failed IA corticosteroid or viscosupplement injections.

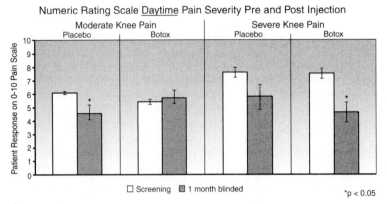

Numeric Rating Scale <u>Daytime</u> Pain Severity Pre and Post Injection

A Bars represent mean value. Error bars represent SEM.

FIGURE 24-6. A, Changes in pain severity 1 month after injection, measured by the Numerical Rating Scale from zero to 10, were significant in those with severe pain at baseline before IA botulinum neurotoxin type A (BoNT/A) injection. **B,** Scores for Sensory Dimension, Affective Dimension, and Total Pain Score on the Short Form McGill Pain Inventory were significantly improved in those patients with severe knee pain at baseline before IA-BoNT/A injection.

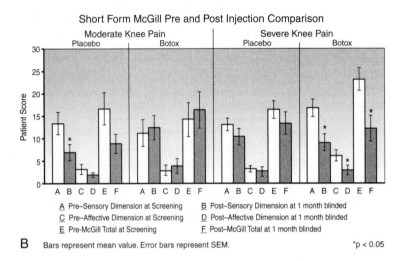

Short Form McGill Pre and Post Injection Comparison

<u>A</u> Pre–Sensory Dimension at Screening   <u>B</u> Post–Sensory Dimension at 1 month blinded
<u>C</u> Pre–Affective Dimension at Screening   <u>D</u> Post–Affective Dimension at 1 month blinded
<u>E</u> Pre–McGill Total at Screening   <u>F</u> Post–McGill Total at 1 month blinded

B Bars represent mean value. Error bars represent SEM.   *$p < 0.05$

WOMAC total score change in the placebo group was 48 (s.d. 3.4) to 38 (s.d. 3.3), $P >.05$, and in the IA-BONT/A group was 53 (5.6) to 54 (5.5) $P >.05$. The only significant changes noted in those with moderate pain was a decrease in daytime pain from 6.1 (0.1) to 4.6 (0.6), $P = .026$ and a 48% decrease in the SF-MQI Sensory Score from 13.3 (s.d. 2.6) to 6.9 (s.d. 1.8), $P = .04$ in the placebo group. Interestingly, IA-BONT/A produced no significant changes in those with moderate pain at baseline. There was no substantial improvement in passive arc of motion or the $10\times$ Timed Stands Test at this early 1-month evaluation point. The trial is ongoing for examinations at the 3- and 6-month time points, which is likely the time needed to show functional improvement. There were no serious systemic or local joint adverse events due to the IA injections. Specifically, there was no significant muscle weakness on manual muscle strength testing of the legs, no new neurologic abnormalities on neurosensory testing for light touch, temperature, vibration, position, and pinprick in the lower extremity. Transient injection site pain, mild joint swelling, or tenderness was reported by four patients who received IA-BoNT/A and five patients who received IA placebo.

This is the first randomized placebo controlled trial of IA injection of BoNT/A for moderate and severe refractory knee joint pain due to osteoarthritis. The 1-month interim analysis demonstrated a statistically and clinically significant reduction in pain and subjective improvement in function in those with severe knee pain using three different pain measures. Maximal pain relief, improvement in function, and duration of effects will be determined in the full 6-month study. These data provide further evidence supporting the efficacy of this novel approach to local treatment of refractory joint pain at one month after IA injection.

EFFECTS OF INTRA-ARTICULAR BOTULINUM NEUROTOXIN TYPE A IN REFRACTORY KNEE PROSTHESIS PAIN

Joint replacement surgery represents one of the most significant advances in the treatment of arthritis in the past 50 years because it results in significant pain relief, increased function, and improved quality of life (QOL).[18] The number of total knee arthroplasty (TKA) procedures performed in the United States is projected to grow by 673% from 450,000 in 2005 to 3.48 million procedures by 2030.[19] Approximately, 1% of prosthetic knee replacements fail every year[20] and are associated with disabling pain, reduced function, and mobility.[21] Even though TKA is associated with excellent outcomes, failed painful prosthetic knees represent a significant public health problem because TKA is a high-volume procedure, joint replacements are being performed in younger patients, and we have an expanding aging population.

The underlying mechanism for a painful prosthesis is not always clear in an individual patient but may be due to infection, loosening of the prosthesis, inflammatory synovitis produced as a reaction to prosthesis wear particles or periarticular problems.[22-24] Neuropeptides and inflammatory cytokines and mediators may play a role in the pain of patients with joint prostheses. The joint fluid SP level was elevated in 73% of replaced knees in 114 patients but not in the normal or asymptomatic contralateral knees.[25] Those with an elevated preoperative joint fluid SP level had significantly greater pain relief than those with normal levels of SP. Nerve fibers in the interface membrane were positive for SP, CGRP and neurokinin A in nine patients undergoing hip prosthesis revision surgery for painful aseptic loosening.[26] Articular tissue nerve fibers had more SP and CGRP immunostaining than tissue removed during surgery for femoral neck fracture and tissue from painless loose prostheses.[27] Tissue culture experiments with the bone-prosthesis interface membrane and studies of macrophages and fibroblasts from the interface membrane produced prostaglandin E_2, collagen, and the cytokines interleukin (IL-1), IL-6, IL-8, and tumor necrosis factor (TNF). The amount of interface membrane IL-1, IL-6, and TNF was greater with osteolysis than without.[24,28,29] Antibodies against TNF-α reduced hyperalgesia in inflammatory models of pain.[30] Treatment of rheumatoid arthritis with TNF blockers produced significant reductions in pain scores.[31] Taken together, these data suggest that cytokines and neuropeptides play an important role in prosthetic joint pain through processes of joint inflammation and periprosthetic bone resorption. Treatment approaches with inhibitors of these mediators may reduce pain and inflammation associated with painful prostheses.

Prosthesis revision surgery was performed in 38,000 patients in 2005, and this number is projected to increase by 601% to 268,200 in 2030.[19] Revision surgery is more complicated and has less predictable outcomes.[32,33] Many patients are reluctant to undergo another surgical procedure. Therefore, there is a pressing, unmet current and growing need for a nonsurgical treatment option for relief of pain in patients with painful knee arthroplasty, which will avoid the systemic adverse effects seen with oral nonsteroidal and opioid analgesics.

We studied six elderly patients (five men and one woman) with seven refractory painful prosthetic knee joints who did not have prosthetic infection, loosening, or other surgically correctable causes of pain. Patients were refractory to oral analgesics or anti-inflammatory drugs, or both, but had not had IA corticosteroid injections. After discussion of off-label use, patients gave informed consent for the procedure. Six joints were injected with 100 U of BoNT/A, and one joint received 200 U of IA-BoNT/A. Patients were evaluated prospectively (under the purview of Quality Assurance/Quality Improvement Initiative approved by Institutional Review Board) at less than 1, 1 to 2, 3 to 4, 5 to 6, and 9 months after IA-BoNT/A. Pain severity was measured on the 0 to 10 Numeric Rating Scale (NRS). Self-reported lower extremity function was measured with the WOMAC[34] Physical Function (PF) subscale. The Timed Stands Test is a validated objective measure of lower extremity function that measures the time to stand up from a chair 10 times. Mean values in 60- to 80-year-old subjects range from 17 to 21 seconds.[35,36] We compared the preinjection values with those at the time of greatest decrease in pain severity after the IA injection because the time to maximal response after IA-BoNT/A was variable between patients (1–4 months). We measured the onset and duration of pain relief. Patient global assessment of change was measured with a validated seven-point verbal descriptor scale: 1, very much improved; 2, much improved; 3, minimally improved; 4, no change; 5, minimally worse; 6, much worse; 7, very much worse.[37] Safety was assessed by inquiry about side effects at each visit, and by manual muscle strength and quantitative sensory testing in the lower extremity at follow-up. Paired one-sided t-tests were used to compare the baseline pain severity on NRS, WOMAC PF scale score, and TST to the observation at the time of maximum improvement because we predicted that IA-BoNT/A would lead to decrease in pain and improvement in function. A P-value less than 0.05 was considered significant.

Median age of patients was 73 years (range, 48–81 years), median pain duration was 2 years (range, 1–10 years), baseline TKA pain was 7 on 0–10 NRS and median follow-up duration was 6 months (range, 3–17 months). Three patients had primary TKA prostheses, and three patients had revised TKA prostheses. No loosening was noted on preinjection radiographs in any patient. Following one or two IA-BoNT/A injections, pain on 0–10 NRS decreased significantly from mean ± SD of 7 ± 1.1 at baseline to 3.8 ± 2.6 at maximum pain decrease representing a 46% reduction in pain severity, $P = 0.009$. The degree of pain relief was variable, as were the onset and duration of relief between patients. Pain relief ranged from none in patient D to almost complete in patient F and a steady worsening of pain severity in patient A. We calculated the proportion of patients with greater than 30% pain relief (a good analgesic response) and greater than 50% (an excellent analgesic response). Four of seven patients had greater than 30% pain decrease and three of seven patients had greater than 50% pain decrease, indicating that IA-BoNT/A injections into a painful prosthetic joint had produced both a clinically significant and clinically meaningful improvement for these patients[37,38] and might be able to obviate the need for revision surgery in some. The WOMAC physical function subscale had a mean maximum improvement from 36.1 ± 10 to 25.7 ± 14.9 (29% reduction, $P = 0.042$). The Timed Stands test improved from 35 ± 13.7 at baseline to 29.6 ± 9 at maximum TST improvement (16% reduction, $P = 0.10$). Five patients reported much improved to very much improved on patient global assessment of change at follow-up visits, and two patients minimal to no improvement. Pain relief began 7 to 11 days after the injection and lasted 1 to 9 months.

No increase in joint inflammation, periarticular muscle weakness, fever or fatigue, or other complications were noted. There were no changes in sensory testing of the lower extremity following IA-BoNT/A injections. In summary, these pilot data suggest that IA-BoNT/A injections can provide significant pain relief in patients with refractory TKA pain. Based on these results, we are conducting a randomized controlled trial to test the efficacy and safety of IA-BoNT/A in patients with chronic TKA pain.

References

1. Schaible HG, Grubb BD. Afferent and spinal mechanisms of joint pain. *Pain*. 1993;55:5-54.
2. Mapp P, Kidd BL. The role of substance P in rheumatic disease. *Semin Arthritis Rheum*. 1994;23:3-9.
3. Matucci-Cerinic M, Konttinen YT, Generini S, Cutolo M. Neuropeptides and steroid hormones in arthritis. *Curr Opin Rheumatol*. 1998;10:220-235.
4. Garrett N, Cruwys SC, Kidd BL, Tomlison DR. Effect of capsaicin on substance P and nerve growth factor in adjuvant arthritic rat. *Neurosci Lett*. 1997;230:5-8.
5. Buma P, Elmans L, van den Berg WB, Schrama LH. Neurovascular plasticity in the knee joint of an arthritic mouse model. *Anat Rec*. 2000;260:51-61.
6. Konttinen YT, Kemppinen P, Segerberg M, Hukkanen M, Rees R, Virta S, et al. Peripheral and spinal neural mechanisms in arthritis, with particular reference to treatment of inflammation and pain. *Arthritis Rheum*. 1994;37:965-982.
7. Lotz M. Experimental models of arthritis: identification of substance P as a therapeutic target and use of capsaicin to manage joint pain and inflammation. *Semin Arthritis Rheum*. 1994;23:10-17.
8. Stein C. The control of pain in peripheral tissues by opioids. *N Engl J Med*. 1995;332:1685-1690.
9. Boyle DL, Moore J, Yang L, Sorkin LS, Firestein GS. Spinal adenosine receptor activation inhibits inflammation and joint destruction in rat adjuvant arthritis. *Arthritis Rheum*. 2002;46:3076-3082.
10. Honore P, Luger NM, Sabino MC, Schwei MJ, Rogers SD, Mach DB, et al. Osteoprotegerin blocks bone cancer-induced skeletal destruction, skeletal pain and pain-related neurochemical reorganization of the spinal cord. *Nat Med*. 2000;6:521-528.
11. Schaible H-G, Schmetz M, Tegeder I. Pathophysiology and treatment of pain in joint disease. *Adv Drug Deliv Rev*. 2006;58:323-342.
12. Schaible HG. Why does an inflammation in the joint hurt? *Br J Rheum*. 1996;35:405-406.
13. Mahowald M, Singh J, Dykstra D. Intra-articular botulinum toxin type A for refractory joint pain: a case series review. *Neurotox Res*. 2006;9:179-188.
14. Dykstra D, Stucky MW, Schimpff SN, Singh JA, Mahowald ML. The effects of intra-articular botulinum toxin on sacroiliac, cervical/lumbar facet and sternoclavicular joint pain and C-2 root and lumbar disc pain: a case series of 11 patients. *Pain Clin*. 2007;19:27-32.

15. Mahowald M, Singh JA, Kushnaryov A, Goelz E, Dykstra D. Repeat injections of intra-articular botulinum toxin A for the treatment of chronic arthritis joint pain—a case series review. *J Clin Rheumatol*. 2008. In press.

16. Singh JA, Mahowald ML. Intra-articular botulinum toxin A as an adjunctive therapy for refractory joint pain in patients with rheumatoid arthritis: a report of two cases. *Joint Bone Spine*. 2008. In press.

17. Mahowald M, Singh J, Dykstra D. Long term effects of intra-articular botulinum toxin type A on refractory joint pain. *Neurotox Res*. 2006;9:179-188.

18. Ethgen O, Bruyère O, Richy F, Dardennes C, Reginster JY. Health-related quality of life in total hip and total knee arthroplasty. A qualitative and systematic review of the literature. *J Bone Joint Surg Am*. 2004;86-A:963-974.

19. Kurtz S, Ong K, Lau E, Mowat F, Halpern M. Projections of primary and revision hip and knee arthroplasty in the United States from 2005 to 2030. *J Bone Joint Surg Am*. 2007;89(4):780-785.

20. Wells V, Hearn T, Heard A, Lange K, Rankin W, Graves S. Incidence and outcomes of knee and hip joint replacement in veterans and civilians. *A N Z J Surg*. 2006;76:295-299.

21. Brander VA, Stulberg SD, Adams AD, Harden RN, Bruehl S, Stanos SP, Houle T. Predicting total knee replacement pain: a prospective, observational study. *Clin Orthop Relat Res*. 2003;416:27-36.

22. Boynton EL, Henry M, Morton J, Waddell JP. The inflammatory response to particulate wear debris in total hip arthroplasty. *Can J Surg*. 1995;38:507-515.

23. Jiranek WA, Machado M, Jasty M, Jevsevar D, Wolfe HJ, Goldring SR, et al. Production of cytokines around loosened cemented acetabular components. Analysis with immunohistochemical techniques and in situ hybridization. *J Bone Joint Surg Am*. 1993;75:863-879.

24. Chiba J, Rubash HE, Kim KJ, Iwaki Y. The characterization of cytokines in the interface tissue obtained from failed cementless total hip arthroplasty with and without femoral osteolysis. *Clin Orthop Relat Res*. 1994;300:304-312.

25. Pritchett JW. Substance P level in synovial fluid may predict pain relief after knee replacement. *J Bone Joint Surg Br*. 1997;79:114-116.

26. Ahmed M, Bergstrom J, Lundblad H, Gillespie WJ, Kreicbergs A. Sensory nerves in the interface membrane of aseptic loose hip prostheses. *J Bone Joint Surg Br*. 1998;80:151-155.

27. Landgraeber S, Toetsch M, Wedemeyer C, Saxler G, Tsokos M, von Knoch F, et al. Over-expression of p53/BAK in aseptic loosening after total hip replacement. *Biomaterials*. 2006;27:3010-3020.

28. Chiba J, Schwendeman LJ, Booth RE, Jr., Crossett LS, Rubash HE. A biochemical, histologic, and immunohistologic analysis of membranes obtained from failed cemented and cementless total knee arthroplasty. *Clin Orthop Relat Res*. 1994;299:114-124.

29. Shanbhag AS, Jacobs JJ, Black J, Galante JO, Glant TT. Human monocyte response to particulate biomaterials generated in vivo and in vitro. *J Orthop Res*. 1995;13:792-801.

30. Woolf CJ, Allchorne A, Safieh-Garabedian B, Poole S. Cytokines, nerve growth factor and inflammatory hyperalgesia: the contribution of tumour necrosis factor alpha. *Br J Pharmacol*. 1997;121:417-424.

31. Maini RN, Breedveld FC, Kalden JR, Smolen JS, Davis D, Macfarlane JD, et al. Therapeutic efficacy of multiple intravenous infusions of anti-tumor necrosis factor alpha monoclonal antibody combined with low-dose weekly methotrexate in rheumatoid arthritis. *Arthritis Rheum*. 1998;41:1552-1563.

32. Kurtz S, Mowat F, Ong K, Chan N, Lau E, Halpern M. Prevalence of primary and revision total hip and knee arthroplasty in the United States from 1990 through 2002. *J Bone Joint Surg Am*. 2005;87:1487-1497.

33. Saleh KJ, Mulhall KJ. Revision total knee arthroplasty: editorial comment. *Clin Orthop Relat Res*. 2006;446:2-3.

34. Bellamy N, Buchanan WW, Goldsmith CH, Campbell J, Stitt LW. Validation study of WOMAC: a health status instrument for measuring clinically important patient relevant outcomes to antirheumatic drug therapy in patients with osteoarthritis of the hip or knee. *J Rheumatol*. 1988;15:1833-1840.

35. Csuka M, McCarty DJ. Simple method for measurement of lower extremity muscle strength. *Am J Med*. 1985;78(1):77-81.

36. Newcomber K, Krug H, Mahowald M. Validity and reliability of the Timed Stands Test for patients with rheumatoid arthritis and other chronic diseases. *J Rheumatol*. 1993;20:21-27.

37. Farrar JT, Young JP, LaMoreaux L, Werth JL, Poole RM. Clinical importance of changes in chronic pain intensity measured on an 11-point numerical pain rating scale. *Pain*. 2001;94:149-158.

38. Dworkin R, Backonja M, Rowbotham MC, Allen RR, Argoff CR, Bennett GJ. Advances in neuropathic pain. *Arch Neurol*. 2003;60:1524-1534.

Botulinum Neurotoxin **25** in the Management of Hyperhidrosis and Other Hypersecretory Disorders

Dee Anna Glaser and Markus Naumann

INTRODUCTION

Botulinum toxins can be used to treat secretory problems such as hyperhidrosis (HH), chromhidrosis, sialorrhea, and Frey syndrome. This chapter focuses on the rationale for and the practical application of using botulinum toxins to treat patients with such problems.

SWEATING

Sweating is a normal physiologic response to increased body temperature and is an important mechanism in releasing heat produced from endogenous as well as exogenous sources. The heat regulatory center is located within the hypothalamus, particularly involving the preoptic and anterior nuclei. Sweating is controlled by the sympathetic nervous system.[1] Nerve fibers exit the preoptic or anterior nuclei and descend ipsilaterally through the spinal cord until they reach the intermediolateral column, where they exit the cord and enter the sympathetic chain. Although the neurotransmitter for the sympathetic nervous system is generally norepinephrine, acetylcholine is the neurotransmitter mainly involved in the sweating response. Other chemical mediators found during sweating, include vasoactive intestinal peptide, atrial natriuretic peptide, galanin, and calcitonin gene peptide.[2]

The eccrine glands, responsible for producing sweat, are distributed around the body, with high concentrations in areas such as the palms, soles, and forehead. They are located at the junction of the dermis and subcutaneous fat, and function is to secrete water while conserving sodium chloride for electrolyte maintenance. Although they continually produce secretions, they are stimulated by heat, exercise, anxiety, and stress.[3,4] Under severe heat stress, up to 10 liters of sweat can be produced in a day; however, the normal rate is 0.5 to 1.0 mL/min. In general, men sweat more than females, although rates vary among individuals.[5]

The apocrine gland opens into the hair follicle and is located mostly in the axillae and perineum. They become functional around puberty and are not important for thermoregulation. The scant viscous secretions are thought to function as chemical attractants or signals, as an odor is produced when the secretions reach the skin surface and interact with bacteria.[1,3,6] The apocrine glands respond to adrenergic stimuli, epinephrine more than norepinephrine.

Hyperhidrosis

HH simply describes excess sweating beyond that necessary for physiologic thermoregulation and homeostasis.[7] Problems can occur

Dr. Glaser reports that she has been a consultant for Allergan and Medicis. Also, she has performed research that has been funded by Allergan and has received unrestricted educational grants from Allergan for research.

within any portion of the system: from the hypothalamus to the sweat gland or duct.[2] The amount of sweat necessary to be considered "excessive" is not well defined and is variable among individuals.

HH may be generalized or focal, bilateral or unilateral, symmetric or asymmetric, or primary or secondary in origin. Generalized HH affects the entire body, whereas focal HH occurs in discrete sections of the body.[8] Generalized HH is usually secondary in nature, and the differential diagnosis is extensive (Table 25-1). Focal or localized HH may result from a secondary process including lesions or tumors of the central or peripheral nervous system.[9] More commonly however, it is idiopathic (primary) focal and is usually referred to simply as HH. It is characterized by excessive sweating of small areas of the skin, usually the axilla, palms, soles, face, or groin (Fig. 25-1). The onset is usually in adolescence to early adulthood but can begin in early childhood, especially the palmar-plantar variants (Table 25-2).[7] The differential diagnosis for excessive sweating is extensive, and an underlying cause must be considered, especially when the HH is generalized, is

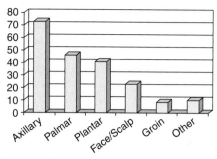

FIGURE 25-1. Sites of hyperhidrosis in patients seeking medical evaluation.

asymmetrically distributed, or has a late onset.[7,10] A detailed history and examination is the first step with careful detail to the review of symptoms. The types or extent of further testing is based on the findings from the history and physical examination.

This chapter focuses on primary focal HH. The prevalence of HH is reported to be 2.8%, although it may be higher. It most commonly presents in the second or third decade of life and a family history has been reported in 30% to 50% of patients.[11] The prevalence is similar for men and women, although interestingly, women are more likely to seek treatment.[12] Patients may sweat on a continuous basis throughout the day, but more commonly, there are episodes of profuse sweating with a sudden onset. Trigger factors include emotional stress, stress at work or the public, higher environmental temperatures, or stimulants such as caffeine and exercise. However, patients also often have episodes without a known trigger factor when they are cool, comfortable, and calm.

TABLE 25-1 Forms of Hyperhidrosis

Generalized	Focal/Localized
Fever	Primary focal hyperhidrosis
Infections	Intrathoracic tumors
Malignancy	Rheumatoid arthritis
Tumors	Spinal cord disease or injury
Thyrotoxicosis	Stroke
Pheochromocytoma	Syringomelia
Diabetes mellitus	Ross syndrome
Diabetes insipidus	Atrioventricular fistula
Hypoglycemia	Gustatory sweating
Hypopituitiarism	Frey syndrome
Endocarditis	Localized unilateral hyperhidrosis*
Gout	Cold-induced hyperhidrosis
Medications	Eccrine nevus
Menopause	Social anxiety disorder
Anxiety	
Drug withdrawal	

*Also referred to as unilateral circumscribed idiopathic hyperhidrosis.

TABLE 25-2 Criteria for Establishing the Diagnosis of Primary Focal Hyperhidrosis[7]

Focal, visible excessive sweating of at least 6 months

No apparent secondary cause

At least two of the following characteristics

    Bilateral and relatively symmetric

    Age of onset younger than 25 years

    Positive family history of primary focal hyperhidrosis

    Cessation of focal sweating during sleep

    Frequency of at least one episode per week

    Impairs daily activities

HH has a negative impact on many aspects of patients' daily living: physically, psychologically, and occupationally.[13-15] The greatest impact of HH is the significant reduction in the quality of life and the alterations it has on daily functioning.[16] Patients report lack of confidence, feeling depressed, refrain from meeting new people, and avoidance of intimate activities. Work limitations are reported because of the sweating, and patients describe having to change clothes during the day.

Measuring Hyperhidrosis

The Minor starch iodine test is a simple way to detect the presence of sweat (Fig. 25-2). The area is dried thoroughly, an iodine solution is

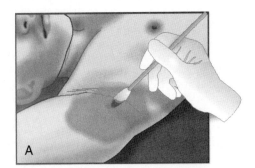

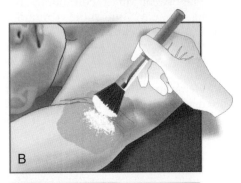

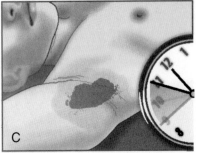

FIGURE 25-2. Starch iodine test is performed to define the area of sweating. **A,** After the area is dried thoroughly, iodine solution is applied to the skin and allowed to dry. **B,** Cornstarch powder is applied to the dried iodine-treated skin. **C,** After several minutes, a purple to black color change occurs in the area of sweating.

painted over the area, and a starch powder such as corn starch is sprinkled on the surface. With the interaction of sweat, a purple to black color develops. Decolorized iodine solutions do not perform the colorimetric change properly and should not be used for this test. The starch iodine test is useful to localize the areas of seat production but is not a quantitative test. For iodine-sensitive patients, alizarin or Ponceau Red dye and starch can be used. The pink powder turns to a bright red color when wet.[17,18] Ninhydrin is another variant, but regardless of which variant is used, they all achieve a colorimetric outline of the sweating area.[19]

Gravimetric testing measures the amount of sweat produced during a given time. It can be performed using a preweighed filter paper that is placed on the affected area (typically for 5 minutes) and then reweighing the paper. Evaporation must be prevented.[20] There is no standard or validated quantity that separates HH from euhidrosis, although it can exceed 30 times that of normal non-hyperhidrotic individuals. Hund suggests a minimum of 100 mg/5 min for men and 50 mg/5 min for women with axillary HH.[5] A study of 60 patients demonstrated that the mean axillary sweat production was 346 mg/5 min for men and 186 mg/5 min for women with HH (healthy control subjects had values of 72 and 46, respectively). Likewise, the mean palmar gravimetric measurement was ~300 mg/5 min.[21]

A third method used to measure disease severity is with questionnaires and quality-of-life scales. Several such tools are available, but two of the more commonly used scales are the Dermatology Life Quality Index (DLQI) and the Hyperhidrosis Disease Severity Scale (HDSS).[22] The HDSS is based on one question that the patient can answer in the office (Table 25-3). The HDSS is a simple tool to use in the clinical setting and is responsive to treatment with a one-point HDSS improvement corresponding with approximately a 50% reduction in sweat. This validated scale can aid in selecting patients appropriate for therapy and for assessing effectiveness of treatment.[23]

Therapy

Many treatments are available for HH, and therapy should be tailored to the needs of the individual based on factors such as age and

TABLE 25-3 Hyperhidrosis Disease Severity Scale[23]

"Which best describes the impact of sweating on your daily activity?"	
1	Never noticeable, never interferes
2	Tolerable, sometimes interferes
3	Barely tolerable, frequently interferes
4	Intolerable, always interferes

health status, location of the disease, occupation, and lifestyle (Table 25-4).

Antiperspirants are used as first-line therapy and function by decreasing sweat secretion through blockage of the distal eccrine ducts. Over-the-counter (OTC) products very rarely control patients with severe disease (HDSS 3 or 4).[12,24-26] Prescription-strength products containing high concentrations of metal salts, most commonly aluminum chloride, are more effective than OTC preparations.[27] Efficacy is still limited, and side effects are frequent with skin irritation, erythema, dryness, and pruritus.

Systemic anticholinergic drugs such as glycopyrrolate, atropine, or oxbutynin provide a generalized acetylcholine blockade.[24,28-30] Adverse effects such as dry eyes, dry mouth, and urinary retention are frequently encountered at the doses required to achieve symptom relief. Additionally, the generalized reduction in sweat production can be dangerous in individuals who engage in exercise, sports, or work in hot environments.

Iontophoresis uses an electric current and tap water. The mechanism of action is unknown but may change the ability of the pores to secrete sweat, or via ions that enter the ducts and physically block the release of sweat. It is most suited for treatment of the hands and feet. Anticholinergic agents can also be added to the tap water.[31] Side effects are relatively minimal but the therapy is relatively time consuming, limiting its use for many patients.[32]

Local surgical excision and liposuction or curettage techniques can be used to remove eccrine units.[33] The outcome is technique dependant and is limited to the axilla. Endoscopic thoracic sympathectomy (ETS) offers long-term improvement but is not universally accepted. The sympathetic chain is interrupted at the T2, T3, and sometimes the T4 ganglion.[34,35] Success rates for palmar disease approximate 95% but is less for axillary HH. Surgical and anesthetic-related adverse events are relatively rare, but the major issue with ETS surgery for HH is the potential for patients to develop compensatory sweating.[36] The incidence varies, but approximately 60% to 70% of patients seem to develop it, with its occurrence and severity being unpredictable.[34,37,38]

Botulinum Toxin Therapy

Because sweating is mediated by acetylcholine, the use of botulinum toxin (BoNT) to treat focal HH is a logical choice. The chemodenervation is localized, reversible, and yet long-lasting. Botulinum toxin type A (BoNT/A) has been most extensively studied and used clinically to treat HH, but botulinum toxin type B (BoNT/B) has also been reported to work.

The basic principle for using botulinum toxins to treat excessive sweating is to treat any underlying etiology as already discussed. Then the area of sweating should be identified using a colorimetric test such as the Minor's Starch Iodine test (see Fig. 25-2). Because the sweat glands are typically located at the junction of the dermis and subcutaneous fat, BoNT is usually placed as a deep intradermal injection. It is important to avoid injecting deeper structures such as muscle to prevent unwanted affects on the underlying muscles and for optimal BoNT interaction at the neuron-eccrine interface. Injections are generally placed 1 to 2 cm apart to allow for diffusion to the entire area. Although this basic technique is used to treat all areas of the body, the more commonly treated sites are covered in more detail. Owing to the differences using the different BoNT/A products, brand names will be listed when necessary.

TABLE 25-4 Therapies Most Commonly Used for Hyperhidrosis

Antiperspirants, over the counter
Antiperspirants, prescription strength
Iontophoresis
Oral medications
Botulinum toxin
Local excision of eccrine glands
Liposuction and/or curettage
Endoscopic transthoracic sympathectomy

Axillary Hyperhidrosis

No areas has been as extensively studied as the axilla,[13,20,39-41] with numerous studies showing the benefit of BoNT/A, including large multi-center randomized, placebo-controlled trials in Europe and the United States. Naumann et al reported on 320 patients with axillary HH who received 50 U of BoNT/A (Botox, Allergan, Inc, Irvine, CA) per axilla or placebo.[42] At 4 weeks, 94% of the BoNT/A group had responded compared with 36% of the placebo group as measured by ≥50% reduction of sweat production from baseline. By 16 weeks, the response rates were 82% and 21%, respectively. Also, repeated injections with BoNT/A over 16 months continued to produce similar results.[39] The mean duration between BoNT/A treatments was approximately 7 months, and patient satisfaction was high. Similar results were published in a large phase III double-blind trial in North America.[43] Subjects with axillary HH were randomized to receive placebo, or 50 U or 75 U of BoNT/A (Botox) into each axilla. The HDSS was the primary efficacy in this study, with gravimetric measurements being secondary. Successful response was seen in 75% of patients in both treatment groups compared with 25% in the placebo group (defined as ≥2 point reduction in HDSS), whereas 80% to 85% of the treated subjects had more than 75% reduction in sweat production. No significant differences were noted between the two doses of BoNT/A and the durability of therapy was ~7 months for both. A 3-year open-label extension study revealed continued effectiveness and with similar duration of results.[44] Specifically, the researchers were able to show a significant sustained improvement in the quality of life of subjects. The DLQI revealed significant improvement in overall quality of life and occupation and work-specific improvements were noted as well.

The efficacy of Dysport (Ipsen, Milford, MA) has been shown in several studies. A multicenter trial of 145 subjects was performed with 200 U BoNT/A in one axilla, whereas the contralateral axilla was injected with placebo.[20] After 2 weeks, the placebo-treated axilla was injected with 100 U BoNT/A. Axillary sweating decreased by 2 weeks in both treatment sides, and results were maintained for 6 months. There were no significant differences gravimetrically between the two doses used. Therapy was well tolerated, and 98% of subjects said they would recommend the therapy to others.

Although studies have consistently shown that 50 U BoNT/A per axilla provides safe and durable results (averaging ~7 months), there is some debate regarding whether higher doses of BoNT/A can provide prolonged efficacy.[45,46] One small open-label study of 200 U BoNT/A per axilla in 47 patients found prolonged results (over 19 months) in half of the patients, although the methodology was very different from other studies; starch iodine and telephone calls were used to assess patients.[45] Likewise, 250 U of BoNT/A (Dysport)[40] in each axilla resulted in prolonged benefit in a small study of 12 patients. Half remained symptom free for 12 months, and 25% of the subjects were symptom free for 9 months.[40] At present, the standard dose in the United States, and that listed in the package insert for Botox, is 50 U per axilla. This achieves excellent results, high patient satisfaction, and helps to keep costs down. There is no such dosing consensus on other brands of BoNT/A products.

To optimize treatment, the area of axillary involvement should be identified (as previously reviewed) so that the BoNT/A can be concentrated into the affected area. The key to performing a high-quality starch iodine test is to thoroughly dry the region before beginning the test. The axilla does not need to be shaved before performing a starch iodine test or to injecting BoNT/A. BoNT/A is injected into the deep dermis at the dermal subcutaneous level and placed 1.5 to 2 cm apart (Fig. 25-3). Because the axillary skin is thin, a wheal may be seen with each injection. An average of 10 to 15 injections per axilla are required, but the number will depend on the size of the hyperhidrodic area.[47] In the event that a starch iodine test cannot be performed before the injection or is equivocal, the physician should treat the hair-bearing areas as described earlier. Should symptoms fail to be alleviated within 2 weeks, the patient can return to the office and a starch iodine test performed to identify any "active" eccrine glands. The skin should be injected with 3 to 5 U BoNT/A for each 1-cm surface area identified.

Pain is minimal, and the procedure is well tolerated. Although the package insert describes the use of unpreserved saline to reconstitute BoNT/A, many physicians have found that the use of preserved saline reduces pain without altering efficacy.[48,49] The use of 2% lidocaine to reconstitute BoNT/A has been reported in one small study to be less painful than the use of unpreserved saline when injecting axillary HH and with equal efficacy.[50] Side effects

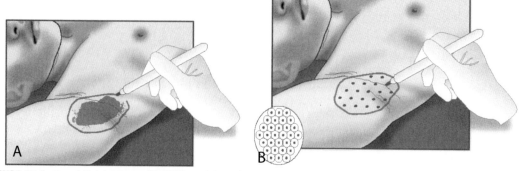

FIGURE 25-3. A and **B,** Injections of BoNT/A are injected approximately every 1.5 to 2 cm. The location of injections is best identified by the starch iodine test.

noted in studies include pain, hematoma, bruising, headache, muscle soreness, increased facial sweating, perceived compensatory sweating, and axillary pruritus.

Treatment intervals are mandated by the longevity of an individual's treatment response but will average every 6 to 7 months. Some clinicians have advocated that patients use a topical therapy twice a week when the sweating starts to return to try and extend the time interval between injections and help to keep costs to a minimum.[51]

Palmar Hyperhidrosis

BoNT injections are useful in the treatment of palmar HH. No large-scale studies have been published, but multiple small studies have demonstrated the ability of BoNT to establish clinical improvement in patients' symptoms.[21,52,53] Several challenges exist when treating hands such as choosing optimal doses, control of pain during injection, and side effects, which include muscle weakness.[54-58]

The optimum dose of BoNT/A to control palmar HH is unknown and the issue is complicated by large variations in hand size. Published data report doses as low as 50 U per hand and as high as 200 U Botox per hand.[59,60] Doses of Dysport have ranged from 120 U per hand to 500 U per hand.[19,52,61] Some authors have suggested using a defined dose per injection, with Swartling's group using 0.8 U/cm², and Naumann's group using 2 U Botox injected every 1.5 cm on the palm but three injections per fingertip and two injections into each of the middle and proximal phalanx, using 1 to 2 U per injection.[59,62] The Canadian advisory committee recommends 1.5 to 2 u/cm² with a mean dose of 100 U Botox per palm.[25] It is unclear whether or not

larger doses add to the duration of symptom relief or increase the risk of developing muscle weakness. When Wollina used 200 U per hand in 10 patients, his relapse time varied from 3 to 22 months.[60] Saadia studied 24 patients: 11 received 50 U Botox per hand and 13 received 100 U per hand. There was higher patient satisfaction reported in the high-dose group, but no difference in terms of duration, (measured as a percentage of the palm area sweating) for the two doses. There were more patients with hand and finger weakness in the high-dose treatment group.[59] Until larger studies are available to address this issue, 75-100 U BoNT/A (Botox) per hand is a good starting point with adjustments being made as needed based on the size of the hand and past responses.[26]

Another challenge with palmar BoNT therapy is an apparent shorter duration of response when compared with axillary injections.[54] Responses range from 3 to 12 months.[63] Aghaei found that anhidrosis lasted up to 5 months for his patients treated with 500 U Dysport per hand, although he observed hypohidrosis lasting an average of 10 months.[61] The reason for this shorter duration is unknown but may be[63] related to a smaller diffusion radius in the thicker palm skin and compartmentalized areas of the phalanges, a higher number of cholinergic nerve endings, or a differential recovery rate of the nerves in the hands compared with the axilla. Backflow of the BoNT solution upon injection can be an issue with palmar injections, and perhaps this plays a role as well.[64]

Injection of the hand can be painful owing to the density of nerve receptors and the large numbers of injections that are required. Pain during injection of the palm has been rated an average 68.1 ± 31.8 compared with

TABLE 25-5 Anesthesia Techniques Used for Palmar Injections

Topical anesthesia
Nerve blocks
Cryoanalgesia
   Dichlorotetrafluoroethane
   Liquid nitrogen spray
   Ice cubes, ice pack, or ice bath
   Cold packs
   Machine-assisted cold air
Vibration
Intravenous regional anesthesia (Bier block)
General anesthesia or sedation anesthesia

29.9 ± 24.5 for axillary treatment (using a visual analogue scale [VAS] of 1–100).[14] Several methods of pain control have been tried (Table 25-5), although a rare patient will not require anesthesia. Topical lidocaine agents and cold packs tend not to provide adequate pain control. More intensive cold exposure can be helpful: the use of dichlorotetrafluoroethane or liquid nitrogen, submersion of the hand in an ice bath, direct application of an ice cube or ice pack.[65,66] Machines that emit chilled air or use a chilled tip can be beneficial but are more expensive. The use of a dermojet to inject BoNT/A was found to be less painful than standard needle injections, but was much less effective in controlling the sweating and thus not recommended as a useful tool to treat the palms.[67] Benohanian has described the use of a pressure unit to inject lidocaine into the palms and soles without the use of needles, before injecting BoNT/A.[68]

Nerve blocks are effective and can be performed in the office.[62] The palm is innervated by three nerves, median, ulnar and radial nerves. All can be anesthetized at the level of the wrist using 1% or 2% lidocaine (Fig. 25-4). Risks of a nerve block include infiltration of the nerve with subsequent nerve injury, and vascular puncture. In addition, temporary hand weakness after the nerve blocks may limit the patients' activities and ability to have both hands treated at one session.

Intravenous regional anesthesia (IVRA), also known as a Bier's block is effective.[69,70] An anesthetic such as prilocaine is injected intravenously following the application of a tourniquet cuff on the forearm. Exsanguination of the extremity is performed, and an electronic double cuff is applied. Complete anesthesia is obtained in 20 minutes using 40 to 60 mL of 0.5% prilocaine. The total tourniquet time for IVRA ranges from 50 to 80 minutes and is well tolerated. Owing to the risk of toxic cardiovascular and central nervous system reactions, blood pressure and electrocardiograms are monitored during the IVRA and for about 30 minutes after the procedure.

Vibratory anesthesia is gaining popularity.[71] The theory is that the nervous system is unable to perceive fully two different types of sensory

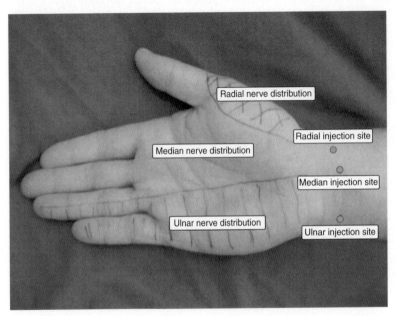

FIGURE 25-4. The palm is innervated by the ulnar, median, and radial nerves.

inputs simultaneously. A hand-held vibrator is applied to the volar and dorsal surface of the hand near the site of BoNT/A injection. This requires an assistant, and there is some movement of the patient's hand, which can make injections challenging. The use of one vibrator to the volar aspect does not diminish pain as much as the use of two vibrators (personal experience). Neither technique results in a pain-free injection, but rather a diminishment of perceived pain. A study by Sherer found that pain threshold is significantly higher during vibration compare with pre- or postvibration, and that vibration applied distal to the site of pain provided better analgesia than vibration applied proximal to the site of pain.[53] The author most commonly combines ice and vibration at this time for palmar injections. An ice cube or ice pack is applied firmly to the planned injection site for 7 to 10 seconds. The vibrator is firmly applied immediately adjacent to the injection site simultaneous to the injection (no more than 2 to 3 seconds). This technique does require an assistant and coordinated timing to optimize pain control.

Bruising is common with palm injections but is temporary. Weakness of the hand or fingers is possible but is usually minor and of limited duration. The incidence varies in published series but ranges from 0 to 77%.[21,52,54,55,59,72] The most commonly affected area of weakness is the thenar eminence and can be measured in the thumb-index finger pinch, whereas gross strength or grip strength of the hand is not usually affected.[56,59] Rarely, patients report numbness, tingling, or decreased dexterity. Injections of BoNT/A should be made in the dermal layer, especially over the thenar eminence to limit the chance that the drug will come in contact with the muscle layer. Subepidermal injections may increase the incidence of hematoma.[55] There is one report of atrophy of the intrinsic musculature of the hands with debilitating weakness associated with BoNT/A injections for palmar HH, after five treatment sessions using 500 U Dysport per palmar basin every 9 months.[73] Patients should be adequately counseled on the risks of weakness, which is usually mild and transient.

In an attempt to prevent muscle weakness, Zaiac advocates the use of the ADG needle, a device designed for the injection of collagen.[74] He found the average depth of the eccrine glands in 10 consecutive palmar biopsies to be 2.6 mm. By adjusting the needle to a

length of 2.6 mm and using a total of 60 to 70 U BoNT/A per palm, he had no weakness in a series of 10 patients. Likewise, Almeida uses an adapter to shorten her 7-mm 30-gauge needle to measure 2.5 to 3.0 mm for palmar injections.[58,75]

Plantar Hyperhidrosis

Very little has been published on BoNT therapy for plantar HH. Like the palms, there is no consensus on the optimal dose, the duration is variable, and the injections are painful. Naumann and colleagues[76] used 42 and 48 U of Botox to treat two soles by injecting 3 U BoNT/A (0.15 mL) into each 2- × 2-cm squares. Blaheta's group used 100 U Botox per sole (100 U/5 mL saline) in a study of eight patients with severe plantar HH.[77] Campanati and associates[78] studied 10 patients with plantar HH using 100 U Botox per foot. All patients had an improvement in symptoms and a "significant decrease of Minor's test" for 12 weeks without significant side effects.

A starch iodine test will delineate the hyperhidrotic area, which can extend up the sides and onto the dorsum of the foot. BoNT/A should be evenly distributed every 1 to 2 cm using a small-gauge needle and injecting into the deep dermis. Injections of the plantar surface can be technically more challenging owing to the thickness of the stratum corneum in some areas, especially if the region is calloused. The physician has to adjust for the variation in depth to accurately place BoNT/A into the appropriate cutaneous level.

The need for pain control has to be addressed as with palmar injections. IVRA can provide sufficient anesthesia for the sole and has been reported to be effective when administering BoNT/A. In a small series of eight patients, IVRA was found to be more effective than nerve blocks in reducing the pain of BoNT/A injections.[77] However, nerve blocks can also be used and are generally performed at the level of the ankle. The tibial and sural nerves need to be blocked, and if the dorsum of the foot must be injected, the superficial peroneal nerve can be anesthetized.[75]

Vadoud-Seyedi[79] reported on using the Dermojet to inject BoNT/A for plantar HH. Ten patients were treated with 50 U Botox/5 mL saline per foot. Fifteen to twenty points were injected per foot, and no analgesia was used. The injections were tolerated well by all patients, although one developed a localized hematoma. The duration of benefit lasted 3 to 6 months; however, 20% of patients reported that the treatment had no effect on their condition.

Bruising and pain with injection are the most common side effects. In the published literature, one patient reported weakness of plantar flexor muscles in both feet following BoNT/A injection, with resolution in 10 days.[80]

Facial Hyperhidrosis

Primary facial HH has several patterns, but most commonly involve the forehead and perhaps the the scalp. Patients with craniofacial HH may present with involvement of the forehead, scalp perimeter, entire scalp, cheeks, nose, upper lip, chin, or a combination of these areas. Gustatory sweating is a relatively common complication after surgery or injury in the region of the parotid gland and is discussed later in the chapter. All forms of facial HH can respond to BoNT/A, with gustatory sweating responding for very long periods of time.

There is a paucity of literature published on craniofacial HH. Kinkelin's group[81] injected a mean of 86 U Botox (3 U BoNT/A per injection site) over the forehead at equidistant locations (1–1.5 cm) in 10 men with frontal HH. The injections were kept 1 cm superior to the eyebrow to help prevent drooping of the eyelid; the injections were intracutaneous. Five of ten patients had partial disability in frowning of the forehead, but the problem was limited to a maximum of 8 weeks. No ptosis was noted, and satisfaction was good or excellent in 90% of the subjects. The benefits were maintained for 5 months in 90% of patients. Similarly, Tan and Solish[14] report that symptoms return on average 4 1/2 months after treatment of the forehead.

Böger treated 12 men suffering from bilateral craniofacial HH with Dysport 0.1 ng per injection.[82] Half of the forehead was treated using a total of 2.5 to 4 ng injected equidistantly, with a total of 25 to 40 injections given. Decreased sweating was seen within 1 to 7 days after injection and lasted a minimum of 3 months, but one patient experienced anhidrosis for 27 months. Side effects were limited to temporary weakness of the frontalis muscle (100%) and brow asymmetry that lasted 1 to 12 months in 17% of subjects.

It is the observation of the author that patients typically present with forehead sweating that may be combined with scalp sweating in a diffuse pattern or in an ophiasis pattern. BoNT/A injections are performed with 2 to 3 U every 1 to 2 cm, avoiding the inferior 2 cm of the forehead to reduce the risk of brow ptosis (Fig. 25-5).[83] Doses range from 50 U (forehead) to 250 to 300 U for the forehead and entire scalp.[83]

Other Sweating Disorders

Inguinal HH affects 2% to 10% of individuals with primary HH.[12] It usually develops in adolescence and can be associated with excessive sweating at other body sites. Intradermal injections of BoNT/A can control symptoms for 6 months or more. Identifying the surface area that needs injection can be

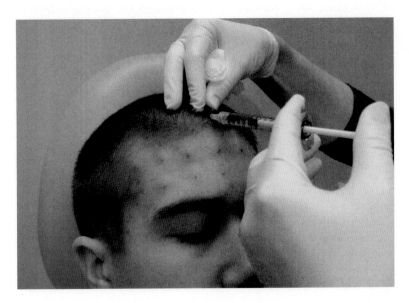

FIGURE 25-5. Injection pattern for craniofacial hyperhidrosis.

technically challenging due to the body location but is valuable. Two to three units BoNT/A are injected every 1 to 2 cm within the affected area; typical doses range from 60 to 100 U per side.[84]

Compensatory sweating is the most common complication of ETS, ranging from 44% to 91%. Treatment has been particularly difficult, but a couple of reports noted success using BoNT/A. Huh and coworkers[85] used 300 U Dysport to treat the chest and abdomen after identifying the area with a starch iodine test. They diluted each 100 U 10 ml^3 saline and injected 0.1 mL into each square centimeter. The effects gradually reduced but were reported to remain for 8 months. Belin and Polo[36] reported good results treating the upper abdomen with BoNT/A, but unfortunately, their patient's compensatory sweating was from the nipple line down to his knees and the entire area was not treated.

Chromhidrosis is a rare disorder characterized by the excretion of colored or pigmented sweat. It is most commonly confined to the face or axilla but has been noted elsewhere on the body. Matarasso[86] used 15 U Botox in the affected area of each cheek, which measured 3 cm in diameter. Within 48 hours, the patient had a marked reduction in the amount of discharged black sweat.

Use of Botulinum Toxin Type B for Hyperhidrosis

Botulinum toxin type B (BoNT/B) use has been primarily limited to treatment of cervical dystonia, but there are a few reports of its use for treating HH. Injection of BoNT/B can induce focal anhidrosis in a dose-dependent fashion. Birklein and colleagues[87] found that a threshold dose of 8 U leads to anhidrotic skin areas greater than 4 cm after 3 weeks. The duration was prolonged for 3 months when 15 U of BoNT/B were injected, and for 6 months when 125 U were injected.

Despite its ability to induce anhidrosis, the use of BoNT/B is limited by the occurrence of systemic adverse events.[88] Dressler and coworkers[89] reported that 100 U Botox, 2000 U Neurobloc, and 4000 U Neurobloc were equally effective in blocking axillary HH when studying 19 patients. The extent of improvement was similar (16 weeks) in all groups, but the onset of action was earlier with the BoNT/B and there was greater discomfort with the BoNT/B compared with BoNT/A. One patient developed severe dryness of the mouth starting 1 week after injection and

lasting 5 weeks; as well as accommodation difficulties and conjunctival irritation that lasted 3 weeks. Likewise, patients treated with 5000 U BoNT/B in each axilla achieved excellent reduction in sweating, but the incidence of side effects was high and included dry mouth, headache, and sensory motor symptoms of the hand.[90]

A patient treated with 2500 U BoNT/B in each palm for HH developed bilateral blurred vision, indigestion, dry sore throat, and dysphagia.[91] The largest published study to date on treating palmar HH with BoNT/B used 5000 U per palm in 20 subjects.[92] Adverse events were common and included dry mouth or throat (90%), indigestion (60%), excessively dry hands (60%), muscle weakness (60%), and decreased grip strength (50%).

Lower dosing may be the key to reducing the high incidence of side effects.[93] However, because of the incidence of systemic side effects when using BoNT/B and the high safety profile in using BoNT/A to treat focal HH, to date, BoNT/A is the neurotoxin of choice.

Gustatory Sweating (Frey Syndrome)

Gustatory sweating occurs on the cheek in response to salivation or anticipation of food (Fig. 25-6). It may result from misdirection of autonomic nerve fibers after surgery and is frequently observed in diseases of the parotid gland and in diabetes.

BoNT is a highly effective treatment option for gustatory sweating, as shown by several uncontrolled studies (Table 25-6).[94-98] In a large open-label study of 45 patients, there was a significant reduction of local facial sweating after injection of BoNT/A (Botox; mean dose 21 MU, range 5–72 MU) and no recurrence of sweating was observed during the follow-up period of 6 months. A marked long-lasting benefit of 11 to 36 months has also been observed by many other physicians.[96-98] Thus, BoNT appears to have a particularly long-lasting effect on gustatory sweating. The reason for this is unclear.

In clinical practice, the Minor iodine test should be performed before injection to visualize the affected area that has to be injected. After that, 2 to 3 MU Botox or 8 MU Dysport are injected intradermally at sites 2.0 to 2.5 cm apart and evenly distributed over the affected area. Specific side effects of the injection of BoNT include pain on injection, local hematomas, and local muscle weakness due to diffusion of the toxin to adjacent muscles (particularly, the zygomatic muscle).

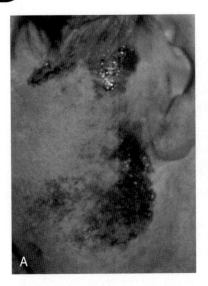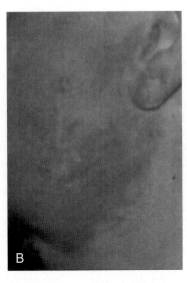

FIGURE 25-6. Gustatory sweating before (**A**) and after (**B**) focal intradermal application of BoNT. The Minor iodine starch test indicates areas of sweating (*dark*).

SIALORRHEA

Sialorrhea is a common and socially disabling symptom in spasticity, cerebral palsy, and degenerative diseases such as motor neuron diseases (e.g., bulbar amyotrophic lateral sclerosis [ALS]) and Parkinson disease. About 70% of patients with Parkinson disease and up to 20% of ALS patients suffer from excessive drooling. It is usually caused by swallowing dysfunction and can lead to choking, aspiration, and chest infections. Drooling can be evaluated subjectively or quantitatively. Conventional treatment options include anticholinergic drugs, surgical treatment, or salivary gland radiation.

Four randomized, double blind, placebo controlled studies evaluated the treatment effect of BoNT on sialorrhea in Parkinson disease. In one study on 20 patients, BoNT/A (450 MU Dysport) or placebo were injected into the parotid and submandibular glands with a follow-up of 3 months. Drooling significantly decreased by 4 points on a drooling score.[99] In another study, 32 patients received BoNT/A (50 MU Botox) or placebo injected into the parotid glands. The treatment effect was measured by the UPDRS-ADL and a VAS on drooling frequency. There was a significant improvement in all measures and no side effects were observed.[100] Another small study evaluated the effect of BoNT/B (Myobloc) or placebo in 16 patients with drooling. BoNT/B was injected into the parotid glands (1000 MU on each side) and into the submandibular glands (250 MU on each side). There was a significant improvement in all measures such as drooling rating scale, drooling severity and frequency scale and VAS. Side effects included dry mouth, among others.[101] Another study evaluated the effect of three different doses of BoNT/A (18.75, 37.5, and 75 MU Dysport) or placebo in 32 patients with Parkinson disease, ALS, MSA, and CBD. There was an improvement of sialorrhea as measured by dental roles and drooling frequency. The study is, however, limited by the small cohort and the high drop out rate of 14 patients.[102]

In clinical practice, both the parotid and submandibular glands are usually injected.

TABLE 25-6 Selected Studies on BoNT/A Treatment of Gustatory Sweating

Author	Year	Design	n	Dose (mean)	Duration (mo)
Naumann et al[95]	1997	Open	45	21 MU Botox	6
Bjerkhoel and Trobbe[96]	1997	Open	15	37 MU Botox	13
Laskawi et al[97]	1998	Open	19	31 MU Botox	11–27
Laccourreye et al[98]	1999	Open	33	86 MU Dysport	12–36

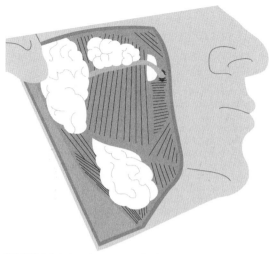

FIGURE 25-7. Local anatomy of salivary glands. (From A. de Almeida and D. Hexsel, 2003)

The parotid gland lies between the mastoid process and the ramus of the mandible (Fig. 25-7). Cranially, it reaches the zygomatic arch; caudally, it ends at the level of body of the mandible, partly covering the dorsal part of the masseter muscle. There is still limited experience with BoNT injections into the salivary glands, and the best dose and way to inject has never been formally evaluated. One way to treat is to inject BoNT at two to three different sites on each parotid gland and at one site of each submandibular gland. Preferably the injection is guided by ultrasound. A retrograde transductal approach is not recommended. As an initial dose not more than 10 to 20 MU Botox or 40 to 60 MU Dysport are injected per parotid gland, at a dilution of 100 MU Botox or 500 MU Dysport/2 mL of sterile 0.9% saline. Depending on the response, the total dose can be slowly increased by injecting the same or a lower amount of BoNT after 8 to 10 weeks (risk of antibody formation if reinjections are given earlier). In the palliative treatment of sialorrhea in ALS, reinjections may be given after a shorter period of time. The submandibular glands can be injected with 5 to 10 MU Botox or 20 to 30 MU Dysport per gland. The highest safe individual dose is not known and may be very low in some patients, particularly in patients suffering from a motor neuron disorder, who may be unusually sensitive to BoNT. We do not know the effect of repeated injections of BoNT over time or the risk of developing antibodies.

Side effects of BoNT injections into the salivary glands include local injection pain, local infection of the salivary gland, dry mouth, deterioration of dysphagia due to diffusion of the toxin into the pharyngeal muscles, and weakness of mouth closing and opening. Other potential adverse effects may include hematomas and salivary duct calculi. The risk for all side effects can be minimized by cautiously increasing the dose and number of treated glands in successive treatment cycles.

Pathologic Tearing (Crocodile Tear Syndrome) and Rhinorrhea

Pathologic tearing (crocodile tears syndrome) is a relatively rare syndrome that is characterized by inappropriate and sometimes excessive lacrimation provoked by eating. It should be distinguished from other local eye disorders associated with increased tearing. The Schirmer test can measure increased tearing. There is no effective conventional treatment of hyperlacrimation. Because the lacrimal glands are innervated by cholinergic fibers, hyperlacrimation in crocodile tears syndrome may be effectively treated by intraglandular injections of BoNT. So far, there are only a few reports on BoNT use.[103-106] In one open-label study,[104] injection of 20 MU Dysport® into the lacrimal gland or subcutaneous injection of a total of 75 MU Dysport® into the orbital part of the orbicularis oculi muscle for treatment of synkinesis produced a marked to moderate improvement of hyperlacrimation. In other reports,[103,106] intraglandular injection of 2.5 or 5 MU Botox® normalized hyperlacrimation for more than 6 months.

In clinical practice, the conjunctival mucosa is anesthetized using eye drops before injecting the lacrimal gland. After ectropionization of the upper lid, 2.5 to 5.0 MU Botox or 10 MU Dysport are injected into the palpebral part of the lacrimal gland. Injections of BoNT into the lacrimal gland may cause dry eye symptoms, local infection, ptosis, or diplopia due to a diffusion of the toxin to the lateral rectus muscle. Based on the few reports published, BoNT injections into the lacrimal gland for hyperlacrimation may be an elegant method to treat this sometimes disabling condition. However, we need larger studies to evaluate the risks and long-term benefits of this treatment.

A single double-blind placebo-controlled study evaluated the effect of BoNT on rhinorrhea in 60 patients with intrinsic rhinitis.[107] The dose of 4 MU Botox given in each nasal cavity significantly improved rhinorrhea as judged subjectively and reduced the number of paper tissues needed per day. No side effects occurred. The benefits lasted 4 weeks.

FUTURE DIRECTIONS

The use of botulinum toxins has revolutionized the treatment of HH and other secretory disorders. Compared with other treatments, it is unmatched in its efficacy, ease of administration, and patient satisfaction. Development of quick, safe, and effective pain control is needed for the treatment of more tender areas such as the palms and soles. New delivery devices are already being researched to help provide the most comfortable and efficient therapy. Kavanagh and colleagues[108] have successfully used a small iontophoresis machine to deliver BoNT/A to two patients with severe palmar HH, sparing them the injections. Glogau[109] demonstrated that Botox can be successfully delivered in the axillary skin when combined with a proprietary transport peptide molecule. Research is ongoing, looking at the clinical applications of different botulinum serotypes. Another area of potential research is with combination therapy. For the present, botulinum toxin therapy is a valuable, well-tolerated therapy and can provide meaningful improvement in the quality of life of patients with HH and other secretory disorders.

References

1. Goldsmith L. Biology of eccrine and apocrine sweat glands. In: Freedberg I, Eisen A, Wolff K, Goldsmith L, Katz S, Fitzpatrick T, eds. *Fitzpatrick's Dermatology in General Medicine.* New York: McGraw-Hill; 1999:157-164.
2. Goldsmith L. Goldsmith disorders of the eccrine sweat gland. In Freedberg I, Eisen A, Wolff K, Goldsmith L, Katz SI, Fitzpatrick T, eds. *Fitzpatrick's Dermatology in General Medicine.* New York: McGraw-Hill; 1999:800-809.
3. Stenn K, Bhawan J. The normal histology of the skin. In Farmer E, Hood A, eds. *Pathology of the Skin.* New York: McGraw-Hill; 2000.
4. Glogau R. Botulinum A neurotoxin for axillary hyperhidrosis: no sweat botox. *Dermatol Surg.* 1998;24:817-819.
5. Hund M, Kinkelin I, Naumann M, Hamm H. Definition of axillary hyperhidrosis by gravimetric assessment. *Arch Dermatol.* 2002;138:539-541.
6. Garcia A, Fulton J. Cosmetic denervation of the muscles of facial expression with botulinum toxin: a dose-response study. *Dermatol Surg.* 1996;22:39-43.
7. Hornberger J, Grimes K, Naumann M, Glaser D, Lowe NJ, Naver H, et al. Recognition, diagnosis, and treatment of primary focal hyperhidrosis. *J Am Acad Dermatol.* 2004;51:274-286.
8. Kreyden O, Scheidegger E. Anatomy of the sweat glands, pharmacology of botulinum toxin, and distinctive syndromes associated with hyperhidrosis. *Clin Dermatol.* 2004;22:40-44.
9. Cheshire W, Freeman R. Disorders of sweating. *Semin Neurol.* 2003;23:399-406.
10. Seline P, Jaskierny D. Cutaneous metastases from a chondroblastoma initially presenting as unilateral palmar hyperhidrosis. *J Am Acad Dermatol.* 1999;40:325-327.
11. Strutton D, Kowalski J, Glaser D, Stang P. US prevalence of hyperhidrosis and impact on individuals with axillary hyperhidrosis: results from a national survey. *J Am Acad Dermatol.* 2004;51:241-248.
12. Lear W, Kessler E, Solish N, Glaser D. An epidemiological study of hyperhidrosis. *Dermatol Surg.* 2007;33:S69-S75.
13. Naumann M, Hamm H, Lowe NJ. Effect of botulinum toxin type A on quality of life measures in patients with excessive axillary sweating: a randomized controlled trial. *Br J Dermatol.* 2002;147:1218-1226.
14. Tan S, Solish N. Long-term efficacy and quality of life in the treatment of focal hyperhidrosis with botulinum toxin A. *Dermatol Surg.* 2002;28:495-499.
15. Kowalski J, Ravelo A, Glaser D, Lowe NJ. Quality-of-Life Effect of Botulinum Toxin Type A on Patients with Primary Axillary Hyperhidrosis: Results from a North American Clinical Study Population. P196. 2-7-2003. American Academy of Dermatology Annual Meeting.
16. Hamm H, Naumann M, Kowalski J, Kutt S, Kozma C, Teale C. Primary focal hyperhidrosis: disease characteristics and functional impairment. *Dermatology.* 2006;212:343-353.
17. Bushara K, Park D. Botulinum toxin and sweating. *J Neurol Neurosurg Psychiatry.* 1994;57:1437-1438.
18. Tugnoli A, Ragona R, Eleopra R, De Grandis D, Montecucco C. Treatment of Frey syndrome with botulinum toxin type F. *Arch Otolaryngol Head Neck Surg.* 2001;127:339-340.
19. Schnider P, Binder M, Auff E, Kittler H, Berger T, Wolff K. Double-blind trial of botulinum A toxin for the treatment of focal hyperhidrosis of the palms. *B J Dermatol.* 1998;138:553-554.
20. Heckmann M, Ceballos-Baumann A, Plewig G. Botulinum toxin A for axillary hyperhidrosis (excessive sweating). *N Engl J Med.* 2002;347:620-621.
21. Lowe N, Yamauchi P, Lask G, Patnaik R, Iyer S. Efficacy and safety of botulinum toxin type A in the treatment of palmar hyperhidrosis: a double-blind, randomized, placebo-controlled study. *Dermatol Surg.* 2002;28:822-827.
22. Swartling C, Naver H, Lindberg M. Botulinum A toxin improves life quality in severe primary focal hyperhidrosis. *Eur J Neurol.* 2001;8:247-252.
23. Glaser D, Kowalski J, Eadie N, Solish N, Ravelo A, Weng Y, et al. Validity and reliability of the hyperhidrosis disease severity scale (HDSS) [poster 198]. American Academy of Dermatology Annual Meeting. Washington DC, February 2004.
24. Stolman L. Treatment of hyperhidrosis. *Dermatol Clin.* 1998;16:863-869.
25. Solish N, Bertucci V, Dansereau A, Hong H, Lynde C, Lupin M, et al. A Comprehensive approach to the recognition, diagnosis, and severity-based treatment of focal hyperhidrosis: recommendations of the Canadian Hyperhidrosis Advisory Committee. *Dermatol Surg.* 2007;33:908-923.
26. Glaser D, Hebert A, Parlser D, Solish N. Palmar and plantar hyperhidrosis: best practice

recommendations and special considerations. *Cutis.* 2007;79(suppl 5):18-28.

27. Benohanian A, Dansereau A, Bolduc C, Bloom E. Localized hyperhidrosis treated with aluminum chloride in a salicylic acid gel base. *Int J Dermatol.* 1998;37:701-703.

28. Praharaj SK, Arora M. Paroxetine useful for palmarplantar hyperhidrosis. *Ann Pharmacother.* 2006;40:1884-1886.

29. Bajaj V, Langtry JAA. Use of oral glycopyrronium bromide in hyperhidrosis. *Br J Dermatol.* 2007;157:118-121.

30. Klaber M, Catterall M. Treating hyperhidrosis: anticholinergic drugs were not mentioned. *Br J Dermatol.* 2000;321:703.

31. Naumann M, Davidson J, Glaser D. Hyperhidrosis: current understanding, current therapy. *www.Medscape.com.* February 28, 2002.

32. Stolman L. Treatment of excess sweating of the palms by iontophoresis. *Arch Dermatol.* 1987;123:893-896.

33. Swinehart J. Treatment of axillary hyperhidrosis: combination of the starch-iodine test with the tumescent liposuction technique. *Dermatol Surg.* 2000;26:392-396.

34. Gossot D, Galetta D, Pascal A, Debrosse D. Long-term results of endoscopic thoracic sympathectomy for upper limb hyperhidrosis. *Ann Thorac Surg.* 2003;75:1075-1079.

35. Kim B, Oh B, Park Y. Microinvasive video-assisted thoracoscopic sympathicotomy for primary palmar hyperhidrosis. *Am J Surg.* 2001;181:540-542.

36. Belin E, Polo J. Treatment of compensatory hyperhidrosis with botulinum toxin type A. *Cutis.* 2003;71:68-70.

37. Andrews B, Rennie J. Predicting changes in the distribution of sweating following thoracoscopic sympathectomy. *Br J Surg.* 1997;84:1702-1704.

38. Kao M, Chen Y, Lin J, Hsieh C, Tsai J. Endoscopic sympathectomy treatment for craniofacial hyperhidrosis. *Arch Surg.* 1996;131:1091-1094.

39. Naumann M, Lowe N, Kumar C, Hamm H. Botulinum toxin type A is a safe and effective treatment for axillary hyperhidrosis over 16 months: a prospective study. *Arch Dermatol.* 2003;139:731-736.

40. Heckmann M, Breit S, Ceballos-Baumann A, Schaller M, Plewig G. Side-controlled intradermal injection of botulinum toxin A in recalcitrant axillary hyperhidrosis. *J Am Acad Dermatol.* 1999;41:987-990.

41. Schnider P, Binder M, Kittler P, Birner D, Starkel K, Wolff K, et al. A randomized, double-blind, placebo-controlled trial of botulinum A toxin for severe axillary hyperhidrosis. *Br J Dermatol.* 1999;140:677-680.

42. Naumann M, Lowe NJ. Botulinum toxin type A in treatment of bilateral primary axillary hyperhidrosis: randomised, parallel group, double blind, placebo controlled trial. *Br Med J.* 2001;323:596-599.

43. Lowe N, Glaser D, Eadie N, Daggett S, Kowalski J, Lai P. Botulinum toxin type A in the treatment of primary axillary hyperhidrosis: a 52-week multicenter double-blind, randomized, placebo-controlled study of efficacy and safety. *J Am Acad Dermatol.* 2007;56:604-611.

44. Glaser DA, Kowalski J, Ravelo A, Weng EY, Beddingfield F. Functional and dermatology-specific quality of life benefits with repeated botulinum toxin type A treatment of primary axillary hyperhidrosis. [poster 409]. American Academy of Dermatology Summer Meeting. San Diego, CA. July 2006.

45. Wollina U, Karamfilov T, Konrad H. High-dose botulinum toxin type A therapy for axillary hyperhidrosis markedly prolongs the relapse-free interval. *J Am Acad Dermatol.* 2002;46:536-540.

46. Karamfilov T, Konrad H, Karte K, Wollina U. Lower relapse rate of botulinum toxin A therapy for axillary hyperhidrosis by dose increase. *Arch Dermatol.* 2000;136:487-490.

47. Glaser D. Treatment of axillary hyperhidrosis by chemodenervation of sweat glands using botulinum toxin type A. *J Drugs Dermatol.* 2004;3:627-631.

48. Alam M, Dover J, Arndt K. Pain associated with injection of botulinum A exotoxin reconstituted using isotonic sodium chloride with and without preservative: a double-blind, randomized controlled trial. *Arch Dermatol.* 2002;138:510-514.

49. Sarifakioglu N, Sarifakioglu E. Evaluating effects of preservative-containing saline solution on pain perception during botulinum toxin type A injections at different locations: a prospective, single-blinded, randomized controlled trial. *Aesth Plast Surg.* 2005;29:113-115.

50. Vadoud-Seyedi J, Simonart T. Treatment of axillary hyperhidrosis with botulinum toxin type A reconstituted in lidocaine or in normal saline: a randomized, side-by-side, double-blind study. *Br J Dermatol.* 2007;156:986-989.

51. Lowe NJ, Campanati A, Bodokh I, Cliff S, Jaen P, Kreyden O, et al. The place of botulinum toxin type A in the treatment of focal hyperhidrosis. *Br J Dermatol.* 2004;151:1115-1122.

52. Simonetta M, Cauhepe C, Magues J, Senard J. Therapeutics: A double-blind, randomized, comparative study of Dysport vs. Botox in primary palmar hyperhidrosis. *Br J Dermatol.* 2003;149:1041-1045.

53. Scherer C, Clelland J, O'Sullivan P, Doleys D, Canan B. The effect of two sites of high frequency vibration on cutaneous pain threshold. *Pain.* 1986;25:133-138.

54. Naver H, Swartling C, Aquilonius S. Treatment of focal hyperhidrosis with botulinum toxin type A. Brief overview of methodology and 2 years experience. *Eur J Neurol.* 1999;6:S117-S120.

55. Vadoud-Seyedi J, Heenen M, Simonart T. Treatment of idiopathic palmar hyperhidrosis with botulinum toxin. *Dermatology.* 2001;203:318-321.

56. Glaser D, Kokoska M, Kardesch C. Botulinum toxin type A in the treatment of palmar hyperhidrosis: the effect of dilution and number of injection sites. American Academy of Dermatology Annual Meeting, Poster, Washington, DC, March 2001.

57. Baumann L, Frankel S, Esperanza W, Halem M. Communications and brief reports: cryoanalgesia with dichlorotetrafluoroethane lessens the pain of botulinum toxin injections for the treatment of palmar hyperhidrosis. *Dermatol Surg.* 2003;29:1057-1062.

58. Trindade de Almeida A, Kadunc B, Martins de Oliveira E. Improving botulinum toxin therapy for palmar hyperhidrosis: wrist block and technical considerations. *Dermatol Surg.* 2001;27:34-36.

59. Saadia D, Voustianiouk A, Wang A, Kaufmann H. Botulinum toxin type A in primary palmar hyperhidrosis: Randomized, single-blind, two-dose study. *Neurology.* 2001;57:2095-2099.

60. Wollina U, Karamfilov T. Botulinum toxin A for palmar hyperhidrosis. *J Eur Acad Dermatol Venereol.* 2001;15:555-558.

61. Aghaei S. Botulinum toxin therapy for palmar hyperhidrosis: experience in an Iranian population. *Int J Dermatol.* 2007;46:212-214.

62. Hund M, Rickert S, Kinkelin I, Naumann M, Hamm H. Does wrist nerve block influence the result of botulinum toxin A treatment in palmar hyperhidrosis. *J Am Acad Dermatol.* 2004;50:61-62.

63. Perez BA, Avalos-Peralta P, Moreno-Ramirez D, Camacho F. Treatment of palmar hyperhidrosis with botulinum toxin type A: 44 months of experience. *J Cosmet Dermatol.* 2005;4:163-166.

64. Glogau R. Treatment of hyperhidrosis with botulinum toxin. *Dermatol Clin.* 2004;22:177-185.

65. Kontochristopoulos G, Gregoriou S, Zakopoulou N, Rigopoulos D. Cryoanalgesia with dichlorotetrafluoroethane spray versus ice packs in patients treated with botulinum toxin A for palmar hyperhidrosis: self-controlled study. *Dermatol Surg.* 2006;32:873-874.

66. Smith K, Comite SL, Storwick GS. Ice minimizes discomfort associated with injection of botulinum toxin type A for the treatment of palmar and plantar hyperhidrosis. *Dermatol Surg.* 2007;33(1 Spec No.):S88-S91.

67. Naumann M, Bergmann I, Hofmann U, Hamm H, Reiners K. Botulinum toxin for focal hyperhidrosis: technical considerations and improvements in application. *Br J Dermatol.* 1998;139:1123-1124.

68. Benohanian A. Needle-free anaesthesia prior to botulinum toxin type A injection treatment of palmar and plantar hyperhidrosis. *Br J Dermatol.* 2007;156: 593-596.

69. Vollert B, Blaheta H, Moehrle E, Juenger M, Rassner G. Intravenous regional anaesthesia for treatment of palmar hyperhidrosis with botulinum toxin type A. *Br J Dermatol.* 2001;144:632-633.

70. Ponce-Olivera RM, Tirado-Sanchez A, Arellano-Mendoza MI, Leon-Dorantes G, Kassian-Rank S. Palmar hyperhidrosis. Safety efficacy of two anaesthetic techniques for botulinum toxin therapy. *Dermatology Online J.* 2006;12:9.

71. Reed M. Surgical pearl: mechanoanesthesia to reduce the pain of local injections. *J Am Acad Dermatol.* 2001;44:671-672.

72. Solomon B, Hayman R. Botulinum toxin type A therapy for palmar and digital hyperhidrosis. *J Am Acad Dermatol.* 2000;42:1026-1029.

73. Glass GE, Hussain M, Fleming ANM, Powell R. Atrophy of the intrinsic musculature of the hands associated with the use of botulinum toxin-A injections for hyperhidrosis: a case report and review of the literature [published online ahead of print January 17, 2008]. *J Plast Reconstr Aesthet Surg.* 2008.

74. Zaiac M, Weiss E, Elgart G. Botulinum toxin therapy for palmar hyperhidrosis with ADG needle. *Dermatol Surg.* 2000;26:230.

75. Trindade de Almeida A, Boraso R. Palmar hyperhidrosis. In: Trindade de Almeida A, Hexsel D, eds. *Hyperhidrosis and Botulinum Toxin.* Sao Paulo: Knowhow Editorial Ltd.; 2004:155-162.

76. Naumann M, Hofmann U, Bergmann I, Hamm H, Toyka K, Reiners K. Focal hyperhidrosis: effective treatment with intracutaneous botulinum toxin. *Arch Dermatol.* 1998;134:301-304.

77. Blaheta H, Deusch H, Rassner G, Vollert B. Intravenous regional anesthesia (Bier's block) is superior to a peripheral nerve block for painless treatment of plantar hyperhidrosis. *J Am Acad Dermatol.* 2003;48:301-303.

78. Campanati A, Bernardini M, Gesuita R, Offidani A. Plantar focal idiopathic hyperhidrosis and botulinum toxin: a pilot study. *Eur J Dermatol.* 2007;17:52-54.

79. Vadoud-Seyedi J. Treatment of plantar hyperhidrosis with botulinum toxin type A. *Int J Dermatol.* 2004;43:969-971.

80. Sevim S, Dogu O, Kaleagasi H. Botulinum toxin-A therapy for palmar and plantar hyperhidrosis. *Acta Neurol Belg.* 2002;102:167-170.

81. Kinkelin I, Hund M, Naumann M, Hamm H. Effective treatment of frontal hyperhidrosis with botulinum toxin A. *Br J Dermatol.* 2000;143:824-827.

82. Boger A, Herath H, Rompel R, Ferbert A. Botulinum toxin for treatment of craniofacial hyperhidrosis. *J Neurol.* 2000;247:857-861.

83. Glaser DA, Herbert AA, Pariser DM, Solish N. Facial hyperhidrosis: best practice recommendations and special considerations. *Cutis.* 2007;79(5 suppl):29-32.

84. Hexsel D, Dal'forno T, Hexsel C. Inguinal, or Hexsel's hyperhidrosis. *Clin Dermatol.* 2004;22:53-59.

85. Huh C, Han K, Seo K, Eun H. Botulinum toxin treatment for compensatory hyperhidrosis subsequent to an upper thoracic sympathectomy. *J Dermatolog Treat.* 2002;13:91-93.

86. Matarasso S. Treatment of facial chromhidrosis with botulinum toxin type A. *J Am Acad Dermatol.* 2005;52(1):89-91.

87. Birklein F, Eisenbarth G, Erbguth F, Winterholler M. Botulinum toxin type B blocks sudomotor function effectively: a 6 month follow up. *J Invest Dermatol.* 2003;121:1312-1316.

88. Schlereth T, Mouka I, Eisenbarth G, Winterholler M, Birklein F. Botulinum toxin A (Botox) and sweating-dose efficacy and comparison of other BoNT preparations. *Auton Neurosci.* 2005;117:120-126.

89. Dressler D, Adib F, Benecke R. Botulinum toxin type B for treatment of axillary hyperhidrosis. *J Neurol.* 2002;249:1729-1732.

90. Nelson L, Bachoo P, Holmes J. Botulinum toxin type B: a new therapy for axillary hyperhidrosis. *Br J Plast Surg.* 2005;58:228-232.

91. Baumann L, Halem M. Systemic adverse effects after botulinum toxin type B (Myobloc) injections for the treatment of palmar hyperhidrosis. *Arch Dermatol.* 2003;139:226-227.

92. Baumann L, Slezinger A, Halem M, Vujevich J, Mallin K, Charles C, et al. Double-blind, randomized placebo-controlled pilot study of the safety and efficacy of Myobloc (botulinum toxin type B) for the treatment of palmar hyperhidrosis. *Dermatol Surg.* 2005;31:263-270.

93. Hecht M, Birklein F, Winterholler M. Successful treatment of axillary hyperhidrosis with very low doses of botulinum toxin B: a pilot study. *Arch Dermatol.* 2004;295:318-319.

94. Drobik C, Laskawi R. Frey's syndrome: treatment with botulinum toxin. *Acta Otolaryngol.* (Stockh) 1995;115:459-461.

95. Naumann M, Zellner M, Toyka K, Reiners K. Treatment of gustatory sweating with botulinum toxin. *Ann Neurol.* 1997;42:973-975.

96. Bjerkhoel A, Trobbe O. Frey's syndrome: treatment with botulinum toxin. *J Laryngol Otol.* 1997;111:839-844.

97. Laskawi R, Drobik C, Schonebeck C. Up-to-date report of botulinum toxin type A treatment in patients with gustatory sweating (Frey's syndrome). *Laryngoscope.* 1998;108:381-384.

98. Laccourreye O, Akl E, Gutierrez-Fonseca R, Garcia D, Brasnu D, Bonan B. Recurrent gustatory sweating (Frey syndrome) after intracutaneous injection of botulinum toxin type A. *Arch Otolaryngol Head Neck Surg.* 1999;125:283-286.

99. Mancini F, Zangaglia R, Cristina S, Sommaruga MG, Martignoni E, Nappi G, et al. Double-blind,

placebo-controlled study to evaluate the efficacy and safety of botulinum toxin type A in the treatment of drooling in parkinsonism. *Mov Disord.* 2003;18: 685-688.

100. Lagalla G, Millevolte M, Capecci M, Provinciali L, Ceravolo MG. Botulinum toxin type A for drooling in Parkinson's disease: a double-blind, randomized, placebo-controlled study. *Mov Disord.* 2006;21: 704-707.

101. Ondo WG, Hunter C, Moore W. A double-blind placebo-controlled trial of botulinum toxin B for sialorrhea in Parkinson's disease. *Neurology.* 2004;62: 37-40.

102. Lipp A, Trottenberg T, Schink T, Kupsch A, Arnold G. A randomized trial of botulinum toxin A for treatment of drooling. *Neurology.* 2003;61:1279-1281.

103. Riemann R, Pfenningsdorf S, Riemann E, Naumann M. Successful treatment of crocodile tears by injection of botulinum toxin into the lacrimal gland. *Ophthalmology.* 1999;106:2322-2324.

104. Boroojerdi B, Ferbert A, Schwartz M, Herath H, Noth J. Botulinum toxin treatment of synkinesia and hyperlacrimation after facial palsy. *J Neurol Neurosurg Psychiatry.* 1998;65:111-114.

105. Hofmann RJ. Treatment of Frey's syndrome (gustatory sweating) and crocodile tears (gustatory epiphora) with purified botulinum toxin. *Ophthal Plastic Reconstruct Surgery.* 2000;16:289-291.

106. Meyer M. Botulinumtoxin-Therapie im Kopf-Hais-Bereich. In: Laskawi R, Roggenkamper P, eds. *XXX.* Munich: Urban and Vogel; 1999:245-255.

107. Kim K, Kim S, Yoon J, Han J. The effect of botulinum toxin type A injection for intrinsic rhinitis. *J Laryngol Otol.* 1998;112:248-251.

108. Kavanagh G, Oh C, Shams K. BOTOX delivery by iontophoresis. *Br J Dermatol.* 2004;151:1093-1095.

109. Glogau R. Topically applied botulinum toxin type a for the treatment of primary axillary hyperhidrosis: results of a randomized, blinded, vehicle-controlled study. *Dermatol Surg.* 2007;33:S76-S80.

Botulinum Neurotoxin **26**
for Dermatologic and
Cosmetic Disorders

Dee Anna Glaser

INTRODUCTION

This century has seen an explosion in the number of individuals seeking out ways to look younger and more beautiful. As the demand for procedures increases, so does the desire for less invasive therapy with shortened down times and "natural" nonsurgical appearance. The injection of botulinum neurotoxin (BoNT) for the treatment of dynamic facial lines is the most popular cosmetic procedure in the United States.[1] Such use has increased by 4700% since 1997, more than any other nonsurgical procedure.[2] Along with the increased use, there has been an expansion in the cosmetic indications for BoNT usage. Initially, treatment was generally limited to the upper one-third of the face, including the glabellar lines, horizontal forehead lines, and crow's feet. Now the midface, lower face, and neck are common areas to be treated, and there has been a shift from pure "wrinkle removal" to reshaping and recontouring the face and body with botulinum toxin. Examples include using BoNT to lift and shape the eyebrows, widen the aperture of the eye, contouring of squared-shape mandibles, and even reshaping the calf areas of legs.

AVAILABLE BOTULINUM NEUROTOXIN PRODUCTS

As noted in previous chapters, two serotypes of BoNT are available currently for clinical use: botulinum neurotoxin type A (BoNT/A) and botulinum toxin neurotoxin type B (BoNT/B) (Table 26-1). Although both inhibit the release of acetylcholine from the motor nerve terminal, each enters the neuron through different pathways and cleaves different proteins, which is covered in more detail in earlier chapters. BoNT/B is not approved for cosmetic uses and is used much less commonly than BoNT/A for cosmetic procedures. The Botox brand (Allergan, Inc, Irvine, CA) is the most commonly used BoNT/A product worldwide for aesthetic procedures. In the United States, Botox has been approved since 2002 for the treatment of glabellar lines and it is approved for multiple facial lines in Canada. Approval of Dysport (Ipsen, Milford, MA) is currently being pursued in the United States under the name Reloxin.

Other BoNT/A products are available in select areas of the world. Xeomin (Merz Pharma, Greensboro, NC) comprises only the naked 150-kDa toxin without other nontoxin proteins.[3] It is approved for cervical dystonia and blepharospasm in Germany. Trials are under way with Xeomin for glabellar lines. Neuronox (Medy-Tox, Inc., Seoul, South Korea) is approved in Korea and is available in parts of North Africa, some European countries, Russia, and Mexico. A Chinese toxin also referred to as Chinese botulinum toxin A (CBTX-A, Lanzhou Institute of Biological Products, Shanghai, China) can be found in some Asian countries and parts of South America (also known as Prosigne).[2] At the time of writing, there are no published studies in the English medical literature on the aesthetic uses of these products.

The various BoNT products are derived from different strains of *Clostridium botulinum*

Dr. Glaser reports that she has been a consultant for Allergan and Medicis. Also, she has performed research that has been funded by Allergan and has received unrestricted educational grants from Allergan for research.

TABLE 26-1 Botulinum Toxins Widely Available Internationally

Names	Manufacturer	BoNT Serotype	Approval for Cosmetic Use	Toxin Complex Size (kDA)	Supplied	Concentration Per Vial	Neurotoxin Protein Content (ng/vial)
Botox Cosmetic, Botox, Vistabel, Vistabex	Allergan, Inc	A	Yes	900	Vacuum-dried powder	100 U	5
Dysport, Reloxin	Ipsen, Ltd	A	Yes*	500-900	Lyophilized powder	500 U	≤12.5
Myobloc, Neurobloc	Solstice Neurosciences, Inc	B	No	700	Solution	2500, 5000, or 10,000 U	38–71

*Excludes approval in the United States.

using different proprietary methods of isolation, purification and manufacturing. Thus, each product is unique. Of the two BoNT/A products most widely used, it is generally reported that 1 U of Botox has the same therapeutic effect as 2.5 to 5 U of Dysport. However, there is no universally applicable safe dose conversion ratio between the two products. Any conversion from one product to another requires "dose finding" on a case-by-case basis. It is clear that Botox and Dysport are not interchangeable products: they differ in critical chemical properties, dose requirements, duration of effect, and adverse event profiles.[4-6] Throughout this chapter, doses of BoNT/A will refer to Botox unless otherwise stated.

TABLE 26-2 Typical Patient Goals Using Botulinum Toxins[49]
Look as good as possible for their age
Look rested
Look natural and relaxed
Avoid looking angry, mad or sad
Maintain some facial movement and animation
Long lasting results
Pain-free procedure
Avoid adverse events
No down time
Cost-efficacy or value for the money; not too expensive

PRINCIPLES OF AESTHETIC USES

A thorough understanding of the anatomy and pathophysiology of the aging process is necessary for the cosmetic use of BoNTs. The major forces responsible for facial aging include gravity, soft tissue maturation, and skeletal remodeling resulting in volume loss, muscular activity resulting in hyperdynamic wrinkles, and solar changes affecting skin color, texture, and elasticity.[7] With this in mind, a multipronged approach is necessary to achieve maximum aesthetic improvement.[8] Fillers, skin rejuvenation, and surgical procedures can all be performed in concert with BoNT, even at the same sitting to enhance patient outcomes and satisfaction.[9-11] It is beyond the scope of this chapter to cover combination therapy, but it is covered in many other articles and textbooks.[9,12,13]

FACIAL AESTHETICS

Because the face is still the most common area to be treated with BoNT, it is critical that the physician have a thorough understanding of the pathophysiology of aging, anatomy, and the desired aesthetic goals of the patient. For cosmetic uses, the target of BoNT is primarily the muscles of facial expression. These generally have soft tissue attachments and, when contracted, move the overlying skin. With repeated muscle contraction, folding and pleating of the skin lead to permanent creases over time. Botulinum toxin temporarily weakens contracting muscles, thereby improving and even eliminating the overlying skin creases. The position and interplay of opposing muscle actions contribute to the appearance of facial aging, and BoNT can be used to alter such relationships.

Patients are often seeking subtle changes, and it is paramount that the injector be able to meet patients' goals (Table 26-2). The undesirable "frozen" look should be replaced by a more "natural and relaxed" appearance. Patients report a change in appearance within 2 weeks of receiving BoNT/A, and 4 weeks after therapy to their upper face, they report looking 3 years younger than baseline.[14]

FACIAL ANATOMY

On the body, muscles typically have bony attachments through tendons, and muscle contraction results in skeletal movement. In contrast, the muscles of facial expression generally have soft tissue attachments, and muscle contraction results in movement of the overlying skin. This unique facial anatomy helps us communicate and express emotional states. The muscles of the face and neck (Fig. 26-1) vary in size and depth beneath the skin. The seventh cranial nerve, the facial nerve, provides motor function of the face. Injection points are determined by the muscles and not the course of the nerve.

Although the locations of the facial muscles is crucial to achieving good outcomes (Table 26-3), understanding the interplay of muscle groups is just as critical.

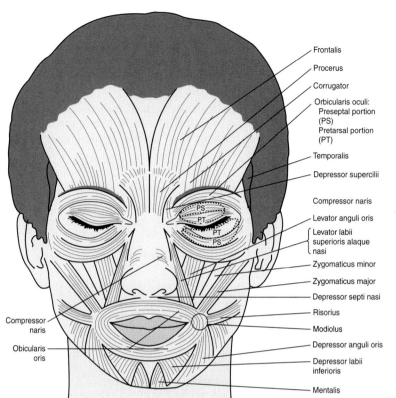

FIGURE 26-1. Muscular anatomy of the face.

Frontalis
Procerus
Corrugator
Orbicularis oculi:
  Preseptal portion (PS)
  Pretarsal portion (PT)
Temporalis
Depressor supercilii
Compressor naris
Levator anguli oris
Levator labii superioris alaque nasi
Zygomaticus minor
Zygomaticus major
Depressor septi nasi
Risorius
Modiolus
Depressor anguli oris
Depressor labii inferioris
Mentalis

Compressor naris
Obicularis oris

GENERAL PRINCIPLES AND TREATMENT GUIDELINES

Reconstitution of Botox can be performed using preserved saline despite the manufacturer's recommendations of the use of nonpreserved saline. The benzyl alcohol preservative in the former decreases the discomfort of the injection without altering the efficacy.[15,16] The amount of diluent used to reconstitute a vial varies among physicians, with a typical range being 1 to 4 mL but it can be as high as 10 mL per 100-unit vial. As the efficacy is high regardless of the amount of diluent used, clinical practice is based on physician preference.[17] Syringe and needle selection also

TABLE 26-3 Anatomic Profile for Botulinum Neurotoxin Aesthetic Use

Treatment Site/Aesthetic Goal	Targeted Muscles
Glabella/frown lines	Procerus, corrugator, and depressor supercilii muscles
Forehead wrinkles	Frontalis muscle
Crow's feet	Orbicularis oculi muscle
Lower eyelid lines	Orbicularis oculi muscle
Bunny lines	Nasalis muscle
Lip lines	Orbicularis oris muscle
Down turned corners of the mouth	Depressor anguli oris muscle
Chin dimpling	Mentalis muscle
Deep horizontal chin groove	Mentalis muscle
Masseter hypertrophy or squared jaw	Masseter muscle
Vertical platysma neck bands	Platysma muscle
Necklace or horizontal neck lines	Platysma muscle

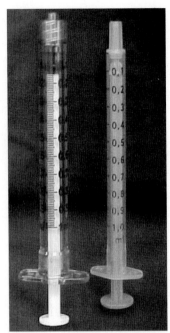

FIGURE 26-2. A standard 1-mL tuberculin syringe versus a 1-mL syringe with a bullet-shaped plunger designed to decrease waste.

varies, with insulin syringes or 1-mL tuberculin type syringes being the most popular (Fig. 26-2). The latter results in waste of product in the tip of the syringe and hub of the needle.[18] Specially designed syringes are available with a bullet-shaped plunger to reduce any waste. Small-gauge needles should be used for cosmetic injections; most commonly 30- to 32-gauge ½-inch needles are used.

To reduce the risk of bruising with injections, patients should stop the use of anticoagulants, nonsteroidal anti-inflammatory agents, aspirin, and supplements such as vitamin E, garlic, gingko, and fish oils 7 days before their injection appointment. Although this is ideal, it is not necessary to postpone injections should the patient fail to stop such agents.

Patients should be placed in a comfortable position, ideally with their head supported. An upright or slightly reclined position is best for cosmetic injections. Pain is usually minimal, but some patients may prefer to use a topical anesthetic cream before injections.[19] This is especially valuable in more sensitive areas such as the upper lip. The application of ice or cold air before injections may also help to reduce any discomfort and at the same time may reduce the risk of bruising secondary to vasoconstriction. The use of cold packs can be particularly useful in areas that are most likely

to bruise, such as the lateral orbital rim and the lower eyelid.

Although there are no controlled studies to support the need for special postoperative instructions, many physicians recommend the following:

- Contract the treated muscles immediately after injection to enhance uptake. Several minutes to several hours have been recommended.

- Do not bend over for 2 to 3 hours such as to pick up objects from the floor, or to try on shoes.

- Do not massage the treated areas for 2 to 3 hours.

- Do not lie down for 2 to 3 hours after treatment.

- Limit heavy physical activities for several hours after treatment.

Treatment should always begin with an accurate assessment of the patient. In particular, the patient's needs and goals should be addressed. Adjuvant therapy with fillers, lasers, resurfacing, or surgery may need to be combined with BoNT to achieve maximum improvement. A signed consent form should be obtained before the procedure, and photographic documentation of the patient in repose and with animation is beneficial.

The following text serves as a guideline for the treatment of the cosmetic patient using BoNT/A. It is always best to customize therapy based on the individual's needs and desires as discussed, with close attention to anatomy, muscle size, and function. Ideally, muscles should be visualized or palpated at rest and with movement before injection. The use of the injector's nondominant thumb and finger can help to localize and stabilize the muscle groups during injection (Fig. 26-3).

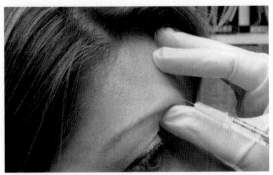

FIGURE 26-3. The nondominant thumb and fingers stabilize the patient and localize the muscle to be injected.

COSMETIC FACIAL INJECTIONS

Glabella

The glabellar frown lines represent one of the most commonly treated cosmetic units. The muscles generally targeted when treating the glabellar frown lines are the corrugator supercilii, procerus, and depressor supercilii.[20] Five injection points are most commonly used, but the treatment area may range from three to seven sites. Doses vary as well, with 20 to 30 units for the average woman and 30 to 50 units for a male glabellar complex, depending on the muscle mass and the desires of the patient.[21-23]

Having the patient frown is the best way to visualize the muscles. The procerus muscle may not be easily visualized and can be injected in the midline at the crossing point of an X that intersects the medial brows and the contralateral medial canthi (Fig. 26-4). It is important that the brow be used as the landmark and not the eyebrows, because the eyebrows can be reshaped and distorted in terms of their anatomic landmarks. Five to ten units of Botox is injected into the procerus muscle, which is secured by the injector's nondominant hand (Fig. 26-5). Massage can help diffusion into the depressor supercilli muscle. The corrugator muscles are identified with animation or frowning. The belly of the muscle is supported by the nondominant thumb, and ~5 units are injected into the muscle (Fig. 26-6). The tail of the corrugator generally needs to be treated as well and is usually located approximately 1 cm above the supraorbital ridge near the midpupillary line. A typical dose is 2.5 to 5 units into each tail of the corrugator (Figs. 26-7 and 26-8).

The efficacy and safety of the Dysport brand of BoNT/A to treat glabellar lines has been studied, and doses of 50 units seem to provide optimal results.[24] The injection pattern used

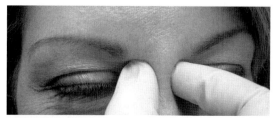

FIGURE 26-5. The procerus muscle is pinched between the thumb and finger of the nondominant hand.

for Dysport is slightly different than for Botox, with three central injection points most crucial (procerus and each corrugator) but lateral injection sites do not appear to improve efficacy.[25]

Horizontal Forehead Lines

Horizontal forehead lines are easily treated by targeting the frontalis muscle. In many individuals, frontalis fibers are not present in the superior midline section of the forehead and are replaced with membranous galea. If this is the case, injection into this area is unnecessary. It is important to remember that the frontalis muscle is the only levator muscle of the upper face that elevates the brow, eyebrows and skin of the forehead. High doses or incorrect placement of BoNT can result in a real or perceived brow or eyebrow ptosis. Injections must be kept well above the brow to avoid brow ptosis and to avoid loss of facial expressivity.

Injections should usually start 2 cm or more superior to the orbital rim, and doses should err on the low side (Fig. 26-9). Doses will vary depending on the height and width of the forehead, muscle mass, and eyebrow placement, as well as on the coadministration of BoNT/A to

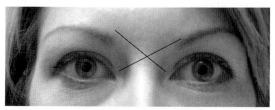

FIGURE 26-4. The procerus muscle is injected at the crossing point of an X that intersects the medial brows and contralateral medial canthi.

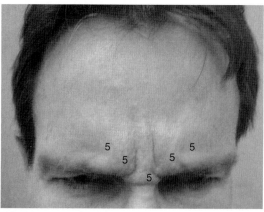

FIGURE 26-6. Male glabellar frown pre Botox 25 U.

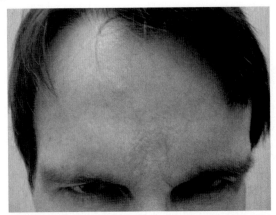

FIGURE 26-7. One month after botulinum neurotoxin type A injections.

the depressor muscles of the upper face. Starting doses of 10 to 20 units for women and 15 to 30 units for men should be considered.

Frontalis muscle fibers can extend laterally, and if not treated adequately, a quizzical appearance can develop unilaterally or bilaterally (Fig. 26-10). If this should develop, an additional 1 to 3 units should be injected to bring the peaked brow down.

Brow Lifting and Shaping

Brow ptosis is common and results in a tired, run-down appearance. When treating the eyebrows, it is necessary to assess for asymmetry of the eyebrows, a very common finding. It is important to review such findings with the patient before injection, because perfect symmetry cannot always be obtained, and patients may not have noticed their asymmetries before treatment.

Treatment of the glabellar complex as described can be combined with injections of the orbicularis oculi muscle or inferior portions of the frontalis muscle to elevate and shape the eyebrows. Initially, this elevation was thought to be purely a result of the effect on the brow depressor muscles, but it has been postulated that the frontalis is the main factor.[26] Placement or diffusion of BoNT A into fibers of the frontalis may induce an increased resting tone in the remainder of the muscle and result in changes in eyebrow position. Treating the superolateral portions of the orbicularis oculi with 2 to 6 units (usually at the lateral brow at the junction with the temporal fusion line) along with injections of the lateral canthus can be very helpful when trying to elevate the eyebrow position.

Eyes

The "crow's feet" or wrinkles at the lateral canthus are caused by contraction of the lateral portion of the orbicularis oculi muscle, and to some degree, the zygomaticus and risorius muscles of the mouth. It is important to examine the patient during smiling to assess the effect of the zygomaticus muscles pushing up the cheek into the periorbital area and contributing to the "crow's feet" (Fig. 26-11). These are difficult to treat without risking facial droop or an unnatural appearance.

At the lateral canthus, the vertically oriented fibers of the orbicularis oculi muscle are injected. Two to four injection sites are typically required with a starting dose of 10 to 15 U

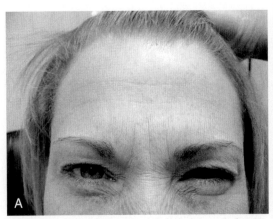
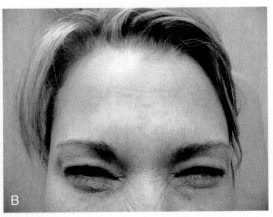

FIGURE 26-8. A and **B,** Female glabella before and after 20 units of Botox.

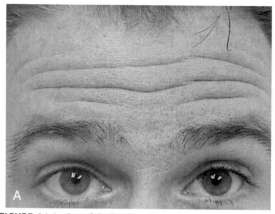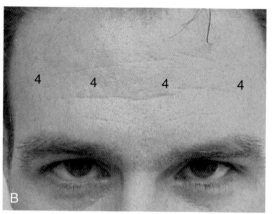

FIGURE 26-9. A and **B,** Forehead injection sites to improve horizontal forehead lines, staying superior to the eyebrows to prevent further ptosis.

per canthus. The patient should smile maximally to locate the injection sites (Fig. 26-12). The center point is usually 1 to 2 cm lateral to the lateral canthus, with injections placed 1 to 1 1/2 cm superior and inferior to this point. It is important to stay above the zygomatic arch to avoid lip ptosis. Injection into the subcutaneous fat and not the muscle may help reduce bruising. Owing to the very thin skin in the canthus, diffusion into the muscle is sufficient. Care should also be used to avoid the vessels in this area to help minimize the risk of bruising as well.

A prominent bulge of the lower eyelid when the patient is smiling or animated is caused by the pretarsal portion of the orbicularis oculi muscle (Fig. 26-13). One injection at the mid-pupillary line about 2 mm inferior to the lid margin can be performed. Small doses using 1 to 2 U is usually sufficient to reduce this bulge,

and a more open, almond-shaped eye can also be produced. Injections medial to the midpupillary line can weaken the blink reflex and result in dry eyes. Injections lateral to the mid-pupillary line increases the risk for lower lid ectropion. A "snap test" should be performed in which the lower eyelid is pulled off the globe by downward pressure on the eyelid skin and then quickly released. Good candidates for lower eyelid BoNT/A treatment will have a quick return of the lower eyelid skin to its original position with the snap test.

Nose

Nasal scrunch or "bunny lines" are produced when wrinkling the nose and can be accentuated with speech, smiling or frowning (Fig. 26-14). These lines result from the contraction of the nasalis muscle, especially the transverse portion, although the levator labii superioris alaeque nasi muscle may contribute to their appearance as well.[27] Very small doses of BoNT/A are needed: usually 1 to 3 U per side are injected superficially into the subcutaneous tissue at the lateral wall of the nasal bridge. Placement is particularly important to avoid drooping of the upper lip or other lip asymmetries because the levator labii superioris alaeque nasi and the levator labii superioris both originate along the medial aspect of the malar prominence.

Mouth

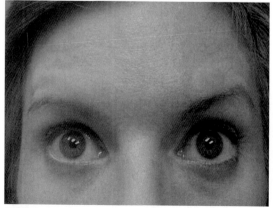

FIGURE 26-10. A unilateral quizzical brow developed after forehead injection due to functioning lateral frontalis muscle fibers.

Rejuvenation of the mouth can be achieved using small doses of BoNT/A; however,

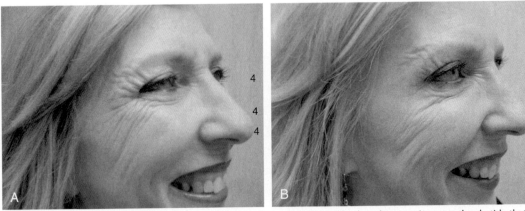

FIGURE 26-11. Injection of 12 U Botox results in diminished crow's feet wrinkles but does not improve the rhytids that are pushed up by the cheek during a smile.

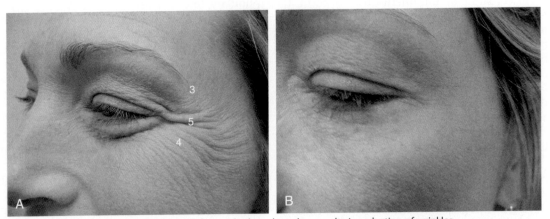

FIGURE 26-12. A and **B,** Injection of 12 U Botox to the lateral canthus results in reduction of wrinkles.

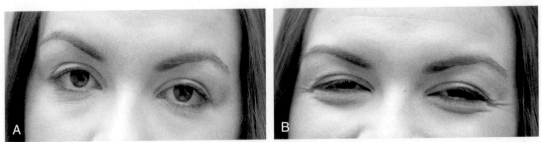

FIGURE 26-13. A and **B,** A prominent bulge of the lower eyelids is seen with smiling. One to two units Botox are injected into the pretarsal portion of the orbicularis oculi muscle at the midpupillary line.

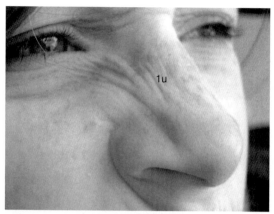

FIGURE 26-14. Nasal scrunch, or "bunny," lines are treated with 1 to 2 U Botox injected into the nasalis muscle.

outcomes are usually optimized when combined with other procedures such as fillers or resurfacing. "Smoker's lines" or radial lip lines are common, especially in women. Repetitive pursing or movement of the orbicularis oris muscle contribute to the development of these lines. The radial lip wrinkles can interfere with the use of lipstick, which may run or "bleed" into them.

Four to 10 U can be used for the upper lip, whereas 3 to 8 U are needed for the lower lip. Injections do not need to be placed into the lines. They should be placed 1 to 2 mm away from the pink border of the lip to help minimize discomfort (Fig. 26-15). I avoid the lateral quadrants of the lip and usually do not inject in cupid's bow. Not only can the wrinkles be reduced with therapy, but enhanced lip fullness and eversion has been reported.[28]

Conservative dosing is recommended to avoid oral incompetence. Patients should be counseled on the possibility of a change in their speech and enunciation, and ability to drink with a straw, or other activities requiring a strong pursing of their lips. Often, patients can perceive a difference in their speech, but it is usually unnoticed by others and resolves within 2 weeks, if it occurs at all. Patient satisfaction can be lower when treating the lip lines compared with other cosmetic units such as the glabella, and proper patient counseling is valuable.

The corners of the mouth represent another very important point of cosmetic enhancement. Because the corners of the mouth turn downward with age, they portray sadness or anger. The depressor anguli oris (DAO) muscle can be injected with 3 to 5 U as a starting dose that can be increased, as needed, to achieve a reduction in the marionette lines and a more neutral or upturned corner of the mouth. Combination therapy with dermal fillers can optimize the results.

Injections should be made directly into the DAO muscle located on the mandibular body.[29] An inferior and lateral approach is recommend to avoid the depressor labii inferioris (DLI) muscle, which lies beneath and slightly medial to the DAO, and the orbicularis oris muscle located around the lips. The DAO muscle can be palpated when the patient makes a sad or disappointed face or with an exaggerated pronunciation of the letter "e" (Fig. 26-16). If not identified with these types of maneuvers, injections should be made ~8 to 10 mm lateral to the oral commissure and ~15 mm inferior to this point.

Nasolabial Folds

Although treating the nasolabial folds (NLFs) is usually accomplished with fillers, some

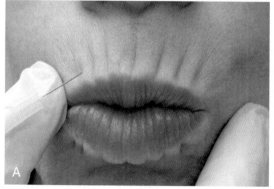

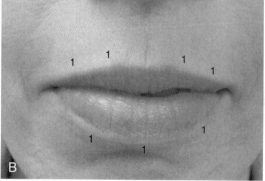

FIGURE 26-15. Perioral wrinkles secondary to movement of the orbicularis oris muscle (**A**) and low doses (**B**) of Botox to reduce the lines without compromising mouth competency.

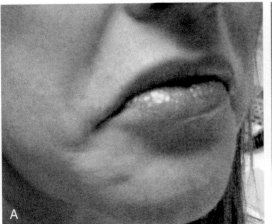
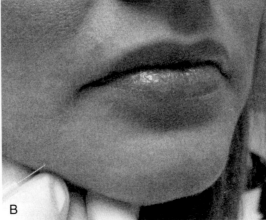

FIGURE 26-16. A, The depressor anguli oris muscle can be accentuated by having the patient make a "sad" face. **B,** Injection should be inferior and laterally to avoid the depressor labii inferioris muscle.

patients may benefit from BoNT/A therapy, usually as an adjuvant to the fillers. Changes in the patient's smile may occur, and the white portion of the upper lip may lengthen. Small doses such as 2 to 5 U are good starting doses and are injected at the nasomaxillary junction, just lateral to the ala (Fig. 26-17). The targeted muscle is the levator labii superioris alaeque nasi, although some physicians prefer to target the zygomaticus muscles.[30]

Patients with a "gummy smile" in which all the incisors and some of the gingivae show are generally considered to be good candidates for BoNT/A therapy. Doses as high as 7.5 U may be used, but starting doses of 2.5 to 3 U are recommended per side.[31] Pretreatment asymmetries are common and require different dosing on each side.

Chin

Chin dimpling is the result of the mentalis muscle and can give the appearance of peau d'orange or golf ball dimpling. It can be seen at rest or with talking and tends to become more pronounced with advancing age and loss of dermal and subcutaneous tissue thickness (Fig. 26-18). Low-dose BoNT/A can give a more relaxed and smooth appearance to the chin. As little as 2.5 to 5 U and up to 10 U should be injected into the central lower portion of the mentalis (Fig. 26-19). A deep mental crease can also be improved with this same technique. Care to avoid the DLI and the orbicularis oris muscles is important.

Neck

Vertical neck bands and cords may be prominent in some individuals at rest or with animation (Fig. 26-20). The superficial platysma muscle is injected into the bands using 2 to 4 U every 1 to 2 cm. It may be helpful to have the patient exaggerate the bands for the physician to grab and then have the patient relax the muscle contraction during the actual injection (Fig. 26-21). The injections are very superficial, and a bleb should be seen at the injection site. Doses of 50 U or more may be needed to treat the entire neck, but high doses can be associated with neck weakness and trouble swallowing.[32,33]

Horizontal neck lines or "necklace" lines can be treated with BoNT/A but are much less responsive than the vertical bands, and patients need to be adequately counseled on the expected outcomes.

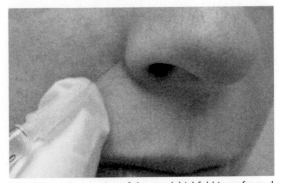

FIGURE 26-17. Injection of the nasolabial fold is performed lateral to the ala.

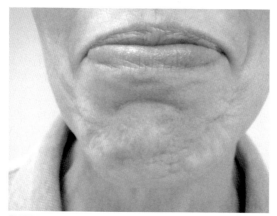

FIGURE 26-18. Dimpled chin is secondary to mentalis muscle hyperfunction.

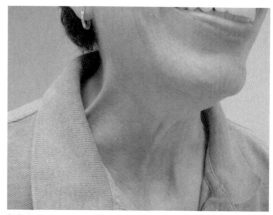

FIGURE 26-20. Vertical neck bands.

Mandibular Contouring

A square-appearing jaw line can widen the lower face and give a more masculine appearance. In some patients, this is secondary to masseter muscle hypertrophy that, with treatment, can return the face to a more oval shape.[34] It is important that patients be appropriately diagnosed, namely, that it is the masseter muscle causing facial widening and not just a prominent bony mandible. Reductions of up to 30% in masseter muscle volume or a decrease in thickness of 2.9 mm have been reported after treatment with BoNT/A.[35]

Before injection, the patient should accentuate the contours of the masseter at the angle of the jaw, which can be done by having the patient strongly clench the teeth. Approximately 6 to 8 injections are required, with doses ranging from 25 to 30 U Botox per side. Kim reported that 100 to 140 U Dysport per side resulted in high patient satisfaction when treating the masseter.[36] A 1-inch needle is used, and the deeper muscle should be injected. Patients may experience localized aching and swelling for 24 to 48 hours postinjection. Ice packs can be beneficial.

COMPLICATIONS WITH AESTHETIC BOTULINUM NEUROTOXIN THERAPY

The overall safety of BoNT in doses used for cosmetic purposes is exceptional. As with all procedures, proper patient selection and technique are crucial to minimize complications and poor outcomes (Table 26-4). Complications are rare, and generally mild and transient in nature (Table 26-5). In clinical

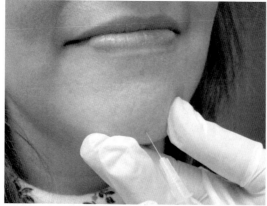

FIGURE 26-19. Injection of the mentalis muscle should be performed into the lower central portion to avoid the orbicularis oris and depressor labii inferioris muscles.

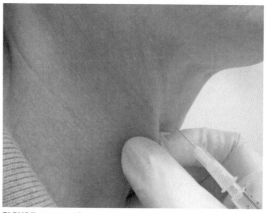

FIGURE 26-21. The injector grabs the platysmal band for injections that are superficial.

TABLE 26-4 Contraindications

Known allergy to any component in botulinum neurotoxin formulation

Pre-existing infection at the site of planned injection

Pre-existing active inflammatory skin condition at the site of planned injection

Unrealistic expectations

Neuromuscular disease (e.g., myasthenia gravis, Lambert-Eaton syndrome)

Pregnant or lactating women

Concomitant use of medications known to interfere with neuromuscular transmission (e.g., aminoglycosides, cholinesterase inhibitors, succinylcholine, curare-like depolarizing blockers, magnesium sulfate, quinidine, calcium channel blockers, lincosamides, polymyxins)

trials of Botox cosmetic, 43.7% of treated subjects reported adverse effects versus 41.5% of the placebo group, with the most common being headache, upper respiratory tract infection, blepharoptosis, nausea, pain, and flu-like symptoms.[37] General side effects related to intramuscular injection include pain, erythema, edema, and bruising. The use of small needles can help as can reconstituting BoNT/A with preserved saline rather than unpreserved saline.[15,16,38] Topical anesthesia can be used, especially for tender areas such as the upper lip, but frequently is not necessary.[19,39] Ice or coolants can be used to reduce discomfort and swelling.[40] Having patients abstain from nonsteroidal anti-inflammatory agents and other agents that affect platelets or the clotting cascade for 1 week before treatment will reduce the risk of bruising.

Physicians should look for and avoid any visible cutaneous vessels.

The majority of undesirable cosmetic events are related to improper injection technique, poor patient selection, or local diffusion of BoNT. Typically, the radius of neurotoxin diffusion is 1 to 3 cm.[41] The diffusion varies depending on the site of injection, the formulation of BoNT used, and the amount of diluent used.[42,43] Clinical mantra states that reconstituting with smaller volumes yields a more concentrated solution, which translates into decreased local toxin spread. However, one study by Carruthers et al[17] did not show any relationship between dilution and clinical response in the glabella. Muscular contraction after injection may also affect the pattern of toxin spread.[44] Patients should avoid massaging the treated site, and contract the muscles

TABLE 26-5 Side Effects are Relatively Uncommon and Vary Depending on the Part of the Face that Is Being Treated

Adverse Events of Short Duration	Adverse Events of Longer Duration	Immediate Hypersensitivity Reaction
Stinging or discomfort with injection	Blepharoptosis	Urticaria
Erythema and edema at injection site	Brow ptosis	Dyspnea
Headache	Diplopia	Angioedema
Bruising	Decreased tearing and xerophthalmia	Anaphylaxis
Asymmetry	Ectropion	
Localized numbness or paresthesias at injection site	Lagophthalmos	
Focal twitching	Oral incompetence	
Mild nausea	Decreased neck strength	
Malaise and myalgias	dysphagia	
	dysarthria	

of the site after injection to expedite toxin uptake.[37]

Dry eyes and even keratitis have been reported following injection of cosmetic BoNT/A but are temporary.[45,46] One case of pseudoaneurysm was reported in a patient 6 months after the injection of 30 units of BoNT/A.[47] Serious adverse events including death and cardiovascular events have been reported to the US Food and Drug Administration after the therapeutic use of BoNT/A, although a causal relationship between the fatalities and BoNT injection could not be established. There have been no fatalities reported with cosmetic use of BoNT/A.[48]

The overall safety and high patient satisfaction with cosmetic BoNT therapy is high but requires physician experience and expertise.

References

1. The American Society for Aesthetic Plastic Surgery. Cosmetic Surgery National Data Bank. 2005 Statistics, multispecialty expanded data for 2005. www.surgery.org. Accessed September 14, 2007.
2. de Boulle K. Botulinum Neurotoxin Type A in Facial Aesthetics. *Expert Opinion On Pharmacotherapy.* London: Ashley Publications; 2007:1059-1072.
3. Jost W, Kohl A, Brinkmann S, Comes G. Efficacy and tolerability of a botulinum toxin type A free of complexing proteins (NT 201) compared with commercially available botulinum toxin type A (BOTOX) in healthy volunteers. *J Neural Transm.* 2005;112: 905-913.
4. Wenzel R, Jones D, Borrego J. Comparing two botulinum toxin type A formulations using manufacturers' product summaries. *J Clin Pharm Ther.* 2007;32:387-402.
5. Sampaio C, Costa J, Ferreira J. Clinical comparability of marketed formulations of botulinum toxin. *Mov Disord.* 2004;19(suppl 8):S129-S136.
6. Chapman M, Barron R, Tanis D, Gill C, Charles P. Comparison of botulinum neurotoxin preparations for the treatment of cervical dystonia. *Clin Ther.* 2007;29:1325-1337.
7. Zimbler M, Kokoska M, Thomas J. Anatomy and pathophysiology of facial aging. *Facial Plast Surg Clin North Am.* 2001;9:179-187.
8. Draelos ZD. Concepts in a multiprong approach to photoaging. *Skin Therapy Lett.* 2006;11:1-3.
9. Coleman K, Carruthers J. Combination therapy with BOTOX and fillers: the new rejuvenation paradigm. *Dermatol Ther.* 2006;19:177-188.
10. Flynn T. Update on botulinum toxin. *Semin Cutan Med Surg.* 2006;25:115-121.
11. Semchyshyn N, Kilmer SL. Does laser inactivate botulinum toxin? *Dermatol Surg.* 2005;31:399-404.
12. Wise J, Greco T. Injectable treatments for the aging face. *Facial Plast Surg.* 2006;22:140-146.
13. Carruthers A, Carruthers J. Upper face treatment. In: Carruthers A, Carruthers J, eds. *Procedures in Cosmetic Dermatology.* Philadelphia: Elsevier Saunders; 2005:31-44.
14. Carruthers J, Carruthers A. Botulinum toxin type A treatment of multiple upper facial sites: patient-reported outcomes. *Dermatol Surg.* 2007;33(suppl 1): S10-S17.
15. Sarifakioglu N, Sarifakioglu E. Evaluating effects of preservative-containing saline solution on pain perception during botulinum toxin type-A injections at different locations: a prospective, single-blinded, randomized controlled trial. *Aesth Plast Surg.* 2005;29:113-115.
16. Alam M, Dover J, Arndt K. Pain associated with injection of botulinum A exotoxin reconstituted using isotonic sodium chloride with and without preservative: a double-blind, randomized controlled trial. *Arch Dermatol.* 2002;138:510-514.
17. Carruthers A, Carruthers J, Cohen J. Dilution volume of botulinum toxin type A for the treatment of glabellar rhytides. *Dermatol Surg.* 2007;33:S97-104.
18. Flynn T, Carruthers A, Carruthers J. Surgical pearl: the use of the Ultra-Fine II short needle 0.3-cc insulin syringe for botulinum toxin injections. *J Am Acad Dermatol.* 2002;46:931-933.
19. Carruthers A, Carruthers J. Single-center, double-blind, randomized study to evaluate the efficacy of 4% lidocaine cream versus vehicle cream during botulinum toxin type A treatments. *Dermatol Surg.* 2005;31:1655-1659.
20. Carruthers J, Lowe NJ, Menter M, Gibson J, Nordquist M, Morgaunt J, et al. A multicenter, double-blind, randomized, placebo-controlled study of the efficacy and safety of botulinum toxin type A in the treatment of glabellar lines. *J Am Acad Dermatol.* 2002;46:840-849.
21. Carruthers A, Carruthers J, Said S. Dose-ranging study of botulinum toxin type A in the treatment of glabellar rhytids in females. *Dermatol Surg.* 2005;31:414-422; discussion 422.
22. Carruthers J, Lowe NJ, Menter M, Gibson J, Eadie N, BOTOX Glabellar Lines II Study Group. Double-blind, placebo-controlled study of the safety and efficacy of botulinum toxin type A for patients with glabellar lines. *Plast Reconstr Surg.* 2003;112:1089-1098.
23. Carruthers A, Carruthers J. Prospective, double-blind, randomized, parallel-group, dose-ranging study of botulinum toxin type A in men with glabellar rhytids. *Dermatol Surg.* 2005;31:1297-1303.
24. Monheit GD, Carruthers A, Brandt F, Rand R. A randomized, double-blind, placebo-controlled study of botulinum toxin type A for the treatment of glabellar lines: determination of optimal dose. *Dermatol Surg.* 2007;33:S51-59.
25. Rzany BD, Ascher B, Fratila A, Monheit GD, Talarico S, Sterry W. Efficacy and safety of 3- and 5-injection patterns (30 and 50 U) of botulinum toxin A (Dysport) for the treatment of wrinkles in the glabella and the central forehead region. *Arch Dermatol.* 2006;142:320-326.
26. Carruthers A, Carruthers J. Eyebrow height after botulinum toxin type A to the glabella. *Dermatol Surg.* 2007;33:S26-S31.
27. Petrus G, Lewis D, Maas CS. Anatomic considerations for treatment with botulinum toxin. *Facial Plast Surg Clin North Am.* 2007;15:1-9.
28. Semchyshyn N, Sengelmann R. Botulinum toxin A treatment of perioral rhytides. *Dermatol Surg.* 2003;29:490-495.
29. Dayan S, Maas C. Botulinum toxins for facial wrinkles: beyond glabellar lines. *Facial Plast Surg Clin North Am.* 2008;15:41-49.
30. Carruthers J, Carruthers A. Periorbital area. In: Carruthers A, Carruthers J, eds. *Using Botulinum Toxins Cosmetically.* United Kingdom: Martin Dunitz Publishing; 2003:39-44.

31. Kane M. The effect of botulinum toxin injections on the nasolabial fold. *Plast Reconstr Surg.* 2003;112(Suppl 5):66S-72S.

32. Brandt F, Boker A. Botulinum toxin for the treatment of neck lines and neck bands. *Dermatol Clin.* 2004;22:159-166.

33. Matarasso A, Matarasso S, Brandt F, Bellman B. Botulinum A exotoxin for the management of platysma bands. *Plast Reconstr Surg.* 1999;103:645-652- (discussion 653-655).

34. Choe SW, Cho WI, Lee CK, Seo SJ. Effects of botulinum toxin type A on contouring of the lower face. *Dermatol Surg.* 2005;31:502-507 (discussion 507-508).

35. To EW, Ahuja AT, Ho WS, King WW, Wong WK, Pang PC, et al. A prospective study of the effect of botulinum toxin A on masseteric muscle hypertrophy with ultrasonographic and electromyographic measurement. *Br J Plast Surg.* 2001;54:197-200.

36. Kim NH, Chung J, Park RH, Park JB. The use of botulinum toxin type A in aesthetic mandibular contouring. *Plast Reconst Surg.* 2005;115:919-930.

37. Carruthers J, Carruthers A. Complications of botulinum toxin type A. *Facial Plast Surg Clin North Am.* 2007;15:51-54.

38. van Laborde S, Dover J, Moore M, Stewart B, Arndt K, Alam M. Reduction in injection pain with botulinum toxin type B further diluted using saline with preservative: A double-blind, randomized controlled trial. *J Am Acad Dermatol.* 2003;48:875-877.

39. Sami M, Soparkar C, Patrinely J, Hollier LM, Hollier LH. Efficacy of botulinum toxin type A after topical anesthesia. *Ophthal Plast Reconstr Surg.* 2006;22: 448-452.

40. Elibol O, Ozkan B, Hekimhan P, Caglar Y. Efficacy of skin cooling and EMLA cream application for pain relief of periocular botulinum toxin injection. *Ophthal Plast Reconstr Surg.* 2007;23:130-133.

41. Krishtul A, Waldorf H, Blitzer A. Complications of cosmetic botulinum toxin therapy. In: Carruthers A, Carruthers J, eds. *Procedures in Cosmetic Dermatology: Botulinum Toxin.* Philadelphia: Elsevier Saunders; 2005:121-132.

42. Flynn T, Clark R 2nd. Botulinum toxin type B (MYOBLOC) versus botulinum toxin type A (BOTOX) frontalis study: rate of onset and radius of diffusion. *Dermatol Surg.* 2003;29:519-522.

43. Trindade de Almeida A, Marques E, De Almeida J, Cunha T, Boraso R. Pilot study comparing the diffusion of two formulations of botulinum toxin type A in patients with forehead hyperhidrosis. *Dermatol Surg.* 2007;33:S37-S43.

44. Hsu T, Dover J, Arndt K. Effect of volume and concentration on the diffusion of botulinum exotoxin A. *Arch Dermatol.* 2004;140:1351-1354.

45. Northington M, Huang C. Dry eyes and superficial punctate keratitis: a complication of treatment of glabelar dynamic rhytides with botulinum exotoxin A. *Dermatol Surg.* 2004;30:1515-1517.

46. Matarasso S. Decreased tear expression with an abnormal Schirmer's test following botulinum toxin type A for the treatment of lateral canthal rhytids. *Dermatol Surg.* 2002;28:149-152.

47. Prado A, Fuentes P, Guerra C, Leniz P, Wisnia P. Pseudoaneurysm of the frontal branch of the superficial temporal artery: an unusual complication after the injection of botox. *Plast Reconstr Surg.* 2007;119: 2334-2335.

48. Cote T, Mohan A, Polder J, Walton MK, Braun MM. Botulinum toxin type A injections: adverse events reported to the US Food and Drug Administration in therapeutic and cosmetic cases. *J Am Acad Dermatol.* 2005;53:407-415.

49. White L, Tanzi E, Alster T. Improving patient retention after botulinum toxin type A treatment. *Dermatol Surg.* 2006;32:212-215.

The Role of Botulinum **27** Toxin in Wound Healing

Holger G. Gassner, David A. Sherris, Kris S. Moe, and Oren Friedman

INTRODUCTION

A visible facial scar may have numerous social and psychological implications for the affected individual, generating a range of social, professional, and psychological problems. Naturally, the creation of a surgical scar is one of the patient's central concerns associated with surgical therapy. Over the past 2 decades, the desire for smaller and less conspicuous scars has driven a notable trend toward less invasive surgical techniques. The introduction of endoscopes has resulted in a substantial reduction of incisions for various surgical procedures ranging from face lifts to thyroidectomies. Nevertheless, a number of procedures still require placement of incisions in visible areas. Moreover, traumatic wounds are frequently located in exposed facial areas. Hence, surgeons continue seeking to enhance the healing of skin wounds and lacerations, and render the resulting scars as cosmetically favorable as possible. A large number of factors have been identified that can affect wound healing positively and negatively. Ideal healing without scar is observed in the fetus but, unfortunately, has never been achieved in humans after birth.[1]

A good understanding of the healing process is crucial to understanding the potential interventions that optimize the appearance of the wound as it progresses through the healing phases. The first inflammatory phase of wound healing is characterized by vasodilatation and cellular response. This phase lasts on the order of days and is prolonged by inflammatory stimuli, most importantly, infectious agents. Thorough irrigation, aseptic technique, and if indicated, the use of topical and systemic antibiotics can contribute to limiting the duration of this phase with its associated inflammatory response. The second proliferative phase of wound healing is marked by re-epithelialization and collagen synthesis. This phase typically lasts weeks and overlaps with the inflammatory phase. Epithelial regeneration is greatly enhanced in wounds closing by primary intention, whereas wounds healing by secondary intention take substantially longer for this process. It has been conclusively shown that epithelial regeneration is also enhanced in a moist environment, and the use of occlusive and semiocclusive dressings has become well established clinical practice until epithelialization is complete. The final stage of wound healing is characterized by the maturation of the scar, which becomes finer and less erythematous, and its collagen content more organized. Avoidance of sun exposure and mechanical irritation should be continued through this phase to minimize scar hypertrophy and untoward pigmentary changes.[2-6]

In clinical practice, measures routinely employed to allow for favorable healing include addressing contamination of the wound, minimizing reactive suture material, performing quality closure, applying occlusive or semiocclusive dressings, avoiding sun exposure, and correcting nutritional deficiencies and systemic metabolic pathologies.[7,8] An even more important factor adversely affecting all phases of healing is tension acting on the wound. Tension exacerbates inflammation,

Dr. Gassner and Dr. Sherris are disclosing that Mayo Medical Ventures has applied for intellectual property on the presented method. The authors have no current or pending financial or other commercial agreement with any company in place at the time of the submission of this manuscript. Dr. Moe and Dr. Friedman have not reported any conflicts of interest.

leads to increased collagen synthesis and deposition of glycosaminoglycans, and prolongs erythema. Even in the presence of otherwise ideal circumstances for wound healing, tension will invariably render scars wider and, frequently, hypertrophic.[9] Tension on healing wounds can be classified as static and dynamic. Static tension is determined by the location, shape and size of the wound, the closure technique, and the inherent biomechanical properties of the healing skin. Studies by Larrabee et al[10,11] have provided us with important insights into the biomechanical characteristics of skin and their surgical implications. Based on these studies, numerous operative techniques have been modified and refined with the goal of minimizing the effects of static tension on healing wounds. These techniques include wide undermining, multilayered closure techniques, local flaps, external dressings, and stenting devices.

DYNAMIC TENSION

Dynamic tension, on the other hand, is exerted on the healing wound by the activity of the underlying musculature. In modern times, the importance of dynamic tension first became evident in the beginning of the 19th century, when Jules Cloquet reported that it is the contraction of the underlying musculature that creates ridges in the skin.[12] Guillaume Dupuytren observed that circular cutaneous wounds inflicted with a round awl eventuate in linear clefts.[13] Using a similar technique, Karl Langer, a Viennese professor of anatomy, created a map of natural cutaneous lines in cadavers.[14] The modern concept of the relaxed skin tension lines (RSTLs) advances Langers' works. The RSTLs are lines that have become inherent to the skin, mainly as a result of repetitive tension of the underlying musculature. In general, RSTLs coincide with wrinkle lines and lie perpendicular to the tension vector of the muscular contraction. Scars aligned with RSTLs are subject to reduced dynamic tension and heal well, whereas scars oriented at obtuse angles with the RSTLs are subject to repetitive tension and distortion and are more prone to scar hypertrophy.[15,16] Surgical techniques including various Z-plasties have been designed to change the direction of wounds and realign them with the RSTLs, thus reducing the effects of dynamic tension on the healing wound. The concept of eliminating rather than reducing or circumventing the effects of muscular activity

on the healing wound has been introduced more recently. With the advent of intramuscular botulinum toxin therapy, it has become possible to paralyze striated muscles with good accuracy and minimal morbidity.

The use of botulinum toxin to eliminate the effects of dynamic tension on the healing wound has been tested in a number of studies. Initial data from a primate model were reported at the Mayo Clinic. Under general anaesthesia, standardized excisions were performed on the foreheads of macaque monkeys in a symmetric fashion. One set of excisions was separated from the other by the midline. The sides of the forehead were randomized to saline versus botulinum toxin injection, and the experimental side was injected with a total of 21 U of botulinum toxin A (Botox, Allergan, Inc, Irvine, CA), 7 U for each of three excisional wounds. Cosmetic closure was performed by a facial plastic surgeon blinded to the randomization scheme. Complete immobilization of the experimental side was observed 72 hours after the procedure (Fig. 27-1). A panel of three facial plastic surgeons evaluated the appearance of the scars 3 months after surgery, using a standardized Visual Analog Scale. The appearance of the pharmacologically immobilized wounds was rated significantly more favorable than the control wounds. The animals were not sacrificed for this study, and the resulting data formed the basis for human use and clinical trials.[17]

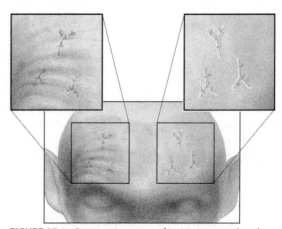

FIGURE 27-1. Symmetric groups of incisions were placed on the primate's forehead and randomized to botulinum toxin injection versus saline injection. Immobilization was complete 1 week postoperatively on the experimental side, and the treated wounds healed with less visible scars.

CASE STUDY OF A FOREHEAD INJURY

As detailed in the literature and highlighted in other sections of this volume, a substantial number of clinical uses of botulinum toxin have been developed from off-label trials.[18] Based on the favorable outcome of the randomized, prospective primate study, chemoimmobilization of traumatic and incisional wounds was offered to patients deemed to be excellent candidates for this treatment,[19] including the following case description of a healthy 17-year-old girl who was involved in a motor vehicle accident. She presented with extensive, complex, traumatic lacerations across her forehead and nose, as well as exposure of the frontal bone. The right upper eyelid was transected along the supratarsal crease, approximately to the midpupillary line (Fig. 27-2). After copious irrigation and minimal débridement under general anesthesia, a total of 40 U of botulinum toxin A was injected into the frontalis, procerus, and corrugator muscles. The right upper lid was spared to prevent lagophthalmos. The wounds were closed in layers using 6-0 Ethilon for skin, 4-0 Vicryl for subcutaneous closure, and 4-0 polydioxanone sutures for muscle (Ethicon, Somerville, NJ; Fig. 27-3). Six days after surgery, her forehead showed complete paralysis, but eyelid movement was not affected. Healing was uncomplicated, and 1 year later, the patient demonstrated better-healed scars over the immobilized parts of the wound (forehead) than over the nonimmobilized part (i.e., the eyelid; Figs. 27-4 and 27-5).

CLINICAL TRIAL

This case represents the body of anecdotal evidence in humans that accumulated at the Mayo Clinic after the macaque monkey study, and it led to the initiation of a prospective, randomized protocol to objectively quantify the potential beneficial effects of chemoimmobilization on human facial wound healing.[20]

Wounds limited to the forehead were to be studied, because animal and preliminary human data were available for this area. In order to make the results of the trial applicable to the routine clinical setting, wound care and closure technique were performed within the variations of usual clinical practice. Criteria for enrollment included randomly selected

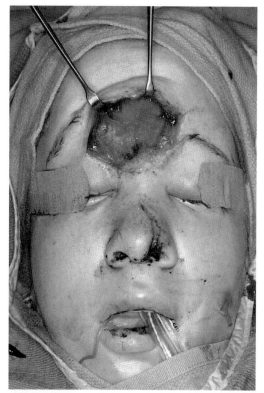

FIGURE 27-2. A 17-year-old patient sustained a complex forehead laceration in a motor vehicle accident. The cut extended through the upper eyelid to the midpupillary line. (From Gassner HG, Sherris DA. Chemoimmobilization: improving predictability in the treatment of facial scars. *Plast Reconstr Surg.* 2003;112:1464-1466.)

patients 18 years and older, who presented to the emergency room with traumatic forehead lacerations, as well as patients undergoing elective excision of cutaneous neoplasms of the forehead. Patients with traumatic forehead lacerations underwent primary closure in the emergency department and were referred to the division of facial plastic surgery for injection of saline or botulinum toxin A according to a predetermined randomized protocol prepared by the department of statistics and implemented through coded vials by the department of pharmacology. Patients undergoing elective excisions of the forehead for removal of skin neoplasms were injected according to the same protocol and randomization method. Close-up photographs were obtained at the time of wound closure and 6 months after wound closure.

After completion of the study, two experienced facial surgeons were asked to assess the photographs in an independent and blinded fashion. In order to limit systematic interrater

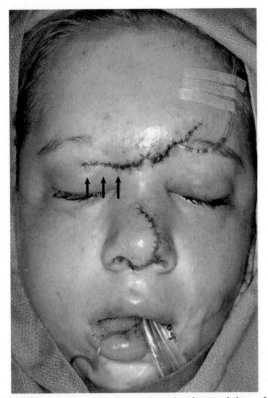

FIGURE 27-3. The wound was injected with a total dose of 40 U of botulinum toxin A (Botox). The injection spared the upper eyelid to avoid post-treatment lagophthalmos (*arrows*). The wound was closed in layers using plastic surgical technique. (Modified from Gassner HG, Sherris DA. Chemoimmobilization: improving predictability in the treatment of facial scars. *Plast Reconstr Surg.* 2003;112:1464-1466.)

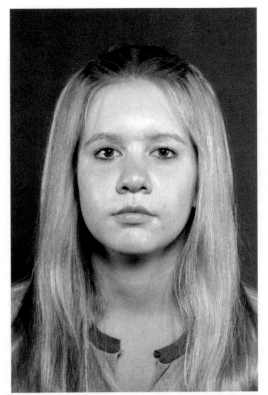

FIGURE 27-4. Appearance of the scar 1 year after surgery.

discordance, these observers were asked to score the first patient together. Considering the condition of the wound at closure and at 6 months, the observers were asked to rate the final cosmetic outcome on a 10-cm Visual Analog Scale.

The Visual Analog Scale results, based on the average of the two physician ratings for each patient, were analyzed. The overall median Visual Analog Scale score for the botulinum-toxin treated group was 8.9, compared with 7.2 for the group treated with normal saline. Based on independent, blinded statistical analysis, this difference was highly significant ($P = 0.003$) and, reflecting clinical experience and observations in the animal model, clinically relevant. Figure 27-6A depicts a representative experimental wound, which was treated with 15 U botulinum toxin (Botox), Figure 27-6B shows the resulting scar 6 months later. Figure 27-7A and B shows a placebo (an equal

volume of saline was injected) control wound at the same intervals.[21]

The reports of favorable outcome data, the remarkable safety profile, and the long-term experiences with facial injections of botulinum

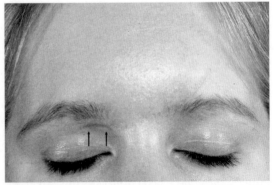

FIGURE 27-5. Close-up photograph reveals hyperpigmentation and more hypertrophic scarring over the nonimmobilized aspect of the scar (*arrows*). (From Gassner HG, Sherris DA. Chemoimmobilization: improving predictability in the treatment of facial scars. *Plast Reconstr Surg.* 2003;112:1464-1466.)

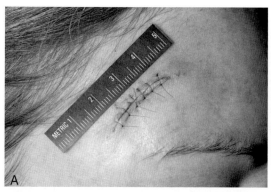 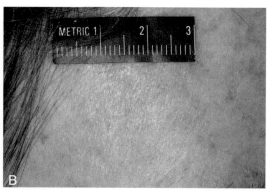

FIGURE 27-6. A, Forty-six-year-old white woman enrolled in a prospective, randomized, placebo-controlled trial underwent excision of a basal cell carcinoma of the right lateral forehead. Postoperative excisional size was 1.0 cm by 0.6 cm. Fifteen units of botulinum toxin were injected, and layered closure was performed with 5-0 Monocryl subcutaneous and 6-0 Nylon simple running sutures. **B,** The resulting scar 6 months after botulinum toxin treatment displays good color match and no hypertrophy or inversion. (**A** and **B** from Gassner HG, Brissett AE, Otley CC, Boahene DK, Boggust AJ, Weaver AL, et al. Botulinum toxin to improve facial wound healing: a prospective, blinded, placebo-controlled study. *Mayo Clin Proc.* 2006;81:1023-1028.)

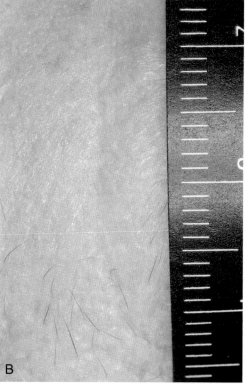

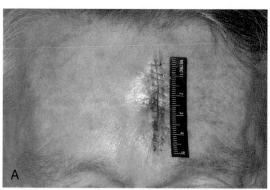

FIGURE 27-7. A, Forty-year-old white woman underwent excision of a cellular neurothekeoma of the central forehead. Postoperative excisional size was 1.0 cm by 0.9 cm. Three milliliters of the placebo medication (1% lidocaine with 1:100,000 epinephrine) were injected, and layered wound closure was performed with 5-0 Monocryl and 6-0 running nylon suture. **B,** The resulting scar at 6 months after placebo treatment shows notable widening and inversion. (From Gassner HG, Brissett AE, Otley CC, Boahene DK, Boggust AJ, Weaver AL, et al. Botulinum toxin to improve facial wound healing: a prospective, blinded, placebo-controlled study. *Mayo Clin Proc.* 2006;81:1023-1028.)

toxin are factors likely contributing to the increasing and widespread acceptance of chemoimmobilization for the treatment of cutaneous scars. Numerous academic centers in the United States, Europe, and Africa have now reported on their experience in the literature. These reports have largely focused on the treatment of forehead and periorbital wounds.[22-26] The forehead is a particularly favorable area to treat because the risk of inducing temporary functional deficits is low. The injection techniques for the forehead are derived from widespread experience with cosmetic injections. In recent years, the indications for treating facial lines and wrinkles have been extended beyond the forehead to include the periorbital and perioral region, as described in Chapter 26.

CASE STUDY OF AN INJURY TO THE LOWER FACE

Analagous to the progression of cosmetic indications in the lower face, treatment of wound healing in the lower third of the face with botulinum toxin has been reported recently.[27] Important functions of the perioral musculature include facial expression, oral closure, and articulation. These functions may be compromised with injection of botulinum toxin. Therefore, transient functional deficits may be anticipated with immobilization of perioral wounds. The perceived risk of inducing such functional deficits may explain the relatively late emergence of reports on perioral and lower facial wound immobilization.

The following case illustrates important aspects of the treatment of lower facial wounds as it differs from the treatment of forehead wounds. A 2-year-old white male sustained a crush injury to the lower lip from a fall. The resulting irregular defect involved the vermillion border. Near complete transection of the orbicularis oris muscle was observed (Fig. 27-8). Under general anesthesia, the orbicularis oris muscle was reapproximated with simple 4-0 Vicryl sutures. The remaining soft tissues were repaired with 5-0 Vicryl sutures, and the epithelium was closed with 6-0 Monocryl simple vertical mattress sutures (Fig. 27-9). The parents had been counseled about risks of transient functional deficits and benefits of reduced tension on the healing wound. Immobilization of the lower lip was requested. A solution of 100 U of botulinum

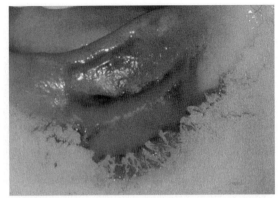

FIGURE 27-8. Two-year-old white boy sustained a crush injury to the lower lip. Near complete transection of the orbicularis oris, vestibular mucosa, and vermillion border was observed.

toxin A (Botox) per 5 mL 1% lidocaine with 1:100,000 epinephrine was injected into the orbicularis oris muscle. This required a total of 10 U of botulinum toxin A. Flaccid paralysis of the injected portion of the lower lip was observed and closely resembled the degree of paralysis predicted by the injection of the local anesthetic agent. The parents were advised to keep the wound moist with petroleum jelly for 10 days. For approximately 6 weeks, mildly reduced oral sphincter tension was observed. Oral competence and sphincter function were not compromised. The eventual cosmetic appearance of the scar is depicted in Figure 27-10A and 10B.

This case illustrates the usefulness of reconstituting botulinum toxin A in a solution of 1% lidocaine with 1:100,000 epinephrine for areas difficult to inject. The simultaneous injection of local anesthetic results in immediate paralysis

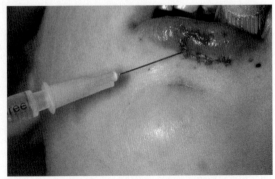

FIGURE 27-9. The wound was closed in layers using 4-0 Vicryl, 5-0 Vicryl, and 6-0 Monocryl (Ethicon, Somerville, NY) sutures using facial plastic technique and loupe magnification.

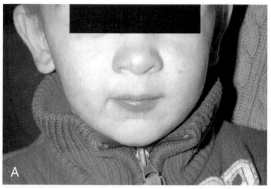
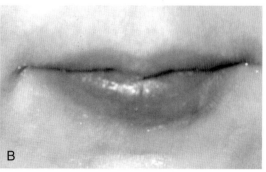

FIGURE 27-10. **A** and **B,** Six months after surgical closure and botulinum toxin A–induced chemoimmobilization of the wound, the resulting scar is barely perceptible.

of the treated muscle. The degree of immediate paralysis has been shown to be predictive of the delayed paralysis resulting from botulinum toxin.[28] This method is particularly useful in nonstandard applications such as treatment of perioral wounds or treatment of the contralateral face in facial paralysis, where the appropriate dosage of botulinum toxin needed for the desired effect is difficult to predict. Published data on this method have described the admixture of 5 mL of 1% lidocaine with 1:100,000 epinephrine and 100 U of botulinum toxin A (Botox).[28] This concentration is suitable for many applications, although higher concentrations on the order of 2 mL per 100 U of botulinum toxin A are more appropriate in cosmetic applications and for the treatment of smaller muscle groups. For these applications, the authors have used a combination of 2 mL 2% lidocaine with 1:100,000 epinephrine per 100 U of botulinum toxin A (Botox). Although the authors have not noted untoward side effects with the use of this formulation, we stress that the patient must be appropriately advised of the off-label use of this formulation. The method is very helpful in difficult cases, including patients with facial paralysis and contralateral compensatory contraction.[29]

OTHER USES FOR BOTULINUM TOXIN IN WOUND HEALING

The application of botulinum toxin to enhance wound healing has been further advanced by Tollefson et al[30] to include its adjunctive use in cleft lip repair. Repair of cleft lip deformities requires meticulous attention to recreating the 3-dimensional characteristics of the lip and nasal structures by re-establishing muscular continuity. An important factor influencing the final result of the cleft lip repair is the amount of wound tension present during healing. Too much tension may result in unacceptably wide scars. In infants between 3 and 6 months of age, the authors inject the denervating agent 1 week before the cleft repair in order to achieve complete flaccid paralysis at the time of surgery. As discussed for the treatment of perioral wounds, temporary compromise of oral sphincter competence must be considered when injecting the orbicularis oris and surrounding musculature. Fortunately, for cleft lip repair, this is less of a factor because these infants start with substantial oral incompetence before surgery. Oral competence is greatly enhanced by the anatomic closure of the cleft, and will further improve as muscle function gradually returns during the ensuing weeks after surgery. Figure 27-11A to C depict a 6-month-old infant with a wide bilateral cleft lip and nasal deformity treated by Tollefson et al.

Similar to broad dosing practice for spasticity in pediatric patients, dosage of botulinum toxin must be highly individualized when injecting facial wounds and lacerations in children. The authors have successfully treated traumatic lacerations including dog bites in children. It is advised that botulinum toxin be available in urgent and emergent care settings to allow for injection at the time of closure of lacerations for both adult and pediatric patients in order to avoid the trauma of a repeat needle stick in the immediate postoperative period.

The status of tetanus immunization should be considered before injection in both the pediatric and the adult population. Important considerations regarding possible simultaneous tetanus vaccination and botulinum toxin therapy are discussed in Chapter 34.

Advancing the use of botulinum toxin in wound healing even further, Moe and colleagues have reported on chemodenervation of the mastication musculature for the treatment of facial fractures.[31] Mandibular fractures are classified as favorable and unfavorable, depending on the vectors of tension acting on the fracture. Favorable fractures tend to get compressed by the action of mastication muscles and generally require conservative or less invasive treatment. Unfavorable fractures are distracted or displaced by the action of the inserting musculature and typically require open reduction with extensive fixation.[32] Midfacial fractures are subject to similar mechanisms, most importantly, fractures of the zygomaticomaxillary complex. The zygomatic arch, origin of the masseter muscle, is subject to massive downward traction by masseter contraction. Hence, zygomaticomaxillary complex fractures usually require internal plate fixation to prevent displacement after successful open reduction. It has been shown that the postoperative complication rate after facial fracture repair increases with the number and thickness of fixation plates that have been used. Adjunctive measures that reduce the number and volume of internal fixation devices required for facial fracture repair, therefore, may reduce the rate of associated complications.

The following case illustrates the use of botulinum toxin as an adjunct to facial fracture repair. A white man sustained a displaced right zygomaticomaxillary complex and orbital floor fracture in an altercation. The patient was taken to the operating room. A stab incision was placed in the cheek skin and an orthopedic bone hook was placed under the zygomatic arch to allow reduction of the fracture, as confirmed by intraoperative computed tomography scanning. A total dose of 100 U of botulinum toxin A (Botox) was then injected into the masseter muscle, and no plate fixation was performed. The orbital floor defect was approached through a transconjunctival incision and repaired with a porous polyethylene (Medpor, Porex Surgical Products Group, Newnan, GA) implant, resulting in correction

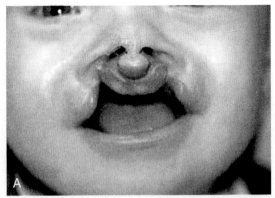
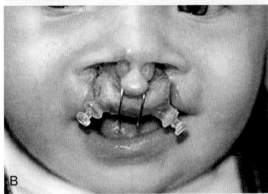
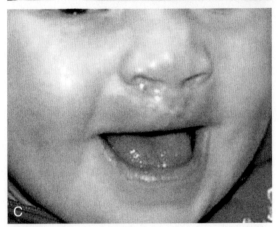

FIGURE 27-11. A to **C,** Six-month-old infant with a wide bilateral cleft lip and nasal deformity. **A,** Appearance after 3 months of presurgical nasoalveolar molding, columellar lengthening, and lip taping. **B,** Appliance in place before injection of 5 U of botulinum toxin into the orbicularis oris at the cleft margins and nasal base. **C,** Three-month postoperative view. (From Tollefson TT, Senders CM, Sykes JM, Byorth PJ. Botulinum toxin to improve results in cleft lip repair. *Arch Facial Plast Surg.* 2006;8:221-222.)

of enophthalmos and hypoglobus. The patient was kept on a soft diet for 4 weeks and healing was uneventful. At 11 months follow-up, the patient presented with normal facial symmetry, midfacial height, smooth orbital contour, and unrestricted jaw mobility.

CONCLUSION

The concept of immobilization in medicine is ancient and firmly established for the treatment of fractures, and tendon and soft tissue injuries. A variety of devices have been developed for this purpose: splints, casts, dressings, wires, screws, internal and external fixators, and others. These devices share a common objective: To minimize the effect of muscular contraction on healing tissues. Therefore, the objective of botulinum toxin injections in wound healing, namely, to eliminate unwanted muscle contractions rather than merely to minimize their effects, is a more definitive treatment concept. The method of injecting facial wounds with botulinum toxin for the purpose of improving the cosmetic appearance of the resulting scar has been introduced and studied in the past decade. Promising experimental data and anecdotal human data have prompted the conduct of a randomized, placebo-controlled study that demonstrated facial wound injection with botulinum toxin to be effective. These data were followed by numerous reports from many institutions describing the application of botulinum toxin in larger series, different sites, and other pathologies, including facial fracture and cleft lip repair. No permanent untoward side effects or complications have occurred in the authors' long-term experience or have been reported in the growing body of peer-reviewed literature in both the adult and the pediatric patient population. Minor temporary deficits should be regarded as a side effect associated with the treatment rather than a complication. These may include brow ptosis, dynamic facial asymmetry, and reduced oral sphincter function. Patients are informed about these predictable temporary deficits, typically accept them, and frequently choose aggressive immobilization in order to maximize the treatment effect. In light of the favorable risk to benefit ratio of this therapy, the authors recommend the use of botulinum toxin injections for the treatment of facial wounds in selected patients who are concerned with the eventual appearance of a resulting scar. Wounds located in functionally sensitive areas such as the periorbital and perioral regions should be injected by physicians who have long-standing experience with facial botulinum toxin injections.

References

1. Hantash BM, Zhao L, Knowles JA, Lorenz HP. Adult and fetal wound healing. *Front Biosci.* 2008;13:51-61.
2. Singer AJ, Clark RA., Cutaneous wound healing. *N Engl J Med.* 1999;341:738-744
3. Woodley DT, Chen JD, Kim JP, Sarret Y, Iwasaki T, Kim YH, et al. Re-epithelialization. Human keratinocyte locomotion. *Dermatol Clin.* 1993;11:641-646.
4. Clark RAF, ed. *The Molecular and Cellular Biology of Wound Repair.* 2nd ed. New York: Plenum Press; 1996.
5. Leibovich SJ, Ross R. The role of the macrophage in wound repair: a study with hydrocortisone and anti-macrophage serum. *Am J Pathol.* 1975;78:71-100.
6. Hunt TK, ed. *Wound Healing and Wound Infection: Theory and Surgical Practice.* New York: Appleton-Century-Crofts; 1980.
7. Due E, Rossen K, Sorensen LT, Kliem A, Karlsmark T, Haedersdal M. Effect of UV irradiation on cutaneous cicatrices: a randomized, controlled trial with clinical, skin reflectance, histological, immunohistochemical and biochemical evaluations. *Acta Derm Venereol.* 2007;87:27-32.
8. Mandal A. Do malnutrition and nutritional supplementation have an effect on the wound healing process. *J Wound Care.* 2006;15:254-257.
9. Sherris DA, Larrabee WF Jr, Murakami CS. Management of scar contractures, hypertrophic scars and keloids. *Otolaryngol Clin North Am.* 1995;28:1057.
10. Larrabee WF Jr, Sutton D. The biomechanics of advancement and rotation flaps. *Laryngoscope.* 1981;91:726-734.
11. Larrabee WF Jr, Trachy R, Sutton D, Cox K. Rhomboid flap dynamics. *Arch Otolaryngol.* 1981;107:755-757.
12. Cloquet JH. *Traité d'Anatomie Descriptive.* Paris: Libraire de Crochard; 1832:313.
13. Dupuytren G: *Traité Théorique et Pratique des. Armes de Guerre.* Vol.2. Paris: Baillère; 1834:60-66.
14. Langer K. On the anatomy and physiology of the skin: I. The cleavability of the skin. *Br J Plast Surg.* 1978;31:3.
15. Larrabee WF Jr, Sherris DA: *Principles of Facial Reconstruction,* Philadelphia: Lippincott-Raven; 1995:7.
16. McCarthy JG: Plastic Surgery. Philadelphia: WB Saunders; 1990:43-44.
17. Gassner HG, Sherris DA, Otley CC. Treatment of facial wounds with botulinum toxin A improves cosmetic outcome in primates. *Plast Reconstr Surg.* 2000;105:1948-1953; discussion 1954-1955.
18. Lee C, Kikkawa D, Pasco N, Granet D. Advanced functional oculofacial indications of botulinum toxin. *Int Ophthalmol Clin.* 2005;45:77-91.
19. Sherris DA, Gassner HG. Botulinum toxin to minimize facial scarring. *Facial Plast Surg.* 2002;18:35-39.
20. Gassner HG, Sherris DA. Chemoimmobilization: improving predictability in the treatment of facial scars. *Plast Reconstr Surg.* 2003;112:1464-1466.
21. Gassner HG, Brissett AE, Otley CC, Boahene DK, Boggust AJ, Weaver AL, et al. Botulinum toxin to improve facial wound healing: A prospective, blinded, placebo-controlled study. *Mayo Clin Proc.* 2006;81:1023-1028.

22. Zimbler MS, Holds JB, Kokoska MS, Glaser DA, Prendiville S, Hollenbeak CS, et al. Effect of botulinum toxin pretreatment on laser resurfacing results: A prospective, randomized, blinded trial. *Arch Facial Plast Surg.* 2001;3:165-169.

23. Bansal C, Omlin K, Hayes C, Rohrer T. Novel cutaneous uses for botulinum toxin type A. *J Cosmet Dermatol.* 2006;5:268-272.

24. Wilson AM. Use of botulinum toxin type A to prevent widening of facial scars. *Plast Recon Surg.* 2006;117:1758.

25. Mann WJ (University of Mainz, Germany), personal communication, March 2007.

26. Laskawi R. Botulinum toxin treatment in the head and neck region: current aspects, developments, and problems. *HNO.* 2007;55:437-442.

27. Gassner HG, Friedman O, Sherris DA. Botulinum toxin A induced immobilization of perioral wounds. *Arch Facial Plast Surg.* 2008. In press.

28. Gassner HG, Sherris DA. Addition of an anesthetic agent to enhance the predictability of the effects of botulinum toxin type A injections: a randomized controlled study. *Mayo Clin Proc.* 2000;75:701-704.

29. Gassner HG, Moe KS: Injuries of the facial nerve. In: Eisele D, ed. *Complications of Head and Neck Surgery.* 3rd ed. St. Louis: Mosby-Year Book. 2008.

30. Tollefson TT, Senders CM, Sykes JM, Byorth PJ. Botulinum toxin to improve results in cleft lip repair. *Arch Facial Plast Surg.* 2006;8:221-222.

31. Moe KS. Personal communication.

32. Champy M, Lodde JP, Jaeger JH, Wilk A. Mandibular osteosynthesis according to the Michelet technique. I. Biomechanical bases. *Rev Stomatol Chir Maxillofac.* 1976;77:569-576.

Understanding Botulinum Neurotoxin Mechanism of Action and Structure to Enhance Therapeutics and Improve Care

28

Keith A. Foster, Emily J. Adams, and Duncan F. Rogers

INTRODUCTION

Botulinum neurotoxins inhibit the release of neurotransmitters from neurons, particularly the release of acetylcholine from peripheral cholinergic nerves, by proteolytic cleavage of specific proteins essential to vesicle fusion and secretion. In the past 3 decades, botulinum neurotoxins have been established as a highly effective therapeutic option for the treatment of a range of neuromuscular and other hyperactivity disorders involving peripheral cholinergic neurotransmission. One of the key features of the neurotoxins' clinical success has been their prolonged duration of activity. Therapeutics that maintain clinical benefit for extended periods of time are particularly advantageous for people suffering from chronic conditions, because they reduce the frequency with which treatment needs to be administered. The use of botulinum neurotoxins for the treatment of chronic diseases is, however, limited both by the neuronal specificity of the toxins and by their extreme toxicity. Based on an understanding of the structural basis of neurotoxin function, it has been possible to design and create recombinant proteins that harness the pharmacologic activity of botulinum neurotoxins, retaining the high potency and long duration of action of the native bacterial

enzymes, while targeting a wider range of cell types. This has enabled the development of therapeutic proteins suitable for treatment of chronic diseases involving secretory processes other than cholinergic neurotransmission. This approach has been exemplified for a number of different secretory cell types, both neuronal and non-neuronal. The initial demonstration of the therapeutic potential of this approach was for inhibition of nociceptive neurotransmission in chronic pain. Non-neuronal use of the technology has been demonstrated for both secretion of hormone from endocrine tumor cells and for mucus release from respiratory epithelial cells. By inhibiting secretion from these target cell types with high levels of biochemical specificity, these novel recombinant proteins have the potential to act as effective therapeutics for the treatment of chronic pain, endocrine disorders, and chronic respiratory conditions such as cystic fibrosis and chronic obstructive pulmonary disease.

Botulinum neurotoxins (BoNTs), together with the other clostridial neurotoxin, tetanus toxin (TeNT), are zinc-dependent metalloproteases that inhibit neurosecretion by highly selective proteolytic cleavage of one of three proteins, the soluble *N*-ethylmaleimide-sensitive factor attachment protein receptor

Dr. Foster is disclosing that he is a founding officer and shareholder in Syntaxin Ltd., Abingdon, UK. Dr. Adams does not report any conflicts of interest. Dr. Rogers is disclosing that he has acted as a consultant for Syntaxin Ltd, Abingdon, UK.

(SNARE) proteins: syntaxin, synaptosomal protein of 25 kDa (SNAP-25) and vesicle-associated membrane protein (VAMP).[1,2] There are seven immunologically distinct serotypes of botulinum neurotoxin, identified as A to G (BoNT/A to BoNT/G). Each of the BoNT serotypes, with the exception of BoNT/C, cleaves just one of the SNARE proteins at a single peptide bond, which is specific to that particular neurotoxin. BoNT/C is unique among the neurotoxins in having two known SNARE substrate proteins, both SNAP-25 and syntaxin, each of which it cleaves at a single peptide bond. The SNARE proteins are essential for synaptic vesicle docking and fusion at the presynaptic membrane, and cleavage of any one by a BoNT prevents formation of a functional SNARE complex, thereby blocking synaptic vesicle docking and fusion at the presynaptic membrane and hence neurotransmitter release. BoNTs exert their effect at the neuromuscular junction, where, by inhibition of acetylcholine release, they bring about a flaccid paralysis.

The clinical application of BoNT was first described by Scott in 1980.[3] He reported that injecting small quantities of toxin into the extraocular muscles of the eye could correct squint (strabismus). The levels of toxin employed were much lower than those that lead to systemic toxicity, and no systemic side effects were observed. The beneficial paralytic effect lasted for several weeks, and there was a controllable dose-response relationship. Following this pioneering report, BoNT/A was used through the 1980s to treat a range of focal dystonias, including blepharospasm. Approval of BoNT/A as an orphan drug for the treatment of strabismus, blepharospasm and hemifacial spasm was given by the US Food and Drug Administration (FDA) in December, 1989. It has subsequently been approved for the treatment of cervical dystonia, and, more recently, for the treatment of glabellar wrinkles and hyperhydrosis. The clinical use of BoNT/A has been explored in a wide range of hyperactivity conditions, many of them off label, and has now been reported to be effective in more than 100 different clinical conditions (for reviews, see references 4 to 7). BoNT/A is manufactured under the trade name Botox by Allergan, Inc. in the United States and as Dysport by Ipsen Ltd. in Europe. Recently, Merz Pharma has received approval in Germany for a purified type A product called Xeomin for the treatment of blepharospasm and dystonia. A preparation of BoNT/B from Solstice Neurosciences, Inc. has also received regulatory approval for use in cervical dystonia, and is available as Myobloc in the United States, and as Neurobloc in Europe. In addition to effects on muscle contraction, recent therapeutic benefits reported for clinical preparations of BoNT have included autonomic conditions and pain relief. A major advantage of BoNTs in clinical use is their prolonged duration of effect.

For many patients with chronic conditions, treatments must be administered on a regular basis to be effective. Being able to use therapeutics that can be administered at a lower frequency without compromising their therapeutic benefit would help to increase the quality of life of patients suffering from a chronic disease. One approach to enable infrequent dosing is to reformulate existing therapeutics to enable sustained release of the active ingredient, for example, sustained-release opioids for chronic pain. An alternative is to identify pharmacologically active agents that can maintain their therapeutic benefit over long periods of time. The clinical BoNT preparations fall into this category of therapeutic agent. Unfortunately, owing to their selectivity for peripheral neurons, particularly cholinergic neurons, the neurotoxins do not affect secretion from other cell types and so are not relevant for the treatment of other chronic diseases. The clinical utility of the neurotoxins is also restricted by their extreme toxicity. BoNTs are the causative agents of botulism and are the most potent acute lethal toxins known, with lethal doses occurring at 10^{-9} g/kg of body weight.[8] The SNARE complex, formed by the SNARE proteins, represents, however, a universal mechanism for vesicle fusion and secretion in eukaryotic cells.[9] Given that the SNARE complex represents a universal mechanism for vesicle fusion and secretion in eukaryotic cells, the endopeptidase activity of clostridial neurotoxins, both BoNTs, and TeNT, is potentially capable of SNARE protein cleavage and inhibition of vesicle fusion and secretion in a wide range of cell types, and hence of bringing therapeutic benefit to a wide range of chronic diseases. Many chronic diseases involve a secretory event as a contributing or causative pathophysiologic factor; for example, the release of hormones in endocrine disorders, inflammatory mediators in inflammatory diseases, and the hypersecretion of airway mucus in chronic respiratory diseases. Protein therapeutics that possessed the pharmacologic activity of the BoNTs, but with a different cellular specificity and without the inherent toxicity of the native toxins, could, therefore, potentially offer long-term relief for patients with chronic conditions. Recent developments in the understanding of the structure and function of the neurotoxins has allowed this opportunity to be explored and developed.

CREATING THERAPEUTIC PROTEINS BASED ON THE NEUROTOXINS

The clostridial neurotoxins, both BoNTs and the closely related TeNT, share a common structure. They are di-chain proteins consisting of a heavy chain (HC) of approximately 100 kDa covalently joined by a single disulfide bond to a light chain (LC) of approximately 50 kDa.[10] The solution of the crystal structures of BoNT/A[11] and BoNT/B[12] and of TeNT H_C[13] revealed a strongly conserved molecular architecture within the clostridial neurotoxins, with very distinct structural domains, each one corresponding to one of the key steps in the mechanism of toxification: binding, translocation, and catalytic activity.[14,15] The HC consists of two domains, each of approximately 50 kDa. The C-terminal domain (H_C) is responsible for the high-affinity neuronal binding of the toxins,[16,17] whereas the N-terminal domain (H_N) is involved in intracellular membrane translocation.[18,19] The binding domain, H_C, further consists of two subdomains, H_{CC} and H_{CN}, and the H_{CC} domain contains key residues responsible for the binding activity of the neurotoxins.[20] It is the LC that is the zinc-dependent endopeptidase that cleaves one of the SNARE proteins essential to synaptic vesicle docking and fusion and thereby inhibits neurotransmitter release.[21] The role of the H_C and H_N domains respectively, therefore, is to deliver the toxin selectively to the target neuron and enable entry of the LC into the neuronal cytosol, where it can proteolytically cleave the substrate SNARE protein.

Given that the neuronal specificity of the clostridial neurotoxins is due to the selectivity of their binding domain, H_C, engineered proteins consisting of the H_N and LC domains of a clostridial neurotoxin, referred to as the LH_N fragment, and a suitably selected ligand could potentially cleave SNARE proteins and thereby inhibit vesicular secretion in a wide range of cell types dependent on the receptor

binding specificity of the selected ligand. Such proteins could be further tailored through the selection of the BoNT serotype employed as the backbone of the protein. This choice will determine which member of the SNARE family will be proteolytically cleaved, which is important because different cell types contain different SNARE protein isoforms. Engineered proteins of the type described have the potential to be of therapeutic value in the treatment of a range of diseases in which SNARE mediated vesicle fusion and secretion is contributing to the pathology of the disease. The potential of such proteins to achieve a sustained inhibition of secretion makes them particularly attractive candidates for the development of therapeutics for the treatment of chronic diseases.

The first description of modifying the cell binding domain of a clostridial neurotoxin was by Bizzini, who reported chemical coupling, via disulfide linkages, of either ricin toxin B-chain or wheat germ agglutinin to the LH_N fragment of tetanus toxin.[22] The LH_N fragment was generated by papain treatment of native toxin. Bizzini described the use of these conjugates to cause mouse lethality by a tetanus-type mechanism and was interested in understanding the mechanism of toxicity, not the potential to develop novel therapeutic agents.

An LH_N fragment (LH_N/A) can also be prepared by limited proteolytic cleavage of BoNT/A,[17] limited treatment of BoNT/A with trypsin degrading the H_C domain, thereby leaving the LC and H_N domains intact and still associated by noncovalent interactions and the single disulfide bond. A chemical conjugate of nerve growth factor coupled to the LH_N/A fragment was demonstrated to be able to cleave the SNARE protein SNAP-25 and inhibit noradrenaline release from PC12 cells in culture.[23] This was the first reported demonstration that the LH_N/A endopeptidase could be delivered into a target cell via a non-native binding ligand and gain access to its substrate SNARE protein. Subsequently, a chemical conjugate of the glucosyl-specific lectin, wheat germ agglutinin, and the LH_N/A fragment was demonstrated to deliver the clostridial endopeptidase into a range of both neuronal and non-neuronal cell types with a consequent cleavage of SNAP-25 and inhibition of secretion.[24] One of the cell lines studied in this latter report was the hamster pancreatic β cell, HIT-T15. A significant concentration-dependent inhibition of stimulated insulin release was observed that correlated with increasing cleavage of SNAP-25. This was an important observation because HIT-T15 cells were known to be resistant to the effects of BoNT/A. Therefore, this result demonstrated that by targeting to a cell via a suitable receptor, it is possible to achieve internalization of the endopeptidase into the cytosol of a cell normally resistant to the effect of BoNT. This presumably reflects the ability of the H_N domain to function correctly in the new target cell following binding and endocytosis. These in vitro data confirmed that it is possible to retarget the LH_N fragment of a clostridial neurotoxin to a cell of interest and so achieve inhibition of stimulated secretion. They also supported the ultimate therapeutic potential of this approach for developing therapeutic proteins.

Preparation of the LH_N fragment from clostridial neurotoxins other than BoNT/A or TeNT by limited proteolytic cleavage has proved very difficult, if not impossible, owing to the susceptibility of the L and H_N domains themselves to proteolytic degradation. Recombinant expression of a catalytically active, stable LH_N fragment of BoNT/A was first reported in 2002.[25] Subsequently, the expression and purification of both catalytically active LH_N/B and LH_N/C from Escherichia coli has been reported.[26] In all cases, the recombinant LH_N fragments were of very low toxicity and, in the case of recombinant LH_N/A, less toxic than highly purified LH_N/A prepared by proteolytic treatment of BoNT/A. The LH_N fragment is effectively nontoxic because it lacks the necessary H_C domain with which to bind to acceptors on the neuronal surface.

CHRONIC PAIN

The foregoing work demonstrates the feasibility of creating hybrid proteins able to deliver a clostridial endopeptidase into cells via a cell surface receptor other than the natural neurotoxin receptor, and thereby cleave SNARE proteins in the target cell and inhibit secretion. The next stage in the development of this approach was to demonstrate the ability to create a molecule able to target and inhibit secretion from a cell type relevant to a disease or medical condition that would benefit from that inhibition. One such opportunity is to target peripheral nociceptive afferents of the pain pathway and thereby develop analgesics for the treatment of chronic pain. The demand for effective treatments for chronic pain that have minimal side effects but long-lasting therapeutic benefits is large. Aside from the significant unmet medical need represented by chronic pain, there is already good clinical evidence from the use of the available therapeutic preparations of BoNTs that these can have analgesic activity.[27] By engineering BoNTs to target peripheral nociceptive neurons, the opportunity exists to develop more effective treatments for this all too prevalent condition.[28,29]

A chemical conjugate of Erythrina cristagalli lectin (ECL) and LH_N/A, $ECL-LH_N/A$, was shown to inhibit the depolarization-stimulated release of both substance P and glutamate from embryonic dorsal root ganglion (DRG) neurons in culture.[30] The inhibition of neurosecretion was very specific for the release from DRG neurons, because $ECL-LH_N/A$ was relatively ineffective at inhibiting depolarization-stimulated glycine release from cultured embryonic spinal cord neurons (SCN) prepared from adjacent embryonic spinal cord to the DRG. Lectins from Erythrina species, such as ECL, bind to galactose-containing carbohydrates, and galactose-containing carbohydrates have been reported to be selectively present on nociceptive afferents relative to other neurons in both the central and peripheral nervous system.[31,32] Importantly, the inhibitory effect of $ECL-LH_N/A$ on neurotransmitter release from DRG neurons is maintained for at least 25 days following a single treatment. Thus, the conjugate demonstrated a duration of action characteristic of the native neurotoxin, confirming that this important property was retained in the hybrid endopeptidase molecules.

The analgesic potential of $ECL-LH_N/A$ demonstrated in vitro by its prolonged inhibition of nociceptive neurotransmitter release from DRG neurons was confirmed in vivo. Nociceptive inputs to convergent dorsal horn neurons by primary sensory afferents of the C-fiber and Ad types were significantly reduced following intrathecal administration of $ECL-LH_N/A$ into the lumbar region of the spinal cord of anaesthetized rats, whereas there was little or no effect on sensory inputs from Aβ-fibers.[30,33] Direct demonstration of analgesic activity of $ECL-LH_N/A$ was provided by measuring withdrawal latency in a 'hotplate' model of acute thermal pain in mice. Latency was significantly prolonged following intrathecal administration of $ECL-LH_N/A$ into the lumbar region of the spinal cord.[33] This effect was sustained for more than 30 days after administration of the conjugate, indicating that, as in the in vitro DRG culture system, ECL-LH$_N$/A has an extended duration of action in vivo characteristic of the native neurotoxin. By contrast, morphine, as expected, ceased to demonstrate analgesic activity in the same model within less than a day. In a formalin model of inflammatory pain in rats, ECL-LH$_N$/A, administered either intrathecally or subcutaneously, inhibited the second phase of inflammatory pain resulting from introduction of formalin into the paw.[30,33] The observation that the conjugate was effective in this model when administered subcutaneously, opens up the possibility of peripheral application for targeted clostridial endopeptidase analgesics. The duration of analgesia observed in response to the conjugate in the inflammatory pain model was again prolonged, being maintained, after an initial peak response, for the duration of the experiment (9 days).

These results clearly demonstrate that the approach of retargeting clostridial endopeptidases to peripheral nociceptive afferent neurons is effective and has the potential to generate analgesic proteins with a prolonged duration of action suitable for the treatment of chronic pain conditions.

Chemical conjugates of LH$_N$ fragments and protein ligands have successfully demonstrated the feasibility of creating hybrid proteins that are able to deliver a clostridial endopeptidase into a selected target cell and achieve a prolonged inhibition of secretion from that cell, and done so in therapeutically relevant systems. There are, however, a number of drawbacks to using chemical conjugation of proteins to produce therapeutic agents. The major one is the inevitable heterogeneous mixture of species that is created using such a process. This inherent heterogeneity of chemical conjugates makes developing a regulatory compliant process based on them very difficult to achieve. Therefore, protein conjugates are not a good basis for developing a pharmaceutical product, and fully recombinant expression is the preferred route for the development of a therapeutic protein. Given the size and complexity of such a fusion protein, developing a fully recombinant chimera protein incorporating the translocation and endopeptidase domains of a clostridial neurotoxin and a targeting ligand is a challenging task. A fully recombinant fusion protein consisting of the LH$_N$-fragment of BoNT/C$_1$ and epidermal growth factor (EGF) has, however, been reported and shown to inhibit stimulated mucus secretion from respiratory epithelial cells.[34]

MUCUS HYPERSECRETION AND CHRONIC RESPIRATORY DISEASE

Hypersecretion of mucus into the airways is an important contributor to morbidity and mortality in many patients with severe chronic lung diseases, such as chronic pulmonary obstructive disease (COPD), asthma, and cystic fibrosis.[35] Excessive mucus in the airways can limit airflow; and its presence is a particular risk factor for those patients with COPD who are prone to chest infections. COPD is a severe chronic inflammatory disease of the respiratory tract that comprises three conditions, namely chronic bronchitis (long-standing airway mucus hypersecretion), small airways disease, and emphysema.[36] It is increasing worldwide in prevalence and economic burden.[37,38] In COPD, patients with chronic mucus hypersecretion have a significantly increased risk of hospitalization and death compared with patients without a marked bronchitic component.[39,40] Current treatments for COPD are palliative and do not halt disease progression,[41] and there is no specific treatment for the mucus hypersecretion.[42] In the absence of effective therapy for any aspect of COPD pathophysiology, development of treatments for mucus hypersecretion is warranted. The ability to clear mucus from the lungs, through airway cilia movement, depends on its viscocity and elasticity. These properties are determined by the proportion of mucin glycoproteins, by weight, that the mucus contains.[43] MUC5AC and MUC5B are the major mucins in both normal and pathologic human airway secretions.[44] In patients with COPD, levels of the mucins MUC5AC and MUC5B are increased in the respiratory mucus, although proportionally more MUC5B is secreted.[45] Mucins are secreted into the airways by goblet cells in the epithelium and seromucous glands in the submucosa.[43] One possibility for inhibiting mucus secretion is to utilize the inhibitory activity of the clostridial neurotoxin endopeptidases on vesicle fusion, targeted to the mucin-secreting cells of the airway using an appropriate targeting ligand.

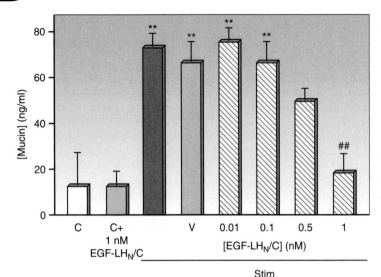

FIGURE 28-1. Effect of EGF-LH$_N$/C on EGF/TNFα-induced mucin secretion in H292 cells. H292 cells were preincubated with EGF-LH$_N$/C for 48 hours, followed by 24 hours of stimulation with EGF/TNFα in the continued presence of EGF-LH$_N$/C and mucin secretion levels determined by lectin assay. C, control; V, highest concentration of vehicle for EGF-LH$_N$/C. Data are mean mucin output (bars = SEM) of four independent experiments. **P < 0.01 vs C; ##P < 0.001 vs Stim.

To investigate whether a suitably targeted clostridial endopeptidase would cleave SNARE proteins in human respiratory epithelial cells, and thereby inhibit mucus secretion, a fusion protein was generated from a recombinant gene encoding the LH$_N$ domain of BoNT/C and EGF, designated EGF-LH$_N$/C, to target EGF receptors on the mucin secreting cells.[34] EGF was selected as the prototype ligand for the creation of such a fusion protein because EGF receptors are present on human respiratory epithelial cells[46,47] and are upregulated in the airway epithelium of patients with asthma and COPD,[48] as well as smokers.[49] The recombinant fusion protein EGF-LH$_N$/C cleaved the relevant SNARE protein syntaxin in a human mucoepidermoid metastatic cell line, H292 cells, in vitro in a concentration-dependent fashion.[34] Pretreating H292 cells with EGF-LH$_N$/C inhibits the stimulated release of mucin in response to a combined stimulus of EGF and tumor necrosis factor-α (TNFα) in a concentration-dependent manner, with an IC$_{50}$ of approximately 0.4 nM (Fig. 28-1). This compares very well with the previously reported inhibitory effect of EGF-LH$_N$/C on stimulated mucin release from another respiratory epithelial cell line, the human type II alveolar cell line A549, in response to the same stimulus.[34] In both cell types, there was no detectable effect of EGF-LH$_N$/C on the basal level of mucin secretion. The inhibition of mucin secretion by EGF-LH$_N$/C is due to the targeted delivery of its endopeptidase activity through the EGF receptor, and is not the result of cell cytotoxicity or receptor antagonism or downregulation.[34] EGF-LH$_N$/C is also able to inhibit stimulated mucin release from A549 cells in response to a stimulatory cocktail of cytokines, a combination of 1 ng/mL interferon (IFN)-γ, TNFα, and interleukin (IL)-1β, called cytomix (Fig. 28-2). Thus, the effect of EGF-LH$_N$/C on stimulated mucin release from respiratory epithelial cells is independent of the precise nature of the stimulus used. Histologic examination shows that the mucin is retained inside the treated cells (Fig. 28-3). Control cells contain stained intracellular mucin, whereas stimulated cells show markedly reduced staining, indicating mucin secretion. Stimulated cells pretreated with EGF-LH$_N$/C show retained intracellular staining, indicating inhibition of secretion by EGF-LH$_N$/C. To assess the response of the cells to such intracellular mucin retention, the effect of EGF-LH$_N$/C pretreatment on MUC5AC mRNA levels was measured as an indicator of mucin synthesis. EGF-LH$_N$/C pretreatment is associated with a concentration-dependent inhibition of EGF-TNFα–induced MUC5AC mRNA expression, with an IC$_{50}$ value of ~0.1 nM (Fig. 28-4). As with the inhibition of stimulated mucin release from the cells, this effect of EGF-LH$_N$/C is due to the targeted delivery of its endopeptidase activity through the EGF receptor, because neither an LH$_N$/C lacking an EGF ligand to target it to the EGF receptor nor a mutated form of the fusion protein in which the endopeptidase domain has been inactivated by three residue changes in the catalytic region (EGF-TE-LH$_N$/C) inhibit MUC5AC mRNA expression. This effect of EGF-LH$_N$/C on MUC5AC mRNA expression suggests the existence of a possible negative feedback mechanism between mucin release

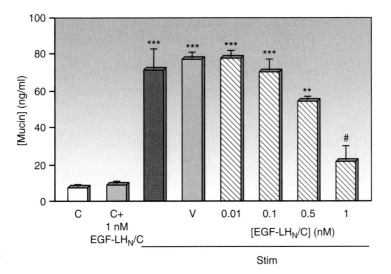

FIGURE 28-2. Effect of EGF-LH$_N$/C on cytomix-induced mucin secretion from A549 cells. Cells were preincubated with EGF-LH$_N$/C for 48 hours, followed by 6 hours of stimulation with cytomix (Stim) in the continued presence of EGF-LH$_N$/C and secreted mucin concentrations determined by lectin assay. C, control; V, highest concentration of vehicle for EGF-LH$_N$/C. Data are mean mucin output (bars = SEM) of three independent experiments. **$P < 0.01$, ***$P < 0.001$ vs C; #$P < 0.05$ vs. Stim.

and mucin synthesis in respiratory epithelial cells, and also that gene expression downregulates in response to inhibition of secretion by a recombinant clostridial endopeptidase.

Recombinant clostridial endopeptidase fusion proteins that can inhibit mucus secretion, as exemplified by EGF-LH$_N$/C, have the potential for development as therapeutic proteins for the treatment of COPD, chronic bronchitis, cystic fibrosis, and other chronic respiratory conditions involving excess airway mucus production. The longevity of the protein's activity would mean that the product

would only need to be inhaled infrequently, making it well suited to the treatment of chronic respiratory diseases of this type.

CONCLUSIONS

The clostridial neurotoxins BoNT and TeNT have evolved a unique mechanism of action that can be harnessed to inhibit secretion in a wide range of cell types. The longevity of inhibition of secretion resulting from the proteolytic cleavage of SNARE proteins by the clostridial

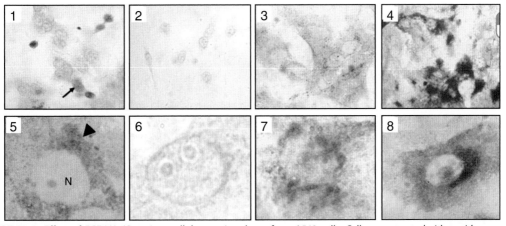

FIGURE 28-3. Effect of EGF-LH$_N$/C on intracellular mucin release from A549 cells. Cells were treated either with serum-free media for 72 hours or serum-free media for 48 hours, followed by stimulation for 24 hours with EGF-TNFα, or were preincubated with EGF-LH$_N$/C for 48 hours, followed by stimulation for 24 hours with EGF-TNFα in the continued presence of EGF-LH$_N$/C. Cells were fixed and stained with AB-PAS for intracellular mucin. Representative images of stained intracellular mucin (*arrow*) in a control cell (*arrowhead*) (1 and 5), a stimulated cell (2 and 6), and in stimulated cells pretreated with either 0.5 nM (3 and 7) or 1 nM EGF-LH$_N$/C (4 and 8). Panels 1, 2, 3 and 4 = × 40 magnification, panels 5, 6, 7 and 8 = × 100 magnification. N, nucleus. *See Color Plate*

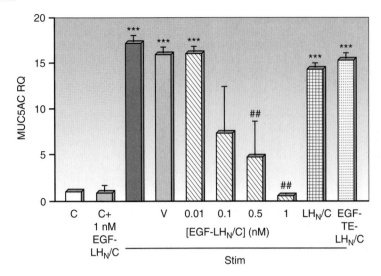

FIGURE 28-4. Effect of EGF-LH$_N$/C on EGF/TNFα-induced MUC5AC mRNA expression. A549 cells were preincubated with EGF-LH$_N$/C for 48 hours, followed by 24 hours of stimulation (Stim) with EGF/TNFα in the continued presence of EGF-LH$_N$/C and MUC5AC mRNA levels determined by Taqman RT-QPCR. C, control; V, highest concentration of vehicle for EGF-LH$_N$/C. Data are mean (bars = SEM) relative quantity (RQ) MUC5AC mRNA, with control (C) set at 1, of 3 independent experiments. ***P < 0.001 vs C; ##P < 0.01 vs. Stim.

endopeptidases means that recombinant proteins that incorporate this activity are ideal candidates for treating chronic diseases, in which effective therapies that need only infrequent administration could greatly enhance patients' quality of life. Preclinical studies have shown that both conjugates and recombinant fusion proteins that possess functional catalytic and translocation domains of derived from clostridial neurotoxins but incorporate novel ligands to target appropriate cell surface receptors can act to inhibit secretion from cell types not sensitive to the native neurotoxins. In particular, this has been demonstrated for both peripheral nociceptive afferent nerve cells and mucin-secreting respiratory epithelial cells, suggesting that such retargeted clostridial endopeptidases could be effective in the treatment of both chronic pain and chronic respiratory diseases. Other diseases that involve secretion could also be tackled using this approach, for example, endocrine cancers. Importantly, removal of the native recognition domain vastly increases the therapeutic index for these proteins, because they no longer target the peripheral cholinergic motor neurons that are the basis for the extreme toxicity of the native neurotoxins.

METHODS

Cell Culture

A549 cells were cultured in 25 mL DMEM supplemented with either 10% fetal bovine serum and 2 mM L-glutamine for complete media, or with no serum for serum-free treatments. Cells were grown in 5% CO^2 in air-humidified incubator at 37°C. The media was replaced every 2 days, and cells were passaged when they were ~80% confluent. All experiments were carried out between passages 88 and 95.

NCI-H292 cells were cultured in 25 mL RPMI 1640, supplemented with either 10% fetal bovine serum and 2 mM L-glutamine for complete media, or with no serum for serum-free treatments. Cells were grown in a 5% CO$_2$ in air-humidified incubator at 37°C. The media was replaced every 2 days, and cells were passaged when they were ~80% confluent. All experiments were carried out between passages 80 and 98.

Mucin Secretion Protocols

A549 or H292 cells were used at ~80% confluency. For baseline control experiments, cells were incubated in serum-free media for 24 hours before treatment (i.e., serum-starved), which was removed and replaced with fresh serum-free media for a further 48 hours (to control for the 48 hours' preincubation with EGF-LH$_N$/C), followed by an additional 24 hours' serum-free incubation (to control for the stimulation period). To examine the effect of drug vehicles on baseline mucin secretion levels, cells were serum-starved for 24 hours before treatment, after which the serum-free media was removed and replaced with serum-free media containing 5 mM v/v HEPES (EGF-LH$_N$/C vehicle) for 48 hours, followed by 24 hours of incubation in serum-free media containing 2.5 nM v/v acetic acid (EGF/TNFα vehicle). For stimulation, cells were serum-starved for 24 hours, followed by a further 48 hours of serum-free media (to account for EGF-LH$_N$/C in inhibition studies), and followed by EGF and TNFα in combination for 24 hours. To examine the effect of EGF-LH$_N$/C vehicle (5 mM HEPES in serum-free media) on stimulation, cells were serum-starved for 24 hours before treatment, after which, the serum-free media was removed and replaced with EGF-LH$_N$/C vehicle for 48 hours. This was followed by a further 24 hours of incubation with EGF/TNFα (stimulation) and vehicle. To examine the effect of EGF-LH$_N$/C on stimulation, cells were serum-starved for 24 hours, and then pre-incubated with EGF-LH$_N$/C for 48 hours, followed by 24 hours of stimulation with EGF/TNFα in the continued presence of EGF-LH$_N$/C. At the end of the experiments, supernatants were removed and tested for mucin content using a lectin assay.

Lectin Assay for Secreted Mucin

Helix pomatia (edible snail) agglutinin (HPA), 6 μg/mL, adhered for 1 hour at 37°C to a 96-well Maxisorp plate was used as a mucin capture lectin. The HPA was decanted, and the plate washed three times in high-salt PBS (HSPBS). Dilutions of 0.78 to 50 ng/mL of a human respiratory mucin standard, purified from spontaneous sputum from a 65-year-old hospitalized male patient according to methods described previously,[50] and cell culture supernatants containing secreted mucin were added to the wells and incubated at 37°C for 30 minutes. The plates were then washed in HSPBS and incubated with horseradish peroxidase conjugated to HPA at 1 μg/mL for 30 minutes. Following a further wash step, the assay was developed using *o*-phenylenediamine dihydrochloride peroxidase (OPD) substrate, and the reaction was terminated with H_2SO_4 and read immediately at 492 nm.

Histologic Staining and Quantification of Intracellular Mucin

A549 cells were grown to ~80% confluency in 4.5 mL complete DMEM on 1-well LabTek system slides. The cells were serum-starved for 24 hours and treated according to the experimental protocol of interest. The treated cells were then fixed in 4% paraformaldehyde for a further 10 minutes. The sections were washed in distilled water for 2 minutes and were immersed in 4% Alcian blue solution, pH 2.5, for 5 minutes. The sections were then washed in running tap water for 5 minutes, followed by a rinse with distilled water. The sections were stained with Schiff's reagent for 4 minutes, washed under running tap water, and dehydrated through graded ethanol before clearing through xylene and mounting in DPX. Slides were viewed under a ×40 objective using a Zeiss Axioplan microscope. Duplicate slides were created for each experimental condition. The amount of staining for intracellular mucin was assessed in each slide in five randomly selected fields, each containing at least ten cells.

TaqMan RT-PCR for MUC5AC mRNA Expression

Total RNA was isolated from respiratory epithelial cells using an RNeasy kit (Qiagen). The total RNAs were then subjected to first-strand cDNA synthesis using hexanucleotide random primers. Relative quantification was then performed using the ABI Prism 7500 sequence detection system (Applied Biosystems, Foster City, CA), using the primers and probe supplied with the MUC5AC gene expression assay. As an internal control, the copy number of GAPDH mRNA was determined using TaqMan GAPDH control reagents (Applied Biosystems, Foster City, CA) and normalized the number of cDNA copies derived from MUC5AC mRNA against corresponding values of GAPDH at the same sample volume. The ΔΔCt method of analysis was employed using the software supplied with the thermal cycling machine (Sequence Detection System—SDS 1.1, Applied Biosystems, Foster City, CA).

Statistical Analysis

Data are mean and SEM for separate experiments performed in duplicate. Significance of differences between experimental groups was evaluated using one-way analysis of variance (ANOVA), followed by examination of specific groups by two-sample t-test (two-tailed), using Prism software. The null hypothesis of no significant difference was rejected at $P < 0.05$.

References

1. Blasi J, Chapman ER, Link E, Binz T, Yamasaki S, De Camilli P, et al. Botulinum neurotoxin A selectively cleaves the synaptic protein SNAP-25. *Nature*. 1993;365:160-163.
2. Montecucco C, Schiavo G. Mechanism of action of tetanus and botulinum neurotoxins. *Mol Microbiol*. 1994;13:1-8.
3. Scott AB. Botulinum toxin injection into extraocular muscles as an alternative to strabismus surgery. *Ophthalmology*. 1980;87:1044-1049.
4. Carruthers J, Carruthers A. Botox: beyond wrinkles. *Clin Dermatol*. 2004;22:89-93.
5. Cordivari C, Misra VP, Catania S, Lees AJ. New therapeutic indications for botulinum toxins. *Mov Disord*. 2004;19:S157-S161.
6. Panicker JN, Muthane UB. Botulinum toxins: Pharmacology and its current therapeutic evidence for use. *Neurol India*. 2003;5:455-460.
7. Thant Z-S, Tan E-K. Emerging therapeutic applications of botulinum toxin. *Med Sci Monit*. 2003;9:RA40-48.
8. Bonifacino JS, Glick BS. The mechanisms of vesicle budding and fusion. *Cell*. 2004;116:153-166.
9. Gill DM. Bacterial toxins: A fable of lethal amounts. *Microbiol Rev*. 1982;46:86-94.
10. Simpson LL. Molecular pharmacology of botulinum toxin and tetanus toxin. *Annu Rev Pharmacol Toxicol*. 1986;26:427-453.
11. Lacy DB, Tepp W, Cohen AC, DasGupta BR, Stevens RC. Crystal structure of botulinum neurotoxin type A and implications for toxicity. *Nat Struct Biol*. 1998;5:898-902.
12. Swaminathan S, Eswaramoorthy S. Structural analysis of the catalytic and binding sites of Clostridium botulinum neurotoxin B. *Nat Struct Biol*. 2000;7:693-699.
13. Umland TC, Wingert LM, Swaminathan S, Furey WF, Schmidt JJ, Sax M. Structure of the receptor binding fragment HC of tetanus toxin. *Nat Struct Biol*. 1997;4:788-792.
14. Hanson MA, Stevens RC. Structural view of botulinum neurotoxin in numerous functional states. In: Brin MF, Jankovic J, Hallett M, eds. *Scientific and Therapeutic Aspects of Botulinum Toxin*. Philadelphia: Lippincott Williams & Wilkins; 2002:11-28.
15. Swaminathan S, Eswaramoorthy S. Crystal structure of Clostridium botulinum neurotoxin serotype B. In Brin MF, Jankovic J, Hallett M, eds. *Scientific and Therapeutic Aspects of Botulinum Toxin*, Philadelphia: Lippincott Williams & Wilkins; 2002:29-40.
16. Halpern JL, Loftus A. Characterisation of the receptor binding domain of tetanus toxin. *J Biol Chem*. 1993;268:11188-11192.
17. Shone CC, Hambleton P, Melling J. Inactivation of Clostridium botulinum type A neurotoxin by trypsin and purification of two tryptic fragments. Proteolytic action near the COOH-terminus of the heavy subunit destroys toxin-binding activity. *Eur J Biochem*. 1985;151:75-82.
18. Shone CC, Hambleton P, Melling J. A 50-kDa fragment from the NH2-terminus of the heavy subunit of Clostridium botulinum type A neurotoxin forms channels in lipid vesicles. *Eur J Biochem*. 1987;167:175-180.
19. Koriazova LK, Montal M. Translocation of botulinum neurotoxin light chain protease through the heavy chain channel. *Nat Struct Biol*. 2003;10:13-18.
20. Herreros J, Lalli G, Montecucco C, Schiavo G. Tetanus toxin fragment C binds to a protein present in neuronal cell lines and motorneurons. *J Neurochem*. 2000;74:1941-1950.
21. Humeau Y, Doussau F, Grant NJ, Poulain B. How botulinum and tetanus neurotoxins block neurotransmitter release. *Biochimie*. 2000;82:427-446.
22. Bizzini B. Investigation of the mode of action of tetanus toxin with the aid of hybrid molecules consisting in part of tetanus toxin-derived fragments. In: Alouf JE, ed. *Bacterial Protein Toxins*. London: Academic Press; 1984:427-434.
23. Chaddock JA, Purkiss JR, Duggan MJ, Quinn CP, Shone CC, Foster KA. A conjugate composed of nerve growth factor coupled to a non-toxic derivative of Clostridium botulinum neurotoxin type A can inhibit neurotransmitter release in vitro. *Growth Factors*. 2000;18:147-155.
24. Chaddock JA, Purkiss JR, Friis LM, Broadbridge JD, Duggan MJ, Fooks SJ, et al. Inhibition of vesicular secretion in both neuronal and non-neuronal cells by a retargeted endopeptidase derivative of Clostridium botulinum neurotoxin type A. *Infect Immun*. 2000;68:2587-2593.
25. Chaddock JA, Herbert MH, Ling RJ, Alexander FCG, Fooks SJ, Revell DF, et al. Expression and purification of catalytically active, non-toxic endopeptidase derivatives of Clostridium botulinum toxin type A. *Protein Expr Purif*. 2002;25:219-228.
26. Sutton JM, Wayne J, Scott-Tucker A, O'Brien SM, Marks PMH, Alexander FCG, et al. Preparation of specifically activatable endopeptidase derivatives of Clostridium botulinum toxins type A, B and C and their applications. *Protein Expr Purif*. 2005;40:31-41.
27. Lang AM. Botulinum toxin type A therapy in chronic pain disorders. *Arch Phys Med Rehabil*. 2003;84(Suppl 1):S69-S73.
28. Foster KA. A new wrinkle on pain relief: re-engineering clostridial neurotoxins for analgesics. *Drug Discov Today*. 2005;10:563-569.
29. Foster KA. The analgesic potential of clostridial neurotoxin derivatives. *Expert Opin Investig Drugs*. 2004;13:1437-1443.
30. Duggan MJ, Quinn CP, Chaddock JA, Purkiss JR, Alexander FCG, Doward S, et al. Inhibition of release of neurotransmitters from rat dorsal root ganglia by a novel conjugate of a Clostridium botulinum toxin A endopeptidase fragment and Erythrina cristagalli lectin. *J Biol Chem*. 2002;277:34846-34852.
31. Streit WJ, Schulte BA, Balentine DJ, Spicer SS. Histochemical localization of galactose-containing glycoconjugates in sensory neurons and their processes in the central and peripheral nervous system of the rat. *J Histochem Cytochem*. 1985;33:1042-1052.
32. Streit WJ, Schulte BA, Balentine DJ, Spicer SS. Evidence for glycoconjugate in nociceptive primary sensory neurons and its origin from the Golgi complex. *Brain Res*. 1986;377:1-17.
33. Chaddock JA, Duggan MJ, Quinn CP, Purkiss JR, Alexander FCG, Doward S, et al. Retargeted clostridial endopeptidases: Inhibition of nociceptive neurotransmitter release in vitro, and antinociceptive activity in in vivo models of pain. *Mov Disord*. 2004;19:42-47.
34. Foster KA, Adams EJ, Durose L, Cruttwell CJ, Marks E, Shone CC, et al. Re-engineering the target specificity of clostridial neurotoxins—a route to novel therapeutics. *Neurotox Res*. 2006;9:101-107.
35. Rogers DF, Barnes PJ. Treatment of airway mucus hypersecretion. *Ann Med*. 2006;38:116-125.
36. Stevenson NJ, Walker PP, Costello RW, Calverley PM. Lung mechanics and dyspnea during exacerbations of

chronic obstructive pulmonary disease. *Am J Respir Crit Care Med.* 2005;172:1510-1516.

37. Halpin DM, Miravitlles M. Chronic obstructive pulmonary disease: the disease and its burden to society. *Proc Am Thorac Soc.* 2006;3:619-623.

38. Hoogendoorn M, Rutten-van Mölken MPMH, Hoogenveen RT, van Genugten MLL, Buist AS, Wouters EFM. et al. A dynamic population model of disease progression in COPD. *Eur Respir J.* 2005;26:223-233.

39. Vestbo J. Epidemiological studies in mucus hypersecretion. *Novartis Found Symp.* 2002;248:3-12.

40. Vestbo J, Hogg JC. Convergence of the epidemiology and pathology of COPD. *Thorax.* 2006;61:86-88.

41. Barnes PJ. Therapy of chronic obstructive pulmonary disease. *Pharmacol Ther.* 2003;97:87-94.

42. Global Initiative for Chronic Obstructive Lung Disease. Global Strategy for the Diagnosis, Management, and Prevention of Chronic Obstructive Pulmonary Disease. www.goldcopd.org (accessed 2007).

43. Jeffery PK. Morphology of the airway wall in asthma and in chronic obstructive pulmonary disease. *Am Rev Respir Dis.* 1991;143:1152-1158.

44. Thornton DJ, Gray T, Nettesheim P, Howard M, Koo JS, Sheehan JK. Characterization of mucins from cultured normal human tracheobronchial epithelial cell. *Am J Physiol Lung Cell Mol Physiol.* 2000;278: 1118-1128.

45. Rose MC, Nickola TJ, Voynow JA. Airway mucus obstruction: mucin glycoproteins, MUC gene regulation and goblet cell hyperplasia. *Am J Respir Cell Mol Biol.* 2001;25:533-537.

46. Polosa R, Puddicombe SM, Krishna MT, Tuck AB, Howarth PH, Holgate ST, et al. Expression of c-erbB receptors and ligands in the bronchial epithelium of asthmatic subjects. *J Allergy Clin Immunol.* 2002;109:75-81.

47. Puddicombe SM, Polosa R, Richter A, Krishna MT, Howarth PH, Holgate ST, et al. Involvement of the epidermal growth factor receptor in epithelial repair in asthma. *FASEB J.* 2000;14:1362-1374.

48. O'Donnell RA, Richter A, Ward J, Angco G, Mehta A, Rousseau K, et al. Expression of ErbB receptors and mucins in the airways of long term current smoker. *Thorax.* 2004;59:1032-1040.

49. Takeyama K, Fahy JV, Nadel JA. Relationship of epidermal growth factor receptors to goblet cell production in human bronchi. *Am J Respir Crit Care Med.* 2001;163:511-516.

50. Carlstedt I, Lindgren H, Sheehan JK, Ulmsten U, Wingerup L. Isolation and characterization of human cervical-mucus glycoproteins. *Biochem J.* 1983;211: 13-22.

Unmet Needs and **29** Challenges in the Therapeutic Use of Botulinum Neurotoxins

David M. Simpson and Yuen T. So

INTRODUCTION

Botulinum neurotoxin (BoNT) has emerged as a major advance in clinical therapeutics. From its early investigations and clinical applications in strabismus and other ocular disorders, BoNT is used in the treatment of diseases in almost every medical specialty. A partial list includes disorders of neurology, ophthalmology, physiatry, otolaryngology, dermatology, plastic surgery, gastroenterology, urology, gynecology, and rheumatology. Although some BoNT indications are supported by randomized, double-blind, placebo-controlled trials, others are reported only in uncontrolled series or anedoctal reports. The enthusiasm generated by results of initial positive case studies has often led to difficulty in mounting and reluctance in accruing to controlled studies of BoNT in some indications. There is a dearth of high-level trials to support the efficacy of BoNT in some disorders, as reported in evidence-based reviews.[1] Thus, there is a chasm between many clinicians' sense of what they consider to be correct information, based on their experience and suboptimal literature, and the scientific community's skepticism, given the lack of high-quality data.

The use of BoNT in some clinical indications arose through serendipity. For example, the potential role for BoNT in the treatment of headache emerged from observations that patients treated with BoNT for cervical dystonia or facial wrinkles had reduction in the incidence of headache.[2] Based on these and other reports that followed, enthusiastic clinicians incorporated BoNT into their headache practices, often with reportedly positive and highly publicized results. It was only later that the academic community, as well as pharmaceutical manufacturers, mounted properly designed, controlled clinical trials. It is notable that the results of the most recent double-blind, placebo-controlled studies of BoNT for the treatment of headache have reported negative results,[3-5] raising questions on the validity of many clinicians' anecdotal experience. An alternative explanation is that limitations of the trials do not reflect the true clinical situation, a phenomenon termed the "failed trial."

Because the evolution of BoNT in clinical therapeutics has not proceeded in a traditional fashion, in comparison to many other pharmaceutical agents, it is not surprising that there are numerous gaps in understanding concerning its optimal use. Examples include imprecision in measures of BoNT potency, inadequate comparisons between different BoNT serotypes and brands, controversy concerning the role of immunogenicity in response failure, lack of dose-response data for most indications, inadequately studied issues concerning injection technique (i.e., volume, dilution, potency, muscle localization, spread of toxin, electromyographic guidance), and lack of consensus

Dr. Simpson is disclosing that he has been a consultant for and received research grant support from Allergan, Merz, and Solstice. Dr. So does not report any conflicts of interest.

on meaningful endpoint measures in clinical trials. Although other sections in this book discuss several of these issues, this chapter reviews open questions that should be addressed in order to advance the state of the art of BoNT in clinical therapeutics.

INJECTION TECHNIQUE

The primary mechanism of action of BoNT is neuromuscular blockade, discussed in other sections of this book. BoNT binds to the presynaptic terminal of the neuromuscular junction, is internalized into cholinergic neurons, and blocks release of acetylcholine, resulting in neuromuscular paralysis. It might be predicted that the degree of muscle weakness induced by BoNT injection is directly related to the number and efficiency of blocked endplates.

There are several factors that might enhance the ability of BoNT to reach the motor endplates. These include the dose, dilution, volume, and proximity of injection to the endplate zone. The effects of varying these factors were examined in an animal model, in which the rat tibialis anterior was injected with BoNT, followed by peroneal nerve stimulation, and histologic determination of muscle paralysis.[6] The most important factor determining the degree of muscle paralysis was the proximity of BoNT injection to the endplate zone. Displacing the injection 0.5 cm superior or inferior to the endplate zone resulted in an approximately 50% reduction in the area of muscle paralysis, whereas displacing the injection 1 cm from the endplate zone resulted in almost no paralysis. The effects of varying other factors produced less dramatic results. For example, it took a 10-fold increase in dose (at a constant volume of injection) to result in twice the degree of paralysis. At a constant dose and injection site, a 100-fold increase in volume resulted in twice the area of muscle paralysis.

There are surprisingly few studies examining these issues in humans. Most recommendations concerning BoNT dosing and technique arose through empirical observations and consensus.[7] For example studies of Botox (Allergan, Inc, Irvine, CA), an agent that must be diluted in 100-U vials, have incorporated wide ranges of volume and potency, even for studies with injection of identical muscles for the same clinical indication. In studies of human spasticity, dilutions of botulinum

neurotoxin type A (BoNT/A) have varied from highly concentrated (100U/mL, e.g., 1 mL of saline per vial of Botox) to highly diluted (20 U/mL, e.g., 5 mL of saline per vials of Botox).[8] Surprisingly, even in those studies investigating the effects of BoNT dilution on outcome, no clear differences emerged.[9,10]

We examined technical injection issues in human studies. There are minimal data providing anatomic localization of neuromuscular endplates in human muscles. We performed a study of endplate mapping in human cadaver specimens.[11] Because the human biceps brachii is a major muscle involved in elbow flexion, commonly injected in patients with spasticity, we focused on endplate mapping in this muscle. The peripheral nerve anatomy, including the fine terminal branches, was identified with a modified Sihler stain, whereas neuromuscular endplates were mapped with whole-mount acetylcholinesterase staining. The results indicated that the major motor endplate band in biceps brachii is an inverted V-shaped band, 1 cm in width, located 7 cm superior to the olecranon laterally, 11 cm superior to the olecranon in the middle, and 8 cm above the olecranon medially. Other studies have attempted to find the anatomic location of the endplates in commonly injected muscles, but the clinical relevance of these observations has not been fully examined.[12]

With the availability of an anatomic map of the motor endplates in human biceps brachii, we then followed with a clinical trial of BoNT injection into this muscle.[13] We hypothesized that injections targeted to the endplate zone would be superior to nontargeted injections, and that high-volume, nontargeted injections would be superior to low-volume injections, similar to the results found in animal studies. In a series of 21 subjects with poststroke upper extremity spasticity, the results supported these hypotheses. BoNT injection into biceps brachii resulted in statistically significant tone reduction in the low-volume, endplate-targeted group, and the high-volume, nontargeted group. Notably the low-volume, nontargeted injection method, an approach that is used commonly in clinical practice, did not result in significant reduction in elbow flexor spasticity.

A series of experiments such as those described earlier pose numerous challenges. The mapping of peripheral nerve and endplate microanatomy in the human cadaver is tedious, time-consuming, and expensive. As noted, the localization of endplates in most human muscles is unknown. There is considerable variability among muscles. For example, although the endplate zone in biceps brachii is well localized to a discrete band, endplates in the gastrocnemius are widely distributed throughout the muscle (Sanders I, unpublished observations). Thus, in order to reach the maximum number of endplates within this muscle, BoNT would need to be injected in multiple sites, preferably with high volume. However, these assumptions have not been clinically tested in muscles other than biceps brachii. Thus, the current approach to BoNT injection location, number of sites, and volume and potency remains empirical. It is possible that variability in these factors has led to the wide range of results reported in clinical trials and found in practice of BoNT therapy.

In addition to the factors noted above, other variables may affect the ability of BoNT to diffuse to adjacent muscles and tissues. Large-bore needles, with resultant increase in local tissue damage, may increase diffusion.[14] Botulinum neurotoxin type B (BoNT/B) has been shown to have greater diffusibility than BoNT/A.[15] In many situations, increased diffusion away from the target muscle will result in a greater incidence of adverse effects. For example, in studies of cervical dystonia, adverse effects of dysphagia and dry mouth are consistently more frequent with BoNT/B than BoNT/A.[16-20] Conversely, in the treatment of other disorders, such as spasticity and hyperhidrosis, in which spread of BoNT is desirable, physicians may harbor increased diffusion capability to their advantage.

Numerous techniques have been employed for the injection of BoNT into the target muscle. These include surface anatomy, electromyographic (EMG) guidance, needle stimulation, endoscopy and fluoroscopy. It is logical to assume that muscles that are easily identified from the surface, such as the biceps brachii and gastrocnemius, might be injected without specific targeting techniques. This is particularly helpful when injecting children with cerebral palsy, in which the speed of the procedure is important. However in small and deep muscles, such as those in the forearm or larynx, electrophysiologic or radiologic techniques are often employed to accurately inject the target muscle. In one study comparing the accuracy of muscle injection, surface localization was correct only 37% of the time as compared with EMG guidance.[21] We have found that electrical stimulation of the target muscle

is preferable to passive EMG localization, particularly in patients with spasticity with poor voluntary muscle control. However, there are few studies that have objectively examined the role of EMG in BoNT application, resulting in wide variability in clinicians' practice in BoNT injection technique.[22]

MEASURES OF TREATMENT RESPONSE

Interpretation of the relevance of clinical trial results is hampered by concerns about the functional significance of outcome measures. For example, most studies of BoNT for the treatment of spasticity used measures of tone as the primary outcome measure. Although placebo-controlled studies have almost all demonstrated that BoNT produces significant reduction in tone scores,[23] such as the Modified Ashworth scale, many authors question whether tone reduction translates into meaningful clinical improvement.[24] Most clinicians agree that tone reduction, and consequent improvement in passive functional activities (i.e., those performed by the caregiver such as cleaning the palm), leads to improvement in quality of life. However, the continued lack of US Food and Drug Administration (FDA) approval of BoNT for the treatment of adult or childhood spasticity suggests that there is not uniformity in this view. Even the demonstration of passive and active functional improvement, as demonstrated on the Disability Assessment Scale,[25] in a large placebo-controlled study of BoNT in poststroke spasticity, has not led to modification of the FDA's position.

Improvement in active function, defined as an ability to voluntarily perform a useful activity with the affected limb, remains difficult to demonstrate in clinical studies. It is possible that outcome measures for active function may not be sensitive enough. Also, it may be difficult to achieve a proper degree of neuromuscular blockade without causing excessive muscle weakness, especially in studies that employed rigid injection protocols. In a study of BoNT/A in the treatment of focal hand dystonia, 80% of subjects experienced weakness in the injected muscles.[26] In treatment of essential hand tremor,[27] BoNT resulted in significant improvement in the tremor rating scale, but functional rating scales did not improve. This may be due to the fact that most subjects injected with BoNT experienced some degree of finger weakness. Notably, the subjects in this study received BoNT injections into both flexors and extensors of the wrist. By reducing dosage or avoiding BoNT in the wrist and finger extensors, it may be possible to eliminate extensor weakness without compromising the benefits in terms of tremor amelioration.[28] Our preliminary observation supports this strategy in that injecting only agonists or antagonists achieves comparable efficacy in tremor reduction, without excessive weakness (Gracies JM, personal communication).

In parallel with a lack of consensus on measures of efficacy for many disorders, there is confusion on how to define treatment failure and attribute its causes. One distinction separates primary from secondary failure. Primary failure is defined as the lack of response following initial treatment with BoNT. Potential explanations include poor injection technique, such as poor muscle targeting, inappropriate muscle selection, inadequate dosing, or misplaced expectations of response. Secondary resistance results from the production of neutralizing antibodies to BoNT.[29,30] Numerous assays have been proposed to detect the presence of neutralizing antibodies, including the mouse lethality assay, enzyme linked immunosorbent assay, and in vivo tests, such as the extensor digitorum brevis, frontalis test, or the more suitable unilateral brow injection.[31,32] However most of these assays lack in optimal sensitivity and specificity, and their role in clinical practice is uncertain.

GAPS IN CLINICAL EVIDENCE

The literature supporting the use of BoNT in many indications is remarkably scanty, in contrast to its acceptance by most clinicians. For instance, BoNT is widely accepted as the treatment of choice in blepharospasm, hemifacial spasm, and laryngeal spasm. The use of BoNT in blepharospasm and hemifacial spasm was supported by only a few small clinical trials, involving a total of less than 20 patients in each disorder.[33-36] There is only one randomized controlled study of BoNT in 13 patients with adductor spasmodic dysphonia.[37] Common to all of these conditions is that none of them have satisfactory treatment alternatives. Dramatic results

using BoNT in the initial open-label studies undoubtedly discouraged efforts to study BoNT in larger and more vigorously designed clinical trials. Given the almost universal acceptance of BoNT as standard of care for these disorders, better data are unlikely to be forthcoming in the near future.

In conditions that have other effective treatments, BoNT has generally not been compared with the treatment alternatives. Examples include disorders such as tremor, cervical and limb dystonia, hyperhidrosis and urologic disorders. Clinicians need data on comparative efficacy, cost, and side effects in order to choose treatment intelligently for patients with these disorders. Valid data will only come from direct comparison studies assessing the existing treatment options under identical clinical settings in the same patient population.

In one of the few available comparative studies, BoNT/A had superior efficacy and less side effects than trihexyphenidyl in cervical dystonia.[38] In another trial, we compared the efficacy and safety of BoNT and tizanadine in a head-to-head, placebo-controlled trial in the treatment of upper extremity spasticity associated with stroke or traumatic brain injury.[39] Results of this 60-patient study revealed that Botox, up to a total dose of 500 U, resulted in superior tone reduction, and with less side effects, than tizanadine (Zanaflex, Acorda Therapeutics, Hawthorne, NY) up to a dosage of 36 mg/day.

In addition to comparison of safety and efficacy, it is important to understand the cost-effectiveness of different treatments. Such analyses are inherently difficult, because in addition to the cost of the treatment of interest, there are many related costs that are difficult to quantitate. These include ancillary medications, office visits, diagnostic tests, hospitalizations, use of physical and occupational therapy, and bracing. Several studies demonstrated the cost-effectiveness of BoNT/A in the treatment of poststroke spasticity.[40]

Treatment of most disorders requires individualized selection of BoNT dose, muscles, and injection sites. Many clinical trials, however, make use of a standardized treatment protocol to ensure uniformity and reproducibility, and to facilitate randomization and blinding. A rigid, fixed site, fixed-dose injection regimen has serious limitations. It may be less effective than an individually customized approach. Even when a treatment paradigm is shown to be successful in a treatment trial, it may not be directly translatable to the care of individual patients. Presumably, a treatment that can be customized to individual patients is likely to be more effective and more representative of the real life clinical situation. Such treatment is difficult to implement in clinical trials, because it magnifies confounding variables such as dosages, injection sites and techniques, and heterogeneity in the clinician's skills, and it complicates the issue of blinding.

Another gap in clinical evidence is the lack of high-quality data on the long-term efficacy and safety of BoNT in most disorders. Given the requirement of a placebo group in controlled studies, they usually must be short-term. The duration of observation ranges from one to several months, which is the typical duration of action of BoNT. The placebo-controlled double-blind period is occasionally followed by an open-label extension period. In one such analysis, the efficacy of BoNT/A in the treatment of poststroke upper extremity spasticity, as shown in the 12-week double-blind, placebo-controlled period, was also present in the 42-week open-label period.[41] However, the quality of data from extension period studies is limited, because there is no placebo control group, and patient dropout is usually difficult to control. Studies of efficacy of BoNT over a longer period are available, but they are primarily retrospective case series. An example of one such study showed that repeated injections of BoNT appeared to maintain efficacy over a 10-year period in the treatment of hemifacial spasm,[42] but there was no control group and the natural history of the disease was unknown.

There is a large unmet need for properly conducted clinical trials to assess the efficacy of BoNT in several disorders. The use of BoNT in the treatment of headache mentioned earlier illustrates this unmistakably. Negative results from recent randomized controlled trials in migraine headache[3,5] have dampened the initial enthusiasm from early anecdotal therapeutic success.[2] Studies of BoNT in the treatment of chronic daily headache have also yielded inconsistent results. Although earlier randomized controlled studies have reported positive results,[43,44] the largest studies fail to find a significant benefit.[45] Similarly most controlled studies of BoNT in the treatment of tension-type headache yielded negative results.[4] It is possible that underdosing or suboptimal muscle selection may have led to treatment failures or falsely negative results. Another potential source of discrepancy may be the variation in study patient characteristics, such as response to past treatments and psychological variables.

FUTURE CLINICAL TRIALS

The difficulty in interpretation of published headache studies highlights several important study design issues that should be addressed in future clinical trials. First, the use of a placebo control group is mandatory. This is important not only in the treatment of pain, where the placebo effect is typically large, but in most other neurologic disorders in which assessments by patients, caregivers, and even experienced clinicians may be biased by expectation of treatment effect. However, it is often difficult to recruit subjects into placebo-controlled studies, in disorders for which clinicians and patients believe that BoNT has demonstrated success. Second, all outcome assessments need to be done without knowledge of the treatment status in order to minimize bias. Third, the treatment allocation has to be randomized, because the clinical course of all of these disorders is typically variable. Fourth, the selection criteria of study patients need to be chosen judiciously. A homogeneous study population is helpful to ensure scientifically vigorous and reproducible results. This consideration, however, has to be balanced against the fact that a restrictive selection of patients will limit the generalizability of study findings.

Finally it is intriguing to consider that BoNT may have benefits beyond symptom control. It is possible that BoNT may have disease-modifying effects, perhaps based on its impact on cortical plasticity. For example, early studies show that BoNT may enhance the effect of constraint-induced movement therapy in improving hand function after stroke.[46] It is possible that future studies of BoNT, using modern neuroimaging techniques, may provide a rationale for early use of BoNT following brain injury, with the aim of improving long-term outcomes.

References

1. Simpson DM, Blitzer A, Brashear A, Comella C, Dubinsky R, Hallett M, et al. Botulinum Neurotoxin for the Treatment of Movement Disorders: An Evidence-Based Review. Report of the Therapeutics and Technology Assessment Subcommittee of the American Academy of Neurology. *Neurology.* In press.
2. Binder WJ, Brin MF, Blitzer A, Schoenrock LD, Pogoda JM. Botulinum toxin type A (BOTOX) for

treatment of migraine headaches: an open-label study. *Otolaryngol Head Neck Surg.* 2000;123:669-676.

3. Evers S, Vollmer-Haase J, Schwaag S, Rahmann A, Husstedt IW, Frese A. Botulinum toxin A in the prophylactic treatment of migraine—a randomized, double-blind, placebo-controlled study. *Cephalalgia.* 2004;24:838-843.

4. Silberstein SD, Gobel H, Jensen R, Elkind AH, Degryse R, Walcott JM, et al. Botulinum toxin type A in the prophylactic treatment of chronic tension-type headache: a multicentre, double-blind, randomized, placebo-controlled, parallel-group study. *Cephalalgia.* 2006;26:790-800.

5. Elkind AH, O'Carroll P, Blumenfeld A, DeGryse R, Dimitrova R. A series of three sequential, randomized, controlled studies of repeated treatments with botulinum toxin type A for migraine prophylaxis. *J Pain.* 2006;7:688-696.

6. Shaari CM, Sanders I. Quantifying how location and dose of botulinum toxin injections affect muscle paralysis. *Muscle Nerve.* 1993;16:964-969.

7. Lim EC-H, Seet RCS. Botulinum toxin: description of injection techniques and examination of controversies surrounding toxin diffusion. *Acta Neurol Scand.* 2008. In press.

8. Gracies JM, Simpson D. Focal Injection Therapy. In: Hallett M, ed. *The Handbook of Clinical Neurophysiology.* Philadelphia: Elsevier Science B.V.; 2003:651-695.

9. Francisco GE, Boake C, Vaughn A. Botulinum toxin in upper limb spasticity after acquired brain injury: a randomized trial comparing dilution techniques. *Am J Phys Med Rehabil.* 2002;81:355-363.

10. Lee LR, Chuang YC, Yang BJ, Hsu MJ, Liu YH. Botulinum toxin for lower limb spasticity in children with cerebral palsy: a single-blinded trial comparing dilution techniques. *Am J Phys Med Rehabil.* 2004;83:766-773.

11. Amirali A, Mu L, Gracies JM, Simpson DM. Anatomical localization of motor endplate bands in the human biceps brachii. *J Clin Neuromusc Dis.* 2008. In press.

12. Deshpande S, Gormley ME Jr, Carey JR. Muscle fiber orientation in muscles commonly injected with botulinum toxin: an anatomical pilot study. *Neurotox Res.* 2006;9:115-120.

13. Gracies JM, Weisz DJ, Yang B, Flanagan S, Simpson D. Impact of botulinum toxin type A (BTX-A) dilution and endplate targeting technique in upper limb spasticity. *Ann Neurol.* 2002;52(Suppl 1):S87.

14. Kennett D. Botulinum toxin A injections in children: technique and dosing issues. *Am J Phys Med Rehabil.* 2004;83(Suppl):S59-S64.

15. Flynn TC, Clark RE 2nd. Botulinum toxin type B (MYOBLOC) versus botulinum toxin type A (BOTOX) frontalis study: rate of onset and radius of diffusion. *Dermatol Surg.* 2003;29:519-522.

16. Lew MF, Adornato BT, Duane DD, Dykstra DD, Factor SA, Massey JM, et al. Botulinum toxin type B: a double-blind, placebo-controlled, safety and efficacy study in cervical dystonia. *Neurology.* 1997;49:701-707.

17. Brin MF, Lew MF, Adler CH, Comella CL, Factor SA, Jankovic J, et al. Safety and efficacy of NeuroBloc (botulinum toxin type B) in type A-resistant cervical dystonia. *Neurology.* 1999;53:1431-1438.

18. Truong D, Duane DD, Jankovic J, Singer C, Seeberger LC, Comella CL, et al. Efficacy and safety of botulinum type A toxin (Dysport) in cervical dystonia: Results of the first US randomized, double-blind, placebo-controlled study. *Mov Disord.* 2005;20:783-791.

19. Comella CL, Jankovic J, Shannon KM, Tsui J, Swenson M, Leurgans S, et al. Comparison of botulinum toxin serotypes A and B for the treatment of cervical dystonia. *Neurology.* 2005;65:1423-1429.

20. Tintner R, Gross R, Winzer UF, Smalky KA, Jankovic J. Autonomic function after botulinum toxin type A or B: a double-blind, randomized trial. *Neurology.* 2005;65:765-767.

21. Molloy FM, Shill HA, Kaelin-Lang A, Karp BI. Accuracy of muscle localization without EMG: implications for treatment of limb dystonia. *Neurology.* 2002;58:805-807.

22. Jankovic J. Needle EMG guidance for injection of botulinum toxin. Needle EMG guidance is rarely required. *Muscle Nerve.* 2001;24:1568-1570.

23. Simpson DM, Alexander DN, O'Brien CF, Tagliati M, Aswad AS, Leon JM, et al. Botulinum toxin type A in the treatment of upper extremity spasticity: a randomized, double-blind, placebo-controlled trial. *Neurology.* 1996;46:1306-1310.

24. Landau WM. Spasticity after stroke: why bother? *Stroke; a journal of cerebral circulation.* 2004;35:1787-1788.

25. Brashear A, Gordon MF, Elovic E, Kassicieh VD, Marciniak C, Do M, et al. Intramuscular injection of botulinum toxin for the treatment of wrist and finger spasticity after a stroke. *N Engl J Med.* 2002;347:395-400.

26. Cole R, Hallett M, Cohen LG. Double-blind trial of botulinum toxin for treatment of focal hand dystonia. *Mov Disord.* 1995;10:466-471.

27. Jankovic J, Schwartz K, Clemence W, Aswad A, Mordaunt J. A randomized, double-blind, placebo-controlled study to evaluate botulinum toxin type A in essential hand tremor. *Mov Disord.* 1996;11:250-256.

28. Sheffield JK, Jankovic J. Botulinum toxin in the treatment of tremors, dystonias, sialorrhea and other symptoms associated with Parkinson's disease. *Exp Rev Neurother.* 2007;7:637-647.

29. Dressler D, Hallett M. Immunological aspects of Botox, Dysport and Myobloc/NeuroBloc. *Eur J Neurol.* 2006;13(Suppl 1):11-15.

30. Jankovic J, Hunter C, Dolimbek BZ, Dolimbek GS, Adler CH, Brashear A, et al. Clinico-immunologic aspects of botulinum toxin type B treatment of cervical dystonia. *Neurology.* 2006;67:2233-2235.

31. Hanna PA, Jankovic J, Vincent A. Comparison of mouse bioassay and immunoprecipitation assay for botulinum toxin antibodies. *J Neurol Neurosurg Psychiatry.* 1999;66:612-616.

32. Cordivari C, Misra VP, Vincent A, Catania S, Bhatia KP, Lees AJ. Secondary nonresponsiveness to botulinum toxin A in cervical dystonia: the role of electromyogram-guided injections, botulinum toxin A antibody assay, and the extensor digitorum brevis test. *Mov Disord.* 2006;21:1737-1741.

33. Girlanda P, Quartarone A, Sinicropi S, Nicolosi C, Messina C. Unilateral injection of botulinum toxin in blepharospasm: single fiber electromyography and blink reflex study. *Mov Disord.* 1996;11:27-31.

34. Jankovic J, Orman J. Botulinum A toxin for cranial-cervical dystonia: a double-blind, placebo-controlled study. *Neurology.* 1987;37:616-623.

35. Park YC, Lim JK, Lee DK, Yi SD. Botulinum a toxin treatment of hemifacial spasm and blepharospasm. *J Korean Med Sci.* 1993;8:334-340.

36. Yoshimura DM, Aminoff MJ, Tami TA, Scott AB. Treatment of hemifacial spasm with botulinum toxin. *Muscle Nerve.* 1992;15:1045-1049.

37. Troung DD, Rontal M, Rolnick M, Aronson AE, Mistura K. Double-blind controlled study of botulinum toxin in adductor spasmodic dysphonia. *Laryngoscope*. 1991;101:630-634.

38. Brans JW, Lindeboom R, Snoek JW, Zwarts MJ, van Weerden TW, Brunt ER, et al. Botulinum toxin versus trihexyphenidyl in cervical dystonia: a prospective, randomized, double-blind controlled trial. *Neurology*. 1996;46:1066-1072.

39. Simpson D, Gracies JM, Yablon S, et al. Botulinum neurotoxin vs oral tizanidine in the treatment of upper limb spasticity: A double-blind, placebo-controlled study (abstr). 59th Annual Meeting of the American Academy of Neurology, Boston, MA. 2007.

40. Ward A, Roberts G, Warner J, Gillard S. Cost-effectiveness of botulinum toxin type A in the treatment of post-stroke spasticity. *J Rehabil Med*. 2005;37:252-257.

41. Gordon MF, Brashear A, Elovic E, Kassicieh D, Marciniak C, Liu J, et al. Repeated dosing of botulinum toxin type A for upper limb spasticity following stroke. *Neurology*. 2004;63:1971-1973.

42. Defazio G, Abbruzzese G, Girlanda P, Vacca L, Curra A, De Salvia R, et al. Botulinum toxin A treatment for primary hemifacial spasm: a 10-year multicenter study. *Arch Neurol*. 2002;59:418-420.

43. Ondo WG, Vuong KD, Derman HS. Botulinum toxin A for chronic daily headache: a randomized, placebo-controlled, parallel design study. *Cephalalgia*. 2004;24:60-65.

44. Mathew NT, Frishberg BM, Gawel M, Dimitrova R, Gibson J, Turkel C. Botulinum toxin type A (BOTOX) for the prophylactic treatment of chronic daily headache: a randomized, double-blind, placebo-controlled trial. *Headache*. 2005;45:293-307.

45. Silberstein SD, Stark SR, Lucas SM, Christie SN, Degryse RE, Turkel CC. Botulinum toxin type A for the prophylactic treatment of chronic daily headache: a randomized, double-blind, placebo-controlled trial. *Mayo Clin Proc*. 2005;80:1126-1137.

46. Levy CE, Giuffrida C, Richards L, Wu S, Davis S, Nadeau SE. Botulinum toxin A, evidence-based exercise therapy, and constraint-induced movement therapy for upper-limb hemiparesis attributable to stroke: a preliminary study. *Am J Phys Med Rehabil*. 2007;86:696-706.

Potential New 30 Therapeutic Indications for Botulinum Neurotoxins

Mark Hallett

INTRODUCTION

The botulinum neurotoxins (BoNTs) are incredible therapeutic agents with a very wide range of accepted indications. Moreover, the indications seem to increase almost daily. This book covers most of the indications that are in common use already and those that seem very promising. This chapter covers a range of indications that are very new or seem to have potential (Table 30-1). It will also note some minor older applications not noted in the other chapters. It is organized by medical discipline. Published literature for an indication, when available, will be quoted, but for many of these indications, there is often other unpublished experience. Most of the reports of the use of BoNT for these new or minor indications are based on anecdotal experience and have not been subjected to rigorous clinical trials.

NEUROLOGY

Movement Disorders

Parkinson Disease
Of all the disorders for which BoNT is currently used, movement disorders represent about half of all the indications. Although dystonia is the most common movement disorder treated with BoNT, there are many other movement disorders that benefit from BoNT treatment. Even within Parkinson disease, the most common movement disorder, BoNT can be used for a variety of symptoms, such as hand and jaw tremor, limb dystonia, blepharospasm and apraxia of eyelid opening, bruxism, camptocormia, freezing of gait, sialorrhea and constipation.[1]

Myoclonus
Myoclonus consists of jerk-like movements produced by quick muscle contractions. When focal, BoNT can suppress the abnormal activity. This has been recognized for many years, and a number of case reports have appeared describing benefit.[2,3] Myoclonus associated with Rasmussen encephalitis has been successfully treated in the face.[4] Hereditary chin tremor has been also reported to respond to treatment with BoNT.[5]

Essential Palatal Tremor
Essential palatal tremor is also referred to as essential palatal myoclonus. Patients with this disorder are often troubled by clicking in the ear due to rhythmic contraction of the tensor veli palatini muscle. The disorder is of unknown origin, and oral therapies have very limited value. Focal injection of the tensor veli palatini muscle can be helpful.[6-8] Approach to the muscle can be transoral or transnasal.

Myokymia
Myokymia is characterized by small, irregular movements in a region, sometimes described

Dr. Hallett is disclosing that he is the Chair of the Neurotoxin Institute Advisory Council (NAC).

TABLE 30-1 New and Less Frequent Applications of Botulinum Toxin

Neurologic indications
    Movement disorders
        Parkinson disease
        Myoclonus
        Essential palatal tremor
        Myokymia
        Stiffperson syndrome
        Scoliosis
    Pain syndromes
        Low back pain
        Postherpetic neuralgia
        Trigeminal neuralgia
        Stump pain
        Plantar fasciitis
        Clubfoot
        Restless legs syndrome
        Carpal tunnel syndrome
    Central nervous system: Epilepsy
Surgery: Immobilization
Otolaryngology: Rhinitis
Dermatology
    Acne
    Psoriasis
    Dupuytren contracture
    Body odor
Other
Veterinary use

as a "bag of worms." There are many causes, but, independent of cause, a focal injection of BoNT can be effective.[9-11]

Stiff Person Syndrome

Stiff person syndrome is a disorder with continuous muscle contraction of truncal and limb muscles. Its manifestations are sufficiently widespread that ordinarily it requires systemic therapy. Because it is an autoimmune disorder, therapies such as intravenous immunoglobin are appropriate, and systemic therapy with drugs like benzodiazepines can be effective. In some circumstances, however, some local therapy can be undertaken with BoNT.[12,13]

Scoliosis

The notion that scoliosis might be helped with injections of BoNT was raised a decade ago.[14] Twelve children with severe additional disorders requiring surgical delay were treated. Short-term results showed that all patients had some reduction in their curves, up to more than 50 degrees. Despite this success, this treatment has not been undertaken very often, perhaps because the effects of BoNT therapy would only be temporary.

Pain Syndromes

The exact method of action of BoNT on pain is not known, and perhaps there are multiple mechanisms, including relief of painful muscle spasm. For example, BoNT, has been found to be very effective in the treatment of cervical muscles spasms that occur after whiplash type injuries.[15]

There is some evidence that BoNT has effects on pain separate from its effects on muscle spasms, but this is still debatable. The principle idea at present is that BoNT prevents the release of peptide neurotransmitters at pain endings, reducing peripheral sensitization and indirectly reducing central sensitization.[16] Despite these theoretical considerations, several studies have failed to provide definitive evidence that BoNT has independent analgesic properties. For example, quantitative sensory testing and measurements of pain thresholds in response to local electrical stimulation showed no statistically significant differences between patients pretreated with subcutaneous injection of botulinum neurotoxin type A (BoNT/A) or placebo.[17,18] A randomized, double-blind, paired study compared the effects of BoNT versus pure saline and found no direct effect on acute, noninflammatory pain produced by ultraviolet B irradiation or any anti-inflammatory effects.[19] Studies are conflicting with a capsaicin model of pain. One study compared intradermal injections of BoNT/A and placebo in a double-blind manner and found that such injections had no effect on thermal or current sensory perception or on flare response to capsaicin.[20] Similar results were seen in another double-blind study in which there was no effect of prior BoNT/A injections on heat, cold, and electrical stimulation pain in response to capsaicin.[21] On the other hand, a suppressive effect of BoNT/A on pain, flare, and hyperalgesia area produced by capsaicin was observed in another double-blind investigation.[22] The strong placebo effect should always be considered when designing and interpreting studies of BoNT treatment of pain disorders.[23]

Low Back Pain

BoNT has been used for treatment in chronic low back pain. It is the chronic condition that is difficult to treat, and most patients with acute low back pain improved relatively rapidly. In an early, randomized, double blind study, 31 patients received either 200 U of Botox (Allergan, Inc, Irvine, CA), 40 U/site at five lumbar paravertebral levels on the side of maximum discomfort or normal saline.[24] At 3 weeks, 11 of 15 patients who received Botox had more than 50% pain relief compared with 4 of 16 in the placebo group. At 8 weeks, 9 of 15 in the toxin group and 2 of 16 in the placebo group had relief. In a more recent report of a two-part study, investigators used up to 500 U of Botox, treating multiple levels of the lumbar paravertebral muscles with 50 U per site.[25] In an initial prospective open-label study, 53% of 75 patients improved, and 91% of the responders continued to respond over 14 months. In a subsequent double-blind, randomized, placebo-controlled study, 60% of patients had significant pain relief.

Postherpetic Neuralgia
One case has been reported of an 80-year-old man who had severe pain, refractory to the usual therapies. The pain was "dramatically relieved" for 52 days after multiple BoNT/A injections.[26]

Trigeminal Neuralgia
There have been a number of case reports about successful treatment of trigeminal neuralgia. Two open-label studies also have favorable outcomes. For eight patients, 100 U BoNT/A (Botox) was injected into the region of the zygomatic arch resulting in improvement.[27] Thirteen patients were treated with BoNT/A, and Visual Analog Scale score, surface area of pain, and therapeutic coefficient were reduced in all patients and for all branch trigeminal nerves studied.[28] The dose of BoNT/A (Botox) was individualized (V_1 received an average of 6.83 units, V_2 received an average of 6.45 units, and V_3 received an average of 9.11 units).

Stump Pain
Two patients with arm amputations and two patients with leg amputations were treated with BoNT/B (Neurobloc, Solstice Neurosciences, Malvern, PA) injections at several trigger points of their stump musculature.[29] A total dose of 2500 units was used in the arm, and 2500 units and 5000 units was used in the two leg stumps. All patients experienced a reduction in stump pain, which lasted for many weeks. There was also a decreased occurrence of involuntary stump movements. Another four patients, one with phantom pain and three with stump pain, were each treated with 100 U BoNT/A (Botox), divided between several trigger points in the distal stump musculature.[30] The pain was reduced in all four patients, and allowed a greater use of the limb prostheses.

Plantar Fasciitis
A randomized, double-blind, placebo-controlled study of 27 patients (43 feet) with plantar fasciitis was done using BoNT/A.[31] In patients with bilateral symptoms of comparable severity, injections of toxin were given in one foot and saline in the other. The treatment group received injections into two sites per foot: (1) 40 U (Botox) into the tender area in the medial aspect of the heel close to the calcaneal tuberosity, (2) 30 U (Botox) in the arch of the foot between an inch anterior to the heel and middle of the foot. The placebo group received normal saline. Compared with placebo injections, the BoNT group improved in several measures of pain and had improved foot function at both 3 and 8 weeks after injection (Fig. 30-1). In another study, nine patients with an average duration of symptoms of 14 months and at least two prior conservative treatments received a one injection of 200 U of BoNT/A (Dysport, Ipsen, Milford, MA) subfascially into the painful area.[32] There was a significant reduction of pain during weight bearing of about 50% at 6 weeks after injection, and the effect

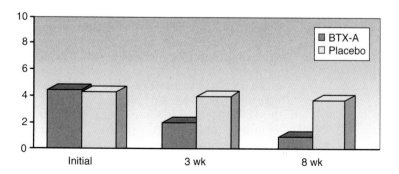

FIGURE 30-1. Treatment response of plantar fasciitis to BoNT/A. Pain Visual Analog Scale scores for the BoNT/A and placebo groups. (From Babcock MS, Foster L, Pasquina P, Jabbari B. Treatment of pain attributed to plantar fasciitis with botulinum toxin A: a short-term, randomized, placebo-controlled, double-blind study. *Am J Phys Med Rehabil.* 2005;84:649-654 with permission.)

persisted at 14 weeks. The pain at rest was reduced to less than half of the initial value at both 6 and 14 weeks.

Other Foot Problems

In a study of 51 patients, mean age 16 months (range 2.5–33 months), affected with 73 clubfoot deformities, BoNT/A injections into the triceps surae muscle complex produced significant improvement in various measures.[33]

Restless Legs Syndrome

Three patients with restless legs syndrome were treated with BoNT/A whose symptoms were refractory to or who refused oral medication.[34] Areas of maximal discomfort were injected. The first patient received injections in both legs and had benefit for 12 weeks. The second patient received injections in both legs and his lumbar paraspinal muscles. He had improvement in the sensory discomfort at 3 days, and by 1 month had improvement also in his Epworth Sleepiness Scale score. The third patient was also injected in both legs, had improvement in 2 days and benefit lasted 10 weeks. In all three, the benefit was repeated in additional injection cycles.

Carpal Tunnel Syndrome

An open-label, prospective study of five women was conducted using 60 units of BoNT/A (Botox) injected into the carpal area.[35] At 3 months, pain was improved in three, remained static in one, and was aggravated in one. The authors noted that the data were difficult to interpret given the lack of placebo control. Another study of 20 patients using BoNT/B was randomized, double blind, and placebo controlled.[23] Here, the agent was injected into three hypothenar muscles anatomically linked or attached to the carpal tunnel and its tentorium, opponens digiti minimi, flexor digiti minimi, and palmaris brevis muscles. Over the course of 13 weeks, there was no statistically significant difference between the two study groups regarding changes from baseline in any study outcome. Although the present conclusion must be that BoNT is not effective for carpal tunnel syndrome, it is not clear in either study that injections were optimally placed.

Central Nervous System Use

Epilepsy

From a theoretical point of view, the focal delivery of BoNT into an epileptic focus could inhibit neurotransmitter release and be antiepileptic. BoNT/E was injected into the rat hippocampus to inhibit glutamate release and consequently block spike activity of pyramidal neurons.[36] This reduced both focal and generalized kainic acid–induced seizures, and prevented neuronal loss and long-term cognitive deficits that are associated with kainic acid seizures. Additionally, it was more difficult to kindle BoNT/E-injected rats. The investigators concluded that BoNT/E can be both anti-ictal and antiepileptogenic. More work will clearly be needed in animal models before human trials could be initiated.

SURGERY

After surgery or in other circumstances, such as after a fracture or athletic injury, it is often valuable to have the healing body part immobilized. Sometimes, this is difficult because of the site of the injury or because of an underlying neurologic problem, such as an involuntary movement disorder. In such circumstances, BoNT could be useful to aid the immobilization.

OTOLARYNGOLOGY

Rhinitis

Thirty-four patients with allergic rhinitis were investigated in a double-blind, placebo-controlled study with BoNT/A (Botox).[37] Patients were randomly divided into three groups: Group A, 20 units was injected into each nasal cavity (total 40 U); Group B, 30 U was injected into each nasal cavity (total 60 U); Group C, 2 mL of isotonic saline was injected as placebo. Rhinorrhea, nasal obstruction, sneezing, and itching were scored by the patients, who were examined at Weeks 1, 2, 4, 6 and 8. There was no statistically significant difference between groups A and B, but rhinorrhea, nasal obstruction and sneezing scores in groups A and B were significantly better than those in group C at all time points. Thirty-five patients with vasomotor rhinitis were treated in a prospective, controlled (but not blinded) investigation.[38] Fifteen patients were injected 10 U of BoNT/A (Botox), and 15 patients were injected 20 units to inferior and middle turbinates. Five patients were controls and were injected with saline solution into the inferior and middle turbinates. Treated patients were statistically better than controls for nasal obstruction, sneezing, nasal discharge, and nasal itching.

DERMATOLOGY

Acne

Two patients with Tourette syndrome have been described, whose acne cleared for 4 to 5 months in the local region where BoNT was injected for tics.[39]

Psoriasis

Anecdotal evidence was presented in a poster at the International Conference on Neurotoxins (ICON) meeting in two patients (Andrews 2006).

Dupuytren Contracture

Use of BoNT therapy for Dupuytren contracture has been hypothetically proposed.[40]

Body Odor

There have been several controlled trials of BoNT for body odor independent of its effect on sweating. Sixteen healthy volunteers were injected with BoNT/A (100 U Dysport) in one axilla and 0.9% sodium chloride solution in the other axilla in a randomized,

double-blinded study.[41] At 7 days, body odor was assessed by a T-shirt sniff test, and there was a significant reduction of odor intensity for the side treated with toxin (Fig. 30-2). The smell was also considered less unpleasant (Fig. 30-3). The authors suggested that the underlying mechanisms may include interference with skin microbes and denervation of apoeccrine sweat glands. In another randomized, double-blind, placebo-controlled study, 51 healthy volunteers were injected with BoNT/A (50 U Botox) in one axilla and placebo in the other.[42] Again the T-shirt sniff test was the primary outcome measure. Samples from the toxin side smelled less intense and even "better" according to self-assessments and those from independent raters. After BoNT injection, the raters preferred "to work together with the respective person" and even found the odor "more erotic."

Genital odor is an uncommon problem characterized by an offensive and malodorous smell. Such a patient was treated with BoNT/A and improved the odor substantially.[43] BoNT is also being used in the treatment of special body odor (referred to as "wakiga") in Japan.[44]

OTHER CONDITIONS

Injection of BoNT guided by computed tomography to inhibit overactivity of the diaphragmatic crus caused by diaphragmatic compression of the renal artery has been reported to alleviate hypertension and may be an alternative to surgery and renal artery stenting.[45] Unilateral injection of the soft

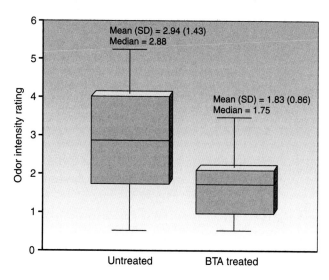

FIGURE 30-2. Treatment response of body odor to BoNT/A. Ratings of body odor intensity, on a numeric scale of 0 (no odor) to 6 (most intense odor) in treated and untreated subjects. Box range represents 50% of all ratings; bar range, 100% of all ratings. $P = .02$ for significance of the difference (Wilcoxon test). (From Heckmann M, Teichmann B, Pause BM, Plewig G. Amelioration of body odor after intracutaneous axillary injection of botulinum toxin A. *Arch Dermatol.* 2003;139:57-59 with permission.)

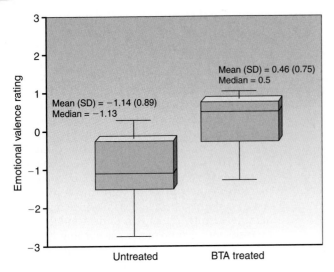

Mean (SD) = 0.46 (0.75)
Median = 0.5

Mean (SD) = −1.14 (0.89)
Median = −1.13

FIGURE 30-3. Treatment response of body odor to BoNT/A. Ratings of emotional valence of body odor, on a numeric scale of −3 (most repulsive) to +3 (most pleasant) in treated and untreated subjects. Box range represents 50% of all ratings; bar range, 100% of all ratings. $P = .01$ for significance of the difference (Wilcoxon test). (From Heckmann M, Teichmann B, Pause BM, Plewig G. Amelioration of body odor after intracutaneous axillary injection of botulinum toxin A. *Arch Dermatol.* 2003;139:57-59 with permission.)

palate (20 U Dysport) has been reported to be effective in ameliorating habitual snoring.[46]

VETERINARY USE

BoNT is beginning to be used also in veterinary medicine for a variety of conditions. For example, the condition of a cat with a tarsal deformity was improved with BoNT.[47] BoNT/A was used successfully to treat essential blepharospasm in a dog over several cycles.[48]

ACKNOWLEDGMENT

Many of the ideas in this chapter came out of a workgroup for the ICON meeting. In addition to the editors of this book, other members of the ICON workgroup were Drs. A. Blitzer, D. Dressler, D. Dykstra, M. Ferrante, D.A. Glaser, M. Mahowald, M. Naumann, S. Silberstein, and L. Smith.

References

1. Sheffield JK, Jankovic J. Botulinum toxin in the treatment of tremors, dystonias, sialorrhea and other symptoms associated with Parkinson's disease. *Expert Rev Neurother.* 2007;7:637-647.
2. Polo KB, Jabbari B. Effectiveness of botulinum toxin type A against painful limb myoclonus of spinal cord origin. *Mov Disord.* 1994;9:233-235.
3. Lagueny A, Tison F, Burbaud P, Le Masson G, Kien P. Stimulus-sensitive spinal segmental myoclonus improved with injections of botulinum toxin type A. *Mov Disord.* 1999;14:182-185.
4. Browner N, Azher SN, Jankovic J. Botulinum toxin treatment of facial myoclonus in suspected Rasmussen encephalitis. *Mov Disord.* 2006;21:1500-1502.
5. Devetag Chalaupka F, Bartholini F, Mandich G, Turro M. Two new families with hereditary essential chin myoclonus: clinical features, neurophysiological findings and treatment. *Neurol Sci.* 2006;27:97-103.
6. Saeed SR, Brookes GB. The use of Clostridium botulinum toxin in palatal myoclonus. A preliminary report. *J Laryngol Otol.* 1993;107:208-210.
7. Penney SE, Bruce IA, Saeed SR. Botulinum toxin is effective and safe for palatal tremor: a report of five cases and a review of the literature. *J Neurol.* 2006;253:857-860.
8. Pal PK, Lakshmi PS, Nirmala M. Efficacy and complication of botulinum toxin injection in palatal myoclonus: experience from a patient. *Mov Disord.* 2007;22:1484-1486.
9. Jordan DR, Anderson RL, Thiese SM. Intractable orbicularis myokymia: treatment alternatives. *Ophthalmic Surg.* 1989;20:280-283.
10. Lou JS, Pleninger P, Kurlan R. Botulinum toxin A is effective in treating trismus associated with postradiation myokymia and muscle spasm [letter]. *Mov Disord.* 1995;10:680-681.
11. Sedano MJ, Trejo JM, Macarron JL, Polo JM, Berciano J, Calleja J. Continuous facial myokymia in multiple sclerosis: treatment with botulinum toxin. *Eur Neurol.* 2000;43:137-140.
12. Davis D, Jabbari B. Significant improvement of stiff-person syndrome after paraspinal injection of botulinum toxin A. *Mov Disord.* 1993;8:371-373.
13. Liguori R, Cordivari C, Lugaresi E, Montagna P. Botulinum toxin A improves muscle spasms and rigidity in stiff-person syndrome. *Mov Disord.* 1997;12:1060-1063.
14. Nuzzo RM, Walsh S, Boucherit T, Massood S. Counterparalysis for treatment of paralytic scoliosis with botulinum toxin type A. *Am J Orthop.* 1997;26:201-207.
15. Freund B, Schwartz M. The role of botulinum toxin in whiplash injuries. *Curr Pain Headache Rep.* 2006;10:355-359.
16. Dolly JO, Aoki KR. The structure and mode of action of different botulinum toxins. *Eur J Neurol.* 2006;13(suppl 4):1-9.
17. Blersch W, Schulte-Mattler WJ, Przywara S, May A, Bigalke H, Wohlfarth K. Botulinum toxin A and the

cutaneous nociception in humans: a prospective, double-blind, placebo-controlled, randomized study. *J Neurol Sci.* 2002;205:59-63.

18. Kramer HH, Angerer C, Erbguth F, Schmelz M, Birklein F. Botulinum toxin A reduces neurogenic flare but has almost no effect on pain and hyperalgesia in human skin. *J Neurol.* 2003;250:188-193.

19. Sycha T, Samal D, Chizh B, Lehr S, Gustorff B, Schnider P, et al. A lack of antinociceptive or antiinflammatory effect of botulinum toxin A in an inflammatory human pain model. *Anesth Analg.* 2006;102:509-516.

20. Voller B, Sycha T, Gustorff B, Schmetterer L, Lehr S, Eichler HG, et al. A randomized, double-blind, placebo controlled study on analgesic effects of botulinum toxin A. *Neurology.* 2003;61:940-944.

21. Schulte-Mattler WJ, Opatz O, Blersch W, May A, Bigalke H, Wohlfahrt K. Botulinum toxin A does not alter capsaicin-induced pain perception in human skin. *J Neurol Sci.* 2007;260:38-42.

22. Gazerani P, Staahl C, Drewes AM, Arendt-Nielsen L. The effects of botulinum toxin type A on capsaicin-evoked pain, flare, and secondary hyperalgesia in an experimental human model of trigeminal sensitization. *Pain.* 2006;122:315-325.

23. Breuer B, Sperber K, Wallenstein S, Kiprovski K, Calapa A, Snow B, et al. Clinically significant placebo analgesic response in a pilot trial of botulinum B in patients with hand pain and carpal tunnel syndrome. *Pain Med.* 2006;7:16-24.

24. Foster L, Clapp L, Erickson M, Jabbari B. Botulinum toxin A and chronic low back pain: a randomized, double-blind study. *Neurology.* 2001;56:1290-1293.

25. Jabbari B. Treatment of chronic low back pain with botulinum neurotoxins. *Curr Pain Headache Rep.* 2007;11:352-358.

26. Liu HT, Tsai SK, Kao MC, Hu JS. Botulinum toxin A relieved neuropathic pain in a case of post-herpetic neuralgia. *Pain Med.* 2006;7:89-91.

27. Turk U, Ilhan S, Alp R, Sur H. Botulinum toxin and intractable trigeminal neuralgia. *Clin Neuropharmacol.* 2005;28:161-162.

28. Piovesan EJ, Teive HG, Kowacs PA, Della Coletta MV, Werneck LC, et al. An open study of botulinum-A toxin treatment of trigeminal neuralgia. *Neurology.* 2005;65:1306-1308.

29. Kern U, Martin C, Scheicher S, Muller H. Effects of botulinum toxin type B on stump pain and involuntary movements of the stump. *Am J Phys Med Rehabil.* 2004;83:396-399.

30. Kern U, Martin C, Scheicher S, Muller H. Does botulinum toxin A make prosthesis use easier for amputees? *J Rehabil Med.* 2004;36:238-239.

31. Babcock MS, Foster L, Pasquina P, Jabbari B. Treatment of pain attributed to plantar fasciitis with botulinum toxin a: a short-term, randomized, placebo-controlled, double-blind study. *Am J Phys Med Rehabil.* 2005;84:649-654.

32. Placzek R, Deuretzbacher G, Meiss AL. Treatment of chronic plantar fasciitis with botulinum toxin A: preliminary clinical results. *Clin J Pain.* 2006;22:190-192.

33. Alvarez CM, Tredwell SJ, Keenan SP, et al. Treatment of idiopathic clubfoot utilizing botulinum A toxin: a new method and its short-term outcomes. *J Pediatr Orthop.* 2005;25:229-235.

34. Rotenberg JS, Canard K, Difazio M. Successful treatment of recalcitrant restless legs syndrome with botulinum toxin type-A. *J Clin Sleep Med.* 2006;2:275-278.

35. Tsai CP, Liu CY, Lin KP, Wang KC. Efficacy of botulinum toxin type a in the relief of carpal tunnel syndrome: A preliminary experience. *Clin Drug Investig.* 2006;26:511-515.

36. Costantin L, Bozzi Y, Richichi C, et al. Antiepileptic effects of botulinum neurotoxin E. *J Neurosci.* 2005;25:1943-1951.

37. Unal M, Sevim S, Dogu O, Vayisoglu Y, Kanik A. Effect of botulinum toxin type A on nasal symptoms in patients with allergic rhinitis: a double-blind, placebo-controlled clinical trial. *Acta Otolaryngol.* 2003;123:1060-1063.

38. Ozcan C, Vayisoglu Y, Dogu O, Gorur K. The effect of intranasal injection of botulinum toxin A on the symptoms of vasomotor rhinitis. *Am J Otolaryngol.* 2006;27:314-318.

39. Diamond A, Jankovic J. Botulinum toxin in dermatology - beyond wrinkles and sweat. *J Cosmet Dermatol.* 2006;5:169.

40. Namazi H, Abdinejad F. Botulinum toxin as a novel addition to the antidupuytren armamentarium. *Med Hypotheses.* 2007;68:240-241.

41. Heckmann M, Teichmann B, Pause BM, Plewig G. Amelioration of body odor after intracutaneous axillary injection of botulinum toxin A. *Arch Dermatol.* 2003;139:57-59.

42. Heckmann M, Kutt S, Dittmar S, Hamm H. Making scents: improvement of olfactory profile after botulinum toxin-A treatment in healthy individuals. *Dermatol Surg.* 2007;33:S81-S87.

43. Lee JB, Kim BS, Kim MB, Oh CK, Jang HS, Kwon KS. A case of foul genital odor treated with botulinum toxin A. *Dermatol Surg.* 2004;30:1233-1235.

44. Jankovic J. Botulinum toxin in clinical practice. *J Neurol Neurosurg Psychiatry.* 2004;75:951-957.

45. Bilici A, Karcaaltincaba M, Ilica AT, Bukte Y, Senol A. Treatment of hypertension from renal artery entrapment by percutaneous CT-guided botulinum toxin injection into diaphragmatic crus as alternative to surgery and stenting. *AJR Am J Roentgenol.* 2007;189:W143-W145.

46. Kuhnel TS, Schulte-Mattler W, Bigalke H, Wohlfarth K. Treatment of habitual snoring with botulinum toxin: a pilot study. *Sleep Breath.* 2007;12:63-68.

47. Bright SR, Girling SL, O'Neill T, Innes JF. Partial tarsal arthrodesis and botulinum toxin A injection for correction of tarsal arthrogryposis in a cat. *J Small Anim Pract.* 2007;48:39-42.

48. Meyer-Lindenberg A, Wohlfarth KM, Switzer EN. The use of botulinum toxin A for treatment of possible essential blepharospasm in a dog. *Aust Vet J.* 2003;81:612-614.

Botulism Vaccines and 31 the Immune Response

Leonard A. Smith and Janice M. Rusnak

INTRODUCTION

Botulinum toxin is a neurotoxin produced by *Clostridium botulinum*, and one of the most potent known toxins. Intoxication from botulinum neurotoxin (BoNT), known as botulism, may result from ingestion of toxin present in improperly preserved foods (food-borne botulism), ingestion of *C. botulinum* organisms or spores (infant botulism and intestinal botulism), infections of wounds with *C. botulinum* (wound botulism), or inhalation of aerosolized toxin as may occur from a laboratory exposure or a bioterrorism event. Symptoms of intoxication begin hours to days after toxin exposure (usually 12 to 36 hours postexposure; range 2 hours to 8 days postexposure), with neurologic symptoms consisting of an acute, symmetric descending paralysis that may result in respiratory failure. With supportive treatment and antitoxin therapy, case fatalities are generally less than 10%.

Individuals working in public health laboratories (who test food sources for BoNT) or who work in research institutions or industries with botulinum toxin or *C. botulinum* cultures are at risk for botulism.[1] Botulinum vaccines have been given to at-risk individuals since 1946. Initially an investigational bivalent (A/B) botulinum toxoid was administered to at-risk individuals in the U.S. Offensive Biological Warfare Program, that was subsequently replaced in 1959 with an investigational botulinum toxoid adsorbed pentavalent (ABCDE) product, currently referred to as the pentavalent (ABCDE) botulinum toxoid (PBT).[2-6] In 1965, the PBT was made available to at-risk persons under Centers of Disease Control and Prevention (CDC) IND 161. More than 20,000 injections of the PBT have been given to date to at-risk individuals under CDC IND 161 (more than 7000 of the doses were given under IND 161 at the United States Army Medical Research Institute of Infectious Diseases [USAMRIID] since 1979). Additionally, more than 8000 doses of the PBT were administered to military troops (mainly during Operation Desert Storm) under the U.S. Army's Office of the Surgeon General IND 3723.[7]

PENTAVALENT (ABCDE) BOTULINUM TOXOID

The PBT, an investigational vaccine, is an aluminum phosphate-adsorbed toxoid derived from formalin-inactivated, partially purified toxin serotypes A to E.[8,9] The PBT was developed by the Department of Defense, and initially manufactured by Parke-Davis Company in 1958.[10] Each of the five toxin serotypes was propagated individually in bulk culture, followed by separation of extracellular toxin from bacterial cell mass, acid precipitation of toxin, filtration, detoxification of the active toxins using formaldehyde, and adsorption of the toxoid onto aluminum phosphate.[11] The five monovalent toxoid products (A–E) were then blended to produce the final PBT product. Formulation for blending the five serotypes was based on concentrations of immunogen that induced protective immunity in guinea pigs against a lethal challenge with 10^5 mouse intraperitoneal (IP) LD_{50} doses of the respective *C. botulinum* toxins. In the 1970s, The Michigan Department of Public Health (MDPH), using Parke-Davis methodologies, produced the monovalent toxoids contained in the PBT product in use today. The monovalent toxoids produced in the 1970s were used to formulate the PBT lots used in recent years (Lots A2, PBP-001, PBP-003, and PBP-004).

374 Dr. Smith is disclosing that he is a consultant for Allergan, Inc. Dr. Rusnak did not report any outside consulting agreements.

The final PBT product is bottled in 5-mL vials, with each 5-mL multidose vial containing 0.22% formaldehyde as a stabilizer and 1:10,000 thimerosal as a preservative. Each 0.5-mL dose of vaccine contains 7 mg of aluminum phosphate and approximately 5 mg of inactivated toxin. The PBT has been administered throughout the years as a primary series of three injections of 0.5 mL subcutaneously (injection given at day 0, 2 weeks, and 12 weeks), followed by a mandatory booster dose at 1 year. Although the dosing of the initial 3 doses of the primary series has remained constant, the regimen for booster doses has varied since 1959.

Animal Studies

The potential protection of the PBT in humans is based on the levels of antitoxin titers observed in vaccinated individuals, which are presumed to be protective based on extrapolation of data from animal studies.[9,12] Animal studies with the PBT demonstrated (1) protection against intraperitoneal challenge with lethal doses of botulinum toxin serotypes A, B, C, D, and E, and (2) correlation of serum antitoxin levels with protection against botulism.[5,7,12,13] Only one study had been performed in nonhuman primates to demonstrate protection of the PBT against aerosol challenge.[14] Five nonhuman primates, following an abbreviated vaccination schedule of PBT Lot PBP-001 (1 and 2 weeks), were protected against aerosol challenge with a lethal dose of toxin serotype A (challenge doses of 13, 24, 26, 27, and 29 LD_{50}). Antitoxin titers in three monkeys at the time of challenge were 0.25 IU/mL, but lower antitoxin levels in the remaining two monkeys (0.06 IU/mL and <0.01 IU/mL) were also protective.

Initial Pentavalent Botulinum Toxoid Study in Humans

The initial PBT study reported by Fiock et al[9] in humans, using the initial three pentavalent toxoid lots produced by Parke-Davis, demonstrated antibody induction with a primary series given as three 0.5-mL subcutaneous injections at 0, 2, and 12 weeks. At week 14 (2 weeks after the primary series), a "measurable titer" to the toxin serotypes with the pentavalent product designated ABCDE-6 was observed in 90%, 93%, 100%, 80%, and 100%

of vaccinated subjects to the five respective toxin serotypes. The other two PBT products (designated ABCDE-7 and ABCDE-8) were associated with somewhat lower response rates at week 14, with measurable antitoxin titers for the five toxin serotypes ranging from 60% to 97% for product ABCDE-7 and 52% to 89% for product ABCDE-8. A "measurable titer" was defined as the level of standardization of each antitoxin that neutralized approximately 30 LD_{50} of its homologous toxin, which was as follows for the individual serotypes: type A (0.02 IU/mL), type B (0.005 IU/mL), type C (0.02 IU/mL), type D (0.16 IU/mL), and type E (0.00125 IU/mL).

Antitoxin titers in vaccinated subjects at week 52 in this study revealed absence of measurable titers in most vaccinated individuals.[9] Measurable antitoxin levels in vaccinated subjects at week 52 for the three pentavalent products were serotype A (29% to 43%), serotype B (4%), serotype C (13% to 25%), serotype D (0 to 7%), and serotype E (20% to 50%), suggesting that perhaps a 6-month dose may be required.

After a 12-month booster dose, nearly 100% of individuals had measurable titers to all five toxin serotypes with all three PBT products. Although measurable antitoxin titers were observed in most vaccinated individuals after completion of the primary series, the higher antitoxin titers (antitoxin titers often 10 times higher than observed after the primary series) were generally not observed until after the 12-month booster dose.[9] Based on the results of this initial PBT study, the PBT dosing was recommended as a primary series at 0, 2, and 12 weeks, with a mandatory 12-month booster dose and yearly booster doses thereafter.

Experience of The United States Army Medical Research Institute of Infectious Diseases with Pentavalent Botulinum Toxoid (1979 to 2004)

Antitoxin titers and sustainability of titers varied with the different PBT lots. Four lots of the PBT were administered to at-risk individuals at USAMRIID between 1979 and 2004: Lot A2 (1979 to 1993), Lot PBP-001 (1991 to 1994), Lot PBP-003 (1994 to 1996), and Lot PBP-004 (1997 to 2004).

In 1988, immunization with three doses of the primary series of PBT with Lot A-2 was demonstrated to result in detectable antitoxin titers in 21/23 (91%) and 18/23 (78%) vaccinated individuals to toxin serotypes A and B, respectively.[10] Similar to the early publication by Fiock et al,[9] antitoxin titers were not detectable in most vaccinated subjects before the 12-month mandatory booster dose, present in only 13/23 (56%) and 9/23 (39%) vaccinated individuals to toxin serotypes A and B, respectively. All 23 vaccinated individuals had measurable antitoxin titers after the 12 month booster dose, with titers that were often 10-fold higher than observed after the primary series.[10] Higher antitoxin levels (antitoxin present at a 1:16 dilution of serum, corresponding to approximately 0.25 IU/mL or greater) were also observed post-booster dose in vaccinated subjects who had received from one to eight previous PBT boosters doses, with 74/77 (96%) and 44/77 (57%) having higher titers to toxin serotype A and B, respectively.

Beginning in 1990, serum was obtained from vaccinated individuals 28 days after dose 3 of the primary series, to confirm the presence of detectable antitoxin before entrance into the laboratory. If no antitoxin antibody was detected (no antitoxin in an undiluted specimen of serum, corresponding to less than 0.02 IU/mL for toxin serotype A), individuals were then given a booster dose of PBT with follow-up serology 28 days post-booster.

Also, in 1990, the recommendation for the annual booster doses at USAMRIID was revised to require only four annual booster doses following the 12-month booster dose. Subsequent booster doses were deferred for another year if antitoxin was present at higher levels (presence of antitoxin on a 1:16 dilution of serum, corresponding to approximately 0.25 IU/mL or greater for toxin serotype A). In 1993, all booster doses subsequent to the mandatory 12-month booster were deferred based on the presence of antitoxin on a 1:16 dilution of serum. This policy differed from the CDC, where antitoxin titers were obtained every 2 years after the 12 month mandatory booster dose, to determine the need for subsequent booster doses.[10,15]

The sustainability of higher levels of antitoxin titers after the 12 month booster dose varied with the PBT lot and among individuals. Antitoxin titers persisted a mean of 724 days (range 16 to 2203 days) after a 12-month booster dose, with Lot A2 given from 1991 to 1993, versus only 395 days (range 28 to 1106 days), with PBT Lot PBP-003 given from 1994 to 1996, and 292 days with PBT Lot PBP-004

(range 28 to 1647 days) given from 1997 to 2001 (P = 0.0161, Sidak; duration of antitoxin titers to Lot A2 greater than Lot PBP-003).[16]

Recent Modifications of Pentavalent Botulinum Toxoid

In 2004, modifications of the PBT dosing regimen and protocol were made based on three sources of data: (1) the MDS Harris Project (sponsored by the Joint Vaccine Acquisition Program, Fort Detrick and performed by MDS Pharma Services, Lincoln, Nebraska and Batelle Memorial Institute Medical Research and Evaluation Facility, Columbus, Ohio) that was designed to determine the need for a 6-month dose of the PBT, as suggested by the initial PBT study by Fiock et al. in 1962, (2) the yearly PBT potency studies showing a recent decline in potency in some of the toxin serotypes, and (3) results of postimmunization antitoxin titers in vaccinated individuals at USAMRIID.[9,16-19]

MDS Harris Project

Results of the MDS Harris Project, conducted from July 1998 to May 2000, supported the addition of a PBT dose at 6 months. After receiving the primary series (0, 2, and 12 weeks) with PBT Lot PBP-003, most vaccinees did not have antitoxin antibody levels above the predetermined "benchmark" levels at 6 months. Only 30.8%, 58.3%, 60.9%, 32.3%, and 18.8% vaccinated subjects had adequate titers at 6 months to the five toxin serotypes A to E, respectively.[12,17,18] The "benchmark" titers in this study were defined as protective levels of antitoxin in guinea pigs, that were achieved by passive transfer of human botulinum toxin immune globulin, and that resulted in 80% survival of the guinea pigs after a lethal aerosol toxin challenge dose of $25 \times LCt_{50}$. The "benchmark" titers to the five toxin serotypes were: toxin serotype A (0.20 IU/mL), B (0.014 IU/mL), C (0.058 IU/mL), D (0.055 IU/mL), and E (0.014 IU/mL).[12] Of note, the benchmark level of 0.20 IU/mL for toxin serotype A was higher than that observed in previously reported studies, where 0.02 to 0.04 IU/mL titers ranges were protective,[5,8,12-14] and attributed to a higher toxin challenge dose with toxin serotype A of $80 \times LCt_{50}$ instead of $25 \times LCt_{50}$. Antitoxin titers with PBT Lot PBP-004 (other PBT lot currently in use at this time) were similar to Lot PBP-003, with the exception that antitoxin titers elicited to toxin serotype B were statistically significantly lower than with Lot PBP-003.

The addition of a 6-month dose of PBT in the MDH Harris study resulted in increased antitoxin levels at 4 weeks post vaccination. However, antitoxin levels declined again by month 12, to levels observed before the 6-month dose. Thereby, the data suggested that a 6-month dose of PBT was necessary to maintain "adequate" antitoxin titers, and that the 12-month booster dose was still required to maintain protective titers.

Annual Potency Studies

The two aspects to the potency testing for the PBT are (1) the animal resistance to challenge testing and (2) the antibody induction component. A decline in potency test results to the PBT was initially noted beginning in 2001. In the animal resistance to challenge aspect of the potency test, guinea pigs are vaccinated with one injection of 1.0 mL (volume of two human doses) of the PBT and then given a lethal IP challenge 4 weeks later with each of the five toxin serotypes. Only toxin serotypes A, B, and C currently pass the potency challenge aspect of the potency testing (pass requires 50% or greater animal survival). Failure of toxin serotype D and E was initially noted beginning in 2001 (< 50% survival).

In the antibody induction component of the potency test, guinea pigs are vaccinated with one injection of 1.0 mL (volume of two human doses) of the PBT. A minimum level of neutralizing antibodies must be present on serum collected 30 days postvaccination, as measured by a mouse bioassay. Induction of antitoxin levels required for the five toxin serotypes are: toxin A (≥ 0.02 IU/mL), toxin B

(≥ 0.01 IU/mL), toxin C (≥ 0.40 IU/mL), toxin D (≥ 0.12 IU/mL), and toxin E (≥ 0.035 IU/mL). PBT Lot PBP-003 currently passes antibody induction potency testing to only toxin serotypes A and B (antibody induction with PBT Lot PBP-004 currently passes only for toxin serotype A). The other toxin serotypes (C, D, and E) initially failed in antibody induction potency testing between 2001 and 2003.

Postimmunization Titers in Pentavalent Botulinum Toxoid–Vaccinated Individuals at the United States Army Medical Research Institute of Infectious Diseases

Antitoxin titers to toxin serotypes A, B, and E obtained from at-risk laboratory workers at USAMRIID were consistent with results of the recent potency testing. Antitoxin titers were obtained at 28 ± 7 days after the primary series or after a booster dose of PBT Lot PBP-004, and also as yearly surveillance titers during the time period from 1999 to 2002, using a mouse neutralization assay (Batelle Laboratories, Columbus, OH).[16]

Nearly all individuals (30/32 [94%] vaccinated subjects) who received the primary series of PBT Lot PBP-004 (2001-02) had detectable antitoxin levels to toxin serotype A (≥ 0.02 IU/mL) obtained between days 21 and 60 after the primary series (Table 31-1).[16] At day 21 to 60 post-booster dose of the PBT, 54/54 (100%) vaccinated individuals had detectable titers to toxin serotype A, with 52/54 (96%) vaccinated individuals having higher antitoxin levels (detectable antitoxin

TABLE 31-1 Percentage of Vaccine Recipients with Detectable Antitoxin (On Undiluted Serum Specimen) to Toxin Serotypes A, B, and E Post Primary Series

Toxin Serotype	Percentage of Vaccine Recipients with Detectable Antitoxin Titer by Time Post-primary Series (undiluted serum)*				
	21-60 days	2-6 months	6–12 months	12–24 months	>24 months
A	30/32	9/12	4/12	3/5	1/5
B	5/7	1/2	0/1	0/0	1/1
E	1/7	1/2	0/1	0/0	0/1

*Presence of antitoxin on an undiluted serum specimen corresponds to antitoxin titer of ≥ 0.02 IU/mL for toxin serotype A, ≥ 0.005 IU/ml for toxin serotype B, and ≥ 0.013 IU/ml for toxin serotype E.

TABLE 31-2 Percentage of PBT Boosters with Antitoxin to Toxin Serotypes A, B, and E Post Booster Dose on Undiluted Serum Specimens

Toxin Serotype	Percentage of Vaccine Recipients with Detectable Antitoxin Titer by Time Post-Booster Dose (undiluted serum)*					
	21–60 days	2–6 months	6–12 months	12–24 months	24–48 months	>48 months
A	54/54	7/7	35/37	11/12	10/10	21/21
B	15/15	7/8	16/24	18/25	14/26	46/49
E	10/15	4/8	10/24	12/25	14/26	33/49

*Presence of detectable antitoxin on an undiluted serum specimen corresponds to antitoxin titer of ≥ 0.02 IU/mL for toxin serotype A, ≥ 0.005 IU/mL for toxin serotype B, and ≥ 0.013 IU/mL for toxin serotype E.

on a 1:16 dilution of serum which corresponded to a titer of ≥ 0.32 IU/mL) that were deemed adequate for delay of the booster for another year (Tables 31-2 and 31-3).

However, results of antitoxin titers to toxin serotype E were consistent with the failing potency testing to toxin serotype E.[16] Detectable antitoxin titers to toxin serotype E (≥ 0.013 IU/mL) were observed in only one of seven vaccinated subjects 21 to 60 days post primary series given from 1999 to 2001 (see Table 31-1). Only 10/15 (67%) vaccinated individuals had detectable titers at 21 to 60 days post booster dose, with only 6/15 (40%) achieving higher antitoxin levels for deferment of the booster dose for another year (corresponding with an antitoxin level of ≥ 0.21 IU/mL) (see Tables 31-2 and 31-3).

For toxin serotype B, detectable antitoxin titers (≥ 0.005 IU/mL) were seen in five of seven vaccinated individuals at day 21 to 60 post primary series from 1999 to 2001

(see Table 31-1). After a booster dose, detectable antitoxin was noted in all 15 vaccinated subjects, with 10 of 15 vaccinated subjects having higher antitoxin titers that would permit deferment of the booster dose (corresponding to a level of ≥ 0.079 IU/mL) (see Tables 31-2 and 31-3).[16]

Antitoxin titers obtained at 6 to 12 months after the PBT, although detectable in 16/24 (67%) and 10/24 (42%) persons to toxin serotypes B and E, respectively, were only present in a small percentage of vaccines at higher titers that would allow for deferment of a booster dose for another year (7/24 and 3/24 to toxin serotypes B and E, respectively) (see Tables 31-2 and 31-3). However, most vaccinated subjects (28/37 [76%]) still had higher titers to toxin serotype A on a 1:16 dilution of serum obtained 6 to 12 months after the booster dose of vaccine, and more than 50% (7/12) had higher titers at 12 to 24 months (see Tables 31-2 and 31-3).[16]

TABLE 31-3 Percentage of Pentavalent Botulinum Toxoid Boosters with Antitoxin to Toxin Serotypes A, B, and E Post Booster Dose on Diluted (1:16) Serum Specimens

Toxin Serotype	Percentage of Vaccine Recipients with Detectable Antitoxin Titer by Time Post-Booster Dose (1:16 diluted serum)*					
	21–60 days	2–6 months	6–12 months	12–24 months	24–48 months	>48 months
A	52/54	6/7	28/37	7/12	5/10	10/21
B	10/15	6/8	7/24	3/25	5/26	20/49
E	6/15	0/8	3/24	2/25	4/26	12/49

*Presence of detectable antitoxin antibody on a 1:16 dilution of serum corresponds to antitoxin titer of ≥ 0.32 IU/mL for toxin serotype A, ≥ 0.079 IU/mL for toxin serotype B, and ≥ 0.21 IU/mL for toxin serotype E.

Revisions to the Pentavalent Botulinum Toxoid Protocol

Based on the results of the MDS Harris project that demonstrated the need for a 6-month PBT dose and the results of the failing potency and immunogenicity studies, the following revisions were made to the PBT protocol (IND 161) in 2004. A 6-month dose of the PBT was added (following the initial 3 injections at 0, 2, and 12 weeks), but the 12-month mandatory booster dose was still maintained, owing to the decline of antitoxin titer by 12 months (decline of titers in MDS Harris study was to levels observed before the 6-month PBT dose). Owing to the declining potency studies, booster doses were now required yearly, and antitoxin titers were no longer required. The resulting PBT dosing regimen was essentially the same as the initial PBT dosing regimen in 1959, with the exception of the addition of a 6-month dose (which was even suggested as a potential requirement in the initial PBT study published by Fiock in 1962). PBT Lot PBP-003 replaced the use of Lot PBP-004 for at-risk laboratory workers at USAMRIID beginning in 2005, owing to the continued passing of Lot PBP-003 to both toxin serotypes A and B on potency testing (PBP-004 passes potency testing to only toxin serotype A). Last, the protocol scientists no longer noted potential protection of PBT against all five toxin serotypes, based on the failing potency studies to some of the toxin serotypes.

Adverse Events

The PBT clinical experience has indicated the PBT to be safe. Ninety percent of vaccinations (330 of 367 vaccinations given to 183 at-risk individuals at USAMRIID between August 2005 and August 2007) were associated with either only mild or no local reactions.[20] The most common local reactions observed were erythema, induration, tenderness or pain, localized pruritus, and warmth. Moderate local reactions (erythema or induration $\geq$30 mm but <120 mm) were associated with only 9% of vaccinations, and severe local reactions (erythema or induration $\geq$120 mm, or axillary lymph node enlargement and/or tenderness) were observed in less than 1% of vaccinations (3 of 367 injections). Systemic adverse events were associated with 38/367 (10%)

vaccinations, and were mild and self-limiting. Most commonly reported systemic reactions were malaise or fatigue, headache, myalgia, light-headedness, and lower back pain.

Data from USAMRIID are consistent with data from the CDC from more than 20,000 vaccinations that also showed local reactions to be the main adverse event, with 91% of vaccinations associated with either only mild or no local reaction.[21] Systemic reactions with the PBT reported by the CDC were also uncommon (5% of vaccinations) and generally mild. Systemic adverse events included fever, malaise, headache, myalgia, stiffness/soreness of neck or back, and hives or pruritus.

Botulinum toxin type A (i.e., Botox and Botox Cosmetic, Allergan, Inc, Irvine, CA) and botulinum toxin type B (Myobloc, Solstice Neurosciences, Malvern, PA) have been approved by the US Food and Drug Administration (FDA) for therapeutic and cosmetic uses. These products have been approved by the FDA for indications such as treatment of strabismus, blepharospasm, cervical dystonia, temporary improvement in the appearance of moderate to severe glabellar lines associated with corrugator and procerus muscle activity, and severe primary axillary hyperhydrosis; but the products have also been used off-label for multiple other indications, including treatment of both migraine and tension headaches.[22-25]

Antitoxin antibodies may develop during treatment with these toxin preparations.[26-29] Studies have reported a correlation with botulinum toxin antibodies and some response failures with botulinum toxin A preparations.[27-29] Thereby, individuals who receive the PBT may theoretically have a decreased or possibly no therapeutic response with the future use of these products. Antitoxin titers to toxin serotype A may persist in individuals who received from one to three doses of PBT in 28% of individuals (serum titers > 0.02 IU/mL) even 18 to 24 months later, and detectable antitoxin titers may be observed in 99% of these individuals after a booster dose given at 18 to 24 months.[7] There are no data concerning induction of memory response in PBT vaccinated individuals after injection with the botulinum toxin type A and B therapeutic products. However, individuals are cautioned on the potential decrease in treatment response to future use of the toxin A and B therapeutic products, before receiving the PBT. Although PBT does not result in cross-neutralizing antibodies to type F botulinum toxin,[30] the decreased duration of therapeutic effect for dystonias with type F toxin (investigational) compared with type A toxins may limit clinical use of type F toxins.[29,33]

Current Status of Pentavalent Botulinum Toxoid

Because of the limited supply of PBT vaccine stocks, compounded by decreasing potency and immunogenicity of the PBT in vaccinated individuals, efforts have been under way to develop a replacement vaccine against botulinum neurotoxin that will be available for (1) at-risk workers for botulinum neurotoxin and (2) volunteers who are vaccinated for the purpose of obtaining protective antibodies for production of human botulinum immune globulin to treat infant botulism (Baby BIG). At-risk individuals for botulinum toxin include laboratory workers and researchers working directly with large quantities of toxin (especially those conducting animal studies or working in manufacturing facilities producing therapeutic botulinum toxin preparations), and a select population of individuals in government agencies responsible for Homeland Security.

STRATEGIES AND PROGRESS TOWARDS DEVELOPING FUTURE VACCINE CANDIDATES

Formalin-Inactivated Toxoids

Production of formalin-inactivated toxoids requires partially purified culture supernatants to be treated exhaustively with formaldehyde within a dedicated high-containment laboratory and by a highly trained staff.[34] Both the need for multiple injections to achieve and sustain antitoxin titers and the relative impurity of formalin-inactivated toxoids are thought to contribute to the local adverse reactions associated with the PBT.

Vaccine candidates for protection against botulinum toxin include formalin-inactivated toxoids (a tetravalent toxoid for toxin serotypes A, B, E, and F and a monovalent toxoid for toxin serotype F) made with similar methodology as the formalin-inactivated PBT.[35,36] Recently, a bivalent AB botulinum toxoid (BBT) was developed, based upon the

experience with the PBT, that optimized the following manufacturing issues: (1) the use of animal protein-free media to eliminate the risk of bovine spongiform encephalopathy, (2) additional filtration steps to reduce bioburden, (3) use of depth filtration to facilitate product recovery and process scale up, (4) improvements in detoxification and adjuvant adsorption steps, and (5) reduction of formaldehyde levels in the final toxoid product to reduce local reactinogenicity.[37] Preclinical studies demonstrated that a single dose (1.0 mL) of the monovalent A and the monovalent B product comprising the BBT was protective in the guinea pig model against intraperitoneal challenge with 10^5 LD_{50} of toxin serotype A and B, respectively, and in the mouse model against challenge with 10^3 LD_{50} of toxin. Immunogencity studies performed in guinea pigs demonstrated neutralizing antibody levels of 8 IU/mL to toxin serotype A after injection with 1.0 mL of the monovalent toxoid (levels 50 to 100 times higher than generally observed with the PBT) and 1.25 IU/mL to toxin serotype B (levels 10 to 20 times higher than observed with the PBT).

Recombinant Subunit Hc Vaccines

Development of recombinant vaccines against clostridial neurotoxins was pioneered by Helting and Nau[38] and Fairweather and his colleagues[39] using tetanus toxin (TeNT) as the model. They demonstrated that a C-terminal fragment from TeNT heavy chain (receptor-binding domain, Hc or fragment C) was able to protect mice from active challenge with tetanus toxin. The high sequence and structural homology between TeNT and BoNT led scientists at USAMRIID to take a similar approach for BoNT recombinant vaccines. The 50-kDa fragment C receptor-binding domain from botulinum toxin serotype A was expressed in *Escherichia coli* using both the native *C. botulinum* gene sequence[40] and a codon-optimized gene[41] and shown to elicit protective immunity in mice against native type A toxin challenges.[40,41] Dertzbaugh and West[42] expressed in *Escherichia coli* overlapping BoNT/A gene fragments (~15 kDa in size) that spanned the entire neurotoxin protein. The recombinant proteins were purified using preparative SDS-PAGE. The denatured fragments were inadequate at eliciting any notable protective immunity in mice, inferring that properly

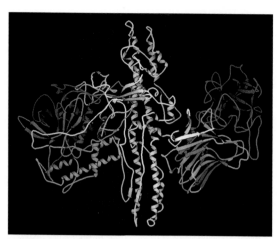

FIGURE 31-1. Botulinum neurotoxin is composed of a ~50-kDa light chain (LC) and a ~100-kDa heavy chain linked by a single disulfide bond. The LC functions as a zinc-dependent endopeptidase, whereas the heavy chain contains two functional ~50-kDa domains: a C-terminal receptor-binding domain (Hc or fragment C) and an N-terminal translocation domain (Hn). The Hc is subdivided into a 25-kDa Hc-C terminal subdomain and an Hc-N amino terminal subdomain. The Hc-C has a single ganglioside-binding site. An amino acid sequence of ~50 amino acid residues (referred to as a belt) makes up the N-terminal region of the Hn and wraps around LC domain. (Rendition of BoNT/A structure was obtained from the Protein Data Base (PDB) website: BoNT/A: *http://www.rcsb.org/pdb/ explore/explore.do?structureId=3BTA* Structure for BoNT/A was from Lacy DB, Tepp W, Cohen AC, DasGupta BR, Stevens RC. Crystal structure of botulinum neurotoxin type A and implications for toxicity. *Nat Struct Biol.* 1998;5:898-902.) *See Color Plate*

folded epitopes were most likely required for obtaining potent neutralizing antibodies.

X-ray crystal structures of BoNT/A[43] (Fig. 31-1) and BoNT/B[44] revealed that the receptor-binding domains were composed of two subdomains, referred to as Hc-N and Hc-C. In an attempt to define the minimal fragment of the Hc domain harboring protective antigenic properties, Tavallaie et al[45] produced the BoNT/A(Hc) domain and each of its two subdomains (A[Hc-N] and A[Hc-C]) in *E. coli* and evaluated their immune response in the mouse model. All three antigens produced varying immunoglobulin levels as detected by enzyme-linked immunosorbent assay (ELISA), with the Hc-C subdomain evoking the highest level of antibody. However, only the full Hc domain protected mice from a challenge of 1000 mouse LD_{50} after a single vaccination with 5 μg of antigen. Even with a single 10-μg dose of the Hc-N or the Hc-C, or a mixture of 5 μg each of the Hc-N and Hc-C, there were no survivors against the 1000 MLD_{50} toxin

challenge as opposed to a 90% survival rate when mice were administered 5 μg of Hc and 100% survival if given a single dose of 10 μg. If mice were administered three 10-μg doses of Hc, Hc-N, or Hc-C antigen and challenged with 10^5 mouse LD_{50} toxin, complete survival was observed with the Hc and the Hc-C vaccinated mice, but only 30% survival with the Hc-N vaccinated mice. The structural integrity at the interface between the Hc-N and Hc-C subdomains appeared to be an important factor in eliciting the most robust protective immune response in the mice. The single ganglioside binding site on the Hc-C subdomain[46,47] and potentially a protein receptor–binding site on the same subdomain are presumably essential components of the immunodominant epitope or epitopes on the C fragment, as judged by the ability of the Hc-C subdomain to elicit a much higher protective antibody response after multiple vaccinations than the Hc-N subdomain.

BoNT Hc antigens were originally produced in *E. coli* to demonstrate proof of concept that they were sufficient for eliciting short and long-term protective immunity in animal models.[48] For pilot lot manufacturing of the BoNT Hc subunit proteins, the yeast expression system *Pichia pastoris* proved to be a superior system for their production.[49,50] BoNT A(Hc),[51-53] B(Hc),[54,55] C(Hc),[56] D(Hc),[56] E(Hc),[57,58] F(Hc)[59,60] antigens were produced in *P. pastoris* in high yields and shown to elicit significant protective immunity in rodent (Table 31-4) and nonhuman primate models.[55,61]

Phase I Clinical Assessment of a rBV A/B Vaccine

Recombinant subunit H_c vaccines for serotypes A and B were combined into a bivalent vaccine (rBV A/B vaccine)[62] and evaluated in a phase I clinical trial. In this study, safety and immunogenicity of the vaccine at three ascending dosage levels (5 μg, 10 μg, and 20 μg for each serotype antigen adsorbed to 0.2% [w/v] Alhydrogel [Brenntag Biosector, Frederikssund, Denmark]) was assessed in 33 healthy adults.[63] Volunteers received 0.5-mL injections intramuscularly (IM) at days 0 and 28, and were followed for 12 months. BoNT neutralizing antibody concentrations were measured using a mouse neutralization assay. The initial (112 days after the second vaccination) study results[62] indicated that the vaccine was well tolerated at all dosage levels tested. The bivalent

TABLE 31-4 Protective Efficacy and Immunological Response of *Pichia pastoris* Produced Botulinum Neurotoxin (H$_c$) Antigens in Mice

Antigen[†]	Number of Doses	% Survival Against Direct Challenge*				GM ELISA titer	Serum neutralization
		10^3 LD$_{50}$	10^4 LD$_{50}$	10^5 LD$_{50}$	10^6 LD$_{50}$		
BoNT A (H$_c$)	1	ND	100	90	60	615	1.16 IU/mL
	2	ND	100	100	100	29,548	20.97 IU/mL
	3	ND	100	100	100	97,776	79.20 IU/mL
BoNT B (H$_c$)	1	100	90	100	ND	1,678	0.13 IU/mL
	2	100	100	100	ND	89,144	28.67 IU/mL
	3	100	100	100	ND	97,776	28.67 IU/mL
BoNT C (H$_c$)	1	90	50	70	ND	4,032	0.11 IU/mL
	2	100	100	100	ND	373,442	284 IU/mL
	3	100	100	100	ND	470,507	451 IU/mL
BoNT D (H$_c$)	3	ND	ND	100	ND	310,419	ND
BoNT E (H$_c$)	1	20	30	0	ND	138	0.06 IU/mL
	2	89[‡]	100	80	ND	74,100	1.41 IU/mL
	3	100	100	100	ND	242,000	48.20 IU/mL
BoNT F (H$_c$)	1	100	90	100	ND	<100	<0.05 IU/mL
	2	100	100	100	ND	10,640	23.74 IU/mL
	3	100	100	100	ND	24,405	70.66 IU/mL

BoNT, botulinum neurotoxin; ELISA, enzyme-linked immunosorbent assay; GM, geometric mean.
*Ten mice per group.
[†]All groups received 1 µg of vaccine except BoNT D (H$_c$) group which received 5 µg vaccine.
[‡]Eight of nine survivors.

vaccine stimulated serotype-specific neutralizing antibodies among the majority of recipients at all dosage levels studied. Geometric mean antibody concentrations, as well as the proportion of volunteers seroconverting, increased for more than 3 months after the second vaccine injection.[63]

In a separate arm of the phase I study, the impact of the Alhydrogel adjuvant on the safety and immunogenicity in vaccinated volunteers was assessed.[64] Healthy volunteers received IM vaccinations on days 0 and 28 with 0.5 mL of rBV A/B containing 20 µg of each BoNT antigen formulated in buffer with 0.2% Alhydrogel, or 20 µg of each BoNT antigen formulated in buffer without Alhydrogel. Again, the rBV A/B vaccine was safe and well tolerated, whether or not it was adsorbed to 0.2% Alhydrogel or devoid of adjuvant. The vaccine, when formulated with Alhydrogel, stimulated serotype-specific neutralizing antibodies among the majority of recipients. Serum geometric mean neutralizing antibody concentrations, as well as the proportion of volunteers seroconverting, increased for at least 3 months after the second vaccine injection. In the absence of adjuvant, each BoNT Hc antigen (20 µg) was poorly immunogenic, especially for the BoNT/B(H$_c$) vaccine component.[64]

Protection from botulism was demonstrated in guinea pigs passively immunized with botulinum immune globulin (BIG) purified from the vaccine recipients in the phase I clinical trial.[65] In this study, guinea pigs were passively immunized by IP injection with hBIG A/B or immune globulin negative for BoNT-neutralizing antibodies. Twenty-four hours later, guinea pigs were challenged by IM injection with BoNT/A or BoNT/B levels that were approximately 10 times greater than the guinea pig IM median lethal dose for both BoNT serotypes. The average circulating neutralizing antibody concentration at the time of challenge in the passively immunized guinea pigs was 0.07 ± 0.017 U/mL for BoNT/A and 0.029 ± 0.028 U/mL for BoNT/B. Nine of 10 of the passively immunized guinea pigs survived challenge with either BoNT/A or BoNT/B and none of the surviving guinea pigs had clinical signs of botulinum intoxication. All guinea pigs in the negative control group died within 48 hours of challenge.[65]

Delivery of Hc Antigens by Intranasal Administration

The route of BoNT Hc vaccination in most of the animal studies described in the literature has been with the traditional IM or subcutaneous injection of antigen adsorbed to an aluminum adjuvant. Recently, monovalent and trivalent A, B, and E BoNT (Hc) vaccines in phosphate-buffered saline were tested in the mouse model using an intranasal delivery to induce both a mucosal and systemic immune response.[66] Two mucosal adjuvants, chitosan and a water-soluble form of vitamin E TPGS (d-alpha tocopheryl polyethylene glycol 1000 succinate), were evaluated as mucosal adjuvants. In one part of this study, mice were vaccinated at 0, 2, and 4 weeks by an intranasal administration of 20 µg of either monovalent or trivalent Hc vaccine devoid of adjuvant or admixed to either chitosan or vitamin E adjuvant. Coadministration of adjuvant with vaccine resulted in a significantly higher level of IgG and IgA than vaccine without adjuvant and vitamin E adjuvant yielded higher immunoglobulin titers (by ELISA) than with the chitosan adjuvant. All animals vaccinated survived a challenge of 3×10^4 mouse LD_{50}, whereas unvaccinated controls succumbed to challenge.[66]

Naked DNA and Recombinant-Vector Hc Vaccines

Presentation of BoNT Hc antigens in animal models has included delivery not only of purified macromolecules but also by naked DNA vaccines[67-70] and by recombinant-vector vaccines.[71-74] Early naked DNA vaccine research inserting the Hc genes for types A, B, and E toxins in plasmids under the control of the CMV promoter[67,68] lead to a fairly inadequate immune response in mice and poor to no protection against toxin challenges. Bennett et al[69] reported more encouraging results using a yeast codon-optimized F(Hc) gene under the control of the cytomegaloviral (CMV) promoter, whereas Jathoul et al[70] demonstrated a more effective DNA vaccine when the F(Hc) gene was under the control of a human ubiquitin gene (UbC) promoter. In this case, two IM injections with 100-µg DNA vaccine afforded 90% protection against a BoNT/F challenge of 10^4 mouse LD_{50}. Saikh et al[75] compared the immune response of

tetanus toxin DNA vaccine using a TeNT Hc gene under the control of the Rous sarcoma virus (RSV) promoter with that of a recombinant tetanus toxin Hc protein and the tetanus toxoid. The DNA vaccine consistently produced a lower neutralizing antibody response in mice than the recombinant purified Hc antigen or toxoid. Although specific T-cell proliferation resulted from all vaccines tested, cytotoxic T-cell responses dominated the DNA vaccinations. Hc and toxoid vaccines elicited T-helper type-2 responses, whereas the DNA vaccine exhibited T-helper type-1 responses. The authors noted that the lower neutralizing antibody response with the DNA vaccine was not due to an insufficient level of Hc being produced in vivo but rather a result most likely of a less efficient mode of antigen presentation for supporting antibody production.

Recombinant-vector BoNT Hc vaccines to include Venezuelan equine encephalitis (VEE) virus vector system,[71,72] attenuated *Salmonella enterica var typhimurium* strains,[73] and an adenovirus-vectored vaccine[74] have demonstrated promise in small animal models, but their efficacy and safety in larger animals and humans is unknown. Lee et al[72] described a multivalent vaccine (against Marburg virus, *Bacillus anthracis* and botulinum neurotoxins serotypes A and C) vectored and delivered by VEE virus replicon particles (VRP). Mice receiving three parenteral inoculations of the VRPs at 10^7 IU (infectious units) were completely protected against a challenge of 10^3 LD_{50} of BoNT/A or BoNT/C. Foynes et al[73] evaluated the feasibility of an orally delivered F(Hc) vaccine using an *Salmonella enterica var typhimurium*. Mice were inoculated intragastrically with two doses (0 and 21 days) of $1-5 \times 10^9$ cells of attenuated *Salmonella* harboring an F(Hc) gene under the control of various promoters and challenged with 10^4 LD_{50} type F toxin. Although vaccinations induce low serum antibody levels, protection from challenge ranged from 40% to 73% depending on the promoter used in the genetic construct. Zeng et al[74] constructed and tested a replication-incompetent adenovirus BoNT/C(Hc) vaccine using a recombinant human serotype 5 adenoviral vector and a codon-optimized gene for C(Hc) protein. After a single IM dose of 2×10^7 plaque forming units (pfu), mice elicited a robust serum antibody response against the C(Hc) antigen and were completely protected against a challenge of 100 LD_{50} of BoNT/C as late as 7 months postvaccination.

Domains Other than Hc as Vaccine Candidates

Undoubtedly, the BoNT Hc domain has been the most thoroughly studied subunit in botulinum neurotoxin in terms of its production capacities in various recombinant host systems and in its quality attributes as a vaccine candidate to include safety, efficacy, potency and stability profiles. Recombinant light chains (LC) for serotype A,[76-79] B,[80] and C[81] were expressed and purified from E. coli in catalytically active forms and their ability to induce protective antibodies in mice assessed. Refolded light chain[76] from E. coli inclusion bodies were enzymatically active against a synaptosomal-associated protein with Mr = 25 kDa (SNAP-25) substrate and functionally inhibited exocytosis-dependent plasma membrane resealing in sea urchin eggs, but failed to elicit any protective immunity in mice when vaccinated with 3 doses of 15 μg A(LC) per dose adsorbed to 0.2% Alhydrogel and challenged with as little as 100 LD_{50} BoNT/A.[76] When A(LC) was solubly expressed and purified from E. coli, the A(LC) again failed to elicit protective immunity when it was stored in an acetate buffer.[79] However, when the A(LC) had its buffer changed to a phosphate buffer, protective immunity in mice was then observed after vaccination.[79] Interestingly enough, when an A(LC + belt) fusion protein was produced recombinantly and stored in an acetate buffer,

it had the ability to elicit protective immunity in the mouse.[79] Three doses of 5 μg of A(LC) in acetate buffer was unsuccessful at protecting mice from a challenge of 10^3 LD_{50} of BoNT/A, whereas 5 μg of A(LC+belt) in acetate buffer fully protected mice from the same challenge level.[79] BoNT B(LC)[80] and C(LC)[81] both elicited protective immunity in mice when administered by parenteral inoculation.

Recombinant A(LC + Hn) fusion protein,[79,82] rHC (heavy chain),[83] and atoxic (genetically inactivated protease) holotoxins for types A[84] and C[81] toxins elicited a formidable protective immunity against homologous toxin challenges in mice. Webb et al[84] used a mouse potency assay[85] to measure and compare the ability of recombinant subtype A1 antigens to elicit protective immunity against other subtype neurotoxins[86,87] from the C. botulinum Hall strain (subtype A1 toxin), C. botulinum FRI-honey strain (subtype A2 toxin), and subtype A3 toxin from C. botulinum Loch Maree strain (Table 31-5). In the potency assay,[85] seven groups of mice (10 mice per group) are administered a single IM injection of antigen adsorbed to 0.2% Alhydrogel adjuvant. Mice receive in a dose escalation, 0.011 μg (Group 1), 0.033 μg (Group 2), 0.1 μg (Group 3), 0.3 μg (Group 4), 0.9 μg (Group 5), 2.7 μg (Group 6), or 8.1 μg (Group 7). Mice are challenged 21 days post-vaccination with 1000 mouse (IP) LD_{50} of A1, A2 or A3 neurotoxin. Survival data were analyzed by Probit analysis,

TABLE 31-5 Effectiveness (ED_{50}) of Recombinant Botulinum Neurotoxin Type A Antigens to Elicit Protective Immunity in Mice Against Serotype A Toxin Subtypes Using a Mouse Potency Assay

Antigen*	BoNT A1[†]	BoNT A2[†]	BoNT A3[†]
BoNT A(LC)	No survivors	ND	ND
BoNT A(LC + Hn)	89 ng	209 ng	192 μg
BoNT A(HC)	52 ng	6 μg	18 μg
BoNT A(LC + Hn) + BoNT A(Hc)	14 ng	254 ng	739 ng
Atoxic BoNT A(HT)	18 ng	132 ng	144 μg

BoNT, botulinum neurotoxin; HC, heavy chain; LC, light chain; ND, not determined.

*Antigens adsorbed to 0.2% Alhydrogel were administered (single intramuscular injection) to 7 groups of 10 mice per group in a dose escalation manner at 0.011 μg (Group 1), 0.033 μg (Group 2), 0.1 μg (Group 3), 0.3 μg (Group 4), 0.9 μg (Group 5), 2.7 μg (Group 6), and 8.1 μg (Group 7).

[†]Mice were challenged 21 days postvaccination with 1000 mouse LD_{50} of either Subtype A1 neurotoxin from Clostridium botulinum Hall strain, subtype A2 neurotoxin from C. botulinum FRI-honey strain, or subtype A3 from C. botulinum Loch Maree strain. Challenges were by intraperitoneal injection of toxin. Survival rates were assessed 4 days postchallenge and survival data was analyzed by Probit analysis (95% confidence limits). Effective antigen dose for 50% survival (ED_{50}) were then noted.

and the effective dose (ED_{50}) to protect 50% of the mice from the challenge was determined. The antigens used in the study were recombinant A1(LC), A1(LC + Hn), A1(Hc), A1(LC + Hn) + (Hc), and an atoxic A1 holotoxin with genetic mutations in the protease active site rendering the catalytic activity inactive. The light chain domain (see Table 31-5) is the least immunogenic domain in BoNT/A, with no survivors after a single vaccination. The atoxic holotoxin and the vaccine combination of LC + Hn fusion and Hc yielded similar ED_{50}s (18 ng vs 14 ng) when mice were challenged with subtype A1 toxin, whereas LC + Hn alone had an ED_{50} of 89 ng. The fragment C (Hc) had an ED_{50} of 52 ng against A1 toxin but was not as good as the LC + Hn, atoxic holotoxin, or LC + Hn/Hc when A2 and A3 were used as the toxin for challenging (see Table 31-5). These studies did not include recombinant heavy chain because it is difficult producing stable heavy chain protein.

Synthetic Peptide Vaccines

Atassi et al[88-93] mapped the antibody and T-cell recognition regions on the N-terminal region of the heavy chain (residues 449–859) and the C-terminal region of the heavy chain (residues 855–1296) using antibodies from human, horse, chicken, and mouse species. Localization of immune recognition regions on the BoNT molecule is an important first step for inclusion in the design of an effective synthetic vaccine against botulism. However, there has been no peptide or combination of peptides reported to have the ability to induce a strong protective immunity in animal models against botulinum toxin. And based on the work of Dertzbaugh and West[42] (described earlier), a synthetic peptide vaccine strategy may be an impossible task.

SUMMARY

All three architecturally sound and correctly folded domains (i.e., the catalytic, translocation and receptor-binding domains) of botulinum neurotoxin have the capacity to elicit varying degrees of protective immunity in animal models and may offer further approaches to the development of recombinant botulinum vaccines. Conformationally correct epitopes appear to be the primary determinant for inducing notable levels of toxin-neutralizing antibodies, highlighting the importance of the B-cell response in adaptive immunity. Botulinum toxin vaccines are necessary to protect a limited population at risk from the toxin and are not vaccines that, in all probability, will be widely distributed to the general population, not only because of the ever-expanding clinical use of the toxins but also because it is hard to imagine any risk assessment that would justify vaccinating an entire population against botulinum toxin.[94]

ACKNOWLEDGMENTS

Denise Clizbe, RN, CCRC, who served as the research protocol nurse specialist for the PBT study at USAMRIID. Jaqueline Cupino, SGT, USA and Evan Hanzlik, SGT, USA who served as research assistants on the PBT study at USAMRIID.

Opinions, interpretations, conclusions, and recommendations are those of the authors and are not necessarily endorsed by the US Army.

Research was conducted in compliance with the Animal Welfare Act and other federal statutes and regulations relating to animals and experiments involving animals and adheres to principles stated in the Guide for the Care and Use of Laboratory Animals, National Research Council, 1996. The facility where this research was conducted is fully accredited by the Association for the Assessment and Accreditation of Laboratory Animal Care International.

References

1. Holzer E. Botulism caused by inhalation. *Med Klin.* 1962;41:1735-1740.
2. Rusnak JM, Kortepeter MG, Hawley RJ, Anderson AO, Boudreau E, Eitzen E. Risk of occupationally acquired illnesses from biological threat agents in unvaccinated laboratory workers. *Biosecur Bioterr.* 2004;2:281-293.
3. Rusnak JM, Kortepeter MG, Aldis J, Boudreau E. Experience in the medical management of potential laboratory exposures to agents of bioterrorism on the basis of risk assessment at the United States Army Medical Research Institute of Infectious Diseases (USAMRIID). *J Occup Environ Med.* 2004;46:801-811.
4. Wedum AG. The Detrick experience as a guide to the probable efficacy of P4 microbiological containment facilities for studies on microbial recombinant DNA molecules. *J Am Biosafety Assoc.* 1996;1:7-25.
5. Reames HR, Kadull PJ, Housewright RD, Wilson JB. Studies on botulinum toxoids, types A and B. III. Immunization of man. *J Immunol.* 1947;55:309-324.
6. Siegel LS. Evaluation to neutralizing antibodies to type A, B, E, and F botulinum toxins in sera from human recipients of botulinum pentavalent (ABCDE) toxoid. *J Clin Microbiol.* 1989;27:1906-1908.

7. Pittman PR, Hack D, Mangiafico J, Gibbs P, McKee KT Jr, Friedlander AM, et al. Antibody response to a delayed booster dose of anthrax vaccine and botulinum toxoid. *Vaccine*. 2002;20:2107-2115.

8. Fiock MA, Devine LF, Gearinger NF, Duff JT, Wright GG, Kadull PJ. Studies on immunity to toxins of Clostridium botulinum. VIII. Immunological response of man to purified bivalent AB botulinum toxoid. *J Immunol*. 1962;88:277-283.

9. Fiock M, Cardella M, Gearinger N. Studies on immunity to toxins of Clostridium botulinum. IX. Immunologic response of man to purified pentavalent ABCDE botulinum toxoid. *J Immunol*. 1963;90:697-702.

10. Seigel LS. Human immune response to botulinum pentavalent (ABCDE) toxoid determined by a neutralization test and by an enzyme-linked immunosorbent assay. *J Clin Microbiol*. 1988;26:2351-2356.

11. Cardella MA. Botulinum toxoids. In Proceedings of the Symposium on Botulism, Lewis KG and Cassel K. Fr, Eds., Public Health Service Publication No. 999-FP-1. U.S. Department of Health, Education and Welfare, Cincinnati, 1964, 113-30.

12. Gelzleichter TR, Myers MA, Menton RG, Niemuth NA, Matthews MC, Langford MJ. Protection against botulinum toxins provided by passive immunization with botulinum human immune globulin: Evaluation using an inhalation model. *J Appl Toxicol*. 1999;19:535-538.

13. Cardella MA, Fiock MA, Wright GG: Immunologic response of animals to purified pentavalent ABCDE botulinum toxoid [abstract M70]. Proc. of 58th General Meeting. Bact Proc. 1958 April 27-May 1 (page 78); Chicago, Illinois.

14. Brown JE, Parker GW, Pitt LM, Swauger JE, Elliott JJ, Ruble DL, et al. Protective efficacy of monkey pentavalent botulinum toxoid vaccine on an abbreviated immunization schedule [abstract]. ASM Int Conf Molec Genet and Pathogen of Clostridia, 1994.

15. Ellis RJ. Immunobiologic agents and drugs available from the Centers for Disease Control: Descriptions, recommendations, adverse reactions, and serologic response, 3rd ed. 1982. Centers for Disease Control. Atlanta.

16. Rusnak JM, Smith LA, Boudreau E, Norris S, Cannon T, Clizbe D, et al. Decreased immunogenicity of botulinum pentavalent toxoid to toxins B and E. [Abstract No. S10]. Sixth Annual Conference on Vaccine Research, Arlington, Va. May 5-7, 2003.

17. Battelle Memorial Institute, Chemical Warfare/Chemical and Biological Defense Information Analysis Center: Evaluation of safety and immunogenicity of pentavalent botulinum development of safe and effective products to exposure to biological chemical warfare agents. March 2001.

18. Battelle Memorial Institute, Chemical Warfare/Chemical and Biological Defense Information Analysis Center. Evaluation of safety and immunogenicity of pentavalent botulinum toxoid (A-E) administered to healthy volunteers - continuation of study for determination of booster vaccination interval. November 2002.

19. Smith LA, Rusnak JM. Botulinum neurotoxin vaccines: past, present, and future. *Crit Rev Immunol*. 2007;27:303-318.

20. Continuing Review Report, USAMRIID Protocol FY04-20; Log A13236, August 2007. A Phase 2, Four-Dose Primary Series and Booster Study. The Human Response to the Administration of Botulinum Toxoid, Adsorbed, Pentavalent (ABCDE), MDPH, IND 161.

21. Centers for Disease Control and Prevention. Information brochure: Pentavalent (ABCDE) Botulinum Toxoid. Atlanta, GA, U.S. Department of Health & Human Services, Public Service, 2000.

22. Cote TR, Mohan AK, Polder JA, Walton MK, Braun MM. Botulinum toxin A injections: Adverse events reported to the US Food and Drug Administration in therapeutic and cosmetic cases. *J Am Acad Dermatol*. 2005;53:407-415.

23. Jankovic J, Brin MF. Therapeutic uses of botulinum toxin. *N Engl J Med*. 1991;324:1186-1194.

24. Troost BT. Botulinum toxin type A (Botox®) in the treatment of migraine and other headaches. *Expert Rev Neurother*. 2004;4:27-31.

25. Cheng CM, Chen JS, Patel RP. Unlabeled uses for botulinum toxins: a review, part 1. *Am J Health Syst Pharm*. 2006;63:145-152.

26. Tsui JK, Wong NLM, Wong E, Calne DB. Production of circulating antibodies to botulinum-A toxin in patients receiving repeated injections for dystonia. *Ann Neurol*. 1988;24:181.

27. Jankovic J, Schwartz KS. Clinical correlates of response to botulinum toxin injection. *Arch Neurol*. 1991;48:1253-1256.

28. Hambleton P, Cohen HE, Palmer BJ, Melling J. Antitoxin and botulinum toxin treatment. *BMJ*. 1992;304:959-960.

29. Jankovic J, Schwartz K. Response and immunoresistance to botulinum toxin injections. *Neurology*. 1995;45:1743-1746.

30. Siegel LS. Evaluation of neutralizing antibodies to type A, B, E, and F botulinum toxins in sera from human recipients of botulinum pentavalent (ABCDE) toxoid. *J Clin Microbiol*. 1989;27:1906-1907.

31. Mezaki T, Kaji R, Kohara N, Fujii H, Katayama M, Shimizu T, et al. A double-blind, controlled study. *Neurology*. 1995;45:506-508.

32. Kaufman JA, Way JF Jr, Siegel LS, Sellin LC. Comparison of the action of types A and F botulinum toxin at the rat neuromuscular junction. *Toxicol Appl Pharmacol*. 1985;79:211-217.

33. Ludlow GL, Hallett M, Rhew K, Cole R, Shimizu T, Sakaguchi G, et al. Therapeutic use of type F botulinum toxin. *N Engl J Med*. 1992;326:349-350.

34. Middlebrook JL. Protection strategies against botulinum toxin. *Adv Exp Med Biol*. 1995;383:93-98.

35. Torii Y, Tokumaru Y, Kawaguchi S, Izumi N, Maruyama S, Mukamoto M, et al. Production and immunogenic efficacy of botulinum tetravalent (A,B,E,F) toxoid. *Vaccine*. 2002;20:2556-2561.

36. Edelman R, Wasserman SS, Bodison SA, Perry JG, O'Donnoghue M, DeTolla LJ. Phase II safety and immunogenicity study of type F botulinum toxoid in adult volunteers. *Vaccine*. 2003;21:4335-4347.

37. Tong X, Ford P, Johnson V, Ionin B, Brazer S, Tranter H, Shane C, Nabors G. Bivalent AB botulinum toxoid (BBT) [Abstract]. 43rd Interagency Botulism Research Coordinating Committee Meeting. Rockville, MD. Nov 14-17, 2006.

38. Helting TB, Nau HH. Analysis of the immune response to papain digestion products of tetanus toxin. *Acta Pathol Microbiol Immunol. Scand*. 1984;92:59-63.

39. Fairweather NF, Lyness VA, Maskell DJ. Immunization of mice against tetanus with fragments of tetanus toxin synthesized in Escherichia coli. *Infect. Immun*. 1987;55:2541-2545.

40. LaPenotiere HF, Clayton MA, Middlebrook JL. Expression of a large, nontoxic fragment of botulinum

neurotoxin serotype A and its use as an immunogen. *Toxicon.* 1995;33:1383-1386.

41. Clayton MA, Clayton JM, Brown DR, Middlebrook JL. Protective vaccination with a recombinant fragment of Clostridium botulinum neurotoxin serotype A expressed from a synthetic gene in Escherichia coli. *Infect Immun.* 1995;63:2738-2742.

42. Dertzbaugh MT, West MW. Mapping of protective and cross-reactive domains of the type A neurotoxin of Clostridium botulinum. *Vaccine.* 1996;14:1538-1544.

43. Lacy DB, Tepp W, Cohen AC, DasGupta BR, Stevens RC. Crystal structure of botulinum neurotoxin type A and implications for toxicity. *Nat Struct Biol.* 1998;5:898-902.

44. Swaminathan S, Eswaramoorthy S. Structural analysis of the catalytic and binding sites of Clostridium botulinum neurotoxin B. *Nat Struct Biol.* 2000;7:693-699.

45. Tavallaie M, Chenal A, Gillet D, Pereira Y, Manuch M, Gibert M, et al. Interaction between the two subdomains of the C-terminal part of the botulinum neurotoxin A is essential for the generation of protective antibodies. *FEBS Lett.* 2004;572:299-306.

46. Fotinou C, Emsley P, Black I, Ando H, Ishida H, Kiso M, et al. The crystal structure of tetanus toxin Hc fragment complexed with a synthetic GT1b analogue suggests cross-linking between ganglioside receptors and the toxin. *J Biol Chem.* 2001;276:32274-32281.

47. Rummel A, Mahrhold S, Bigalke H, Binz T. The Hcc-domain of botulinum neurotoxins A and B exhibits a singular ganglioside binding site displaying serotype specific carbohydrate interaction. *Mol Microbiol.* 2004;51:631-643.

48. Smith LA, Jensen MJ, Montgomery VA, Brown DR, Ahmed SA, Smith TJ. Roads from vaccines to therapies. *Mov Disord.* 2004;19:48-52.

49. Smith LA. Development of recombinant vaccines for botulinum neurotoxin. *Toxicon.* 1998;36:1539-1548.

50. Byrne MP, Smith LA. Development of vaccines for prevention of botulism. *Biochimie.* 2000;82:955-966.

51. Byrne MP, Smith TJ, Montgomery VA, Smith LA. Purification, potency, and efficacy of the recombinant vaccine candidate botulinum neurotoxin type A binding domain from Pichia pastoris. *Infect Immun.* 1998;66:4817-4822.

52. Potter KA, Zhang W, Smith LA, Meagher MM. Production and purification of the heavy chain fragment C of botulinum neurotoxin, serotype A, expressed in the methylotrophic yeast Pichia pastoris. *Protein Expr Purif.* 2000;19:393-402.

53. Zhang W, Smith LA, Plantz BA, Schlegel VL, Meagher MM. Design of methanol feed control in Pichia pastoris fermentations based upon a growth model. *Biotechnol Prog.* 2002;6:1392-1399.

54. Potter KJ, Bevins MA, Vassilieva EV, Chiruvolu VR, Smith TJ, Smith LA, et al. Production and purification of the heavy chain fragment C of botulinum neurotoxin, serotype B, expressed in the methylotropic yeast Pichia pastoris. *Protein Expr Purif.* 1998;13:1357-1365.

55. Boles J, West M, Montgomery V, Tammariello R, Pitt ML, Gibbs P, et al. Recombinant C fragment of botulinum neurotoxin B serotype (rBoNTB (HC)) immune response and protection in the rhesus monkey. *Toxicon.* 2006;47:877-884.

56. Webb RP, Smith TJ, Wright PM, Montgomery VA, Meagher MM, Smith LA. Protection with recombinant Clostridium botulinum C1 and D binding domain subunit (Hc) vaccines against C and D neurotoxins. *Vaccine.* 2007;25:4273-4282.

57. Loveless BM. *Clostridium botulinum* neurotoxin type E binding domain from *Pichia pastoris* as a recombinant vaccine candidate, Master of Science Thesis, Hood College, Frederick, MD, 2001.

58. Dux MP, Barent R, Sinha J, Gouthro M, Swanson T, Barthuli A, et al. Purification and scale-up of a recombinant heavy chain fragment C of botulinum neurotoxin serotype E in Pichia pastoris. *Protein Expr Purif.* 2006;45:359-367.

59. Byrne MP, Titball RW, Holley J, Smith LA. Fermentation, purification, and efficacy of a recombinant vaccine candidate against botulinum neurotoxin serotype F from Pichia pastoris. *Protein Expr Purif.* 2000;18:327-337.

60. Johnson SK, Zhang W, Smith LA, Hywood-Potter KJ, Swanson ST, Schlegel VL, et al. Scale-up of the fermentation and purification of the recombinant heavy chain fragment C of botulinum neurotoxin serotype F expressed in Pichia pastoris. *Protein Exp. Purif.* 2003;32:1-9.

61. Morefield GL, Chapman J, Tammariello RT, Purcell BK, Worsham PL, Smith LA, et al. Protection from multiple bacterial and toxin-mediated diseases using an intradermal vaccine array. *Proc Natl Acad Sci U S A.* 2008;In press.

62. Smith LA, Henderson I. Vaccines to protect against neurotoxins. In: Foster KA, Hambleton P, Shone CC, eds. *Treatments from Toxins.* Boca Raton, FL: CRC Press; 2006:75-106.

63. Mckee Jr. KT, Greenberg RN, Swiderski W, et al. Initial evaluation of a recombinant *Clostridium botulinum* A/B vaccine (rBV A/B) in healthy volunteers. Presented at the 45th Interscience Conference on Antimicrobial Agents and Chemotherapy (ICAAC) 2005, Washington, DC. G-918.

64. Swiderski W, Greenberg RN, Hoover DL, et al. Impact of adjuvant and immunogenicity of a recombinant botulinum vaccine A/B in healthy adult volunteers. Presented at the 42nd Annual Interagency Botulinum Research Coordinating Committee Meeting (IBRCC) 2005. Baltimore, MD. P26.

65. Henderson I, Shearer J, Swiderski W, et al. Protection against botulinum neurotoxin exposure in guinea pigs passively immunized with immune globulin purified from human volunteers vaccinated with recombinant botulinum vaccine (rBV A/B). Presented at the Ninth Annual Conference on Vaccine Research 2006, Baltimore, MD. S19.

66. Ravichandran E, Al-Saleem FH, Ancharski DM, Elias MD, Singh AK, Shamim M, et al. Trivalent vaccine against botulinum toxin serotypes A, B, and E that can be administered by the mucosal route. *Infect Immun.* 2007;75:3043-3054.

67. Clayton J, Middlebrook JL. Vaccination of mice with DNA encoding a large fragment of botulinum neurotoxin serotype A. *Vaccine.* 2000;18:1855-1862.

68. Shyu RH, Shalo MF, Tang SS, Shyu HF, Lee CF, Tsai MH, et al. DNA vaccination using the fragment C of botulinum neurotoxin type A provided protective immunity in mice. *J Biomed Sci.* 2000;7:51-57.

69. Bennett AM, Perkins SD, Holley JL. DNA vaccination protects against botulinum neurotoxin type F. *Vaccine.* 2003;21:3110-3117.

70. Jathoul AP, Holley JL, Garmory HS. Efficacy of DNA vaccines expressing the type F botulinum toxin Hc fragment using different promoters. *Vaccine.* 2004;22:3942-3946.

71. Lee JS, Pushko P, Parker MD, Dertzbaugh MT, Smith LA, Smith JF. Candidate vaccine against

botulinum neurotoxin serotype A derived from a Venezuelan equine encephalitis virus vector system. *Infect Immun.* 2001;69:5709-5715.

72. Lee JS, Groebner JL, Hadjipanayis AG, Negley DL, Schmaljohn AL, Welkos SL, et al. Multiagent vaccines vectored by Venezuelan equine encephalitis virus replicon elicits immune responses to Marburg virus and protection against anthrax and botulinum neurotoxin in mice. *Vaccine.* 2006;24:6886-6892.

73. Foynes S, Holley JL, Garmony HS, Titball RW, Fairweather NF. Vaccination against type F botulinum toxin using attenuated Salmonella enterica var Typhimurium strains expressing the BoNT/F Hc fragment. *Vaccine.* 2003;21:1052-1059.

74. Zeng M, Xu Q, Pichichero ME, Simpson LL, Smith LA. Protective immunity against botulism provided by a single dose vaccination with an adenovirus-vectored vaccine. *Vaccine.* 2007. In press.

75. Saikh KU, Sesno J, Brandler P, Ulrich RG. Are DNA-based vaccines useful for protection against secreted bacterial toxins? Tetanus toxin test case. *Vaccine.* 1998;16:1029-1038.

76. Ahmed SA, Smith LA. Light chain of botulinum A neurotoxin expressed as an inclusion body from a synthetic gene is catalytically and functionally active. *J Protein Chem.* 2000;19:475-487.

77. Ahmed SA, Byrne MP, Jensen M, Hines HB, Brueggemann E, Smith LA. Enzymatic autocatalysis of botulinum A neurotoxin light chain. *J Protein Chem.* 2001;20:221-231.

78. Ahmed SA, McPhie P, Smith LA. Autocatalytically fragmented light chain of botulinum a neurotoxin is enzymatically active. *Biochemistry.* 2003;42:12539-12549.

79. Jensen MJ, Smith TJ, Ahmed SA, Smith LA. Expression, purification, and efficacy of the type A botulinum neurotoxin catalytic domain fused to two translocation domain variants. *Toxicon.* 2003;41:691-701.

80. Gilsdorf J, Gul N, Smith LA. Expression, purification, and characterization of Clostridium botulinum type B light chain. *Protein Expr Purif.* 2006;46:256-267.

81. Kiyatkin N, Maksymowych AB, Simpson LL. Induction of an immune response by an oral administration of recombinant botulinum toxin. *Infect Immun* 1997;65:4586-4591.

82. Chaddock JA, Herbert MH, Ling RJ, Alexander FCG, Fooks SJ, Revell DF, et al. Expression and purification of catalytically active, non-toxic endopeptidase derivatives of Clostridium botulinum toxin type A. *Protein Expr Purif.* 2002;25:219-228.

83. Arimitsu H, Lee JC, Sakaguchi Y, Hayakawa Y, Hayashi M, Nakaura M, et al. Vaccination with recombinant whole heavy chain fragments of Clostridium botulinum type C and D neurotoxins. *Clin Diagn Lab Immunol.* 2003;11:496-502.

84. Webb RP, Smith TJ, Wright P, Brown J, Smith LA. Efficacy of botulinum neurotoxin A1 domains to elicit protective immunity against subtype A1, A2 and A3 neurotoxins. Submitted to Vaccine (2008).

85. Smith LA, Byrne MP. Vaccines for preventing botulism. In: Brin MF, Jankovic J, Hallett M, eds. *Scientific and Therapeutic Aspects of Botulinum Toxin.* Philadelphia: Lippincott Williams & Wilkins; 2002:27-37.

86. Smith TJ, Lou J, Geren IN, Forsyth CM, Tsai R, LaPorte SL, et al. Sequence variation within botulinum neurotoxin serotypes impacts antibody binding and neutralization. *Infect Immun.* 2005;73:5450-5457.

87. Hill KK, Smith TJ, Helma CH, Ticknor LO, Foley BT, Svensson RT, et al. Genetic diversity among botulinum neurotoxin-producing clostridial strains. *J Bacteriol.* 2007;189:818-832.

88. Atassi MZ, Dolimbek BZ, Hayakari M, Middlebrook JL, Whitney B, Oshima M. Mapping of the antibody-binding regions on botulinum neurotoxin H-chain domain 855-1296 with antitoxin antibodies from three host species. *J Protein Chem.* 1996;15:691-700.

89. Oshima M, Hayakari M, Middlebrook JL, Atassi MZ. Immune recognition of botulinum neurotoxin type A: Regions recognized by T cells and antibodies against the protective Hc fragment (residues 855-1296) of the toxin. *Mol Immunol.* 1997;34:1031-1040.

90. Rosenberg JS, Middlebrook JL, Atassi MZ. Localization of the regions on the C-terminal domain of the heavy chain of botulinum toxin A recognized by T-Lymphocytes and by antibodies after immunization of mice with pentavalent toxoid. *Immunol Invest.* 1997;26:491-504.

91. Oshima M, Middlebrook JL, Atassi MZ. Antibodies and T cells against synthetic peptides of the C-terminal domain (Hc) of botulinum neurotoxin type A and their cross-reaction with Hc. *Immunol Lett.* 1998;60:7-12.

92. Atassi MZ, Oshima M. Structure, activity, and immune (T and B cell) recognition of botulinum neurotoxins. *Crit Rev Immunol.* 1999;19:219-260.

93. Atassi MZ, Dolimbek BZ. Mapping of the antibody-binding regions on the HN-domain (residues 449-859) of botulinum neurotoxin A with anti-toxin antibodies from four host species. Full profile of the continuous antigenic regions of the H-chain of botulinum neurotoxin A. *Protein J.* 2004;23:39-52.

94. Smith L.A. Bioterrorism: what level is the threat and are vaccines the answer? *Expert Rev Vaccines.* 2004;3:493-495.

Hans Bigalke

INTRODUCTION

Botulinum neurotoxins (BoNT, terminology proposed by Niemann[1]) are produced by several *Clostridia* species including *C. barati*[2] and *C. butyricum*.[3] The neurotoxins (M_R 150,000) are embedded within a complex of various sizes depending on the serotype. Botulinum neurotoxin type A (BoNT/A)–complex may have an M_R of 900,000 (LL), 600,000 (L), and 300,000 (M). The complexing proteins consist of hemagglutinins with M_R between 17,000 and 52,000, as well as of a nontoxic nonhemagglutinating protein (NTNH) with a M_R of 120,000. The latter protein is the connecting link between the neurotoxin and the various hemagglutins. In case NTNH is nicked, the hemagglutinins dissociate out of the complex and the M-complex emerges consisting of the neurotoxin and the NTNH (see later). The complexing proteins enhance oral toxicity by stabilizing the neurotoxins, protecting them from the hostile environment in the stomach and upper gut and, most likely, facilitate their absorption from the intestine as shown for types A and C1 neurotoxins.[4,5] The complex is stable at acidic conditions, which only makes sense from the view of the *clostridium*. The toxin, produced in organic matter, must withstand the acidic and protease-rich environment after ingestion. When pH increases higher than 7, the neurotoxin desintegrates from the complex.[6] This neurotoxin is the active ingredient that causes botulism. BoNT/A proteins produced by the same species are almost identical; however, when the same serotype proteins are produced by a different group of organisms, their amino acid sequence can differ,[7,8] as seen in the cases of Botox (Allergan, Inc, Irvine, CA) and Dysport (Ipsen, Milford, MA) (see later).

The clostridial neurotoxins belong to the so-called AB class of toxins. They consist of two separate parts with different functions. The larger (B, or binding) part (M_R 100,000) navigates the smaller (A, or active) part, the enzymatic part (M_R 50,000), through the plasma membrane into the compartment, where its substrate is localized. The organism produces the toxin as an inactive single chain protein, which, to become active, must be cleaved by limited proteolysis at a distinct nicking site. Physiologically, nicking is performed by coreleased clostridial proteases, which can, however, be replaced by trypsin or various other proteases.[9] The resulting two proteins are still connected by an inter-chain disulfide bond and ionic interactions. This so-called di-chain protein represents the actual neurotoxin (M_R 150,000). Inside the neurons, the two chains have to be cleaved by endogeneous redox systems, because it is only the free enzyme that is proteolytically active.[10,11] Thus, intracellular enzymes that physiologically protect cells from the destructive action of free radicals are used to convert the prodrug, the inactive di-chain molecule into the active drug, the light chain enzyme.

As a result of Dr. Scott's original recognition of their therapeutic value, which gave rise to the remarkable success of these otherwise deadly poisons, botulinum neurotoxins have

Dr. Bigalke is disclosing that he has given lectures in workshops sponsored by Allergan, Ipsen, and Merz, respectively.

389

been used for therapeutic purposes for more than three decades.[12] At present, four different pharmaceuticals containing BoNT/A are on the market: Botox, Dysport, Xeomin (Merz Pharma, Greensboro, NC), Hengli (Chinese BoNT/A complex [CBTX-A], Lanzhou Institute of Biological Products, Shanghai, China). There is one product on the market that contains BoNT/B: Neurobloc/Myobloc (Solstice Neurosciences, Malvern, PA). They are approved for various indications. With respect to the growing market, it can be expected that other products will be available soon with the same or different properties and qualities. In this chapter, the commercially available products are described with respect to content, potencies, and immunologic properties.

MANUFACTURING OF BOTULINUM TOXIN CONTAINING PHARMACEUTICALS

Because of proprietary concerns, only scarce information is available about the manufacturing process of the different pharmaceuticals containing botulinum toxin. In general, the production of the drug substance (active pharmaceutical ingredient) starts with the fermentation of the respective type of *Clostridium botulinum*. The Hall strain is used for the production of BoNT/A-containing products Botox, Xeomin, and the CBTX-A, whereas Dysport is derived from strain NCTC 2916. The production of Neurobloc/Myobloc starts with the fermentation of *C. botulinum* type B ("bean" strain isolated at Fort Detrick).

After fermentation of *Clostridium botulinum*, the toxin is harvested by acid preparation,

followed by extraction, precipitation with ethanol, and the toxin is finally crystallized in 0.9 M ammonium sulfate.[6] This procedure provides a toxin complex with a molecular weight of 900 kD (the so-called LL complex, see later), which is the active toxin product in Botox. Instead of the ethanol precipitation and crystallization steps used to produce Botox, an anion exchange chromatography step (DEAE), followed by final precipitation with ammonium sulfate is used to produce the active substance for Dysport.[13,14] The production of the active substance of Xeomin employs the same initial steps as the other products. Contaminating clostridial proteins including the complexing proteins are separated by ion exchange chromatography. In contrast to the other products, Xeomin is free of any complexing proteins. To produce the active substance of Myobloc/Neurobloc, the toxin is also harvested after fermentation by acid precipitation, followed by extraction of the toxin and a series of ammonium sulfate precipitations. The toxin is finally purified by anion exchange chromatography (DEAE) and size exclusion chromatography.[15,16]

This short overview shows that there are several differences in the manufacturing processes that might affect the properties of the drug substances, for example, the structure of the active substance and the presence of other proteins.

DRUG SUBSTANCE

The characteristics of the active substance (drug substance, active pharmaceutical ingredient) are summarized in Table 32-1.

The active substance of all botulinum neurotoxin products is the neurotoxin with a molecular weight of approximately 150 kD.

TABLE 32-1 Characteristics of the Active Substance of Botulinum Toxin Containing Therapeutics

	Botox	Dysport	CBTX-A	Xeomin	Neurobloc/ Myobloc
Clostridial strain	Hall A	NCTC 2916	Hall A	Hall A	"Bean" strain
Molecular composition	900 kD neurotoxin complex	Mixture of 600-kD and 300-kD neurotoxin complexes	900-kD neurotoxin complex (probably)	150-kD neurotoxin	700-kD neurotoxin complex
Clostridial protein per mouse LD50 unit	48 pg	25 pg	47 pg	6 pg	11 pg

The neurotoxin is synthesized by the *clostridia* as a single polypeptide, which is cleaved by an endogeneous protease into two subunits that remain linked by an interchain disulfide bond. Whereas the cleavage in the type A neurotoxin is almost complete (> 95%),[17] the type B neurotoxin is only partially severed.[18] In Myobloc/Neurobloc, the proportion of uncleaved neurotoxin is between 22% and 26%.[19] Only the dichain molecule exhibits its full biologic activity. The single chain neurotoxins are almost inactive.

Only under slightly acid conditions as in the fermenter broth is the 150-kD neurotoxin associated with the other clostridial proteins, forming toxic complexes of various compositions.[20] The complexing proteins protect the neurotoxin after oral ingestion against the harsh conditions in the intestinal tract and allow the resorption of the active neurotoxin[21,22]; they do not contribute to the active mechanism of the neurotoxin at the motor endplate. In Table 32-2, the different forms of the complexes are summarized and the commercial products are related to the respective forms.

The sizes of the complexes are determined by sedimentation in a sucrose gradient and given by the sedimentation constant.[23] The 19S (900-kD) complex is found only in cultures of *C. botulinum* type A and not in type B or the other serotypes. The 900-kD and the 600-kD complexes consist of the neurotoxin, the nontoxic nonhemagglutin protein (molecular weight 120 kD) and four hemagglutinins (molecular weight 17 kD to 52 kD).[24]

The stoechiometric composition of the complexes is not known. It was speculated that the 900-kD complex is a dimer and contains two neurotoxin molecules,[24] but there is no experimental proof supporting this hypothesis. In contrast, it was shown by structural analysis of the respective hemagglutinin that this hemagglutinin cannot function as a link to build a dimer.[25]

As shown in Table 32-2, the products contain different forms of the neurotoxin complexes or the neurotoxin alone. Botox contains solely the 900-kD complex. According to Hambleton,[14] the active substance of Dysport consists of a mixture of toxin complexes with molecular weights of 300 kD (M complex) and 600 kD (L complex). The composition of CBTX-A is not published. Because a similar production process is used as for Botox, it can be assumed that CBTX-A contains also the 900-kD complex. The drug substance of Myobloc/Neurobloc consists of the 700-kD (600-kD) complex of *C. botulinum* type B.[19] Xeomin is based on the 9S neurotoxin lacking any complexing proteins.[26]

Although the complexing proteins have no impact on the active mechanism of the neurotoxin, it was hypothesised that the form of the complex influences the diffusion of the toxin, that is, that according to Fick's law, the 900-kD complex in Botox diffuses less than the smaller complexes in Dysport.[27,28] This should be even more apparent for the complex protein-free neurotoxin. A faster diffusion out of the treated muscle could induce more systemic adverse effects. There is, however, no experimental proof for this hypothesis, in contrast, Dodd et al[29] have demonstrated that after injection into the *m. tibialis anterior* of rats, the spread of Botox, Dysport, and pure neurotoxin into an adjacent muscle did not differ. More recently, it was demonstrated that diffusion of radiolabeled complexed toxin and complexing protein-free neurotoxin, both type A, did not differ either when injected into rats' *gastrocnemius* muscle.[30] These results could be expected because the complexes are stable only under slightly acidic conditions (pH < 7).[6,23] At physiologic pH (7.4), the neurotoxin dissociates

TABLE 32-2 Different Forms of Botulinum Neurotoxin Type A According to Sugyama[23] 1980

Type of Complex/ Neurotoxin		Composition	Molecular Weight	Specific Activity (LD50 Units/mg protein)	Product
19 S	LL	NT, NTNH, HAs	900 kD	4.0 - 4.8 × 10⁷	Botox CBTX-A
16 S	L	NT, NTNH, HAs	600 kD	4.0 - 4.8 × 10⁷	Myobloc Dysport
12 S	M	NT, NTNH*	300 kD	7.2 - 8.0 × 10⁷	Dysport
9 S	S	NT	150 kD	1.6 - 2.0 × 10⁸	Xeomin

HAs, hemagglutinins; NT, neurotoxin; NTNH, nontoxic nonhemagglutinating protein; NTNH*, nicked NTNH.

from the other complexing proteins[31] and diffuses as a single molecule in exactly the same way as the complexing protein-free neurotoxin into the tissue to the motor endplate.

Although data about the purity of the active substance of Botox, Xeomin, CBTX-A and Myobloc/Neurobloc are not published, there is some information in the public domain about the active substance of Dysport. Pickett et al[32] showed that beside the neurotoxin with heavy and light chains, the other complexing proteins are present. The bulk of the NTNH protein is nicked by limited proteolysis into two fragments of lower molecular weight (115 kD and 5 kD). Neither fragment is able to bind the other hemagglutinins, leading to dissociation of the LL complex into a mixture of M complexes and hemagglutinins.[33] It can, therefore, be concluded that Dysport consists predominantly of the M complex (300 kD). This is also suggested by the fact that the hemagglutinins are present only in a small amount. In addition to the known complex proteins Dysport contains further clostridial proteins: a *clp* protease and flagellin, a protein that forms the flagella of motile bacteria.[32]

CBTX-A is presumably produced according to the procedure described by Schantz and Johnson[6] and consists of the 900-kD complex.

DRUG PRODUCT

The drug products are manufactured according to similar procedures. After assessing the potency of the drug substance solution, a defined volume (calculated form the potency of the solution) is diluted into different excipients.[14] A volume that contains the respective activity of the end product is filled into vials and the solution is lyophilized, vacuum dried (Botox), or is not further processed and provided as a solution (Myobloc/Neurobloc). The characteristics of the drug products are summarized in Table 32-3.

All neurotoxin products contain a protein as a stabilizer that serves especially to prevent the adsorption of the toxin to glass and plastic surfaces. CBTX-A formulation contains gelatin whereas the other products use human serum albumin in different amounts. Compared with the other products, Dysport contains the lowest

TABLE 32-3 Characteristics of the Botulinum Toxin Therapeutics

Feature	Botox	Dysport	CBTX-A	Xeomin	Neurobloc/ Myobloc
Manufacturer	Allergan Inc	Ipsen Biopharm Ltd	Lanzho Institute of Biological Products	Merz Pharma	Solstice
Type of toxin	Type A	Type A*	Type A	Type A	Type B
Dose in units per vial	100 or 50	500	100	100	5000, 10000, or 20000
Protein stabilizer	0.5 mg HSA	0.125 mg HSA	20 mg gelatin	1 mg HSA	0.5 mg/mL HSA
Other excipients	0.9 mg NaCl	2.5 mg Lactose	25 mg Dextran 25 mg Sucrose	25 mg Sucrose	10 nM sodium succinate 100 nM sodium chloride, sodium octanoate pH=5.6
Type of formulation	Vaccum dryed powder	Lyophilisate	Lyophilisate	Lyophilisate	Liquid
Storage	2-8°C	2-8°C	-5°C to -20°C	Room temperature	2-8°C
Stability	2 y	1 y	3 y	2 y	3 y
Stability after opening	24 h at 2-8°C	8 h at 2-8°C	4 h at 2-8°C	24 h at 2-8°C	8 h at room temperature

CBTX-A, Chinese BoNT/A complex.
*The amino acid sequence of this neurotoxin type A is slightly different from the other type A neurotoxins (Pickett et al. 2005).

TABLE 32-4 Content of Drug Substance in Drug Product

Feature	Botox	Dysport	CBTX-A	Xeomin	Neurobloc/ Myobloc
Molecular composition	900-kD complex	Mixture of 600-kD and 300-kD complex	900-kD complex ?	150-kD neurotoxin	700-kD complex
Clostridial protein per vial	5 ng	12.5 ng	4.7 ng	0.6 ng	55 ng (5000 U)
Clostridial protein per unit	50 pg	25 pg	47 pg	6 pg	11 pg

CBTX-A, Chinese BoNT/A complex.

amount of albumin. Using an in vitro activity assay (mouse hemidiaphragm) Bigalke et al[34] showed that at higher dilutions of Dysport (500 U in >5 mL) the concentration of albumin is not sufficient to prevent the loss of toxin completely. This might explain why an apparently higher dose of Dysport than that of the other type A products has to be injected to achieve a comparable therapeutic effect.

Other excipients (e.g., sugars) act as bulking agents in the freeze-drying process and may also stabilize the toxin. The use of sodium chloride is detrimental in a lyophilization procedure.[35] Botox contains sodium chloride, which may be the reason why the toxin is vaccum dried.

The products are stored in different conditions. Xeomin is stored at room temperature. The other products are stored at 2° to 8°C or frozen like the Chinese product CBTX-A.

PROTEIN LOAD AND SPECIFIC POTENCY

The amount of clostridial protein in a vial cannot be quantified experimentally because of the tremendous surplus of human serum albumin. Based on its specific potency, the active substance (in mg/mL) is diluted several thousand fold to end up with the respective concentration (e.g., few nanograms per milliliter). Therefore, the amount of clostridial protein in a vial can be calculated only from the specific potency and the dilution factor of the active substance. Because there is no international standard, each company uses its own standard to determine botulinum toxin

activity. Moreover, variations in the bioassay that is used for determination of activity is large when different laboratories were compared.[36] Thus, the units marked on the label of the different products might not be equivalent.

The content of clostridial protein in a vial depends on the specific potency of the active substance and is different in the products, as can be seen in Table 32-4.

The specific potency is defined by the mouse LD50 U related to the amount of clostridial protein. Schantz and Johnson[6] described the specific potency for the 900-kD complex with 3×10^7 LD50 ± 20% U per mg protein. This would correspond with 2.4 to 3.6 ng clostridial protein per 100-U vial. The actual amount published by Allergan for Botox is 5 ng. Presumably a part of the neurotoxin is denatured during the formulation process. This assumption is confirmed by a recent patent application filed by Allergan,[37] in which the average specific potency of the active substance is reported to be 28 pg/LD50 U. Therefore, 2.8 ng would suffice to provide 100 LD50 U per vial. Because considerably more toxic complex must be formulated, a part of the neurotoxin seems to be inactivated during the formulation process and is present as a toxoid.

The information about the protein content of Dysport is contradictory. Until 2005, an amount of 12.5 ng clostridial protein per vial was communicated by Ipsen (company leaflet for Dysport published in 1994). But a poster presentation by Pickett et al[32] indicated that the amount was 5 ng/vial, and in a subsequent article by Pickett et al,[38] the protein load of Dysport was reported to be 4.35 ng. The authors do not provide any explanation for the discrepancy. Thus, it is hard to calculate from these conflicting statements the actual specific activity.

The toxin B complex represented by Myobloc/Neurobloc exhibits a higher potency than the type A complex[16] if determined in mice. Approximately 11 pg represents the median lethal dose.

The neurotoxin in Xeomin shows relatively high specific potency, corresponding to 6 pg/MLD, possibly reflecting the low mass of the protein (see Table 32-2).

IMMUNOLOGIC PROPERTIES

Treatment with biologic drugs can cause an immune response. Even an active substance with the same amino acid sequence as the native human protein (e.g., insulin, human growth hormone, and erythropoietin) may elicit antibodies.[39] Several product-specific factors influence the immunogenicity of therapeutic proteins, for example, impurities, aggregation, formulation, and degradation (oxidation, deamidation). Impurities and contaminants were identified as the main cause for immunogenicity of human insulin and growth factor.[39] In addition, host-specific factors also determine the immunologic response, for example, frequency of treatment and genetic predisposition of the patient.[39] As a foreign protein, botulinum toxin is inherently immunogenic. Because this therapeutic protein is administered only in extremely small quantities and in long intervals, most patients do not develop antibodies. Nevertheless, botulinum neurotoxin elicits antibodies in some patients that can neutralize the neurotoxin and terminate the therapy.

Although Botox, Dysport, CBTX-A, and Xeomin are based on the same active substance, the 150-kD botulinum neurotoxin type A substance, the products are not identical. Differences between the products can influence the immune response against the active substance. The products differ in their manufacturing process and their formulation and, furthermore, they contain a different set of other (complexing) proteins. These differences could affect the immune response to the neurotoxin. The complexing proteins (especially the hemagglutinins) elicit antibodies in 40% to 60% of patients treated with the complex-containing products Botox and Dysport.[40,41] In contrast, the proportion of patients with antibodies against the neurotoxin

remains small. It was demonstrated that patients with antibodies only against the complexing proteins still respond to the therapy, that is, antibodies against the complexing proteins are non-neutralizing, whereas antibodies against the neurotoxin can prevent the therapeutic effect, that is, they cause secondary nonrespose.[40] Besides the NTNH protein (responsible for binding the neurotoxin into the complex), the other complexing proteins are hemagglutinins. These proteins act as lectins with high specificity to galactose-containing glycoporteins or glycolipids.[42] Lectins are known to function as immune adjuvants. For example, the cell-binding subunit of ricin, which resembles one of the C. botulinum hemagglutinin (HA 1), stimulates the antibody production against a virus antigen.[43]

From vaccination experiments, it is known that the magnitude of an immune response against an antigen is predominantly determined by the concomitant administration of such an adjuvant.[41] Lee et al[44] could show that the hemagglutinins act as adjuvants, which enhance the antibody titer against the neurotoxin type B. Atassi,[45] however, pointed out that a formalin inactivated toxin (toxoid) was used in much higher doses (about 100,000 fold) than the therapeutic dose, and therefore, the results were not relevant for the clinical situation. Furthermore, the injections were made in weekly intervals, which does not reflect current therapeutic recommendations. Although the hemagglutinins acted as adjuvants in these experiments, it is not clear yet if they enhance the immune response against the neurotoxin administered in therapeutic doses.

The antibody response is also influenced by the amount of protein applied to the patient. This amount depends on the specific potency of the active substance. Botox consists of the 900-kD complex, and it contains relatively high amount of other clostridial proteins (complexing proteins); the neurotoxin represents approximately only 20% of the complex. As mentioned earlier, the specific potency of Botox seems to be diminished in the formulation process, that is, a part of the neurotoxin (about 40%) is denatured and could act as an antigen.[37] Despite these theoretical concerns, the current Botox product, however, is associated with very low risk of blocking antibodies,[46] suggesting that factors other than complexing proteins determine the products' immunogenicity.

Dysport contains predominantly the 300-kD complex besides the 600-kD complex.[14]

TABLE 32-5 Amount of Botulinum Toxin for the Treatment of Cervical Dystonia

Feature	Botox	Dysport	Xeomin	Myobloc/Neurobloc
Average dose in LD50 units	200	600	200	8000
Amount of administered clostridial protein (ng)	10	15	1	88
Calculated amount of neurotoxin* (ng)	2	5	1	22

*Based on the calculated proportion of the neurotoxin in Botox of approximately 20% (150 kD/900 kD) in Dysport of 33% (150 kD/ [300 kD + 600 kD]/2 and 25% in Myobloc/Neurobloc 150 kD/600 kD). Because of lack of information, data on CBTX-A have been omitted.

This might be the reason why the specific potency of Dysport (1U = 25 pg) is higher than that of Botox (1U = 50pg) because the proportion of the neurotoxin in the lower molecular weight complexes is higher. It is difficult to estimate, however, the actual amount of neurotoxin that reaches the patient's tissue when Dysport is applied. Because the concentration of albumin in this product varies depending on the volume of the solvent and is not sufficient at larger volumes, the neurotoxin binds irreversibly to glass and plastic surfaces and a part of the neurotoxin is lost before it reaches the patients' tissue. Although the dose of Dysport is often 3 to 5 times higher than that of Botox, the actual amount of neurotoxin injected into the muscle might be similar to the respective amount of Botox.[34]

The active substance of Dysport contains some impurities not related to the complexing protein.[32] Besides other clostridial proteins, a flagellin, a protein that is known for its immunostimulatory properties, is present.[47] It reacts with Toll-like receptor 5 and induces the maturation of dendritic cells. Lee et al[48] showed that the addition of flagellin to tetanus toxoid in a vaccination experiment enhanced the antibody titer against tetanus toxin. However, it is difficult to estimate the immunologic effect of flagellin in Dysport because the dose of flagellin in vaccination experiments was much higher than the amount of flagellin in a therapeutic dose of Dysport.

It is not known whether the immunologic potential of the neurotoxin type B is different from that of the BoNT/A. A vaccine based on the pentavalent botulinum toxoid induced a markedly higher antibody titer against BoNT/A than against the BoNT/B.[49] But the antigenic potential might be influenced by the fact that the neurotoxins were inactivated by treatment with formalin. When comparing the BoNT/A with BoNT/B, it has to be considered that BoNT/B contains a proportion of nonactivated neurotoxin (single-chain toxin), which could act as a toxoid.[50] In terms of mouse LD50 units, the specific activity of Myobloc is remarkably higher (1 U = 11 pg) than the specific activity of the type A–containing products. However, a substantially higher dose of Myobloc/Neurobloc than the doses of toxin A–containing products has to be injected to achieve a similar therapeutic effect. Thus, the specific potency in human is much lower (estimated 40-fold lower[51]). Table 32-5 gives an overview of the average protein load for the treatment of cervical dystonia.

The higher amount of BoNT/B applied with Myobloc/Neurobloc might be the reason why patients develop antibodies and become nonresponders to the neurotoxin after only a few treatments.[52,53] The proportion of patients treated with Botox or Dysport who develop antibodies against the neurotoxin type A is in the range of 1%.[46,54,55] Because Xeomin has been in clinical use for a relatively short time compared with the other products, data about the immunologic potential of this product are not yet available.

References

1. Niemann H. Clostridial neurotoxins—Proposal of a common nomenclature. *Toxicon.* 1992;30:223-225.
2. Hall JD, McCroskey LM, Pincomb BJ, Hatheway CL. Isolation of an organism resembling Clostridium baratii which produced type F botulinal toxin from an infant with botulism. *Clin Microbiol.* 1985;21: 654-655.
3. Aureli P, Fenicia L, Pasolini B, Gianfranceschi M, McCroskey LM, Hatheway CL. Two cases of type E infant botulism caused by neurotoxigenic Clostridium butyricum in Italy. *J Infect Dis.* 1986;154:207-211.
4. Fujinaga Y, Inoue K, Watanabe S, Yokota K, Hirai Y, Nagamachi E, et al. The haemagglutinin of

Clostridium botulinum type C progenitor toxin plays an essential role in binding of toxin to the epithelial cells of guinea pig small intestine, leading to the efficient absorption of the toxin. *Microbiology.* 1997;143:3841-3847.

5. Sharma SK, Singh BR. Hemagglutinin binding mediated protection of botulinum neurotoxin from proteolysis. *J Nat Toxins.* 1998;7:239-253.

6. Schanz EJ, Johnson EA. Properties and use of botulinum toxin and other microbiol neurotoxins in medicine. *Microbiol Rev.* 1992;56:80-99.

7. Henderson I, Davis T, Elmore M, Minton N. The genetic basis of toxin production in Clostridium botulinum and Clostridium tetani. In Rood J, McClane D, Souger J, Titball R, eds. *The Clostridia: Molecular Biology and Pathogenesis.* Philadelphia: Academic Press; 1997:261-284.

8. Arndt JW, Jacobson MJ, Abola EE, Forsyth CM, Tepp WH, Marks JD, et al. A structural perspective of the sequence variability within botulinum neurotoxin subtypes A1-A4. *J Mol Biol.* 2006;362:733-742.

9. Dekleva ML, Dasgupta BR. Purification and characterization of a protease from Clostridium botulinum type A that nicks single-chain type A botulinum neurotoxin into the di-chain form. *J Bateriol.* 1990;172:2498-2503.

10. Erdal E, Bartels F, Binscheck T, Erdmann G, Frevert J, Kistner A, et al. Processing of tetanus and botulinum A neurotoxins in isolated chromaffin cells. *Naunyn Schmiedebergs Arch Pharmacol.* 1995;351:67-78.

11. Kistner A, Habermann E. Reductive cleavage of tetanus toxin and botulinum neurotoxin A by the thioredoxin system from brain. Evidence for two redox isomers of tetanus toxin. *Naunyn Schmiedebergs Arch Pharmacol.* 1992;345:227-234.

12. Scott AB, Rosenbaum A, Collins CC. Pharmacologic weakening of extraocular muscles. *Invest Ophthalmol.* 1973;12:924-927.

13. Melling J, Hambleton P, Shone CC. Clostridium botulinum toxins: nature and preparation for clinical use. *Eye.* 1988;2:16-23.

14. Hambleton P. Clostridium botulinum toxins: a general review of involvement in disease, structure, mode of action and preparation for clinical use. *J Neurol.* 1992;239:16-20.

15. Callaway JE, Grethlein AJ. Production, quality, and stability of botulinum type b (Myobloc) for clinical use. In: Brin MF, Hallet M, Jankovic J, eds. *Scientific and Therapeutic Aspects of Botulinum Toxin,* Baltimore, MD: Lippincott Williams & Williams; 2002:115-122.

16. Callaway JE. Botulinum toxin type B (Myobloc): pharmacology and biochemistry. *Clin Dermatol.* 2004;22:23-28.

17. DasGupta BR, Sathyamoorthy V. Purification and amino acid composition of type A botulinum neurotoxin. *Toxicon.* 1984;22:415-424.

18. DasGupta BR, Sugiyama H. Molecular forms of neurotoxins in proteolytic Clostridium botulinum type B cultures. *Infect Immun.* 1976;14:680-686.

19. Callaway JE, Arezzo JC, Grethlein AJ. Botulinum toxin type B: an overview of its biochemistry and preclinical pharmacology. *Dis Mon.* 2002;48:367-383.

20. Sakaguchi G. Clostridium botulinum toxins. *Pharmac Ther.* 1983;19:165-194.

21. Ohishi I, Suggii S, Sacaguchi G. Oral toxicities of clostridium botulinum toxins in response to molecular size. *Infect Immun.* 1977;16:107-109.

22. Chen F, Kuziemko GM, Stevens RC. Biophysical characterization of the stability of the 150-kilodalton botulinum toxin, the nontoxic component, and the 900-kilodalton botulinum toxin complex species. *Infect Immun.* 1998;66:2420-2425.

23. Sugiyama H. Clostridium botulinum neurotoxin. *Microbiol Rev.* 1980;44:419-448.

24. Inoue K, Fujinaga Y, Watanabe T, Ohyama T, Takeshi K, Moriishi K, et al. Molecular composition of Clostridium botulinum type A progenitor toxins. *Infect Immun.* 1996;64:1589-1594.

25. Arndt JW, Gu J, Jaroszewski L, Schwarzenbacher R, Hanson MA, Lebeda FJ, et al. The structure of the neurotoxin-associated protein HA33/A from Clostridium botulinum suggests a reoccurring beta-trefoil fold in the progenitor toxin complex. *J Mol Biol.* 2005;346:1083-1093.

26. Jost WH, Blümel J, Grafe S. Botulinum neurotoxin type A free of complexing proteins (XEOMIN) in focal dystonia. *Drugs.* 2007;67:669-683.

27. Aoki KR, Ranoux D, Wissel J. Using translational medicine to understand clinical differences between botulinum toxin formulations. *Eur J Neurol.* 2006;13(suppl 4):10-19.

28. Wenzel R, Jones D, Borrego JA. Comparing two botulinum toxin type A formulations using manufacturers' product summaries. *J Clin Pharm Ther.* 2007;4:387-402.

29. Dodd SL, Rowell BA, Vrabas IS, Arrowsmith RJ, Weatherill PJ. A comparison of the spread of three formulations of botulinum neurotoxin A as determined by effects on muscle function. *Eur J Neurol.* 1998;5:181-186.

30. Tang-Liu DD, Aoki KR, Dolly JO, de Paiva A, Houchen TL, Chasseaud LF, et al. Intramuscular injection of 125I-botulinum neurotoxin-complex versus 125I-botulinum-free neurotoxin: time course of tissue distribution. *Toxicon.* 2003;42:461-469.

31. Friday D, Bigalke H, Frevert J. In vitro stability of botulinum toxin complex preparations at physiological pH and temperature. *Naunyn-Schmiedebergs Arch Pharmacol.* 2002;46:S365.

32. Pickett A, Shipley S, Panjwani N, O'Keeffe R, Sing BR. Characterisation and consistency of botulinum A toxin-hemagglutinin complex used for clinical therapy. Posterpresentation International conference 2005, Basic and Therapeutic Aspects of Botulinum and Tetanus Toxins, Denver, Co, 23-25 June 2005.

33. Fujita R, Fujinaga Y, Inoue K, Nakajima H, Kumon H, Oguma K. Molecular characterization of two forms of nontoxic-nonhemagglutinin components of Clostridium botulinum type A progenitor toxins. *FEBS Lett.* 1995;376:41-44.

34. Bigalke H, Wohlfarth K, Irmer A, Dengler R. Botulinum A toxin: Dysport improvement of biological availability. *Exp Neurol.* 2001;168:162-170.

35. Goodnough MC, Johnson EA. Stabilization of botulinum toxin type A during lyophilization. *Appl Environ Microbiol.* 1992;58:3426-3428.

36. Sesardic D, Leung T, Gaines Das R. Role for standards in assays of botulinum toxins: international collaborative study of three preparations of botulinum type A toxin. *Biologicals.* 2003;31:265-276.

37. Hunt TJ. Botulinum toxin composition. US Patent application 2007/0025019.

38. Pickett A, O'Keeffe R, Panjwani N. The protein load of therapeutic botulinum toxins. *Eur J Neurol.* 2007;14:e11.

39. Kromminga A, Schellekens H. Related articles. Antibodies against erythropoietin and other protein-based therapeutics: an overview. *Ann N Y Acad Sci.* 2005;1050:257-265.

40. Göschel H, Wohlfarth K, Frevert J, Dengler R, Bigalke H. Botulinum A toxin therapy: neutralizing and non-neutralizing antibodies—therapeutic consequences. *Exp Neurol.* 1997;147:96-102.

41. Critchfield J. Considering the immune response to botulinum toxin. *Clin J Pain.* 2002;18(6 suppl): S133-S141.

42. Inoue K, Fujinaga Y, Honke K, Arimitsu H, Mahmut N, Sakaguchi Y, et al. Clostridium botulinum type A haemagglutinin-positive progenitor toxin (HA(+)-PTX) binds to oligosaccharides containing Gal beta1-4GlcNAc through one subcomponent of haemagglutinin (HA1). *Microbiology.* 2001;147:811-819.

43. Choi NW, Estes MK, Langridge WH. Ricin toxin B subunit enhancement of rotavirus NSP4 immunogenicity in mice. *Viral Immunol.* 2006;19:54-63.

44. Lee JC, Yokota K, Arimitsu H, Hwang HJ, Sakaguchi Y, Cui J, et al. Production of anti-neurotoxin antibody is enhanced by two subcomponents, HA1 and HA3b, of Clostridium botulinum type B 16S toxin-haemagglutinin. *Microbiology.* 2005;151(Pt 11):3739-3747.

45. Atassi MZ. On the enhancement of anti-neurotoxin antibody production by subcomponents HA1 and HA3b of Clostridium botulinum type B 16S toxin-haemagglutinin. *Microbiology.* 2006;152(Pt 7):1891-1895.

46. Jankovic J, Vuong KD, Ahsan J. Comparison of efficacy and immunogenicity of original versus current botulinum toxin in cervical dystonia. *Neurology.* 2003;60:1186-1188.

47. Honko AN, Sriranganathan N, Lees CJ, Mizel SB. Flagellin is an effective adjuvant for immunization against lethal respiratory challenge with Yersinia pestis. *Infect Immun.* 2006;74:1113-1120.

48. Lee SE, Kim SY, Jeong BC, Kim YR, Bae SJ, Ahn OS, et al. A bacterial flagellin, Vibrio vulnificus FlaB, has a strong mucosal adjuvant activity to induce protective immunity. *Infect Immun.* 2006;74:694-702.

49. Siegel LS. Evaluation of neutralizing antibodies to type A, B, E, and F botulinum toxins in sera from human recipients of botulinum pentavalent (ABCDE) toxoid. *J Clin Microbiol.* 1989;27:1906-1908.

50. Aoki KR. Immunological and other properties of therapeutic botulinum toxin serotypes. In: Brin MF, Jankovic J, Hallet M, eds. *Scientific and Therapeutic Aspects of Botulinum Toxin.* Baltimore, MD: Lippincott Williams & Wilkins; 2002:103-113.

51. Dressler D. Pharmacological aspects of therapeutic botulinum toxin preparations. *Nervenarzt.* 2006;77:912-921.

52. Dressler D, Hallett M. Immunological aspects of Botox, Dysport and Myobloc/NeuroBloc. *Eur J Neurol.* 2006;13(suppl 1):11-15.

53. Jankovic J, Hunter C, Dolimbek BZ, Dolimbek GS, Adler CH, Brashear A, et al. Clinico-immunologic aspects of botulinum toxin type B treatment of cervical dystonia. *Neurology.* 2006;67:2233-2235.

54. Kessler KR, Skutta M, Benecke R. Long-term treatment of cervical dystonia with botulinum toxin A: efficacy, safety, and antibody frequency. German Dystonia Study Group. *J Neurol.* 1999;246:265-274.

55. Herrmann J, Geth K, Mall V, Bigalke H, Schulte Mönting J, Linder M, et al. Clinical Impact of antibody formation to botulinum toxin in children. *Ann Neurol.* 2004;55:732-735.

Comparative Clinical Trials of Botulinum Toxins

33

Dirk Dressler and Cynthia Comella

INTRODUCTION

Edward Schantz and Alan B. Scott pioneered the use of botulinum toxin (BoNT) as a therapeutic agent in the 1970s.[1] In 1979, Schantz and colleagues at the University of Wisconsin prepared 150 mg of twice-crystallized botulinum toxin serotype A, which was approved for human use in the United States in 1989 for the indications of strabismus, blepharospasm (BEB), and other disorders of the seventh cranial nerve. The original batch of botulinum toxin serotype A (BoNT/A; Botox, lot 79-11) was the only commercially available botulinum toxin for human use until the year 2000. From 2000 to present, four brands of BoNT have become available. There are three brands of BoNT/A (Botox [Allergan, Irvine, CA], Dysport [Ipsen, Milford, MA], and Xeomin [Merz, Greensboro, NC]) and one brand of BoNT/B, Myobloc/NeuroBloc (Solstice Neurosciences, Malvern, PA).

Despite the widespread use of the various brands and serotypes, the comparability of the different formulations of BoNT remains an open question. BoNT is a complex biologic molecule. In contrast to other medicinal products, each serotype has a distinct pharmacology and mechanism of action. There are no equivalent plasma concentrations to compare.[2] Within a single serotype, pharmacologic differences may arise from differences in preparation, type and quantity of associated proteins, and varied methods in assessing potency (see Chapter 32). Comparability is further complicated by widely differing injection schemes (including target muscle selection, dosages, injection sites), dilutions, application techniques, and treated patient population.[3] Finally, the standard clinical outcomes used to assess severity of dystonia may not be sensitive to small differences between groups. Given the multiplicity of these factors, comparative trials of different brands may show conflicting results. At this time, there is no definitive information to guide the clinician in choosing one toxin over the other. This chapter focuses on the electrophysiologic effect of BoNT brands in humans and highlights clinical comparisons among the different BoNT brands for dosing, clinical efficacy, and adverse effects.

BOTULINUM NEUROTOXIN BRANDS: MOUSE UNITS

In making comparisons of BoNT brands and serotypes, it is important to understand the concept of BoNT dose in mouse units (mu). The mouse lethality assay is a biologic assay used to define the activity of BoNT. The potency of BoNT is indicated as mouse units. One mouse unit is defined as the amount of BoNT required to kill 50% (LD50) of a certain weight, strain, and sex of mice.[4] Although it is well defined, potency as defined by this biologic assay may vary

Dr. Dressler is disclosing that he has acted as a consultant for Allergan, Ipsen, Merz, Desitin, Medtronic, and Cephalon. Dr. Comella is disclosing that she has acted as a consultant for Allergan, Merz, UCB, and Boehringer. Also, she has received contracted research support from Boehringer, Ipsen, Solstice, Solvay, and Allergan.

from one particular test system to another.[5] Hence, it is not surprising that dosages of botulinum toxin may vary depending on the preparation of the toxin. For the three brands of serotype A commercially available, doses of Botox for cervical dystonia (CD) range from 100 to 300 U per injection series,[6] Xeomin appears to have the same dose range as Botox,[7] and Dysport dosing ranges from 500 to 1000 U.[8] Not surprisingly given the basic differences among serotypes, the dosing of BoNT/B as Myobloc/NeuroBloc has a much different dose range than do the brands of BoNT/A. The usual dosing of Myobloc/NeuroBloc for CD ranges from 2500 to 10000 U, with some extending the maximum dose as high as 25,000 U.[9]

COMPARATIVE EFFECTS OF BOTULINUM NEUROTOXIN IN A SINGLE MUSCLE

Direct comparisons of BoNT/A (Botox) and BoNT/B (Myobloc/NeuroBloc) have been conducted in single muscles and in patients. In normal extensor digitorum brevis muscle (EDB M), M wave amplitudes were compared following injections of BoNT/A and BoNT/B.[10] In this study, the outcome measure was the postexercise facilitation of the EDB M wave following 10 seconds of exercise. Measures were obtained at baseline and 2, 6, 9, and 14 days following injection. Subjects were followed using the same measure at 7, 11, 15, 27, 42, and 57 weeks following injection to determine duration of effect. The decrement in M wave amplitude in the EDB occurred 2 weeks following a dose of 320 to 480 U of BoNT/B and 7.5 to 10 U of BoNT/A and was greater with BoNT/A than with BoNT/B. Whether M wave amplitude is a reliable measure of clinical response or whether the doses of BoNT/A (7.5–10 U) and BoNT/B (320–480 U) used in this study are comparable is not clear. In the BoNT/B-treated muscle, M wave amplitude returned to normal after 11 weeks. In BoNT/A injected muscle, there was a sustained reduction in M wave amplitude that was still present at 57 weeks following injection.[10] It may be that increasing the dose of BoNT/B would have prolonged the duration of this effect, but this cannot be accurately extrapolated from the data available in the study.

COMPARATIVE BoNT EFFECTS IN BLEPHAROSPASM AND HEMIFACIAL SPASM

Three studies have compared BoNT brands for the treatment of BEB and hemifacial spasm (HFS) (Table 33-1). Two studies compared Dysport and Botox. Both studies compared a conversion ratio of Botox to Dysport of 1:1.4.[11,12] In one study, a single-blind, parallel-group design in 91 BEB and HFS patients was used with duration of effect as the primary outcome. Maximal benefit is not given. In this study, 24% of the Dysport group and 12% of the Botox group required booster treatments. Overall, the duration of effect did not differ between the groups (Dysport 12.8 ± 5.6 weeks versus Botox 13.1 ± 11.8 weeks), although there was marked variability in the outcome. The frequency of adverse effects was similar for the two brands.[11]

A second study in 212 patients with BEB used a randomized, double-blind crossover study design. Again no efficacy data are provided. The duration of effect was similar for Dysport and Botox (8 weeks), but the frequency of side effects, particularly ptosis, was reduced in those receiving Botox (Dysport 6.6% versus Botox 1.4%).[12] A third study compared Botox and Xeomin in 302 BEB patients enrolled in 42 study sites. This study used a conversion ratio of Botox to Xeomin of 1:1 and was designed as a noninferiority study. Both treatment groups showed similar efficacy on the Jankovic Rating Scale sum score, as well as other efficacy measures. Duration of effect (110 days) and adverse effects did not differ between the groups.[13]

COMPARATIVE EFFECTS OF BOTULINUM NEUROTOXIN IN CERVICAL DYSTONIA

Botulinum Neurotoxin Type A (Botox) and Botulinum Neurotoxin Type B (Myobloc/ NeuroBloc) for Cervical Dystonia

There are two clinical trials that have compared BoNT/A with BoNT/B in the treatment of CD (Table 33-2). The ABCD trial evaluated efficacy, adverse effects, and duration of benefit in

TABLE 33-1 Controlled Studies Comparing Brands of BoNT for Treatment of Blepharospasm (BEB) or Hemifacial Spasm (HFS)

Study	Disorder, Study Aim	BoNT Comparison Ratio and Dose	Study Design	Results	Comments
Sampaio et al[11]	BEB n = 42 HFS n = 49 Comparison of duration of benefit, booster injections needed, efficacy and side effects	Botox:Dysport = 1:4 Botox: 25 mu Dysport: 100 mu	Randomized, parallel group, single blind 3 centers	No efficacy data Duration of benefit: Botox 11.2 weeks Dysport 13.3 weeks Adverse effects: Botox: 47% Dysport: 50%	High variability in patient responses in both groups Endpoint for duration of benefit defined as a patient reported waning of effect
Nüssgens et al[12]	BEB n = 212 Prior treatment with BoNT Comparison of efficacy, duration of effect, and side effects	Botox:Dysport = 1:4 Botox: 45.4 mu Dysport: 182 mu	Randomized, crossover, double blind, single site	No efficacy data Duration of benefit: Botox: 8 weeks Dysport: 8 weeks All adverse effects: Botox: 17% Dysport: 24% (p <.05) Ptosis: Botox: 1.4% Dysport: 6.6% (p <.01)	Botox dilution 4 mL/100 mu Dysport dilution 5 mL/500 mu No defined endpoint for duration of benefit
Roggenkämper et al[13]	BEB n = 304 Previous response to Botox Comparison of efficacy, duration of benefit and side effects	Botox:Xeomin = 1:1 Botox: 41 mu Xeomin: 40 mu	Randomized, parallel group, double blind 42 centers in Europe, Israel	Similar improvement in Jankovic Rating Scale sum Botox: 2.65 Xeomin: 2.83 p < 0.0001 for change from baseline p >.05 Xeomin compared with Botox Duration: Similar duration: (median 110 days) Adverse effects: Similar frequency and type	Duration of effect determined through patient interview Adverse effects, mild to moderate in 90% in both groups Similar outcomes with either toxin.

TABLE 33-2 Controlled Studies Comparing Brands of BoNT for Treatment of Cervical Dystonia (CD)

Study	Disorder, Study Aim	BoNT Comparison Ratio and Dose	Study Design	Results	Comments
Comella et al[14]	CD n = 139 Previous response to Botox Comparison of efficacy, duration of benefit and adverse effects	Botox:Myobloc/ NeuroBloc = 1:40 Botox: 205 mu Myobloc/NeuroBloc: 8520 mu	Randomized, parallel group, double blind 19 centers in the United States	Improvement in total TWSTRS (21%) and subscales of TWSTRS similar between groups Duration in those with benefit Botox: 14.0 weeks Myobloc/NeuroBloc: 12.1 weeks $p = .033$ Adverse effects: % change dry mouth Botox: 9% ($p = .70$) Myobloc/NeuroBloc: 43% ($p \leq 0.0001$) % change dysphagia Botox: 4% ($p = 0.25$) Myobloc/NeuroBloc: 34% ($p = 0.0009$)	Duration if assessed in all patients (those with and without benefit at week 4) did not differ
Pappert et al[18]	CD n = 111 in ITT n = 93 in analysis Naïve to BoNT Non-inferiority trial comparing efficacy, duration of benefit and side effects	Botox:Myobloc/ NeuroBloc = 1 mu:67 mu Botox: 150 mu Myobloc/NeuroBloc: 10,000 mu	Randomized, parallel group, double blind 24 sites in Europe	Improvement in total TWSTRS 21% and TWSTRS subscales similar between groups. Duration: 13.4 weeks; no difference between groups Adverse effects: Dry mouth Botox: 7.3% Myobloc/NeuroBloc: 39.3% $p = 0.0001$ Dysphagia: Botox: 14% Myobloc/NeuroBloc: 16% $p = 1.0$	Noninferiority study showed no differences other than dry mouth. Did not collect adverse effects at baseline prior to injection. Did not systematically interview for side effects. Did not include 13 patients from 1 site for protocol violations
Tintner et al[17]	CD n = 20 Previously treated Comparison of autonomic dysfunction	Botox:Myobloc/ NeuroBloc = 1:50 Botox: 227 ± 83 mu Myobloc/NeuroBloc: 12,083 ± 5899 mu	Randomized, parallel group, double blind 1 site	Overall improvement TWSTRS approximately 29% (not analyzed) No change in orthostatic hypotension, blood pressure, heart rate, respiration, papillary reactions Dysphagia: Botox: 28% Myobloc/NeuroBloc: 55% Not significant: Constipation Botox: 0%	Major limitation is small number of patients (10 in each group)

Continued

TABLE 33-2 Controlled Studies Comparing Brands of BoNT for Treatment of Cervical Dystonia (CD)—Cont'd

Study	Disorder, Study Aim	BoNT Comparison Ratio and Dose	Study Design	Results	Comments
Odergren et al[20]	CD (Rotational) n = 73 Previous response to Botox To find dose equivalence of Dysport and Botox	Dysport:Botox = 3:1 Botox: 152 M (range 70–240) Dysport: 477 mu (range 240–720)	Randomized, parallel group, double blind 7 study sites	Myobloc/NeuroBloc: 33% p = .037 Improvement in Tsui scale at week 4: Dysport: 35% Botox: 32% Similar improvement in pain, patient and investigator assessment of improvement Similar type and percent of adverse events: Dysphagia: 12% Pharyngitis: 11%	Adverse effects determined by spontaneous report. Botox responsive patients
Ranoux et al[21]	CD (n = 54) Previous response to Botox	Dysport:Botox = 3:1 and 4:1	Randomized, double blind, 3 period crossover: Dysport:Botox = 3:1 Dysport:Botox = 4:1	% change in Tsui scale: Botox: 38% Dysport: 1:3: 49% Dysport: 1:4: 55% % change in TWSTRS pain scale: Botox: 46% Dysport: 1:3: 68% Dysport: 1:4: 79% Duration of effect: Botox: 89 Dysport: 1:3: 97 Dysport: 1:4: 114 Adverse events: Dysphagia Botox: 3% Dysport: 1:3: 15.6% Dysport: 1:4: 17.3% Percent with adverse effects: Botox: 17.6% Dysport: 1:3: 33% Dysport: 1:4: 36%	Conclude that Dysport more effective than Botox at either 3:1 or 4:1, but higher frequency of side effects.
Benecke et al[7]	CD (n = 420) Previous response to Botox	Xeomin:Botox = 1:1 Xeomin: 140 mu Botox: 139 mu	Randomized, parallel group, double blind Noninferiority 51 study sites	Improvement comparable in two groups TWSTRS severity 33% improved Cannot approximate for other scores % with adverse events: Botox: 24% Xeomin: 28%	Data for TWSTRS difficult to interpret, small changes for TWSTRS subscales

TWSTRS, Toronto Western Torticollis Rating Scale.

BoNT/A (Botox) and BoNT/B (Myobloc/NeuroBloc) using a blinded, randomized study design in patients with CD, with responsiveness to BoNT established through prior treatments and continued clinical responsiveness.[14] Patients were treated using doses and muscle selection previously shown to be effective, evaluated 4 weeks following injection for maximal benefit, and followed at 2-week intervals until loss of 80% of benefit to estimate duration of effect. The treating investigator and rating investigator were not the same to prevent unblinding. Side effects were systematically obtained using a directed interview. In this study, a conversion ratio of Botox to Myobloc/NeuroBloc of 1:40 was used. There were 139 patients randomized, two patients (1%) were lost to follow-up, and 16 patients (11%) showing no change in the Toronto Western Torticollis Rating Scale (TWSTRS)[15] score at week 4. This study showed equivalent improvement in both treatment groups, with an approximate 24% reduction in TWSTRS score at week 4. Side effects were more frequent in the Myobloc/NeuroBloc group for dysphagia and dry mouth. The duration of effect in those with improvement in TWSTRS following injection was longer in the Botox group by approximately 2 weeks.[14] The major limitation of this study was the inclusion of patients previously and successfully treated with Botox. Increased frequency of systemic autonomic adverse effects in the Myobloc/NeuroBloc treated group supported previous observations, suggesting different sensitivities of the motor and the autonomic nervous systems to BoNT/A and to BoNT/B.[16,17]

A recent noninferiority study using a parallel-arm, blinded study design randomized 111 BoNT-naïve patients with CD to either Botox or Myobloc/NeuroBloc.[18] In this study, a conversion ratio of Botox to Dysport of 1:4-5 was used. Patients were assessed for maximal improvement at week 4, and followed subsequently at 4-week intervals. Following adjustments for differences in baseline TWSTRS, both groups showed improvement of approximately 19% in total TWSTRS scores. The Myobloc/NeuroBloc patients had an increased frequency of mild dry mouth but did not differ from the Botox group for moderate to severe dry mouth or dysphagia. The duration of effect was 13.1 weeks for Botox and 13.7 weeks for Myobloc/NeuroBloc, and did not differ between groups. This study had several limitations. There were 18 patients (16% of those randomized) not included in the analysis (13 patients were excluded from one site due to lack of appropriate training); the evaluations for the duration of effect occurred at intervals of 4 weeks; adverse effects were not systematically obtained, relying on spontaneous reports by the subjects; and the treating investigator was also the rating investigator, which may have been a source of unblinding.[18]

Dysport and Botox for Cervical Dystonia

In an open label study, 48 patients with BEB, CD, or HFS were switched from Dysport to Botox using a conversion ratio of Botox to Myobloc/NeuroBloc of 1:67. This study found that Botox provided greater improvement, fewer adverse effects, and a longer duration of benefit (62 to 65 days for Botox versus 42 to 47 days for Dysport). However, these findings must be interpreted cautiously given the limited number of patients, the lack of blinding, and the possibility that the patient sample enrolled was biased toward those not currently experiencing sufficient benefit from Dysport.[19]

In contrast, a double-blind, randomized study compared outcomes in 73 patients with rotational CD, evaluating Botox and Dysport at a conversion ratio of Botox to Dysport of 1:3. Patients returned for assessment 2, 4, 8, and 12 weeks after treatment. These investigators reported similar benefit, adverse effects, and duration of benefit for the Dysport group (mean dose of 477 mu, range 240 to 720 mu) and the Botox group (mean dose of 152 mu, range 70 to 240 mu).[20]

A second double-blind, randomized, three-period crossover study involving 54 patients with CD reported a different outcome. In this study, CD patients received Botox at the usual dose; Dysport at a conversion ratio of Botox to Dysport of 1:3 and Dysport at a conversion ratio of Botox to Dysport of 1:4. Patients receiving Dysport at either conversion ratio had increased improvement over Botox, but also had increased frequency of adverse effects, although these were generally mild. They concluded that the conversion ratio between Botox and Dysport might be as low as 1:2.[21]

The REAL study was a retrospective study that included six international study sites and evaluated the doses of BoNT/A as Dysport or Botox administered in a clinical setting without pre-established guidelines that would be used in a clinical trial. The study included 70 patients CD and 44 with BEB patients who had received at least 1 year of either Dysport or Botox before switching to the other brand for at least 1 year. The overall conversion ratio of Botox to Dysport was 1:4.5, but it ranged from 1:2 to 1:11. Although adverse events were more frequent during treatment with Dysport (11% of Dysport versus 4% of Botox), the mean total toxin dose was lower in those reporting adverse events. Although this study was not controlled and efficacy was not systematically collected, it shows that in clinical practice conversion between Botox and Dysport varies greatly. Given the fact that dosages influence the therapeutic effect as well as the adverse effects, it is not surprising that the variability of the conversion factor used directly influences both factors.

It may be that the use of clinical scales to assess differences in effect among the BoNT brand is an insensitive measure. Using voluntary electromyographic activity (M-EMG) following BoNT injections into the sternocleidomastoid muscle in 34 patients, one study found that Botox at doses of 20 to 60 mu showed reduction in M-EMG of 80% to 85%. With Dysport at doses of 100 to 500 mu, M-EMG activity was reduced from 70% to 91%. Equivalent reductions in M-EMG were found for 200 to 300 mu Dysport to 40 to 60 mu of Botox, suggesting dose ratios between 5:1 and 7.5:1 may be equivalent.[22]

Xeomin and Botox for Cervical Dystonia

There is only one study that directly compares Xeomin and Botox in the treatment of CD. In this double-blind, noninferiority study, 463 patients with CD were randomized to either Xeomin or Botox, using a 1:1 conversion ratio. There were 420 patients included. The study demonstrated similar benefit from both brands, and a similar side effect profile. The investigators concluded that Xeomin was not inferior to Botox at the doses administered.[7]

CONCLUSION

There are now four brands of BoNT available for clinical use; three are based on BoNT/A and one on BoNT/B. Each brand of BoNT is a complex mixture of components, with BoNT being the therapeutically active one. Each of these components may influence the therapeutic efficacy, adverse effects profile and antigenicity of the particular BoNT preparation.[6] Comparative studies among these brands in the treatment of CD, BEB, and HFS have not been able to establish simple dose equivalencies that can be used in a clinical setting. Although studies to date appear to support a dose ratio of 1 mu:1 mu between Botox and Xeomin, confirmatory studies are needed. At present, clinicians should consider each brand and serotype individually, and not apply specific dose ratios when switching from one brand to another. It is likely that the first choice of brand will not depend on efficacy or side effect profile but may rest with other issues including long term antigenicity.

References

1. Schantz E, Johnson E. Botulinum toxin: the story of its development for the treatment of human disease. *Perspect Biol Med.* 1997;40:317-327.
2. Sampaio C, Costa J, Ferreira JJ. Clinical comparability of marketed formulations of botulinum toxin. *Mov Disord.* 2004;19(suppl 8):S129-S136.
3. Lim EC, Seet RC. Botulinum toxin: description of injection techniques and examination of controversies surrounding toxin diffusion. *Acta Neurol Scand.* 2008;117:73-84.
4. Schantz E, Kautter D. Microbiological methods: Standardized assay for clostridium botulinum toxins. *J Assoc Official Analytical Chemists.* 1977;61:96-99.
5. Pearce LB, Borodic GE, First ER, MacCallum RD. Measurement of botulinum toxin activity: evaluation of the lethality assay. *Toxicol Appl Pharmacol.* 1994;128:69-77.
6. Jankovic J. Botulinum toxin therapy for cervical dystonia. *Neurotox Res.* 2006;9:145-148.
7. Benecke R, Jost WH, Kanovsky P, Ruzicka E, Comes G, Grafe S. A new botulinum toxin type A free of complexing proteins for treatment of cervical dystonia. *Neurology.* 2005;64:1949-1951.
8. Poewe W, Deuschl G, Nebe A, Feifel E, Wissel J, Benecke R, et al. What is the optimal dose of botulinum toxin A in the treatment of cervical dystonia? Results of a double blind, placebo controlled, dose ranging study using Dysport. German Dystonia Study Group. *J Neurol Neurosurg Psychiatry.* 1998;64:13-17.
9. Lew MF, Brashear A, Factor S. The safety and efficacy of botulinum toxin type B in the treatment of patients with cervical dystonia: summary of three controlled clinical trials. *Neurology.* 2000;55(suppl 5):S29-S35.
10. Sloop RR, Cole BA, Escutin RO. Human response to botulinum toxin injection: type B compared with type A. *Neurology.* 1997;49:189-194.
11. Sampaio C, Ferreira JJ, Simoes F, Rosas MJ, Magalhaes M, Correia AP, et al. DYSBOT: a single-blind, randomized parallel study to determine whether any differences can be detected in the efficacy and tolerability of two formulations of botulinum toxin type A—Dysport and Botox—assuming a ratio of 4:1. *Mov Disord.* 1997;12(6):1013-1018.
12. Nüssgens Z, Roggenkamper P. Comparison of two botulinum-toxin preparations in the treatment of essential blepharospasm. *Graefes Arch Clin Exp Ophthalmol.* 1997;235:197-199.

13. Roggenkämper P, Jost WH, Bihari K, Comes G, Grafe S. Efficacy and safety of a new botulinum toxin type A free of complexing proteins in the treatment of blepharospasm. *J Neural Transm.* 2006;113:303-312.

14. Comella CL, Jankovic J, Shannon KM, Tsui J, Swenson M, Leurgans S, et al. Comparison of botulinum toxin serotypes A and B for the treatment of cervical dystonia. *Neurology.* 2005;65:1423-1429.

15. Consky E, Lang AE. *Clinical Assessments of Patients with Cervical Dystonia.* New York: Marcel Dekker; 1994.

16. Dressler D, Benecke R. Autonomic side effects of botulinum toxin type B treatment of cervical dystonia and hyperhidrosis. *Eur Neurol.* 2003;49:34-38.

17. Tintner R, Gross R, Winzer UF, Smalky KA, Jankovic J. Autonomic function after botulinum toxin type A or B: a double-blind, randomized trial. *Neurology.* 2005;65: 765-767.

18. Pappert EJ, Germanson T. Botulinum toxin type B vs. type A in toxin-naive patients with cervical dystonia: Randomized, double-blind, noninferiority trial. *Mov Disord.* 2007.

19. Bihari K. Safety, effectiveness, and duration of effect of BOTOX after switching from Dysport for blepharospasm, cervical dystonia, and hemifacial spasm dystonia, and hemifacial spasm. *Curr Med Res Opin.* 2005;21:433-438.

20. Odergren T, Hjaltason H, Kaakkola S, Solders G, Hanko J, Fehling C, et al. A double blind, randomised, parallel group study to investigate the dose equivalence of Dysport and Botox in the treatment of cervical dystonia. *J Neurol Neurosurg Psychiatry.* 1998;64:6-12.

21. Ranoux D, Gury C, Fondarai J, Mas JL, Zuber M. Respective potencies of Botox and Dysport: a double blind, randomised, crossover study in cervical dystonia. *J Neurol Neurosurg Psychiatry.* 2002;72:459-462.

22. Dressler D, Rothwell JC. Electromyographic quantification of the paralysing effect of botulinum toxin in the sternocleidomastoid muscle. *Eur Neurol.* 2000;43: 13-16.

Tetanus Toxin 34

Paul S. Fishman

INTRODUCTION

Clostridia tetani are anaerobic gram-negative bacteria. Although the organism is sensitive to heat and oxygen, its spores are highly resistant and are capable of surviving boiling as well as household disinfectants. The spores are ubiquitous worldwide and can be found especially in agricultural areas. Individuals may harbor organisms in the gut, and the spores can be found on the skin. In low oxygen environments such as a wound, the spores will germinate.[1]

Tetanus toxin, also known as tetanospasmin, is one of two toxins elaborated by the organism. The other, tetanolysin, is a hemolysin with no known function or pathology. Under anaerobic conditions, the bacteria can be cultured in bulk. These bulk cultures allow for high-yield production of toxin protein for use as the starting product for tetanus toxoid needed in the vaccine industry.

CLINICAL TETANUS

Signs and Symptoms

Four forms of clinical tetanus have been well described. Generalized tetanus, localized tetanus, cephalic tetanus, and neonatal tetanus.

Generalized Tetanus

Generalized tetanus is the most commonly described form of clinical tetanus, accounting for up to 80% of cases in which symptoms commonly develop in a descending pattern.[2] Difficulty opening the mouth due to tetanic spasms of the masseter, known as trismus or lockjaw, is the most common initial symptom. Lockjaw is usually followed by neck stiffness and difficulty swallowing. This is followed by stiffness and spasms of the back, abdominal and chest muscles, as well as flexion and extension of the limbs. The muscular spasms can be extremely forceful, resulting in hyperthermia,

rhabdomyolysis, and even vertebral fractures. Although the toxin is epileptogenic and the spasms may resemble seizure activity, true seizures appear to be rare, except in the circumstance of hypoxia.[3] Tachycardia and hypertension due to autonomic instability are also commonly seen in generalized tetanus and are a major source of morbidity and mortality. Classic descriptions of generalized tetanus note distortion of the face by muscle spasms, resulting in risus sardonicus, as well as opistotonic posturing of the back. Death due to generalized tetanus is usually due to hypoxia secondary to chest wall spastic immobility, hyperthermia, and autonomic instability, and the rate has dramatically declined in the modern era in developed nations.[4] The onset of symptoms, although variable, is usually about 8 days after an identified injury (range 3–21 days), but in 10% to 20% of cases, a wound or other portal for the bacteria cannot be identified. The incubation period has a direct relation to prognosis, with more rapid onset of symptoms a harbinger of a more serious disease due to greater elaboration of toxin. The course of generalized spasms is usually 3 to 4 weeks, but milder and more localized spasms can occur for up to several months.

Localized Tetanus

Although many patients develop spasms around the site of elaboration or a wound during the course of their disease, in a minority of cases (10% to 15%), these spasms remain restricted without the appearance of symptoms of generalized tetanus.[5] These patients are referred to as having localized or local tetanus. Although the contractions can involve an entire limb and be sustained for many weeks, it is a milder form of the disease in which mortality is rare (1%). Localized tetanic spasm as an initial presentation of generalized tetanus is also relatively rare in humans. Cases of localized tetanus have been seen in previously but apparently inadequately vaccinated persons and in

Dr. Fishman is disclosing that has received lecture fees from Allergan, Irvine, CA and consulting fees from Lisa Labs, CA.

individuals who received hyperimmune antitetanus antisera early after the appearance of
localized symptoms, likely aborting the progression to generalized tetanus.[6]

Cephalic Tetanus

The rarest and most poorly understood form of
tetanus is cephalic tetanus, which is usually
associated with wounds to the face or neck.[7]
Facial weakness, rather than active spasms,
occurs as well as dysphagia, diplopia, and
oculomotor paresis. Some of these symptoms
(facial weakness) are a result of a direct botulinum neurotoxin–like effect on release of acetylcholine at the neuromuscular junction, which
is rarely apparent in other forms of tetanus.[8]
Oculomotor dysfunction appears to be a
result of interference with neurotransmission
both of the neuromuscular junction and
within oculomotor nuclei of the brainstem.[9]
This syndrome can have the briefest incubation
period of adult forms of tetanus (1–2 days) and
can progress to generalized tetanus with a high
mortality rate if left untreated.

Neonatal Tetanus

The ubiquitous distribution of *Clostridia tetani*
spores in soil is the likely source of infection in
clinical neonatal tetanus. As with adult tetanus,
this form of generalized tetanus that occurs in
newborns is a result of a lack of maternal
immunity. Such infants are born without
any passive immunity, which would have
been derived from an adequately vaccinated
mother. The usual source of infection is the
umbilicus, usually through severing it during
childbirth with an unsterile instrument.[10]
This situation is compounded in some
cultures where soil is placed on the infant's
cut umbilicus. Mortality can be as high
as 90%, especially when symptoms occur
within 48 hours of infection.[11] Although with
adequate ventilatory support full recovery can
occur, both cognitive and motor residua have
been reported.[12]

PREVENTION OF CLINICAL TETANUS

Epidemiology

In spite of the proven protective benefit of
vaccination against tetanus, there continues to
be significant morbidity and mortality from
clinical tetanus worldwide with more than
300,000 deaths per year. Lack of widespread
vaccination is the major factor driving the
persistent incidence of the disease in developing nations, whereas lack of access to mechanical ventilatory support contributes to its high
mortality rate, particularly in the case of
neonatal tetanus. In the United States, there
are currently only 50 to 70 cases of tetanus
per year with comparable number of cases in
other developed nations.[13] In some parts of the
world, practices in which the umbilicus is
exposed to earth, along with poor sterilization
of surgical instruments, contribute to a high
incidence and mortality of neonatal tetanus.
The mortality rate associated wtih clinical tetanus also increases in the elderly. Declining
immune resistance to the toxin with age leads
to more severe and prolonged disease in a more
frail population, with mortality rising to 50%
in patients older than 65 years.[14] Routine
re-vaccination has been considered for this
population, which accounts for more than
80% of tetanus-related deaths in a developed
country. Factors relating to treatment such as
inadequate wound débridment, and access
to antibiotics and hyperimmune antitetanus
immunoglobulin also contribute to the high
(25% to 75%) mortality rate of adult tetanus
in developing countries.

Vaccination

Shortly after the discovery of the spores of
C. tetani as the causative agent of clinical tetanus in 1889, tetanus toxin was identified and
injected into animals. It was noted that sera
from animals that survived the clinical effects
of the toxin could confer immunity on other
individuals exposed to the toxin. This observation led by the 1920s to the development of
vaccination with an inactive form of the toxin
(toxoid) to raise antibodies that would be protective against the active toxin. Passive immunization with hyperimmune sera was
introduced for both prevention of tetanus
after a potential wound exposure as well as
for treatment of clinical tetanus (where much
higher doses are required). In an effort to
reduce the incidence and severity of immune
reaction from equine antitoxin, human hyperimmune tetanus gamma globulin (TIG) was
introduced in the 1960s.[15] This product is in
use today and is titered in international units
(IU), which measure the ability of the antisera
to precipitate a standard amount of toxin protein. A serum level of 0.01 IU/mL of antitoxin

is considered the minimal protective level in humans.

Current treatment of wounds includes not only local débridement (if evidence of an infected wound) and antibiotics, but administration of TIG, with the dose depending on the type and severity of the wound and the history of past TIG administration. Because of the relative safety of TIG, its administration (usually 250 U) is recommended if the history of previous TIG exposure is unknown.[16]

C. tetani is currently grown in bulk for the production of tetanus toxin (TTX) that can be then inactivated with formaldehyde for use as a toxoid in active immunization. Toxoid protein is expressed as limits of flocculation (Lf), a measure of antigen that can be precipitated by a fixed amount of antitoxin. Administration of tetanus toxoid is recommended as a series during childhood in combination with vaccines against diphtheria and pertussis (DTP). Tetanus toxoid vaccination is also recommended as a booster immunization at the time of treatment of a potentially tetanus-contaminated wound, along with administration of TIG.[17] Because of the declining immune protection with age, boosting with tetanus toxoid has been recommended in adults every 10 years. Although serious immune-related side effects to tetanus toxoid injection are rare, both local reactions and systemic allergic reactions have been reported, leading some experts to question current recommendations for routine use of tetanus toxoid after wounds.

Treatment

The administration of a high dose of TIG (3000–6000 IU) is recommended at the time of suspicion of signs or symptoms of clinical tetanus, along with appropriate antibiotics and treatment of a wound source. These treatments address toxin currently produced in a wound and in the circulation. However, by the time clinical signs of tetanus develop, a significant amount of toxin has been internalized within the central nervous system (CNS). This active toxin is not only within the blood brain barrier, which limits the benefits of systemic antibody but is internalized within a neuronal cellular compartment. As is the case with most intracellular protein toxins including botulinum neurotoxins, once the toxin has been internalized, it cannot be neutralized by antibody. Unlike botulinum toxin, tetanus toxin, although internalized by presynaptic motor terminals of the neuromuscular junction, does not have its primary site of action at this location. Tetanus toxin must be transferred from the motor neuron cell body in the spinal cord to the surrounding presynaptic terminals to express its physiologic action. This transfer requires passage across the extracellular synaptic cleft, a location potentially accessible to neutralizing antibody. This potential has been the rationale for studies with intrathecal anti-tetanus antibody or Fab fragments. However, clinical studies of intrathecal TIG have not shown clear superiority to high-dose intramuscular TIG.[18] A tetanus toxoid booster is also recommended as initial treatment. The combination of TIG with a half-life of approximately 1 month and tetanus toxoid boost when antibody levels rise within 2 to 4 weeks after injection provides both short-term and long-term immune protection.

The major focus of treatment of clinical tetanus is control and relief of symptoms.[19] Escalating amounts of intravenous benzodiazepines that enhance inhibitory neuronal activity within the spinal cord are widely used to suppress the spasms of localized and generalized tetanus as well as possible seizure activity. Muscle relaxation is the primary goal in spite of the possibility of respiratory depression. In the setting of clinical tetanus, mechanical ventilation will likely be needed regardless of treatment owing to spasm of respiratory muscles. Intrathecal baclofen has also been used to control the spasms of generalized tetanus, which also have a spinal neuronal site of action. If these centrally acting agents fail to control muscular spasms, neuromuscular paralytics such as vecaronium are recommended.[20] In the setting of mechanical ventilation, autonomic instability is the major cause of mortality in clinical tetanus. Intravenous labetolol is useful in controlling the resulting hypersympathetic activity. Hypotension and bradycardia are treated with standard methods such as fluids and intravenous pressors, and if needed, temporary cardiac pacemaker placement.

TETANUS TOXIN

Structure

As with most potent protein toxins from plants and bacteria, including the somewhat homologous (35%) botulinum neurotoxins, tetanus toxin is a toxic enzyme. Similar to the botulinum neurotoxins, tetanus toxin is a zinc-dependent endopetidase.[21] The toxin is elaborated by a single clostridial gene as a single polypeptide, which undergoes proteolytic cleavage within the bacteria into two chains (heavy and light) connected by a disulfide linkage. The amino acid sequence has been elucidated, and its three-dimensional structures have been partially determined, along with identification of three functional domains common to most bacterial protein toxins: a membrane-binding domain, a membrane-translocation domain and a catalytic (protease) domain.[22]

The toxin's heavy chain contains the binding domain of the toxin within its carboxyl terminal region. Current nomenclature for this domain is Hc, but this domain is virtually equivalent to a peptide originally described from papain digestion of the toxin that has been known as C-fragment or tetanus toxin fragment C (TTC).[23] The availability of this 50-kD peptide both originally as a toxin cleavage product and later in recombinant form has been a major asset in the study of binding, internalization, and transport of tetanus toxin.[24] This binding domain is highly neural specific and contains multiple putative binding sites. For many years, the nature of the neural membrane receptor for tetanus toxin was highly controversial. Kinetic binding studies identified highly prevalent low-affinity receptors, along with far less prevalent high-affinity membrane receptors.[25] A large body of evidence demonstrated that complex membrane gangliosides, in particular GD_{1B} and GT_{1B}, act as the low-affinity receptor.[26] A second membrane receptor thought to be a protein was also hypothesized primarily on the basis of the observation that binding was protease sensitive.[27] This membrane protein component of the tetanus toxin receptor remains without definitive identification, but recent evidence has shown a role for clathrin-associated glycophosotidylinositol (GPI)–anchored proteins within lipid rafts.[28] It is likely that simultaneous binding of the toxin to both multiple residues of the highly prevalent membrane gangliosides along with the protein receptor accounts for high affinity and physiologically meaningful binding of the toxin. Crystallography studies have determined the three-dimensional structure of the Hc domain, and it is similar to that of the botulinum neurotoxin.[29] The carboxyl terminal domain forms a

beta-trefoil cleft where the terminal five amino acids appear essential for ganglioside binding. There are also three surface regions that have carbohydrate pocket-binding features and are also essential for high affinity binding.[30] The amino terminal region of the binding domain has a so called jelly roll configuration, similar to the carbohydrate binding plant lectin proteins, with the two regions linked by an alpha helical segment.

The Hc (TTC) domain has been widely studied as a nontoxic surrogate for the holotoxin in investigations of binding and transport. Because TTC has both neural binding, retrograde transport, and transsynaptic transport properties, it has been useful for several purposes. Its neuronal selective binding has made it useful in the identification of neurons in culture using either direct fluorescence or immunohistochemistry with commercially available reagents.[31] Immunohistochemical studies after intramuscular injection of TTC have allowed for identification of not only the innervating motor neurons but also of their synaptic neuronal partners, although the degree of specificity of this identification has been questioned.[32,33] More recent studies have taken a more contemporary approach to the use of TTC to map synaptic connectivity within the CNS. Transgenic mice have been created that overexpress a TTC-GFP recombinant gene. When this gene is driven by a promoter with selectivity for a particular neuronal subtype, not only are the original expressing neurons labeled but their synaptic partners are also labeled through transsynaptic movement of TTC-GFP.[34]

The amino terminus of the heavy chain (H_N) is linked to the catalytic light chain (LC) and is involved in translocation of the LC across the vesicle membrane. The domain is highly homologous with the botulinum neurotoxins and has structural similarities to the hemagglutinin proteins of influenza virus. H_N has two antiparallel alpha helices that are likely involved in membrane association, but it remains the domain of tetanus toxin, whose three-dimensional structure has not yet been determined.[35] Although well studied for other toxins such as diphtheria toxin, the translocation process remains the most poorly understood aspect of tetanus toxin action. Acidification of the vesicles is essential for translocation with reduction of the interchain disulfide linkage. Also, acidification is believed also to induce a conformational change in H_N and LC, exposing hydrophobic regions of the protein to allow for insertion of LC into the lipid bilayer of the membrane. Early studies of H_N have demonstrated pore-forming properties, but the mechanism of LC translocation and the role of pore formation remain uncertain.[37]

The 50k-D LC of tetanus toxin is referred to as the catalytic domain and possesses zinc-dependent protease function. X-ray crystallography reveals that the active protease site is located within a deep cavity containing a highly conserved zinc-binding motif.[37] All of the clostridial LCs share structural similarity in spite of modest (35%) sequence homology. As expected, the LCs of tetanus toxin and botulinum neurotoxin type B show more homology (50%) because they not only share vesicle-associated membrane protein (VAMP) as the target substrate but also cleave at the same peptide bond (Gln 76–Phe77).[38] The central position of the active site is compatible with mutational analysis in which deletions of part of the carboxyl terminus of the peptide have relatively small effects on toxicity. The surface of the LC molecule likely plays a major role in docking of VAMP, which contains two SNARE motifs known to be essential for binding all clostridial neurotoxins.

Pathogenesis of Intoxication

Overview

Tetanus toxin has a unique mechanism of action (Fig. 34-1). In a manner similar to the botulinum neurotoxins, tetanus toxin is initially bound at the presynaptic terminals of the neuromuscular junction. Unlike botulinum neurotoxin, it is then transported by motor neurons to the spinal cord. In the spinal cord, tetanus toxin is then transferred to inhibitory presynaptic terminals surrounding those motor neurons. The toxin then destroys a vesicular synaptic membrane protein (VAMP, or synaptobrevin), resulting in *in*activation of inhibitory neurotransmission that normally suppresses motor neuron and muscle activity. This action results in enhanced excitability and activation of the affected motor neurons. Widespread intoxication through the systemic circulation results in continuous involuntary muscle contraction of clinical generalized tetanus, whereas local internalization and transport of toxin can result in a localized state of muscle hyperexcitability.

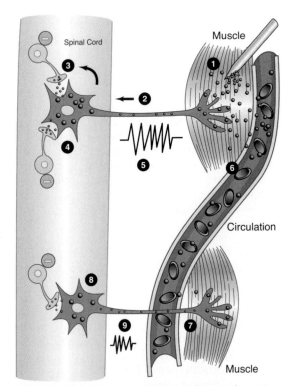

FIGURE 34-1. Tetanus toxin uptake and action. (1) Internalization of toxin at the neuromuscular junction from a nearby wound (or local injection). (2) Retrograde transport to motor neuron cell bodies in the spinal cord. (3) Transsynaptic transfer to presynaptic terminals (inhibitory). (4) Cleavage of vesicle-associated membrane protein with failure of transmitter release. (5) Increased motor neuron excitability, firing rate, and local muscle tetanic contraction. (6) Spread of toxin into the bloodstream. (7) Toxin uptake by all motor neurons. (8) Widespread inactivation of spinal motor inhibition. (9) General increase in motor neuron excitability—generalized tetanus. *See Color Plate*

Binding and Internalization

Tetanus toxin produced by bacteria in the wound is liberated into the bloodstream, where it is able to bind to presynaptic terminals primarily at the neuromuscular junction. The 150-kD toxin is too large to pass through the CNS endothelial tight junctions but has access to the extracellular space including all of the neuromuscular junctions and postganglionic autonomic motor terminals that are not protected by a blood-nerve or blood-brain barrier. The concentration of toxin may be particularly high at neuromuscular junctions near the wound site. The pattern of toxin spread from the site of its elaboration to either nearby muscles or to the systemic circulation, as well as the relative susceptibility of motor neurons and muscles to the action of the toxin, likely accounts for the patterns of localized, generalized, or cephalic tetanus that occur in individual patients. At the neuromuscular junction, tetanus toxin binds to presynaptic nerve terminals because its neuronal receptors are enriched at synapses.[39] As noted earlier, this binding is mediated by the C-terminal domain of the heavy chain. The toxin is then internalized into membrane-bound endosomes of the presynaptic terminal. At this point, the pathogenic processes diverge from that of the botulinum neurotoxins. Although tetanus toxin is capable of blocking transmitter release at the neuromuscular junction, this action occurs at high toxin concentrations and is usually not a significant aspect of the physiologic or clinical action of the toxin.[40] Although a study of hippocampal neurons in culture showed uptake of toxin directly into synaptic vesicles, uptake at the neuromuscular junction is into clathrin-mediated endosomes.[41,42] Tetanus toxin–laden endosomes, unlike those of botulinum neuron toxins, are trafficked to the motor neuron cell body in the spinal cord by the retrograde form of fast axoplasmic transport.[43] This compartment is used by normal regulatory molecules and makes tetanus toxin one of the most efficiently transported known exogenous proteins into the CNS. Up to 2% of the toxin injected systemically into experimental animals can later be detected in the spinal cord, even though the toxin uses only the narrow portals of neuromuscular junction.[44] Tetanus toxin travels in a specific endosomal compartment of retrograde axonal transport that is not acidified, probably accounting for lack of toxin translocation within the motor neuron.[45,46] Retrograde transport of tetanus toxin appears to be similar to that of the neurotrophins and their receptors. Binding of TTC can activate the neurotrophin receptor tyrosine kinase pathway, and TTC is transported in the same axonal organelles as nerve growth factor (NGF) and its P75 NTR receptor.[47] Unlike botulinum neurotoxins, uptake of the tetanus toxin at the neuromuscular junction is not activity dependent, but can be enhanced by the neurotrophin brain derived neurotrophic factor (BDNF).[48] Once toxin-containing vesicles reach the motor neuron cell body, they are trafficked in a highly unusual fashion. The majority of substances, particularly exogenous proteins that undergo retrograde axonal transport, undergo lysosomal degradation in the cell soma.

Tetanus toxin not only evades motor neuronal degradation but also is involved in a process called trans-synaptic transport shared by very few substances including growth factors and neurotropic viruses (herpes virus, rabies virus, glial-derived neurotrophic factor [GDNF] and NGF).[49,50] In this process, toxin-containing vesicles likely fuse with the motor neuron cell body plasma membrane, resulting in exocytosis, emptying their contents into the extracellular space.[51] Toxin release appears to occur preferentially at motor neuron synaptic regions. Tetanus toxin liberated into the synaptic cleft diffuses across and binds to adjacent synaptic membrane of presynaptic terminals. Toxin bound to membrane of these presynaptic terminals within the brain and spinal cord (surrounding the originally transporting motor neurons) undergoes a second round of endocytosis by vesicles that appear to be part of the synaptic vesicle compartment. Once within these second-order presynaptic terminals, the toxin behaves in an analogous manner to that of botulinum neurotoxin at the neuromuscular junction, with translocation of the toxin across the vesicle membrane and liberation of the LC into the cytosol of the presynaptic terminal.

Physiologic Action

It is within the presynaptic terminals of spinal interneurons that the LC cleaves VAMP (predominantly the VAMP2 isoform) in a manner similar to the action of botulinum neurotoxin type B at the neuromuscular junction.[52] Failure of neurotransmitter release and loss of neurotransmission affects predominantly inhibitory synaptic inputs onto motor neurons, although suppression of excitatory synaptic activity onto motor neurons also has been demonstrated.[53,54] Motor neurons, particularly those innervating limb muscles in general, have low resting spontaneous firing rates, reflecting a predominance of inhibitory transmission on limb motor neurons.

The preference for inactivation of inhibitory neurotransmission is not only the hallmark of the action of tetanus toxin but is also the most poorly understood aspect of its mechanism of action. Neither the receptors for tetanus toxin or its substrate VAMP appear to have any preferential concentration within inhibitory synapses. One explanation given for the preference for inhibitory transmission relies on the known cytoarchitecture of the spinal cord. In this model, inhibitory presynaptic terminals are known to be concentrated around motor neuron axon hillock and soma regions, where they can act as an inhibitory brake on excitatory synaptic potentials coming from presynaptic terminals on more distal dendrites. Endosomes containing tetanus toxin are transported from the neuromuscular junction by retrograde axonal transport and would fuse with motor neuron postsynaptic membrane on a first come, first serve basis. This process would result in preferential transfer of tetanus toxin to axonal and somal presynaptic terminals, and preferential inactivation of inhibitory neurotransmission. The model is supported by ultrastructural studies localizing toxin preferentially in presynaptic terminals of the spinal cord that were judged to be inhibitory on anatomic criteria.[55] The strongest evidence against the spinal cytoarchitecture model are experiments showing that the preference of tetanus toxin for blocking inhibitory neurotransmission is evident even in tissue cultures derived from dissociated spinal cord neurons.[56] This work in spinal cord neuronal cultures also illustrates that the toxin's preference for inhibitory transmission is not absolute, because continuous incubation with tetanus toxin results eventually in blockade of all synaptic transmission, similar to incubation with botulinum neurotoxin. The physiologic preference of tetanus toxin for inactivating inhibitory neurotransmission has also been demonstrated after intracerebral injection of toxin into the hippocampus in rodents, resulting in a model of focal epilepsy.[57]

DELIVERY VECTORS FROM TETANUS TOXIN

The determination that H_c of tetanus toxin retained most of the uptake and transport properties of tetanus toxin led to the rapid recognition of its potential use as a delivery vector to the nervous system. Systemically administered holotoxin toxin binds to neuronal surfaces that lie outside the BBB, particularly synaptic membranes, where their receptors are enriched. These limited surfaces include the sites of clinically important binding at the presynaptic terminals of the neuromuscular junction and peripheral autonomic endings. Toxin also binds brain surfaces where the blood-brain barrier (BBB) is incomplete such as the area postrema of the brainstem, periventricular areas, particularly in the

region of the hypothalamus. H_c shows a similar distribution of uptake from the periphery of the holotoxin, although its uptake from systemic routes has not been formally quantitated.[58] Experiments that have quantified uptake of H_c from an intramuscular injection find it to be inferior to the holotoxin, although these early experiments used forms of H_c produced through enzymatic digestion of holotoxin rather than the recombinant form of the protein used in contemporary research.[59] In spite of its possible inferiority to holotoxin in CNS uptake, H_c has been shown to dramatically enhance the CNS uptake of a wide array of passenger proteins. Studies of H_c have shown that it has many useful qualities as a delivery vector for macromolecules to the CNS including (1) highly avid and also high-capacity binding to neurons, (2) neuron specific binding and internalization, (3) transsynaptic passage between neurons of the CNS, and (4) prolonged persistence within the nervous system. In many instances, these properties are fully preserved when coupled to a passenger protein.

The potential of H_c as a carrier molecule was demonstrated quickly after its original characterization. Toxicity of TTX in animals could be re-established by chemically coupling H_c with the other domains of the toxin. Toxicity was correlated with the capacity of this engineered toxin to be transported to the spinal cord.[60]

The first potential therapeutic use of H_c to be considered was an antidote to TTX intoxication. As with clinical botulism, circulating antibody has little impact on the course of clinical tetanus after the disease is established. This is likely caused by the inability of circulating antitetanus antibody to neutralize toxin after internalization by neurons. Conjugates linking H_c to antitetanus antibody directed at the other toxic domains have been created to intercept and neutralize internalized toxin in experimental animals.[61]

The development of conjugates of H_c with horseradish peroxide (HRP) for use as a neuronal tracer, emphasized the potential utility of coupling an enzyme to H_c.[62] The first successful use of an H_c-enzyme conjugate as a potential therapeutic involved hexosaminidase (HEX A).[63] The conjugate enhanced the uptake of HEX A by neuronal cells in culture more than 15-fold than that seen with unmodified enzyme. When exposed to H_c-HEX A conjugates, these HEX A–deficient cells demonstrated a marked reduction in stores of its accumulated substrate (GM$_1$ ganglioside).

This physiologic effect was correlated with internalization of conjugated protein into cellular vesicles. Similar chemical conjugates of H_c with other enzymes also demonstrate clearly enhanced uptake and retrograde axonal transport in vivo from intravenous or intramuscular injection (both HRP and glucose oxidase).[64,65]

The availability of H_c in a recombinant form stimulated the development of H_c enzyme hybrids. H_c has been expressed as a hybrid protein with the major free radical detoxifying enzyme superoxide dismutase (SOD1). The hybrid enhances the delivery of SOD1 to cultured neurons by approximately 1000-fold.[66] The hybrid also undergoes retrograde and transneuronal transport from an intramuscular injection site in vivo.[67] Similar results have been obtained after injection of an H_c–beta-galactosidase hybrid, which demonstrates preserved enzyme activity within the CNS as well as transsynaptic transport.[68]

Tests of physiologic and therapeutic efficacy of such H_c-enzyme hybrids have been somewhat disappointing thus far. An H_c-SOD1 hybrid has a modest beneficial effect that is not seen with free enzyme in a rodent stroke model.[69] The larger hybrid molecule also showed improved pharmacokinetic properties after intravenous injection as compared with rapidly cleared free SOD1. It is unclear whether the beneficial effects seen reflected improved serum SOD1 levels or an H_c specific effect.

Incubation with H_c-SOD1 can substantially raise enzyme levels associated with neuronal cells in culture. These cells, however, were not protected from the cytotoxic effects of starvation, which produces a form of oxidative injury.[70] Absolute SOD1 levels did not predict the lack of beneficial effect of H_c-SOD1 in this model. Neuroprotection was observed when enzyme levels were raised to comparable levels (two to three times control) with transfection or transgenic overexpression of SOD1.

These disappointing physiologic tests of H_c-enzyme hybrids are highly illustrative of both the limitations and potential strengths of this form of vector. H_c-linked enzyme has a very different intracellular distribution from enzymes delivered by overexpression of introduced genes. Gene delivery generally leads to a cytostolic distribution that can be modified if the natural or recombinant gene includes a domain that directs the protein to a specific subcellular target (i.e., mitochondria or secretory vesicles). As discussed earlier, H_c-linked enzymes remain tightly associated with synaptic membranes and vesicles. In the case of SOD1, it is likely that a cystolic location with intimate contact with important structures such as mitochondria is needed for protection from oxidative injury.

Enzymes linked to H_c can escape into the cytosol if the hybrids also contain an appropriate translocation domain. The entire tetanus toxin molecule can even be functionally reconstituted after expression and purification of recombinant light and heavy chains.[71] A three-domain hybrid has also been created that contains H_c as its binding domain, as well as the translocation and catalytic domains from diphtheria toxin. Although it is also a toxic enzyme, the substrate for diphtheria toxin is associated with ribosomes, a more distant cytosolic target than synaptic vesicles. This hybrid protein is extremely neurotoxic in vitro, a property not seen with native diphtheria toxin.[72] Cellular specificity of this toxin is mediated by its neuronal specific H_c-binding domain, whereas its cytotoxicity reflects the ability of its diphtheria domain to inhibit cellular protein synthesis. This hybrid toxin has been proposed as a potential means of selectively killing motor neurons driving abnormal contractions when used in a manner similar to long-lasting, but reversible, inactivation of neuromuscular transmission obtained with botulinum toxin. However its potential of irreversible neurocytotoxicity of nontarget motor neurons with accidental overdosage limits its use in vivo.

Tetanus toxin derived vectors share goals and weaknesses to a number of other vectors that attempt to translocate across the cell membrane in order to reach a cytosolic or nuclear location. There is a large and controversial literature on a group of small cationic peptides referred to as protein translocation domains (PTDs) or cell penetrating peptides (CPPs).[73] These peptides are originally derived from naturally occurring proteins, which like the bacterial toxins, are capable of translocating a passenger peptide or protein across a cell membrane. The most common are derived from the Tat protein of HIV or the homeobox transcription factor antennapoedia from drosophila.[74,75] All of these vectors illustrate the restrictive nature of the cell or endosomal membrane to the translocation process with regard to passenger proteins. In the case H_c, translocation of the survival motor neuron (SMN) protein, (whose absence leads to an inherited motor neuron disease, spinal muscular atrophy) could not be demonstrated even though the fusion protein included a translocation domain from diphtheria toxin.[76] Peptides such as toxin LCs that normally undergo translocation appear to be the most suitable passenger protein for cytosolic delivery.

Recombinant proteins have been created to direct a TTC vector to the appropriate cellular compartment. Although TTC does not normally localize to the endoplasmic reticulum, a fusion protein has been created linking TTC to the lysosomal enzyme beta glucoronidase, which contains sequences directing insertion into a membrane-bound compartment. Expression of this protein in mammalian cells leads to a fusion protein that has appropriate post-translational modification, has neuronal binding properties, and is secreted into the media.[77]

Nanoparticles made from polymers of polyethylglycol (PEG) have been linked to TTC using a avidin-biotin binding strategy. These particles could be selectively targeted to neuroblastoma cells. The goal of this work is to use the particles as a drug delivery system in which diffusion from even an intravesicular cellular location would be useful.[78]

Another class of proteins that has been coupled to TTC in an effort to improve therapeutic properties has been the neurotrophic factors. In some cases, the goal was to enhance neuronal specificity. Cardiotrophin (CT-1) is neurotrophic for motor neurons but also binds to heart and liver. A TTC–CT-1 recombinant protein has shown both preserved motor neuron survival properties and enhanced neuron selective binding.[79] Insulin-like growth factor 1 (IGF1) is another growth factor that shows a trophic effect on motor neurons but little motor neuron selectivity of binding. A recombinant IGF1-TTC shows preserved neurotrophic activity but, unlike IGF1, shows readily detectable retrograde uptake from an intramuscular injection.[80] This protein is one of the rare instances in which a TTC fusion protein showed an enhanced physiologic effect over the native protein. IGF1-TTC injected animals showed evidence of preserved muscle innervation over control animals in aged mice.[81] A fusion protein linking TTC to GDNF also shows preserved activity of both domains. The fusion protein showed enhanced spinal cord uptake from an intramuscular injection compared with native GDNF and comparable (although not superior) protection of motor neurons in the neonatal rat axotomy model.[82]

Although the majority of studies have exploited the capacity of TTC to enter the CNS from the periphery, it also has useful properties when injected directly into the CNS. Although clearly invasive methods, both intraventricular and intracerebral injection have been used in experimental studies in both animal models and humans of protein, gene- and cell-based therapy. These forms of therapies have frequently encountered difficulties during translation from animal models to clinical trials. Issues of penetration, retention, and clearance of protein are clearly more problematic when dealing with a much larger volume human brain. TTC and TTC fusion proteins show substantially superior penetration and retention after intracerebral injection than non-neuronal binding proteins such as SOD1 or albumin.[83] This unusual combination of high tissue penetration along with high tissue retention may relate to the large number of low-affinity receptors within the CNS, with movement of TTC fusion protein resembling transsynaptic transport. Linkage of TTC also improved delivery of SOD1 from an intracerebral ventricular infusion. Although native SOD1 was limited to periventricular regions of brain, the hybrid protein was detected in a perineuronal location throughout both the brain and spinal cord. TTC-SOD1 was retained for at least a day after the infusion was stopped.[84]

It is not surprising that TTC has been considered as a vector to enhance gene therapy in which similar issues of specificity and tissue penetration within brain tissue have been raised. Initial experiments demonstrated that linkage to TTC could enhance to efficiency and neural specificity of transduction of a nonspecific nonviral gene vector such as polylysine.[85] TTC has been linked to antiviral antibody with the goal of masking the normal surface protein of adenoviral vectors and substituting the neural binding properties of TTC.[86] Although this modified vector shows substantially improved selectively for neuronal cells and gene transfer to motor neurons in vivo, the efficiency of neuronal transfection was not enhanced.

Translocation across the cell membrane or the endosomal membrane is likely the major factor limiting the effectiveness of TTC-based gene vectors. To enhance the efficacy of transfection, recombinant multidomain proteins have been expressed that include TTC, a yeast-derived DNA-binding protein (GAL4 transcription factor), along with the translocation domain from diphtheria toxin.[87] Proteins that contained the translocation domain had the highest transfection efficiency for delivery of plasmid DNA expressing the green fluorescent protein as well as a high specificity for neuronal cells. Although much of the DNA was either bound to the cell surface or internalized into endosomes, the efficiency of transfection was increased with incubation of cells in chloroquine whose action is known to enhance membrane translocation.[88]

Through phage library screening methods, a small peptide (12 amino acids) has been identified with many of the neuronal binding features of tetanus toxin but does not have sequence homology to TTC.[89] This peptide has advantages over TTC as a gene vector through its reduced size, high level of expression, and reduced immunogenicity. This peptide (TET1) has been linked to the nonspecific gene transduction agent polyethylenimine (PEI).[90] The modified complexes preferentially transduced both neuroblastoma cells and primary neurons in culture using plasmid DNA. Although this peptide shows retrograde transport in vivo as well, quantification of its efficiency of uptake and direct comparison with TTC have not yet been performed.[91]

TTC's properties of retrograde and transsynaptic transport have also made been explored in gene therapy studies. Intramuscular injection of viral or nonviral vectors containing TTC fusion results in gene expression of TTC hybrid proteins within muscle. This allowed injected muscles to act as a reservoir of TTC linked to GFP or beta-galactosidase. The hybrid proteins not only underwent retrograde transport to motor neurons but were transferred to their synaptic partner neurons as well.[92]

Gene delivery within the CNS is also usually performed by intracerebral injection. A common problem is the limited penetration of large viral vectors into brain tissue, with expression of the target genes and protein frequently limited to regions close to the injection site. Expression of the recombinant gene as a fusion protein with TTC results in transsynaptic spread of the TTC-linked target protein in transgenenic mice. TTC-hybrid proteins can be visualized in neurons connected to cells transfected by adeno-associated viral vectors containing the recombinant gene (JH Wolfe, personal communication) in a manner similar to the transneuronal spread of Tat-linked hybrid proteins after intracerebral viral vector injection.[93] As with TTC-linked protein delivery, these hybrid genes may allow for an enhancement of the distribution of injected gene therapeutic.

TETANUS TOXIN AS A POTENTIAL THERAPEUTIC

Overcoming Immunity to Tetanus Toxin

Although Botulinum neurotoxin has a wide range of clinical indications, the potential clinical use of tetanus toxin has been ignored in the scientific and medical literature. This disregard can be traced to the view that antitetanus antibodies, which are present in the vast majority of individuals in developed countries, would effectively block the biological action of the toxin.[94] Similar concerns regarding the potential clinical use of TTC-linked proteins have been expressed.[95]

Evidence from vaccinated animals and humans challenges the assumption that vaccination precludes local intramuscular use of tetanus toxin. Clinically effective titers in actively vaccinated animals are designed to provide protection from at least 100 times a lethal dose of toxin, but this amounts to only nanogram quantities rather than absolute protection against the toxin.[96] In contrast, uptake of microgram amounts of TTC and its transport from an intramuscular site to the CNS can occur in fully actively immunized animals (Fig. 34-2).[97] This result is consistent with a previous study by Fezza et al[98] in passively immunized rabbits. That study used a model of cephalic tetanus in which the toxin causes flaccid muscular weakness rather than typical spastic tetanus seen in limbs. The rabbits developed a localized muscle effect with high doses of the toxin without signs of systemic toxicity.

These studies demonstrate that following intramuscular injection, a small but physiologically effective amount of the toxin can evade immune inactivation. It is likely that dose-dependent uptake into local presynaptic motor nerve terminals makes the toxin inaccessible to antibodies. The work of Fezza, along with the earlier work of Scott with botulinum neurotoxin/A and Wiley with the plant toxin ricin, further suggests that vaccination may actually enhance the safety of local injection of these toxins.[99,100] Circulating antibodies, by neutralizing toxin that has not been locally internalized, may decrease the amount of active toxin that diffuses from the injected target muscle, producing unwanted effects on neighboring and distant muscles.

We have completed a study evaluating the response to tetanus toxin of animals that have

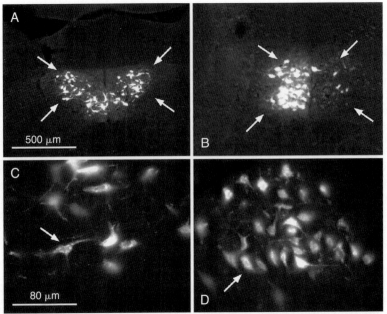

FIGURE 34-2. Photomicrographs from sections through the brainstem of mice injected into the tongue with rhodamine-labeled tetanus toxin fragment C and then allowed to survive for another 24 hours. Numerous fluorescent cells are visible in low-magnification views (**A, B**) of the hypoglossal nucleus (*bounded by arrows*) from both control/naive (**A**) and vaccinated (**B**) mice. The distribution of fluorescent cells was commonly asymmetric (as seen in **B**) in animals from either group. Higher magnification views show that labeled cells in both control (**C**) and vaccinated (**D**) animals were equally fluorescent, with comparable intensities and had morphologies typical of motor neurons (*arrows*). (From Fishman PS, Matthews CC, Parks DA, Box M, Fairweather NF. Immunization does not interfere with uptake and transport by motor neurons of the binding fragment of tetanus toxin. *J Neurosci Res.* 2006;83:1540-1543.)

been either passively immunized with TIG or actively vaccinated against with toxoid in a manner comparable to clinical practice in humans (Fig. 34-3). We wished to determine the extent and duration of localized clinical tetanus in these animals as a preliminary exploration toward the clinical use of the toxin in vaccinated humans. One group of mice was vaccinated with tetanus toxoid (Sanovi Aventis) by IP injection with 1/50th of the recommended human dose and underwent a second (booster) vaccination 30 days later. Passively immunized animals in another group received IP TIG at the time of toxin injection. Initial injection of toxin (List Laboratories) into the gastrocnemius muscle occurred 30 days after the booster vaccination in the active vaccination group or at the time of TIG injection in the passively immunized group. Clinical tetanus was evaluated using a motor behavior scale modified from Webster, in which 5 = generalized tetanus, 4 = sustained spontaneous localized limb tetanus characterized by extension at the knee, ankle, and toes, 3 = intermittent spontaneous limb tetanus, 2 = limb tetanus consistently

evoked on attempted limb movement and usually involving the entire limb, and 1 = limb tetanus that involved only part of limb (usually toe extension/spreading) or that was observed inconsistently with movement.[101] Sera for determination of antitetanus titers were obtained at the time of euthanasia in the actively vaccinated group.

The motor responses of passively immunized mice are shown in Figure 34-3A. All animals developed prolonged localized tetanus with some degree of generalization within the first 1 to 2 weeks. The dose response of animals within each group was highly consistent. Protection from the effects of toxin was substantial, with animals surviving doses of toxin more than 2000-fold, a uniformly lethal dose in naïve animals (data not shown).

Actively vaccinated mice were also dramatically more resistant to the toxin, with only one animal with generalized tetanus requiring euthanasia at a dose of 2.5 μg (see Fig. 34-3B). Unlike the unvaccinated and passively immunized animals, actively vaccinated mice had a more variable dose response to the toxin, although this variability was less apparent at

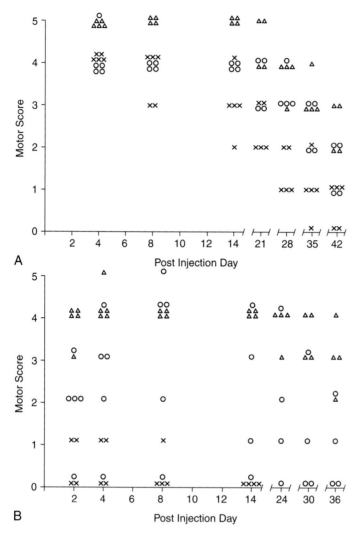

FIGURE 34-3. Scatter plots of motor score and postinjection day of observation for passively (**A**) and actively (**B**) immunized mice. **A,** X-animals injected with 1.25 μg tetanus toxin (TTX) and 20 IU tetanus gamma globulin (TIG). Circles with 2.5 μg TTX and 20 IU TIG: Triangles: with 5.0 μg TTX and 40 IU TIG: (**B**) actively vaccinated mice. X, animals injected with 1.25 μg TTX: Circles with 2.5 μg TTX: Triangles with 5.0 μg TTX.

the highest dose, with all animals showing moderate to severe prolonged localized tetanus. Although there were limited numbers of samples from each dose group, sensitivity to the toxin was not strongly correlated with anti-tetanus antibody titers among actively vaccinated animals (mean titer 1:20,000, range of titers 1:8000–1:46,000).

Because tetanus toxin is one of the most potent biologic toxins known, its effective dose in even vaccinated animals is still within the single microgram range. The duration of response in mice with higher doses was over 1 month, which is consistent with earlier literature in humans in which symptoms and signs of local clinical tetanus lasted from a few weeks to many months, even in patients with historical and serologic evidence of previous vaccination.[102] In agreement with earlier studies,

localized tetanus of a moderate degree is well tolerated in both humans and experimental animals. In humans with localized tetanus of a moderate degree, resting tone may be normal with exaggerated contraction of the involved muscles with attempts at voluntary movement.[103] In our study, mice that developed only localized tetanus showed no signs of distress.

The literature on the effects of tetanus toxin on nerve and muscle suggest that localized tetanus has no significant long-term deleterious effects.[104] Motor neuron and muscle pathology induced by local tetanus is generally mild and of limited duration.[105,106] An electrophysiologic study of 40 patients who recovered from tetanus had evidence of only mild axonal neuropathy.[107] More significant muscle pathology, such as myonecrosis and interstitial fibrosis, has been described after local tetanus but only in the setting of prolonged forced stretching of the tetanically contracted muscle.[108]

It may be a significant challenge to determine an optimal dose in a vaccinated individual. Even in an inbred strain of animals with a standardized vaccination and injection protocol, actively vaccinated mice still had considerable variability in sensitivity to the toxin. In the US population with mandatory antitetanus vaccination, there is a great deal of heterogeneity in antitetanus antibody levels and clinical immunoresistance to the toxin.[109] The number of toxoid vaccinations, age, and duration since the last toxoid booster can contribute to the variability of antitetanus titers and physiologic immunoresistance.[110]

There are potential strategies for determining the appropriate dose of toxin for a particular individual in the setting of a wide variation in immunoresistance to tetanus toxin. The first would be to assess the immune status before toxin injection. The most convenient and widely used assays are enzyme-linked immunosorbent assays (ELISAs) that measure binding to tetanus toxoid, the formaldehyde denatured form of the toxin used for active vaccination.[111] This binding assay is converted to international units (IU) of antitetanus antibody by comparing the patient's sera with standardized commercial antitetanus hyperimmune gamma globulin. The second antitetanus assay is a functional bioassay of protection called the mouse neutralization assay (MNA). In this assay, the patient's sera is mixed with a standard amount of tetanus toxin and injected into mice, which are observed for the development of clinical tetanus. The antitetanus titer is determined by the extent to which the patient's sera can be diluted and still protect the mouse from tetanus toxin–induced death.[112] In general, there is a correlation between antitetanus immunity by ELISA and by MNA.[113] However, there have been several cases reports of patients who developed clinical tetanus in spite of "protective" levels of antitetanus titers by ELISA or other in vitro assays.[114,115] Although they are more convenient, there is reason to believe that the capacity of antitetanus ELISAs to predict physiologic resistance to the toxin may be poor. ELISA measures antibody binding to epitopes of denatured toxin regardless of the importance of these epitopes to function of the toxin in its native confirmation. As with botulinum neurotoxins, a subject's antitetanus titer by MNA may show a stronger correlation with

functional immunoresistance than with antibody levels by ELISA.

There is little previous literature regarding the immunologic effects of repeated injections of an antigen for therapeutic purposes in previously immune individuals. In general, an immune response to a protein therapeutic is associated with a declining physiologic response, with a need for increasing doses to attain the same desired effect. However, in most well-studied settings (bovine insulin, interferons, botulinum neurotoxins A and B), protein therapy is initiated in immunologically naïve individuals.[116-118] Antitetanus titers show an initial dramatic increase with initial and booster vaccinations, but a plateau of maximal antitetanus titers after a limited number of injections, suggesting that immunoresistance to tetanus toxin may stabilize in spite of repeated toxin injection.[119]

Although there is potential for deleterious effects of tetanus toxin injection in vaccinated individuals, there is also enormous clinical experience with administration of tetanus protein in its toxoid form in this population. It is standard practice in the United States to administer a booster vaccination of tetanus toxoid to individuals receiving wound treatment who do not have a documented previous vaccination within the past 3 years. Many of these individuals, however, do in fact have a recent but undocumented tetanus toxoid booster, as well as protective antitetanus titers.[120] This policy reflects the low risk of an adverse vaccination reaction even in a recently boosted individual compared with the risk of clinical tetanus in a patient of unclear vaccination status. Vaccination reactions to a tetanus toxoid booster, although common, are generally mild and localized to the site of injection, with serious local reactions occurring at a rate of less than 1% of patients.[121] Local reactions are associated with high antitetanus antibody levels, although protein load of toxoid and aluminum adjuvants have also been implicated.[122] Systemic allergic reactions are rare (1/60,000), but skin testing is recommended for patients with a history of sensitivity to the toxoid.[123]

The Path to Clinical Development

Observations in humans as well as studies of experimental tetanus in animals support the hypothesis that tetanus toxin could be used to produce a state of hyperexcitability and overactivity in a targeted population of motor neurons in fully and actively vaccinated animals and humans. Although a large number of agents including the botulinum neurotoxins are capable of reducing motor neuron or muscular activity, tetanus toxin is the only substance described that has the potential for selective enhancement of motor function.[124]

In a published patent application, Sanders[125] described the potential uses of tetanus toxin coupled with simultaneous antitoxin injection for a wide range of disorders of inadequate muscle tone, including sleep apnea. To date, the only published report of an attempt at treatment has been of an unvaccinated bulldog (an animal model of sleep apnea) with gradually escalating doses of tetanus toxin injected into pharyngeal muscles. This resulted in improvement of sleep apnea without any observable adverse effects.[126]

One can envision the use of tetanus toxin to enhance inadequate muscle activity in a manner analogous to the clinical use of botulinum neurotoxin to suppress excessive activity. Current state-of-the-art evaluation of patients with motor deficits from conditions such as stroke or cerebral palsy involves both clinical and electrophysiologic analysis of attempts at functionally important movements such as grasping and walking. In this manner, one can discover the pattern of muscle activation during these acts and determine the degree of inappropriate overactivation, as well as inadequate activation of specific muscles. For muscles in which this analysis determines that overactivity of particular muscles as occurs in spasticity interferes with normal posture and movement, those muscles can be injected with botulinum neurotoxin.[127] Injection of botulinum neurotoxin can result in reduction of muscle activity, tone, improvement in limb posture, and to some extent, improvement in use of the limb. Although several strategies, including the use of botulinum neurotoxin, are available to treat spasticity, their capacity to improve motor function and voluntary movement is limited.[128] This limitation is explained by studies in patients after stroke demonstrating that rather than spasticity, inadequate voluntary muscle activation is the major source of weakness and motor disability.[129] The reduced population of surviving cortical motor neurons after stroke and other forms of brain injury generates a reduced voluntary motor signal, resulting in minimal activation of the target spinal motor neurons and inadequate muscle contraction. Although the many muscles with inadequate activation can be identified in patients affected by conditions such as stroke, multiple sclerosis (MS), brain or spinal cord injury, there is no current medical therapy to enhance their activation. These muscles potentially could be injected with an appropriate dose of tetanus toxin. The anticipated effect would be the enhancement of voluntary contraction of the target muscles resulting in an increase in strength. Like botulinum neurotoxin, tetanus toxin has a long duration of action, with the opportunity for repeated treatments and long-term benefit. Tetanus toxin may be the only substance with the potential for selective enhancement of muscle activation in brain- or spinal cord–injured patients. The immunologic consequences of repeated injections of this protein into vaccinated individuals will need to be determined before its use in chronic conditions such as weakness or hypotonia after stroke.

Disuse Muscle Atrophy: An Initial Target for Tetanus Toxin Therapy

Although tetanus toxin has clear therapeutic potential for a wide range of indications, most are persistent conditions that would likely require repeated series of toxin treatments in a manner similar to current botulinum neurotoxin treatment. A condition of limited duration, in which a single course of treatment could have a significant impact is disuse muscle atrophy.

Muscle atrophy after limb immobilization is a major obstacle in the rehabilitation of patients after limb trauma or surgery.[130] In spite of current therapy, a large number of patients have prolonged and significant loss of muscle mass and strength. This is particularly true for fragile and cognitively impaired patients who are unable to comply with early and intensive exercise rehabilitation protocols. A new form of therapy that could prevent or reverse muscle atrophy associated with immobility would significantly compliment current rehabilitation regimens for patients with limb trauma.

We have performed a pilot experiment in unvaccinated rats to assess the capacity of tetanus toxin to prevent disuse atrophy.[131] To induce muscle atrophy, one hindlimb was surgically immobilized (HI) at the knee. At the time of immobilization, the tibialis anterior (TA) muscle was injected with saline (HI/Saline) or tetanus toxin (HI/Tet; 2.5 ng/5 µl).

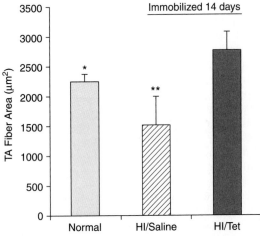

FIGURE 34-4. A, TA myofiber areas from normal and HI (saline- or tetanus toxin–injected) rats. Six to eight TAs per group and 100 fibers/TA were measured. *P < 0.05 versus HI/Tet; **P < 0.01 versus normal.

TAs from normal rats were injected with saline (N/Saline) as a control. After 2 weeks, the muscles were removed, weighed, and processed for histology.

As expected, hindlimb immobilization produced substantial atrophy in the saline injected TAs. HI/Saline TA muscles had a wet weight normalized to body weight of 1.71 ± 0.16 (mean ± SD; N = 6), which was significantly different from wet weight of TAs from normal rats that were injected with saline but not immobilized (2.42 ± 0.30; P < 0.001; N = 6). Most promising, TAs that were immobilized and injected with tetanus toxin (2.20 ± 0.24; P < 0.01; N = 7) were significantly larger than the immobilized, saline injected TAs, the same muscles used to determine fiber cross-sectional areas. Figure 34-4A shows that the fiber cross-sectional areas of the HI/Saline TAs (1522 ± 462 μm^2) were smaller than those from the HI/Tet (2759 ± 306 μm^2; P < 0.05) and N/Saline (2249 ± 125 μm^2; P < 0.01) groups.

With the goal of muscle rehabilitation being the return of function, we were interested in determining whether the HI/Tet rat TAs could produce more force than the HI/Saline TAs. Our preliminary results suggest that they do. Figure 34-4B shows representative tracings of twitch and tetanic (Po) tensions obtained from HI/Saline (N = 3) and HI/Tet (N = 3) rats. The TAs from HI/Tet rats produced 63% greater twitch and 48% greater tetanic tension than those from the HI/Saline rats.

All of the tetanus toxin–injected animals showed clinical signs of localized tetanus of

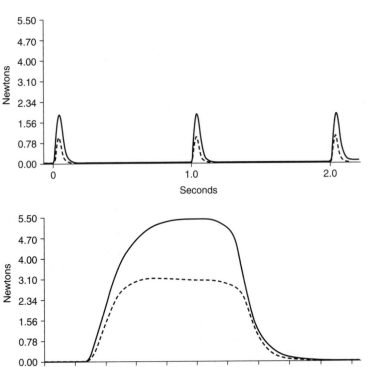

FIGURE 34-4 cont'd. B, Traces of twitch and tetanic tensions after nerve stimulation (in Newtons) from the TA of HI/Saline (*dashed line*, 3.22+/-0.24 mean and SD of three rats) and HI/Tet (*solid black line*, 4.77+/-0.32 mean and SD of three rats) immobilized 14 days.

the injected muscle. All of the injected animals otherwise showed normal behavior, with no signs of distress or of generalized tetanus. These results are encouraging for the further development of tetanus toxin as a treatment to prevent disuse muscle atrophy. This condition with its well-validated animal model, expected effects from only a single course of treatment, and its high clinical importance makes it a logical first target for tetanus toxin therapy

ACKNOWLEDGMENTS

I would like to thank Dr. Christopher Matthews for his assistance in preparation of the manuscript and for contributing his original data. Seth Crawford of Medical Media Service of the Baltimore VAMC created Figure 34-1. This work was supported by the Research Service of the Department of Veterans Affairs.

References

1. Hatheway CL. Toxigenic clostridia. *Clin Microbiol Rev.* 1990;3:66-98.
2. Edlich RF, Hill LG, Mahler CA, Cox MJ, Becker DG, Horowitz JH, Nichter LS, Martin ML, Lineweaver WC. Management and prevention of tetanus. *J Long Term Eff Med. Implants.* 2003;13:139-154.
3. Farrar JJ, Yen LM, Cook T, Fairweather N, Binh N, Parry J, et al. Tetanus. *J Neurol. Neurosurg. Psychiatry.* 2000;69:292-301.
4. Sanya EO, Taiwo SS, Olarinoye JK, Aje A, Daramola OO, Ogunniyi A. A 12-year review of cases of adult tetanus managed at the University College Hospital, Ibadan, Nigeria. *Trop Doct.* 2007;37:170-173.
5. Goonetilleke A, Harris JB. Clostridial neurotoxins [review]. *J Neurol Neurosurg Psychiatry.* 2004;75(suppl 3):iii, 35-39.
6. Berger SA, Cherubin CE, Nelson S, Levine L. Tetanus despite pre-existing antitetanus antibody. *JAMA.* 1978;240:769-770.
7. Jagoda A, Riggio S, Burguieres T. Cephalic tetanus: a case report and review of the literature. *Am J Emerg Med.* 1988;6:128-130.
8. Garcia-Mullin R, Daroff RB. Electrophysiological investigations of cephalic tetanus. *J Neurol Neurosurg Psychiatry.* 1973;36:296-301.
9. Gonzalez-Forero D, Morcuende S, Alvarez FJ, de la Cruz RR, Pastor AM. Transynaptic effects of tetanus neurotoxin in the oculomotor system. *Brain.* 2005;128(Pt 9):2175-2188.
10. Ogunlesi TA, Okeniyi JA, Owa JA, Oyedeji GA. Neonatal tetanus at the close of the 20th century in Nigeria. *Trop Doct.* 2007;37:165-167.
11. Vandelaer J, Birmingham M, Gasse F, Kurian M, Shaw C, Garnier S. Tetanus in developing countries: an update on the Maternal and Neonatal Tetanus Elimination Initiative. *Vaccine.* 2003;21:3442-3445.
12. Anlar B, Yalaz K, Dizmen R. Long-term prognosis after neonatal tetanus. *Dev Med Child Neurol.* 1989;31:76-80.
13. Rushdy AA, White JM, Ramsay ME, Crowcroft NS. Tetanus in England and Wales, 1984-2000. *Epidemiol Infect.* 2003;130:71-77.
14. Quinn HE, McIntyre PB. Tetanus in the elderly—An important preventable disease in Australia. *Vaccine.* 2007;25:1304-1309.
15. McCracken GH Jr, Dowell DL, Marshall FN. Double-blind trial of equine anitoxin and human immune globulin in tetanus neonatorum. *Lancet.* 1971;1:1146-1149.
16. Blake PA, Feldman RA, Buchanan TM, Brooks GF, Bennett JV. Serologic therapy of tetanus in the United States, 1965-1971. *JAMA.* 1976;235:42-44.
17. Weinstein L. Tetanus. *N Engl J Med.* 1973;289:1293-1296.
18. Ernst ME, Klepser ME, Fouts M, Marangos MN. Tetanus: pathophysiology and management. *Ann Pharmacother.* 1997;31:1507-1513.
19. Bleck TP. Management of tetanus. *J R Soc Med.* 1994;87:719-720.
20. Fassoulaki A, Eforakopoulou M. Vecuronium in the management of tetanus. Is it the muscle relaxant of choice? *Acta Anaesthesiol Belg.* 1988;39:75-78.
21. Rossetto O, Seveso M, Caccin P, Schiavo G, Montecucco C. Tetanus and botulinum neurotoxins: turning bad guys into good by research. *Toxicon.* 2001;39:27-41.
22. Turton K, Chaddock JA, Acharya KR. Botulinum and tetanus neurotoxins: structure, function and therapeutic utility. *Trends Biochem Sci.* 2002;27:552-558.
23. Neubauer V, Helting TB. Structure of tetanus toxin: the arrangement of papain digestion products within the heavy chain-light chain framework of extracellular toxin. *Biochim Biophys Acta.* 1981;668:141-148.
24. Lalli G, Bohnert S, Deinhardt K, Verastegui C, Schiavo G. The journey of tetanus and botulinum neurotoxins in neurons. *Trends Microbiol.* 2003;11:431-437.
25. Rogers TB, Snyder SH. High affinity binding of tetanus toxin to mammalian brain membranes. *J Biol Chem.* 1981;256:2402-2407.
26. Sinha K, Box M, Lalli G, Schiavo G, Schneider H, Groves M, et al. Analysis of mutants of tetanus toxin Hc fragment: ganglioside binding, cell binding and retrograde axonal transport properties. *Mol Microbiol.* 2000;37:1041-1051.
27. Schiavo G, Ferrari G, Rossetto O, Montecucco C. Tetanus toxin receptor. Specific cross-linking of tetanus toxin to a protein of NGF-differentiated PC 12 cells. *FEBS Lett.* 1991;290:227-230.
28. Herreros J, Lalli G, Montecucco C, Schiavo G. Tetanus toxin fragment C binds to a protein present in neuronal cell lines and motoneurons. *J Neurochem.* 2000;74:1941-1950.
29. Emsley P, Fotinou C, Black I, Fairweather NF, Charles IG, Watts C, et al. The structures of the H(C) fragment of tetanus toxin with carbohydrate subunit complexes provide insight into ganglioside binding. *J Biol Chem.* 2000;275:8889-8894.
30. Louch HA, Buczko ES, Woody MA, Venable RM, Vann WF. Identification of a binding site for ganglioside on the receptor binding domain of tetanus toxin. *Biochemistry.* 2002;41:13644-13652.
31. Mirsky R, Wendon LM, Black P, Stolkin C, Bray D. Tetanus toxin: a cell surface marker for neurones in culture. *Brain Res.* 1978;148:251-259.
32. Evinger C, Erichsen JT. Transsynaptic retrograde transport of fragment C of tetanus toxin demonstrated by immunohistochemical localization. *Brain Res.* 1986;380:383-388.

33. Perreault MC, Bernier AP, Renaud JS, Roux S, Glover JC. C fragment of tetanus toxin hybrid proteins evaluated for muscle-specific transsynaptic mapping of spinal motor circuitry in the newborn mouse. *Neuroscience.* 2006;141:803-816.

34. Maskos U, Kissa K, St Cloment C, Brulet P. Retrograde trans-synaptic transfer of green fluorescent protein allows the genetic mapping of neuronal circuits in transgenic mice. *Proc Natl Acad Sci U S A.* 2002;99:10120-10125.

35. Lacy DB, Stevens RC. Sequence homology and structural analysis of the clostridial neurotoxins. *J Mol Biol.* 1999;291:1091-1094.

36. Slade AL, Schoeniger JS, Sasaki DY, Yip CM. In situ scanning probe microscopy studies of tetanus toxin-membrane interactions. *Biophys J.* 2006;91:4565-4574.

37. Rao KN, Kumaran D, Binz T, Swaminathan S. Structural analysis of the catalytic domain of tetanus neurotoxin. *Toxicon.* 2005;45:929-939.

38. Breidenbach MA, Brunger AT. 2.3 A crystal structure of tetanus neurotoxin light chain. *Biochemistry.* 2005;44:7450-7457.

39. Lazarovici P, Yavin E. Affinity-purified tetanus neurotoxin interaction with synaptic membranes: properties of a protease-sensitive receptor component. *Biochemistry.* 1986;25:7047-7054.

40. Dreyer F, Becker C, Bigalke H, Funk J, Penner R, Rosenberg F, et al. Action of botulinum A toxin and tetanus toxin on synaptic transmission. *J Physiol. (Paris).* 1984;79:252-258.

41. Matteoli M, Verderio C, Rossetto O, Iezzi N, Coco S, Schiavo G, et al. Synaptic vesicle endocytosis mediates the entry of tetanus neurotoxin into hippocampal neurons. *Proc Natl Acad Sci U S A.* 1996;93:13310-13315.

42. Roux S, Colasante C, Saint Cloment C, Barbier J, Curie T, et al. Internalization of a GFP-tetanus toxin C-terminal fragment fusion protein at mature mouse neuromuscular junctions. *Mol Cell Neurosci.* 2005;30:572-582.

43. Price DL, Griffin J, Young A, Peck K, Stocks A. Tetanus toxin: direct evidence for retrograde intraaxonal transport. *Science.* 1975;188:945-947.

44. Habermann E, Dimpfel W. Distribution of 125 I-tetanus toxin and 125 I-toxoid in rats with generalized tetanus, as influenced by antitoxin. *Naunyn Schmiedebergs Arch Pharmacol.* 1973;276:327-340.

45. Deinhardt K, Berninghausen O, Willison HJ, Hopkins CR, Schiavo G. Tetanus toxin is internalized by a sequential clathrin-dependent mechanism initiated within lipid microdomains and independent of epsin1. *J Cell Biol.* 2006;174:459-471.

46. Bohnert S, Schiavo G. Tetanus toxin is transported in a novel neuronal compartment characterized by a specialized pH regulation. *J Biol Chem.* 2005;280:42336-42344.

47. Gil C, Chaib-Oukadour I, Aguilera J. C-terminal fragment of tetanus toxin heavy chain activates Akt and MEK/ERK signalling pathways in a Trk receptor-dependent manner in cultured cortical neurons. *Biochem J.* 2003;373(Pt 2):613-620.

48. Roux S, Saint Cloment C, Curie T, Girard E, Mena FJ, Barbier J, et al. Brain-derived neurotrophic factor facilitates in vivo internalization of tetanus neurotoxin C-terminal fragment fusion proteins in mature mouse motor nerve terminals. *Eur J Neurosci.* 2006;24:1546-1554.

49. Schwab ME, Suda K, Thoenen H. Selective retrograde transsynaptic transfer of a protein, tetanus toxin, subsequent to its retrograde axonal transport. *J Cell Biol.* 1979;82:798-810.

50. Rind HB, Butowt R, von Bartheld CS. Synaptic targeting of retrogradely transported trophic factors in motoneurons: comparison of glial cell line-derived neurotrophic factor, brain-derived neurotrophic factor, and cardiotrophin-1 with tetanus toxin. *J Neurosci.* 2005;25:539-549.

51. Fishman PS, Savitt JM. Transsynaptic transfer of retrogradely transported tetanus protein-peroxidase conjugates. *Exp Neurol.* 1989;106:197-203.

52. Schiavo G, Benfenati F, Poulain B, Rossetto O, Polverino de Laureto P, et al. Tetanus and botulinum-B neurotoxins block neurotransmitter release by proteolytic cleavage of synaptobrevin. *Nature.* 1992;359:832-835.

53. Benecke R, Takano K, Schmidt J, Henatsch HD. Tetanus toxin induced actions on spinal Renshaw cells and Ia-inhibitory interneurones during development of local tetanus in the cat. *Exp Brain Res.* 1977;27:271-286.

54. Takano K, Kirchner F, Terhaar P, Tiebert B. Effect of tetanus toxin on the monosynaptic reflex. *Naunyn Schmiedeberges Arch. Pharmacol.* 1983;323:217-220.

55. Schwab ME, Thoenen H. Electron microscopic evidence for a transsynaptic migration of tetanus toxin in spinal cord motoneurons: an autoradiographic and morphometric study. *Brain Res.* 1976;105:213-227.

56. Bergey GK, Bigalke H, Nelson PG. Differential effects of tetanus toxin on inhibitory and excitatory synaptic transmission in mammalian spinal cord neurons in culture: a presynaptic locus of action for tetanus toxin. *J Neurophysiol.* 1987;57:121-131.

57. Nilsen KE, Walker MC, Cock HR. Characterization of the tetanus toxin model of refractory focal neocortical epilepsy in the rat. *Epilepsia.* 2005;46:179-187.

58. Fishman PS, Carrigan DR. Motoneuron uptake from the circulation of the binding fragment of tetanus toxin. Arch Neurol 1988;45(5):558-561.

59. Weller U, Taylor CF, Habermann E. Quantitative comparison between tetanus toxin, some fragments and toxoid for binding and axonal transport in the rat. *Toxicon.* 1986;24:1055-1063.

60. Bizzini B, Grob P, Glicksman MA, Akert K. Use of the B-IIb tetanus toxin derived fragment as a specific neuropharmacological transport agent. *Brain Res.* 1980;193:221-227.

61. Kenimer JG, Habig WH, Hardegree MC. Monoclonal antibodies as probes of tetanus toxin structure and function. *Infect Immun.* 1983;42:942-948.

62. Schwab M, Thoenen H. Selective trans-synaptic migration of tetanus toxin after retrograde axonal transport in peripheral sympathetic nerves: a comparison with nerve growth factor. *Brain Res.* 1977;122:459-474.

63. Dobrenis K, Joseph A, Rattazzi MC. Neuronal lysosomal enzyme replacement using fragment C of tetanus toxin. *Proc Natl Acad Sci U S A.* 1992;89:2297-2301.

64. Beaude P, Delacour A, Bizzini B, Domuado D, Remy MH. Retrograde axonal transport of an exogenous enzyme covalently linked to B-IIb fragment of tetanus toxin. *Biochem J.* 1990;271:87-91.

65. Fishman PS, Savitt JM, Farrand DA. Enhanced CNS uptake of systemically administered proteins through conjugation with tetanus C-fragment. *J Neurol Sci.* 1990;98:311-325.

66. Francis JW, Hosler BA, Brown RH Jr, Fishman PS. CuZn superoxide dismutase (SOD-1):tetanus toxin fragment

C hybrid protein for targeted delivery of SOD-1 to neuronal cells. *J Biol Chem*. 1995;270:15434-15442.

67. Figueiredo DM, Hallewell RA, Chen LL, Fairweather NF, Dougan G, Savitt JM, et al. Delivery of recombinant tetanus-superoxide dismutase proteins to central nervous system neurons by retrograde axonal transport. *Exp. Neurol*. 1997;145(2 Pt 1):546-554.

68. Coen L, Osta R, Maury M, Brulet P. Construction of hybrid proteins that migrate retrogradely and transynaptically into the central nervous system. *Proc Nat Acad Sci U S A*. 1997;94:9400-9405.

69. Francis JW, Ren J, Warren L, Brown RH Jr, Finklestein SP. Postischemic infusion of Cu/Zn superoxide dismutase or SOD:Tet451 reduces cerebral infarction following focal ischemia/reperfusion in rats. *Exp Neurol*. 1997;146:435-443.

70. Matthews CC, Figueiredo DM, Wollack JB, Fairweather NF, Dougan G, Hallewell RA, et al. Protective effect of supplemental superoxide dismutase on survival of neuronal cells during starvation. Requirement for cytosolic distribution. *J Mol Neurosci*. 2000;14:155-166.

71. Li Y, Foran P, Lawrence G, Mohammed N, Chan-Kwo-Chion CK, Lisk G, et al. Recombinant forms of tetanus toxin engineered for examining and exploiting neuronal trafficking pathways. *J Biol Chem*. 2001;276:31394-31401.

72. Francis JW, Brown RH Jr, Figueiredo D, Remington MP, Castillo O, Schwarzschild MA, et al. Enhancement of diphtheria toxin potency by replacement of the receptor binding domain with tetanus toxin C-fragment: a potential vector for delivering heterologous proteins to neurons. *J Neurochem*. 2000;74:2528-2536.

73. Kueltzo LA, Middaugh CR. Nonclassical transport proteins and peptides: an alternative to classical macromolecule delivery systems. *Science*. 2003;92:1754-1772.

74. Schwarze SR, Ho A, Vocero-Akbani A, Dowdy SF. In vivo protein transduction: delivery of a biologically active protein into the mouse. *Science*. 1999;285:1569-1572.

75. Derossi D, Joliot AH, Chassaing G, Prochiantz A. The third helix of the Antennapedia homeodomain translocates through biological membranes. *J Biol Chem*. 1994;269:10444-10450.

76. Francis JW, Figueiredo D, vanderSpek JC, Ayala LM, Kim YS, Remington MP, et al. A survival motor neuron: tetanus toxin fragment C fusion protein for the targeted delivery of SMN protein to neurons. *Brain Res*. 2004;995:84-96.

77. Jiang K, Watson DJ, Wolfe JH. A genetic fusion construct between the tetanus toxin C fragment and the lysosomal acid hydrolase beta-glucuronidase expresses a bifunctional protein with enhanced secretion and neuronal uptake. *J Neurochem*. 2005;93:1334-1344.

78. Townsend SA, Evrony GD, Gu FX, Schulz MP, Brown RH Jr, Langer R. Tetanus toxin C fragment-conjugated nanoparticles for targeted drug delivery to neurons. *Biomaterials*. 2007;29:5176-5184.

79. Bordet T, Castelnau-Ptakhine L, Fauchereau F, Friocourt G, Kahn A, Haase G. Neuronal targeting of cardiotrophin-1 by coupling with tetanus toxin C fragment. *Mol Cell Neurosci*. 2001;17:842-854.

80. Payne AM, Zheng Z, Messi ML, Milligan CE, Gonzalez E, Delbono O. Motor neurone targeting of IGF-1 prevents specific force decline in ageing mouse muscle. *J Physiol*. 2006;570(Pt 2):283-294.

81. Payne AM, Messi ML, Zheng Z, Delbono O. Motor neuron targeting of IGF-1 attenuates age-related external Ca2+-dependent skeletal muscle contraction in senescent mice. *Exp Gerontol*. 2007;42:309-319.

82. Larsen KE, Benn SC, Ay I, Chian RJ, Celia SA, Remington MP, Bejarano M, et al. A glial cell line-derived neurotrophic factor (GDNF):tetanus toxin fragment C protein conjugate improves delivery of GDNF to spinal cord motor neurons in mice. *Brain Res*. 2006;1120:1-12.

83. Francis JW, Bastia E, Matthews CC, Parks DA, Schwarzschild MA, Brown RH Jr, et al. Tetanus toxin fragment C as a vector to enhance delivery of proteins to the CNS. *Brain Res*. 2004;1011:7-13.

84. Benn SC, Ay I, Bastia E, Chian RJ, Celia SA, Pepinsky RB, et al. Tetanus toxin fragment C fusion facilitates protein delivery to CNS neurons from cerebrospinal fluid in mice. *J Neurochem*. 2005;95:1118-1131.

85. Knight A, Carvajal J, Schneider H, Coutelle C, Chamberlain S, Fairweather N. Non-viral neuronal gene delivery mediated by the HC fragment of tetanus toxin. *Eur J Biochem*. 1999;259:762-769.

86. Schneider H, Groves M, Muhle C, Reynolds PN, Knight A, Themis M, et al. Retargeting of adenoviral vectors to neurons using the Hc fragment of tetanus toxin. *Gene Ther*. 2000;7:1584-1592.

87. Box M, Parks DA, Knight A, Hale C, Fishman PS, Fairweather NF. A multi-domain protein system based on the HC fragment of tetanus toxin for targeting DNA to neuronal cells. *J Drug Target*. 2003;11:333-343.

88. Barati S, Chegini F, Hurtado P, Rush RA. Hybrid tetanus toxin C fragment-diphtheria toxin translocation domain allows specific gene transfer into PC12 cells. *Exp Neurol*. 2002;177:75-87.

89. Liu JK, Teng Q, Garrity-Moses M, Federici T, Tanase D, Imperiale MJ, et al. A novel peptide defined through phage display for therapeutic protein and vector neuronal targeting. *Neurobiol*. 2005;19:407-418.

90. Park IK, Lasiene J, Chou SH, Horner PJ, Pun SH. Neuron-specific delivery of nucleic acids mediated by Tet1-modified poly(ethylenimine). *J Gene Med*. 2007;9:691-702.

91. Miana-Mena FJ, Munoz MJ, Roux S, Ciriza J, Zaragoza P, et al. A non-viral vector for targeting gene therapy to motoneurons in the CNS. *Neurodegener Dis*. 2004;1:101-108.

92. Kissa K, Mordelet E, Soudais C, Kremer EJ, Demeneix BA, Brulet P, et al. In vivo neuronal tracing with GFP-TTC gene delivery. *Mol Cell Neurosci*. 2002;20:627-637.

93. Cachón-González MB, Wang SZ, Lynch A, Ziegler R, Cheng SH, Cox TM. Effective gene therapy in an authentic model of Tay-Sachs-related diseases. *Proc Natl Acad Sci U S A*. 2006;103:10373-10378.

94. Johnson EA. Clostridial toxins as therapeutic agents: benefits of nature's most toxic proteins. *Ann Rev Microbiol*. 1999;53:551-575.

95. Fishman PS. Neuronal delivery vectors derived from tetanus toxin. In: Brin M, Jankovic J, Hallet M, eds. *Scientific and Therapeutic Aspects of Botulinum Toxin*. Baltimore, MD: Lippincott, Williams and Wilkins; 2002:485-493.

96. Chargelegue D, Drake PM, Obregon P, Prada A, Fairweather N, Ma JK. Highly immunogenic and protective recombinant vaccine candidate expressed in transgenic plants. *Infect Immun*. 2005;73:5915-5922.

97. Fishman PS, Matthews CC, Parks DA, Box M, Fairweather NF. Immunization does not interfere with uptake and transport by motor neurons of the binding fragment of tetanus toxin. *J Neurosci Res*. 2006;83:1540-1543.

98. Fezza JP, Howard J, Wiley R, Wesley RE, Klippenstein K, Dettbarn W. The effects of tetanus toxin on the orbicularis oculi muscle. *Ophthal Plast Reconstr Surg.* 2002;16:101-113.

99. Scott AB. Antitoxin reduces botulinum side effects. *Eye.* 1988;2:29-32.

100. Wiley RG, Oeltmann TN. Anti-ricin antibody protects against systemic toxicity without affecting suicide transport. *J Neurosci Methods.* 1989;27:203-209.

101. Webster RA, Laurence DR. The effect of antitoxin on fixed and free toxin in experimental tetanus. *J Pathol Bacteriol.* 1963;86:413-420.

102. Risk WS, Bosch EP, Kimura J, Cancilla PA, Fischbeck KH, Layzer RB. Chronic tetanus: Clinical report and histochemistry of muscle. *Muscle Nerve.* 1981;4:363-366.

103. Struppler A, Struppler E, Adams RD. Local tetanus in man. Its clinical and neurophysiological characteristics. *Arch Neurol.* 1963;8:162-178.

104. Tarlov IM. Rigidity and primary motoneuron damage in tetanus. *Exp Neurol.* 1974;44:246-254.

105. Chou SM, Mizuno Y. Induction of spheroid cytoplasmic bodies in a rat muscle by local tetanus. *Muscle Nerve.* 1986;9:455-464.

106. Huet de la Tour E, Tardieu C, Tabary JC, Tabary C. Decrease of muscle extensibility and reduction of sarcomere number in soleus muscle following a local injection of tetanus toxin. *J Neurol Sci.* 1979;40:123-131.

107. Luisto M, Seppalainen AM. Electroneuromyographic sequelae of tetanus, a controlled study of 40 patients. *Electromyogr Clin Neurophysiol.* 1989;29:377-381.

108. Mizuno Y, Chou SM. Soleus-specific myopathy induced by passive stretching under local tetanus. *Muscle Nerve.* 1990;13:923-932.

109. Gergen PJ, McQuillan GM, Kiely M, Ezzati-Rice TM, Sutter RW, Virella GA. Population-based serologic survey of immunity to tetanus in the United States. *N Engl J Med.* 1995;332:761-766.

110. Crossley K, Irvine P, Warren JB, Lee BK, Mead K. Tetanus and diphtheria immunity in urban Minnesota adults. *JAMA.* 1979;242:2298-3000.

111. Fairweather NF, Lyness VA, Maskell DJ. Immunization of mice against tetanus with fragments of tetanus toxin synthesized in Escherichia coli. *Infect Immunol.* 1997;55:2541-2545.

112. Christiansen G. Quantification of tetanus antitoxin by toxin neutralization test in mice. A comparison between lethal and paralytic techniques. *J Biol Stand.* 1981;9:453-460.

113. Hagenaars AM, van Delft RW, Nagel J. Comparison of ELISA and toxin neutralization for the determination of tetanus antibodies. *J Immunoassay.* 1984;5:1-11.

114. Passen EL, Andersen BR. Clinical tetanus despite a protective level of toxin-neutralizing antibody. *JAMA.* 1986;255:1171-1173.

115. Crone NE, Reder AT. Severe tetanus in immunized patients with high anti-tetanus titers. *Neurology.* 1992;42:761-764.

116. Chance RE, Root MA, Galloway JA. The immunogenicity of insulin preparations [review]. *Acta Endocrinol. Suppl (Copenh).* 1976;205:185-198.

117. Atassi MZ. Basic immunological aspects of botulinum toxin therapy. *Mov Disord.* 2004;19(suppl 8):S68-S84.

118. Farrell RA, Giovannoni G. Measuring and management of anti-interferon beta antibodies in subjects with multiple sclerosis. *Mult Scler.* 2007;13:567-577.

119. Simonsen O, Bentzon MW, Kjeldsen K, Venborg HA, Heron I. Evaluation of vaccination requirements to secure continuous antitoxin immunity to tetanus. *Vaccine.* 1987;5:115-122.

120. Peebles TC, Levine L, Eldred MC, Edsall G. Tetanus-toxoid emergency boosters: a reappraisal. *N Engl J Med.* 1969;280:575-581.

121. Deacon SP, Langford DT, Shepherd WM, Knight PA. A comparative clinical study of adsorbed tetanus vaccine and adult-type tetanus-diphtheria vaccine. J Hyg. (Lond). 1982;89:513-519.

122. Collier LH, Polakoff S, Mortimer J. Reactions and antibody responses to reinforcing doses of adsorbed and plain tetanus vaccines. *Lancet.* 1979;1:1364-1368.

123. Mansfield LE, Ting S, Rawls DO, Frederick R. Systemic reactions during cutaneous testing for tetanus toxoid hypersensitivity. *Ann Allergy.* 1986;57:135-137.

124. Brooks VB, Curtis DR, Eccles JC. The action of tetanus toxin on the inhibition of motoneurons. *J Physiol.* 1957;135:655-672.

125. Sanders I. 2004 Method for using tetanus toxin for beneficial purposes in animals (mammals). US Patent Application Publication. Pub No. US2004/248188A1, Dec 9, 2004.

126. Sasse A, Conduit R, Ryan D, Woods W, Tucker AP. A pharmacotherapy for obstructive sleep apnea. *Sleep.* 2005;28:1015-1016.

127. Esquenazi A, Mayer NH. Instrumented assessment of muscle overactivity and spasticity with dynamic polyelectromyographic and motion analysis for treatment planning. *Am J Phys Med Rehabil.* 2004;83(suppl):S19-S29.

128. Sheean G. Botulinum toxin treatment of adult spasticity: a benefit-risk assessment. *Drug Saf.* 2006;29:31-48.

129. Fellows SJ, Kaus C, Thilmann AF. Voluntary movement at the elbow in spastic hemiparesis. *Ann Neurol.* 1994;36:397-407.

130. Dillingham TR. Musculoskeletal rehabilitation: current understandings and future directions. *Am J Phys Med Rehabil.* 2007;86:S19-S28.

131. Matthews CC, Fishman PS, Bowen T. Prevention of disuse muscle atrophy after immobilization with tetanus toxin. Society for Neuroscience 37th Annual Meeting, San Diego CA, November, 2007.

Bungarotoxins **35**

Florenta Aura Kullmann, William Chet de Groat, and Debra Elaine Artim

INTRODUCTION

Alpha-bungarotoxin (α-BTX) is a neurotoxin contained in the venom of the Taiwanese many-banded krait. It produces paralysis of striated muscles by blocking cholinergic receptors in the neuromuscular junction. The toxin also blocks a subtype of neuronal cholinergic receptor (α7) located in the central and peripheral nervous systems. Although α-BTX is not used clinically, it is an important experimental tool for studying the properties of cholinergic receptors. This chapter reviews (1) the structure and actions of α-BTX and related toxins, (2) the location and function of cholinergic receptors sensitive to α-BTX and (3) the role of α-BTX–sensitive cholinergic mechanisms in disease, and the potential clinical uses of drugs that target these mechanisms.

HISTORY

Venom from snakes (and other animals) contains many peptide toxins targeting a multitude of ion channels and receptors with high affinity and remarkable specificity. Many of the peptide toxins isolated from snake venom target the peripheral nervous system, especially the neuromuscular junction, where they block neuromuscular transmission, leading to paralysis of skeletal muscles. The focus of this chapter is on α-BTX from the many-banded krait (*Bungarus multicinctus*). Like most snake venoms, krait venom is a combination of many proteins together producing an impressive combination of toxic neurologic effects. Krait venom has numerous effects on neuromuscular transmission, mediated by both presynaptic and postsynaptic actions.

In order to determine the precise mechanism of action of krait venom, it had to be separated into its individual toxic constituents. Based on electrophoretic mobility, the crude venom was separated into four distinct fractions, three toxic fractions named α-, β- and γ-BTX and one nontoxic fraction that was not named.[1] Subsequent studies that explored the mechanisms of action of the toxins revealed that α-BTX binds to the postsynaptic nicotinic acetylcholine receptor (nAChR) at the neuromuscular junction. On the other hand, β- and γ-BTX act presynaptically to reduce acetylcholine (ACh) release.[2] After the initial studies, another BTX fraction, named κ-BTX, was isolated and found to have a postsynaptic mechanism of action. In contrast to α-BTX, κ-BTX has little effect on muscle nAChRs but is a potent antagonist of α3 and α4 containing neuronal nAChRs. Interestingly, even though the original naming of the BTX fractions was based on their electrophoretic mobility, neurotoxins are now named according to their site of action but using the original terminology.[1] Those that have a postsynaptic mechanism of action are categorized 'α' neurotoxins and those with a presynaptic mechanism of action 'β' neurotoxins. α-Neurotoxins are found in the venoms of snakes from the families *Elapidae* (elapids) and *Hydrophiidae* (sea snakes). To date, more than 100 α-neurotoxins have been purified and characterized.[3] The α-neurotoxins are often called curare-mimetic toxins because of the similarity of their effect to the arrow poison tubocurarine. However, unlike curare alkaloids that bind reversibly to the nAChR, the α-neurotoxins bind irreversibly to the nAChR at the neuromuscular junction. Thus, α-BTX has been a very useful tool to study the neuromuscular junction, and to

Dr. Kullman does not report any conflicts of interest. Dr. de Groat is disclosing that he has acted as a consultant for Allergan, Irvine, CA; Ethicon, Somerville, NJ; Procter and Gamble Pharmaceuticals, Mason, OH; Dynogen, Boston, MA; Puretech Ventures, Boston, MA; Hydra, Boston, MA; Medtronic, Minneapolis, MN. Dr. Artim does not report any conflicts of interest.

identify subtypes and localization of nAChRs. The toxin has revolutionized the study of neuromuscular transmission.

CHEMISTRY

Structure of Alpha-Bungarotoxin

Three-Finger Family of α-Neurotoxins

X-ray crystallographic studies and nuclear magnetic resonance (NMR) techniques revealed that all α-neurotoxins share a tertiary structure known as the three-finger fold, consisting of three adjacent β sheet-loops (loop I, II, III) that emerge from a four-disulfide globular hydrophobic core and a C-terminal tail (Fig. 35-1A-D).[3] Consequently, they are referred to as the three-finger family of neurotoxins. Based on the number of amino acids and tertiary structure, α-neurotoxins have been classified as: short-chain, long-chain, atypical long-chain, and non-conventional α-neurotoxins.[3,4] The short-chain α-neurotoxins, like toxin-α (from *Naja nigricollis*) (see Fig. 35-1A), contain 60 to 62 amino acids and target primarily

muscle nAChRs with high affinity ($K_d=10^{-9}$-10^{-11}). The long-chain toxins, which include α-BTX (see Fig. 35-1B), are composed of 66 to 75 amino acids and target muscle ($K_d=10^{-9}$-10^{-11}) and neuronal α7 nAChR subtype ($K_d=10^{-8}$-10^{-9}). The atypical long-chain toxins, like Lc-a and Lc-b (*Laticauda colubrine*) are composed of 69 amino acids and target muscle nAChRs ($K_d \cong 10^{-11}$). The nonconventional α-neurotoxins, like candotoxin (from *Bungarus candidus*) (see Fig. 35-1C), are composed of 65 to 67 amino acids and target muscle with low and high affinity ($K_{d\ muscle} > 10^{-6}$ or 10^{-9}) and neuronal nAChRs with high affinity ($K_{d\ neuronal} \cong 10^{-9}$).[3] Almost all α-neurotoxins have about the same equilibrium dissociation constant for the nAChR, but they differ in their binding kinetics. The short-chain toxins bind to and dissociate from the nAChR five to nine times faster than the long-chain toxins. Thus, the binding of the short-chain toxins can be reversed by washing, while binding of the long-chain toxins is almost irreversible.[3] The relative irreversibility of the long-chain α-neurotoxins binding to the nAChR, especially α-BTX, has made them

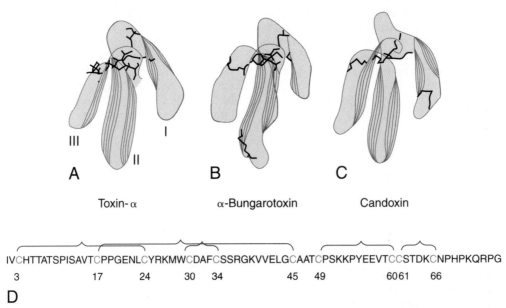

FIGURE 35-1. Three-finger structure of α-neurotoxins. The three-dimensional structures are averaged nuclear magnetic resonance structures shown in similar orientation and in line ribbon representation. Disulfide bridges are shown in black. I, II, III denote loop numbers. Protein Data Bank accession codes are 1NEA, 1IK8, 1JGK, and 2NBT for A, B, C, D, respectively. **A.** Three-dimensional structure of the short-chain toxin-α (from *Naja nigricollis*). **B,** Three-dimensional structure of the long-chain α-bungarotoxin (from *Bungarus multicinctus*). **C,** Three-dimensional structure of the non-conventional long-chain candotoxin (from *Bungarus candidus*). **D,** Amino acid composition of α-BTX. Cysteine residues are in gray, and the links between them are illustrated. Numbers underneath the residues indicate their position. (With permission from Nirthanan S, Gwee MC. Three-finger alpha-neurotoxins and the nicotinic acetylcholine receptor, forty years on. *J Pharmacol Sci.* 2004;94:1-17.)

valuable tools for the purification and characterization of nAChRs.

Domains and Residues Important for Folding, Function, and Binding to the Target

The amino acid structure of α-BTX, an 8000 Da molecular weight long-chain α-neurotoxin, is illustrated in Figure 35-1D. The crystal structure was elucidated initially at 0.25-nm resolution[5] and recently at 1.94 Å.[6] Solution NMR structure further confirmed the three-finger structure (see Fig. 35-1B) and identified flexible and/or mobile parts of the protein that could be involved in binding.[7] Crystallography, NMR, mutagenesis, and chemical modification studies indicated that the amino acid sequence contains several invariant residues that are conserved in most α-neurotoxins and are believed to play a role in folding and binding to nAChRs.[8] Among these, the disulfide bridges, the hydrophobic core, and the COOH-terminal are discussed here.

The disulfide bridges are critical in maintaining the proper folding of the toxin (see Fig. 35-1A to C). In fact, the three-finger structure is determined by disulphide bonds. Short-chain and atypical long-chain α-neurotoxins have four disulfide bonds located at the hydrophobic core of the toxins (see Fig. 35-1A). α-BTX and long-chain toxins have an additional bond located at the tip of loop II (see Fig. 35-1B), whereas the nonconventional α-neurotoxins have an additional bond located at the tip of loop I (see Fig. 35-1C).[3] When these bonds are reduced in cobrotoxin (a long-chain α-neurotoxin similar to α-BTX), both the native structure and the toxicity of the toxin are lost. However, the native structure can be restored after reoxidation.[8]

The hydrophobic core is believed to contribute to protein folding and also to enhance thermal stability of long-chain neurotoxins.[8] The core contains several aromatic residues, for example, Tyr-25, that are conserved in most α-neurotoxins. Nitration (introduction of a NO_2 group at Tyr-25) of this residue in α-BTX results in changes in conformation associated with loss of function.[9]

The COOH-terminal is involved in α-BTX binding to the nAChR. When five residues in the COOH-terminal of α-BTX (residues 71–75) were removed, proton NMR and circular dichroism techniques indicated that the deletion did not induce a significant conformational change of the protein. However, competition binding studies using tritium labelled (^3H) toxin-α and $^3Hα$-BTX showed that the ability of α-BTX to bind to nAChRs was greatly reduced.[10] The toxicity and potency of the toxin to block the neuromuscular transmission were also reduced.[11] Therefore, it was concluded that the COOH terminal plays a role in binding to AChRs rather than in maintaining the proper conformation of the structure.

Specific high-affinity binding of α-BTX to the nAChRs involves not only residues in the COOH-terminal but also several other conserved amino acids including Trp-29, Asp-31, Arg-37, and Lys-53 located near the end of loop II.[8,11] Recent NMR studies comparing the structure of free α-BTX and α-BTX bound either to a 14 amino acid synthetic peptide mimicking the nAChR binding site or to a 18 amino acid peptide derived from the α1 subunit of the Torpedo electric organ, indicated that the interaction with the peptide induced conformational changes mainly at loop II and the COOH terminus of the protein,[7,12] validating the conclusion of earlier studies that these sites play a major role in receptor binding.

Nicotinic Acetylcholine Receptors

General Discussion of Nicotinic Acetylcholine Receptors

AChRs are the primary postsynaptic targets of the toxins found in the venom of snakes. There are two types of AChRs, nicotinic (nAChRs; ionotropic) and muscarinic (mAChRs; metabotropic) receptors, located in the peripheral nervous system (PNS), the central nervous system (CNS) and various target organs. The nAChRs are in general excitatory (i.e., depolarizing the membrane) and are further divided into muscle and neuronal type nAChRs, based on their structure and localization. They are activated by the endogenous ligands ACh and choline, a metabolite of ACh produced by acetylcholinesterase.

The muscle nAChR is the most extensively studied ligand-gated ion channel and was the first to be purified and sequenced.[13] In order to characterize the biochemical and biophysical properties of the receptors, a rich source of receptors had to be found. Early studies around 1920 to 1940, aimed at the discovery of the source of the electric discharge of the *Torpedo* and *Electrophorus* electric fish, suggested that ACh is the neurotransmitter responsible for the discharge. This was demonstrated by the following: (1) the denervated organ was unable to discharge, (2) there was a latency between the stimulation and discharge, and (3) there was an abundance of acetylcholinesterase.[14] After it was realized that the electric organ had a rich cholinergic innervation, it became the source of nAChRs, used for characterizing the biochemical properties of the receptors.[14] The nAChR protein was initially isolated and purified from the membranes of the electric organ of the electric fish *Electrophorus electricus*[15] and *Torpedo marmorata*[14,16] with the aid of radiolabeled $^{125}I\alpha$-BTX. The technique to obtain nAChRs started with solubilization of membranes with appropriate detergents to form micelles containing membrane proteins. nAChRs were then isolated through affinity columns containing $^{125}I\alpha$-BTX or other neurotoxins, which yielded two $^{125}I\alpha$-BTX molecules per each 250-kDa molecule of protein.

Because of the discovery of the high-affinity, almost irreversible binding of the α-BTX, the nAChR became the most intensely studied ligand-gated ion channel and, therefore, a model for understanding the structure and function of related receptors such as glycine, γ-aminobutyric acid type A (GABA$_A$), γ-aminobutyric acid type C (GABA$_C$), and type 3 serotonin receptors, which function as ligand-gated ion channels.

Structure of Nicotinic Acetylcholine Receptors

nAChRs are pentameric structures (mw ~250 kDa) consisting of five subunits arranged to create a cylindrical complex forming an ion channel (Fig. 35-2A to C).[13] To date, five muscle-specific nAChR subunits, named α1, β1, γ, δ, and ϵ, and 12 neuronal specific nAChR subunits named α2 to 10 and β2 to 4, have been identified and cloned. Each subunit is encoded by a different gene. The α8 subunit is found only in avian tissue.[17] The muscle nAChRs are heteromers composed of two α1 subunits, and one of each γ, β1, and δ subunits in the neonatal muscle (see Fig. 35-2A). In the adult muscle, δ subunit is replaced by ϵ subunit.[13] The neuronal nAChRs assemble as homomers composed of α7 to α9 subunits, or heteromers composed of combinations of α2 to α6 and β2 to 4 or α10 and α9 subunits (see Fig. 35-2B, C).[17] It has been shown that α7 can combine with β2 to form a functional channel in heterologous systems, although this combination has not been found in native cells or tissue.[18] It also has been proposed that native α7 heteromers

exist in cultured embryonic chick sympathetic neurons.[19]

Each subunit of nAChR is composed of four membrane-spanning segments (M1–M4; see Fig. 35-2D), a large extracellular N-terminal involved in agonist binding, a large cytoplasmatic loop between M3 and M4 that confers specificity to each subunit, and a short extracellular C-terminus. The second transmembrane region, M2, from each subunit contributes to the formation of the wall lining the channel pore and is involved in gating and ion selectivity properties of the channel. The muscle and neuronal receptors have high homogeneity in the N-terminus and in the pore region.[13]

Alpha-Bungarotoxin and Agonist-Binding Sites

The properties of muscle nAChRs were initially studied by taking advantage of the binding properties of α-BTX and tubocurarine (i.e., tubocurarine binding is reversible, whereas α-BTX binding is almost irreversible). In early studies, the binding site of α-BTX was investigated using muscle preparations treated with tubocurarine followed by α-BTX. On washout, the function of AChRs was recovered, suggesting that tubocurarine and α-BTX competed for the same binding site.[1] Experiments using photoaffinity labeling and site-directed mutagenesis revealed that the binding sites for ACh and α-BTX partially overlap and that they are located at the interface of the α subunit with an adjacent subunit (see Fig. 35-2A-C). There is a principal and a complementary binding site for ACh. In muscle and heteromeric neuronal receptors, the principal binding site is located in the α subunit and the complementary site in the γ, δ, β subunits, respectively, whereas in the homomeric receptors, each α subunit contributes to both principal and complementary binding sites. The α5 and β3 subunits have no binding sites.[20]

Studies using proteolytic fragments of the α1 subunit from the *Torpedo* electric organ or synthetic peptides mimicking the proteolytic fragments have been employed to determine the α-BTX binding site on the α subunit of the nAChR. They have shown that the binding sites of α-BTX are located between the positions 173 and 204 on the α1 or α7 subunit, a region that is situated in the N-terminus and that contains highly conserved aromatic residues (i.e., Tyr190, Tyr198, and Cys192, Cys193; relative to α1 numbering).[6,12,21] Placing residues 184 to 191 of the α-BTX–sensitive α1 and α7 subunits into the corresponding

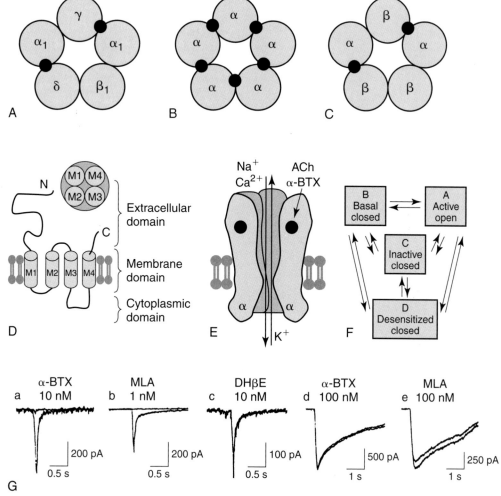

FIGURE 35-2. Structure of the nicotinic acetylcholine receptor. **A** to **C,** Subunit composition of the neonatal muscle (α1,δ,β1, α1,γ) neuronal homomeric (α7, α8, α9, α10) and neuronal heteromeric (α2–6, β2–4) acetylcholine receptors (AChRs). Black dots represent binding sites for acetylcholine (ACh). **D,** Structure of a subunit of a nicotine acetylcholine receptor (nAChR) illustrating the main components: the transmembrane domains M1 to M4, N-terminus, cytoplasmic loop between M3 and M4, and C-terminus. Inset shows the arrangement of the M1-M4 segments within a subunit. **E,** Schematic of the ion channel pore. Ions flowing through the channel are Na^+, Ca^{2+} and K^+. Black dots represent binding sites for ACh and α-BTX. **F,** Schematic of the ion channel states. **G,** Whole cell recordings from rat hippocampal neurons illustrating the difference between α-BTX–sensitive and insensitive currents. a to c, Fast desensitizing ACh-evoked responses sensitive to (a) α-BTX (b) MLA (α7-selective blocker) but not to (c) DHβE (α4β2-selective blocker). d to e, Slow desensitizing ACh-evoked responses insensitive to (d) α-BTX or to (e) MLA. Pairs of traces were obtained in response to 3 mM ACh (in a–d) and 30 μM ACh (in e) before and 10 to 15 minutes after antagonist application. For more details, see reference 27. (**F** adapted from Mazurov A, Hauser T, Miller CH. Selective alpha7 nicotinic acetylcholine receptor ligands. *Curr Med Chem.* 2006;13:1567-1584; **G** printed with permission from Alkondon M, Albuquerque EX. Diversity of nicotinic acetylcholine receptors in rat hippocampal neurons. I. Pharmacological and functional evidence for distinct structural subtypes. *J Pharmacol Exp Ther.* 1993;265:1455-1473.)

positions of the α3, α-BTX–insensitive subunit of nAChRs resulted in nAChRs sensitive to α-BTX.[22] Mutation of the aromatic residues Tyr-187 and Tyr-194 of α7 to phenylalanine decreases the affinities to α-BTX of receptors expressed in *Xenopus* oocyte.[23] In summary, it is believed that the α-BTX–binding sites correspond to the residues 189 to 195 in the *Torpedo* α1 subunit and to 187 to 197 in the human α7 subunit. The binding site for ACh involves several overlapping key residues Tyr190, Tyr198, Cys192, and Cys193, located in the N-terminus.[13] There are two ACh binding sites per receptor for muscle and neuronal heteromeric nAChRs, and both of them have to be occupied for the channel to be functional. Binding of ACh induces conformational changes in the receptors, which allow the opening of the channel. There are five binding sites for neuronal homomeric nAChRs.[13]

α-BTX was found to bind with high affinity to muscle α1 subunit ($K_d=10^{-9}-10^{-11}$) and to neuronal α7 to α10 subunits ($K_d=10^{-8}-10^{-9}$).[3] The binding of α-BTX can be displaced by several competitive agonists of nAChRs. In a study of neuronal α7 receptors expressed in oocytes, it was shown that 1 nM α-BTX was displaced by ACh with an IC_{50} value of 11 μM and by epibatidine with IC_{50} value of 0.25 μM.[24] In addition, 0.2 mM NaCl was used to terminate the binding reaction between α-BTX and nAChRs from crude rat brain preparations, indicating that inorganic cations can compete effectively for the binding sites. Other proteins that bind to neuronal nAChRs include horse heart cytochrome c and hen egg white lysozyme, but they have affinities about six orders of magnitude lower than that of α-BTX.[25]

Ion Channel Structure-Function Relationship

Current models of the nAChR ion channel indicate that the receptor undergoes conformational changes between four states: closed (B), open (A), inactive (C), and desensitized (D) (see Fig. 35-2F). In the absence of the agonist, the receptor is in a basal closed state. On agonist binding, there is a fast transition to an active open state, followed by a fast transition to an inactive closed state. With the agonist still present, the receptor undergoes further conformational changes to a desensitized closed state. On agonist unbinding, the receptor returns to the basal state.[26] The ACh receptor channel can also open spontaneously at a very low rate in the absence of bound agonist. Opening of the channel results in membrane depolarizations and Ca^{2+} influx because the channel is permeable to Na^+, Ca^{2+}, and K^+. The relative permeability of Ca^{2+} to Na^+ is approximately 0.1 to 0.2 for muscle nAChRs, approximately 1 to 1.5 for heteromeric neuronal nAChRs, and 10 to 20 for homomeric α7, α9 or heteromeric α9/α10 nAChRs.[17,18]

The best characterized α-BTX–sensitive receptor in the brain is the α7 homomeric receptor, which comprises a small proportion of the CNS nAChRs, the predominant receptor being the heteromeric combination. There are two particular features that distinguish the α7 homomeric channel from other nAChRs: high permeability to Ca^{2+} and rapid and pronounced desensitization (see Fig. 35-2G).[18,27] The physiologic implications of these properties are discussed in later sections. The high permeability to Ca^{2+} is due to a particular arrangement of charged residues, including glutamate at the inner mouth of the ion channel and to some polar residues in the outer part of the channel.[17] The desensitization is a complex process that reflects conformational transitions of the receptor. The M2 domain is involved in these conformational states because it has been shown that in the α7 subunit from chick brain, mutations of some conserved residues (Leu and Thr) in the M2 domain decreased the rate of desensitization, increased the affinity for ACh, and allowed antagonists to act as agonists, suggesting that this mutant channel can conduct ions in the desensitized state.[28]

Channel activity is also altered by phosphorylation and allosteric modification. The main target for phosphorylation is the cytoplasmic loop between M3 and M4. This region has the most diverse sequence among nAChR subunits and confers the receptor specific kinetic properties and subcellular localization. Src-family kinases play a role in modulation of nAChRs by phosphorylating the receptor. In SH-SY5Y neuroblastoma cells, *Xenopus* oocytes, rat hippocampal interneurons, and neurons from the supraoptic nucleus, phosphorylation of the α7 subunit causes a decrease in ACh-evoked current without altering the surface expression of the receptors, as assessed using ^{125}Iα-BTX.[29] In addition to altering channel activity, phosphorylation can affect receptor expression, assembly, and turnover. For example, in mammalian muscle, α-BTX–isolated nAChRs were found to directly interact with Src kinases via β subunits, and this interaction played a role in clustering of nAChRs at the endplate. α7-containing nAChRs are also candidates for allosteric modulations. Several allosteric modulators including dimethylphenylpiperazinium or ivermectin have been shown to alter the amplitude of the ACh-induced current and response time course.[17]

TOXICOLOGY

Snake envenomation is a major clinical issue, with an estimated 2.5 million cases worldwide annually.[3] It is a particularly devastating problem in Asia and Africa, where the annual mortality rate due to snake bites is estimated at 100,000 and 20,000, respectively. In the United States, there are approximately 8000 venomous snake bites per year, resulting in 5 to 10 deaths. Victims of envenoming bites by krait snakes have a wide spectrum of symptoms. A retrospective study[30] of a large number of subjects (n=210) envenomed by the common krait, *Bungarus caeruleus*, reported that most patients exhibited ptosis, exophthalmoplegia, dysphagia, dyspnea, and neuromuscular weakness. In severely poisoned patients (representing approximately 50% of the study population) who had tidal volumes less than 200 mL, cyanosis and failing speech, mechanical respiration was required. The time between the bite and the initiation of ventilation ranged between 30 minutes and 50 hours (mode 6 hours), and the duration of ventilation ranged between 12 hours and 29 days (mode 2 days). The decision to withdraw ventilation was based on return of neck strength and tidal volume. However normal muscle function usually did not return for 8 to 9 days. Neither anticholinesterase agents nor polyvalent antivenom were effective in reversing symptoms. Approximately 20% of patients exhibited delayed neurologic signs such as nerve conduction deficits.[31]

Because the venom of kraits contains four major types of neurotoxin (α-BTX, β-BTX, γ-BTX and κ-BTX), there has been interest in determining which toxins are responsible for the prolonged neuromuscular paralysis. κ-BTX, like α-BTX, acts on postsynaptic nAChRs but has weak effects on receptors located at the neuromuscular junction and is a minor component of venom.[4] κ-BTX also has a greater affinity for $\alpha3\beta2$ type neuronal nAChRs and, therefore, is not thought to be involved in neuromuscular paralysis. On the other hand, β-BTXs, which constitute greater than 20% of the protein content of krait venom, act presynaptically and are believed to be the most toxic components of the venom.[32] β-BTXs have phospholipase activity that hydrolyzes phosphoglycerides. The toxins belong to the A2 class of phosphatases. The presynaptically active neurotoxins produce neuromuscular blockade by inhibiting the release of acetylcholine from the motor nerve terminals.[33-35] These neurotoxins appear to have a triphasic effect on ACh release. First, there is a decrease, followed by a transient increase, and then a complete block of release. The initial two phases are reported to be independent of phospholipase A2 activity; however, the late phase is directly related to enzymatic activity.

In vivo studies in rats revealed that within 1 hour after injection of β-BTX, nerve terminals exhibited signs of irreversible physical damage and were devoid of synaptic vesicles.[35] Large numbers of terminals were totally destroyed by 24 hours, leaving up to 70% of muscle fibers denervated. Taipoxin, a presynaptic toxin from snakes of the *Elapidae* family irreversibly interferes with the formation of synaptic vesicles by arresting vesicle membrane recycling at the plasma membrane.[36] Neuromuscular block occurs when pre-existing stores of ACh-containing vesicles are depleted by nerve activity. In vitro, the rate of neuromuscular block by β-BTX depends on the frequency of nerve activity and temperature, the onset of block slowing as frequency of nerve stimulation and temperature are lowered.[37] In general, there is a lag period of between 5 and 20 minutes before effects on transmission occur. This lag is thought to represent the time during which the toxins are binding to the presynaptic membrane. After the lag period in vitro, removal of excess toxin by washing has no effect on the rate or degree of neuromuscular blockade. These observations demonstrate why envenomation with β-BTX causes severe and prolonged paralysis that is refractory to antivenom therapy as well as drugs such as anticholinesterases that block the metabolism of ACh. Recovery is dependent on regeneration of motor nerve terminals or formation of new synaptic vesicles, or both.[35,38]

Although β-BTX acting presynaptically is thought to be the major contributor to the toxicity of krait bites, the α-BTX could also be involved in the prolonged neuromuscular paralysis because these toxins are thought to bind irreversibly to the postjunctional cholinergic receptors.[3] However, there are clinical reports that treatment with appropriate antivenom can result in rapid reversal of paralysis. Based on these findings, it has been proposed that in vivo antivenom accelerates the dissociation of toxin-receptor complex, leading to reversal of paralysis.

In an attempt to develop more effective treatments for α-BTX toxicity, knowledge of the chemical structure of the toxin has been used to design short-chain peptides similar to certain amino acid sequences in the nAChRs that can bind to α-BTX with high affinity, preventing the toxin from blocking the receptor and perhaps speeding dissociation of bound toxin. These peptides are thought to offer promise as antivenom agents.[3] A 13-residue–long lead-peptide has been identified from a combinatorial phage-display library that inhibited α-BTX binding with low-micromolar affinity.[39] This led to the creation of a new peptide library and the development of systematic residue replacement, a method for the design and synthesis of high-affinity peptides.[40] Peptides binding α-BTX with high affinity (IC_{50} ~2nM) developed using these methods were better inhibitors of α-BTX binding to muscle nAChRs than peptides derived from natural amino acid sequences of the muscle nAChR itself. In vivo experiments demonstrated that injection of this peptide (peptide No. 50) along with α-BTX prevented all toxic effects, including paralysis and death.[39] Thus, this method of peptide design and synthesis has potential for developing effective antidotes against α-BTX poisoning.

TARGETS AND PHYSIOLOGIC EFFECTS OF ALPHA-BUNGAROTOXIN

Neuromuscular Junction

As described earlier, α-BTX binds to the muscle nAChR with high affinity, effectively blocking neurotransmission at the neuromuscular junction. This leads to muscular weakness and paralysis, resulting in death due to paralysis of the respiratory muscles. α-BTX dissociates from the nAChR very slowly, resulting in a virtually irreversible block of the receptor, although it may be very slowly reversible in vivo.[3] The long-lasting physiologic properties and high-affinity binding of α-BTX make it an ideal tool for studying the localization and function of nAChRs at the neuromuscular junction. It has been used to determine morphologic localization of muscle nAChR, and because it binds stoichiometrically to the nAChR, the number of receptors can be estimated by the number of α-BTX binding sites, allowing for the detection of relatively small changes in receptor numbers in the membrane. Furthermore, among the α-neurotoxins, α-BTX has the least species difference in its affinity for the muscle nAChR, so it can be used effectively in a variety of preparations. Muscle-type nAChRs have been studied using radioactive, fluorescent, or biotinylated derivatives of α-BTX to determine morphologic localization

or qualitative and quantitative identification of the receptors.[3]

Muscle nAChRs on the postjunctional membrane have been labeled with radioactive α-BTX and visualized with autoradiography. These studies allowed for calculation of total binding sites per endplate and the number of receptor sites per squared micrometer of membrane.[41] The precise distribution of nAChRs on the postjunctional membrane was determined using ^{125}Iα-BTX and autoradiography at the electron microscopic level.[42] This method convincingly demonstrated that nAChRs are not evenly distributed on the postjunctional membrane but are localized to the crests of the junctional folds (Fig. 35-3). Clustering of high densities of nAChRs at the junctions is induced by the motor nerves during development and is retained after denervation.[43]

Bambrick and Gordon[44] refer to the discovery and isolation of α-BTX as a revolution in the field of neuromuscular transmission. α-BTX allowed researchers to make quantitative comparisons between the amount of receptors expressed in muscle at various ages or states of innervation and to determine how nerves regulate muscle chemosensitivity. For example, denervated muscles become supersensitive to ACh, responding to concentrations approximately 1000 times less than those needed to activate normally innervated muscle.[45] The distribution of junctional and extrajunctional nAChRs was examined in whole-mount preparations of normal and denervated rat

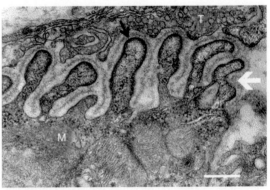

FIGURE 35-3. Electron micrograph of the neuromuscular junction. Figure shows an electron micrograph of a cross section through the neuromuscular junction. T is the axon terminal, M is the muscle fiber. The white arrow shows junctional folds. The black arrow indicates postsynaptic densities, which contain high density clusters of nAChRs. Scale is 0.3 µm. (Source: Synapse Web, Kristen M, Harris PI. http://synapses.clm.utexas.edu/)

hemidiaphragm muscles using $^{125}I\alpha$-BTX autoradiography.[46] These studies revealed that the increased sensitivity to ACh of denervated muscles was due to increased density of extrajunctional nAChRs with no change in the number of receptors in the junctional membrane. Additionally, muscle fiber strips teased from large hindlimb muscles were labeled with $^{125}I\alpha$-BTX and used to measure changes in nAChRs following denervation or postsynaptic blockade of neuromuscular transmission.[47,48] These studies demonstrated that extrajunctional nAChRs are down-regulated by neuromuscular activity and that postsynaptic blockade of neuromuscular transmission, whether by denervation or blocking postsynaptic nAChRs, increases extrajunctional nAChR expression.

Development of the Neuromuscular Junction

In the study of nervous system development, the neuromuscular junction, owing to its large size, accessibility and simplicity, has provided a preparation with which scientists have been able to learn a great deal about critical developmental phenomena. Advances were possible in large part due to the use of α-BTX to label and visualize changes in the numbers and distribution of postjunctional nAChRs during development and in response to changes in neuromuscular transmission.[49] One striking change that occurs in the neuromuscular junction during development is the clustering of nAChRs at the junctional folds of the muscle fiber membrane (see Fig. 35-3).[50] Newly formed myotubes express functional pentameric nAChRs in the membrane with α-BXT binding sites distributed over the entire surface of the myotubes at a density of 200 to 1000 sites/μm^2. In contrast, adult muscle has a very steep gradient in the density of nAChRs with a density of more than 10,000 μm^{-2} directly beneath the motor nerve terminal, declining to less than 10 μm^{2-} in the extrasynaptic membrane. During postnatal development, the density of extrajunctional receptors declines, resulting in a gradient of receptors within a distance of several micrometers from directly under the nerve terminal to the extrajunctional membrane. This gradient becomes very steep in the mature neuromuscular junction.[42] The turnover time of nAChRs also changes during development, whereby adult receptors have increased metabolic stability compared with embryonic receptors. The residence time in the membrane of embryonic receptors is about 1 day, whereas in the adult muscle, synaptic nAChRs reside in the membrane for about 14 days. The degradation rate of nAChRs is reduced shortly after the muscle fiber receives innervation by the motor neuron and is coincident with the receptors becoming resistant to dispersal.

Clustering of nAChRs on the postjunctional membrane is triggered by contact with the motoneuron terminal. Neurites contact myotubes and new nAChR clusters are formed at the sites of contact. Although modulated by synaptic activity, the process of receptor clustering does not require neurotransmission to occur. Instead, it is mediated by agrin, a large heparin sulfate proteoglycan. Isolated by McMahan and colleagues,[51,52] agrin is synthesized by motor neurons, transported down motor axons, released from nerve terminal, and associated with basal lamina of the synaptic cleft. Agrin activates muscle-specific receptor tyrosine kinase (MuSK), which is essential to nAChR clustering in vivo. The activation of the agrin-MuSK pathway results in clustering and anchoring of nAChRs at the postjunctional folds of the muscle fiber membrane.

A series of elegant studies by Lichtman and colleagues has provided an in vivo examination of nAChRs during development after other experimental manipulations. For example, Balice-Gordon and Lichtman[43] used fluorescently tagged α-BTX to label nAChRs at the mouse sternomastoid muscle and analyzed changes in the distribution of nAChRs in the postsynaptic muscle fiber membrane that occur during growth. With this technique, the same neuromuscular junctions could be visualized from 2 weeks to 18 months of age. This study demonstrated that the growth of postsynaptic regions is directly related to the expansion of the muscle fiber. Previously labeled nAChRs spread apart in the muscle membrane as the muscle fibers grew, while simultaneously, new receptors were inserted into the membrane throughout the postsynaptic area.[43]

Plasticity of Nicotinic Acetylcholine Receptors

Denervation of skeletal muscle causes changes in the distribution and properties of nAChRs.[50] Following denervation, receptor synthesis is stimulated and the density of extrajunctional receptors increases to embryonic levels (200–900 μm^{2-}) throughout the muscle surface. However, the receptor distribution at postjunctional membrane initially remains the same. Receptors remain clustered and immobile at the junctional folds for 8 to 16 days after denervation. One property of junctional receptors that does change following denervation is the turnover rate, reverting to the embryonic rate (1/2-life of 17–24 hours).

Acute or chronic blockade of neuromuscular transmission with α-BTX treatment affects the distribution of nAChRs on the postjunctional membrane. In a study by Akaaboune and colleagues,[53] mouse sternomastoid muscle was saturated with a single dose of α-BTX, and the receptors viewed from 2 hours to 7 days later. Even 2 hours after exposure to α-BTX, the half-life of the receptors had been greatly reduced, from approximately 14 days to less than 24 hours, and the lost receptors were not replaced. Thus, the number of receptors in the membrane was significantly reduced 2 hours after α-BTX treatment. Chronic blockade of neuromuscular transmission with α-BTX resulted in a high rate of receptor loss that continued for 7 to 9 hours following α-BTX treatment. Extracellular stimulation of the muscle fibers during saturation with α-BTX prevented the receptor loss, and slowed the rate of receptor loss in previously α-BTX–treated muscle fibers. The receptors lost from the junctional membrane migrated into the perijunctional membrane and were eventually internalized.[53] Taken together, these data suggest that neuromuscular transmission is required to maintain the high-density clusters of nAChRs at the junctional folds.

Myasthenia gravis (MG) is an autoimmune syndrome in which autoantibodies to nAChRs in the muscle, or other postsynaptic proteins involved in skeletal muscle transmission, cause muscular weakness and fatigability due to failure of neuromuscular transmission.[54] The first effective treatment of MG was developed in the 1930s, when Mary Walker recognized the similarities between the symptoms of MG and those of curare poisoning, which had been treated with the cholinesterase inhibitor physostigmine. Administration of physostigmine promptly improved the muscle symptoms in MG patients.[55] Analysis of the neuromuscular junction of patients with MG using α-BTX–binding methods revealed that the motor dysfunction was related to a decreased density of postjunctional nAChRs. Today, MG is treated with acetylcholinesterase inhibitors like neostigmine, as well as steroidal or nonsteroidal immunosuppressants.[13] However, the efficacy of anticholinesterase agents can decrease over time; the phenomenon is called drug tolerance.

Chang and colleagues[56] were the first to investigate the mechanism underlying the development of drug tolerance to anticholinesterase agents in clinical situations. Armed with a radiolabeled α-BTX derivative, Chang and colleagues had the tools needed to evaluate the possibility that drug tolerance was mediated by changes in nAChR numbers on the postjunctional membrane of the neuromuscular junction. The study showed that 7 days of neostigmine treatment caused a 42% decrease in the number of nAChRs in the rat diaphragm muscle. In contrast, treatment with drugs that decrease neuromuscular transmission (such as hemicholinium-3 and β-BTX) increased the number of nAChRs in the muscle.[56] Chang's studies using radiolabeled α-BTX to measure numbers of nAChRs at the neuromuscular junction provide a clear demonstration of the homeostatic mechanism that serves to maintain normal transmission that has been disrupted by chronic drug treatment. Since these studies, there have many examples of chronic drug treatment causing upregulation or downregulation of receptors in a variety of neuronal systems.

Neuronal Alpha-Bungarotoxin–Sensitive Nicotinic Acetylcholine Receptors in the Peripheral Nervous System

In the PNS, α-BTX–sensitive nAChRs, which consist of α7, α8 and α9 subunits, are located in autonomic and dorsal root ganglia, as well as on autonomic postganglionic nerve terminals and motor nerve terminals.[57-60] The α7-containing homomeric receptors are the major α-BTX–sensitive nAChR subtype, and are located presynaptically, postsynaptically, and extrasynaptically. In autonomic ganglia, ACh, which is the main neurotransmitter released by preganglionic nerves, acts on postsynaptic α3-containing nAChRs (κ-BTX–sensitive and α-BTX–resistant receptors) to initiate fast synaptic transmission, and on postsynaptic muscarinic receptors to mediate slow synaptic transmission. Thus, the role of α7 nAChRs in ganglionic transmission is uncertain.

Presynaptically, α7 receptors function as autoreceptors in sympathetic and parasympathetic ganglia, and at the neuromuscular junction, where they are activated by synaptically released ACh and act to increase subsequent evoked and spontaneous ACh release.[58] Presynaptic α7 receptors may also mediate heterosynaptic modulation. For example, α-BTX–sensitive nAChRs have been detected at the postganglionic nerve terminals of adrenergic ganglion cells. Nicotine is known to activate these receptors and stimulate the release of norepinephrine. At some sites in the vascular system, norepinephrine then acts in an autofeedback manner via β2 receptors on the nerve terminals to release nitric oxide, which then elicits vasodilation.[61] α-BTX blocks this effect of nicotine, indicating that α7 nAChRs are likely to be involved.

Postsynaptically, α7 receptors can contribute to evoked and spontaneous nicotinic synaptic currents in autonomic ganglia, for example, in the chick parasympathetic ciliary ganglion.[62] However, in most cases, α7 receptors are not components of the postsynaptic density and are not essential for ganglionic transmission, because transmission is not blocked by α-BTX.[60] In autonomic ganglia, most postsynaptic α7 receptors are localized on the periphery of the synapse (i.e., perisynaptically). Although the precise physiologic function of these receptors has not been determined, they are postulated to contribute to cellular signaling via regulation of calcium-dependent events.[62] Activation of α7 receptors leads directly to increased intracellular calcium levels owing to the high calcium permeability of the receptor and via depolarization-induced opening of voltage-gated calcium channels. Furthermore, because choline, a metabolic product of ACh, is an agonist of α7 receptors, breakdown of ACh released at the synapse may activate perisynaptic α7 receptors by diffusion of choline from the synaptic region. This suggests an additional possible modulatory role for ganglionic α7 receptors.

In the chick parasympathetic ciliary ganglion, which has on average 10^6 nAChRs per cell, early studies revealed that ^{125}Iα-BTX binding sites were located extrasynaptically.[63] Subsequent experiments using biotinylated α-BTX showed that α7 receptors were also localized to perisynaptic somatic spines, which are in close proximity to presumed presynaptic sites of transmitter release.[64] Nevertheless, the α7 receptors do not appear to be essential for synaptic transmission because incubation of the ganglion in α-BTX does not block transmission.[65] However, an α-BTX–sensitive, rapidly desensitizing current

induced by nicotine has been recorded in isolated ciliary ganglion neurons or by stimulating the preganglionic nerve. In addition, activation of α7 receptors on isolated ciliary ganglion neurons raises intracellular calcium levels, suggesting a possible modulatory role of extrasynaptic α7 receptors.[66] Although the α7 receptors are not necessary for transmission through the adult ganglia, early in ganglionic development, they are necessary to ensure reliable and synchronous firing of synaptically evoked action potentials in ciliary neurons at frequencies as low as 1 Hz, likely by contributing directly to the total synaptic current.[56] This suggests a developmental role of α7 receptors in the ciliary ganglion. Although this requirement of α7 for reliable transmission is temporary, ciliary ganglion neurons later in development express greater numbers of α7 receptors that are maintained throughout adulthood. Thus, although both the soma and nerve terminals of autonomic ganglion cells express α7 receptors, the physiologic role of these receptors has not been definitively established.

Non-neuronal Alpha-Bungarotoxin–Sensitive Nicotinic Acetylcholine Receptors

α7 receptors are also found in many types of non-neuronal tissues, including adipocytes, lymphoid tissue, macrophages, keratinocytes, astrocytes, and endothelial cells and epithelial cells of the intestine, lung, and bladder.[20,67] In keratinocytes, α7-containing receptors regulate chemotaxis.[68] Endothelial and bronchial epithelial cells express several neuronal nAChRs subtypes, including α7, and contain the machinery to synthesize and store ACh, suggesting the possibility that ACh may act as an autocrine/paracrine factor in the lung or in the cardiovascular system. A study of α7 receptors in human umbilical vein endothelial cells (HUVECs) investigated the involvement of α7-mediated cholinergic signaling in angiogenesis. The α7 receptor agonist choline increased intracellular calcium concentration, cell proliferation, and tube formation by endothelial cells, as well as the expression of α7 nAChRs.[69] Application of α-BTX produced the opposite effects, suggesting that ACh may be involved in regulation of endothelial cell function as an autocrine factor. Additionally, activation of α7 receptors increased capillary density in ischemic tissues in a rat model of myocardial infarction, suggesting that α7

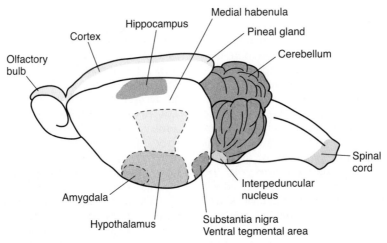

FIGURE 35-4. Distribution of alpha-bungarotoxin–sensitive receptors in the rodent brain.

receptors may be a target for revascularization in treatment of ischemic heart disease.

Neuronal Alpha-Bungarotoxin–Sensitive Nicotinic Acetylcholine Receptors in the Central Nervous System

Localization of Nicotinic Acetylcholine Receptors Using Alpha-Bungarotoxin

Radiolabeled or fluorescently labeled α-BTX has been used for mapping the nAChRs in the CNS. In early studies in rats, the distribution of α-BTX-sensitive receptors was assessed by either injecting radioactive ^{125}Iα-BTX intraventricularly in vivo, followed by a survival period of 1 to 8 days before removal of the tissue and autoradiography or by incubating fresh tissue sections in dilute solutions of radioactive toxin.[70] Comparisons of α-BTX distribution with the distribution of other radioligands for cholinergic receptors (i.e., ^{3}H-nicotine or ^{3}H-epibatidine) resulted in mismatches. Later, it became evident that these mismatches were due to different types of nAChRs, some sensitive to α-BTX and some not. Further studies using mRNA for specific nAChRs subunits indicated that the α-BTX-labeled receptors corresponded mostly to the α7 containing nAChRs, whereas the other nicotine-labeled receptors have different subunit structure (i.e., α4β2 α-BTX–insensitive receptors that comprise the majority of nAChRs in the brain) (see Fig. 35-2A-C).[4,13,17] In addition, studies using brain tissue from α7

knockout mice showed that although there was no ^{125}Iα-BTX binding, the ^{3}H-nicotine binding was unchanged, thus validating that the α-BTX binding sites are equivalent to the α7-containing nAChRs.[71] In several species including human and rodent, α-BTX staining is localized predominantly in (1) areas associated with sensory processing, including cerebral cortex, olfactory bulb, superior colliculus, ventral lateral geniculate nucleus, cochlear nuclei, substantia gelatinosa in spinal cord, spinal trigeminal nucleus, the principal sensory nucleus of the trigeminal, and the dorsal column nuclei; (2) limbic areas including the hippocampus, amygdala, olfactory tubercle, medial mammillary nucleus, cingulate cortex; and (3) other areas including the cerebellum, hypothalamus, thalamus, substantia nigra.[20,70] Thus, α-BTX–sensitive receptors are widely expressed in the CNS (Fig. 35-4).

Function of Alpha-Bungarotoxin–Sensitive Nicotinic Acetylcholine Receptors

α-BTX–sensitive α7 nAChRs, have been implicated in many CNS functions including synapse formation and remodeling, Ca^{2+}-dependent regulation of gene expression, cognitive functions (learning and memory), nicotine and drug addiction, and various neurologic diseases (Alzheimer disease [AD], schizophrenia). The role of α7 receptors varies in different brain areas depending on the cellular localization of the receptors (presynaptic, postsynaptic and perisynaptic) and on the type of neurons where they are expressed (i.e., GABAergic, glutamatergic, dopaminergic, serotonergic, adrenergic, cholinergic neurons).

α7 nAChRs located at the presynaptic terminals or on the axon close to the terminal (perisynaptic) act as autoreceptors or heteroreceptors modulating the release of several neurotransmitters including ACh, dopamine, norepinephrine, glutamate, GABA, and serotonin. Although the release of many neurotransmitters is regulated by α7 as well as other nAChRs (i.e., α4β2), it appears that the release of glutamate is strictly under the control of α7 nAChRs.[18] Activation of presynaptic α7 nAChRs enhances neurotransmitter release, but depending on the neurotransmitter type, it can produce postsynaptic inhibition (i.e., GABA) or excitation (i.e., glutamate). The mechanisms of modulation involve enhancement of Ca^{2+}-dependent exocytosis via increases in the intracellular Ca^{2+} concentration due to high Ca^{2+} permeability of these receptors. Influx of Ca^{2+} can cause release of Ca^{2+} from ryanodine-dependent intracellular stores as shown at the hippocampal glutamatergic terminals[72] or membrane depolarization that activates voltage-gated calcium channels. as shown in the case of glutamate release from the prefrontal cortex synaptosomes.[73] At postsynaptic sites, α7 nAChRs mediate fast excitatory synaptic transmission; this occurs at a small proportion of the CNS synapses, and the physiologic role of these receptors is thought to be less significant than that of the presynaptic receptors.[17]

Developmental Changes in the Expression of Alpha-Bungarotoxin–Sensitive Nicotinic Acetylcholine Receptors

High levels of α-BTX–sensitive receptors are transiently expressed during prenatal and postnatal development, suggesting that α7 receptors may be involved in synapse formation and maturation.[74] In human fetal brain, ^{125}Iα-BTX receptors are present from 5 to 7 weeks of gestation and their expression increases steadily until birth. After birth and throughout life the expression decreases slowly, especially in the hippocampus (CA1 region), entorhinal cortex, thalamus, and striatum. Similarly, in fetal rat brain (hippocampus, dorsal motor nucleus of the vagus nerve) the number of ^{125}Iα-BTX–labeled receptors and mRNA for α7 subunit increase from prenatal day 13 or 14 until birth and then decrease to adult levels in the first few postnatal days. On the other hand, in the somatosensory and auditory cortex of rats,

α-BTX staining (and α7 mRNA) appears at P0, peaks in the second postnatal week (P10–14), and decreases to adult levels in the third postnatal week (by ~P20), a period that overlaps with critical period for onset of sensory function (i.e., rat hearing and vision start at ~P12). Because brain development is dependent on synaptic activity,[75] a mechanism by which presynaptic α7 nAChRs may participate in developmental functions is by converting silent synapses into mature synapses by enhancing glutamate release from the presynaptic terminals.[74]

Postsynaptic α7 receptors may also play an important role during development. Extensive research in the auditory brainstem nuclei indicates that α-BTX staining and mRNA for α7 subunit decline through the first postnatal week, a developmental period characterized by extensive morphologic and functional changes of these neurons. It is believed that Ca^{2+} entry through these receptors contributes to synapse formation, refinement, and maturation.[76] Indeed, in vitro studies in cultured ciliary ganglion neurons[77] or PC12 cells,[78] have demonstrated that nicotinic agonists (nicotine or ACh) induce retraction of neurites, an effect that is blocked by α-BTX, implicating α7 receptors in controlling neurite outgrowth. Other in vitro studies have shown that activation of α7 receptors and particularly Ca^{2+} entry through these receptors can rescue cultured motor neurons destined to die in the absence of neurotrophic factors,[79] thus implicating α7 in neuronal survival. In summary, α7 receptors clearly play a crucial role during development.

Physiologic Functions of Alpha-Bungarotoxin–Sensitive Nicotinic Acetylcholine Receptors

Although the α7 receptors comprise a minority of CNS nAChRs, they seem to play a crucial role in modulating many cognitive functions including attention, learning, and memory. Dysfunctions in the cholinergic system are also thought to underlie some neurologic diseases such as AD and schizophrenia.

α7 in Attention, Learning and Memory

Smoking has been shown to enhance certain cognitive functions in humans, including attention, working memory, and learning.[80] α7 receptors have been shown to play a role in these functions. Systemic administration of α7 agonists such as (3-[2,4-dimethoxybenzylidene] anabaseine (DMXBA) or AR-R17779 improve working memory and reverse the working memory impairment caused by fimbria-fornix lesions in rats. Conversely, impaired working memory occurred after local infusions of the α7 antagonist methyllycaconitine citrate (MLA) into the hippocampus, one of the main brain areas involved in learning and memory.[80] The mechanism of α7-mediated enhancement of memory involves synaptic plasticity in brain areas such as hippocampus and prefrontal cortex. In rodent brain slices containing these areas, it has been shown that acute and chronic nicotine exposure facilitates the induction of long-term potentiation (LTP) due to stimulation of presynaptic nAChRs and enhancement of neurotransmitter release.[81] In addition, Ca^{2+}-dependent downstream activation of signaling pathways (ERK/MAPK kinase activation) contribute to plasticity.[13]

α7 in Nicotine and Other Drug Addiction

The dopaminergic synapses in the nucleus accumbens (NA) arising from neurons in the ventral tegmental area (VTA) are a major component of the brain reward system. An increase in dopamine release at these synapses is believed to play a crucial role in drug addiction.[82] In vitro studies in rodent brain slices have shown that presynaptic α7 receptors increase glutamate release in the VTA, which, in turn, activates N-methyl-D-aspartic acid (NMDA) glutamatergic receptors and leads to LTP. In vivo infusion of the α7 antagonist MLA in the VTA prevented nicotine-induced dopamine release in the VTA-NA pathway in rats.[83,84] Together, these studies suggested that α7 may play a role in nicotine and other drug addiction.

α7 in the Treatment of Cannabis Use

Recently, α7 receptors located in the VTA and striatum have been proposed as new targets for the treatment of cannabis abuse.[85] Behavioral experiments in rats revealed that systemic administration of MLA reduced the ability of rats to discriminate between the active ingredient in cannabis, delta-9-tetrahydrocannabinol (THC), and vehicle, reduced self-intravenous administration of a synthetic cannabinoid CB1 receptor agonist, and reduced the THC-induced elevations of dopamine in the nucleus accumbens.[85] These experiments raise the possibility of using α7 specific inhibitors for the treatment of cannabis addiction.

ROLE OF α7-RECEPTORS IN PATHOLOGY

Schizophrenia

The relationship between nAChRs and schizophrenia has attracted attention because the incidence of tobacco smoking is elevated in schizophrenics and they are heavier smokers who tend to extract more nicotine per cigarette smoked than the general population. One symptom of schizophrenia is the inability to focus attention, resulting in cognitive impairment and overwhelming amounts of sensory stimuli that may perhaps contribute to auditory hallucinations.[86] This is thought to reflect an impairment in auditory sensory gating, specifically indicated by a biologic measurement called P50 suppression, indicative of the ability to suppress the evoked response to the second of two auditory stimuli. P50 suppression, which is impaired in schizophrenics, involves the α7 nAChR-mediated GABA release by hippocampal interneurons resulting in decreased glutamate release, thus preventing hippocampal neurons from responding to the second stimulus in the sensory gating paradigm. DBA/2 mice, an animal model of P50 suppression impairment, have genetically decreased levels of α7 receptors in the hippocampus and impaired auditory gating.[87] Activation of nAChRs with nicotine can improve P50 suppression and normalize sensory gating in DBA/2 mice,[87] and in immediate relatives of people with schizophrenia.[88] Also, clozapine, an atypical neuroleptic that is most effective in treatment of refractory schizophrenia, normalizes P50 suppression. In animal models, clozapine's effect on auditory gating is blocked by α-BTX, implicating an α7 receptor-dependent mechanism.

Because many relatives of people with schizophrenia also have poor P50 suppression, a genetic link was sought. The α7 receptor gene (CHRNA7) is at 15q13-14 locus, and the P50 suppression failure phenotype has been linked to the chromosome 15q14 locus of CHRNA7.[89] Although no polymorphisms have been found in an amino acid coding region of CHRNA7, multiple single-nucleotide polymorphisms in the promoter region have been characterized. These are present more frequently in schizophrenics and their family members, and are associated with decreased promoter region activity and with impaired P50 suppression.

α7-selective agonists have shown promise for the treatment of schizophrenia.[86] One well-characterized compound, DMXBA, which was developed by Kem and colleagues, is a partial agonist at the α7 receptor and normalizes inhibition of auditory response in DAB/2 mice. DMXBA has been evaluated in a Phase I trial in normal human subjects, and was shown to significantly improve performance on tasks of simple reaction time and test of working memory.[90] The drug induces less tachyphylaxis than nicotine, and animal studies suggest that abuse and dependence are less likely than with nicotine. Thus, α7-selective agonists such as DMXBA seem to be good candidates for the treatment of cognitive and perceptual disturbances in people with schizophrenia.

Alzheimer's Disease

Alzheimer's disease (AD), the most common cause of dementia in the elderly, is a neurodegenerative disease characterized by the preferential loss of cholinergic neurons in the brain. α7 receptors have been implicated in the pathology of AD: a reduction in α7 protein levels in the cerebral cortex and hippocampus of patients with AD is seen early in the disease and correlates well with progressive loss of cognitive functions.[91] Amyloid plaques composed of accumulations of beta amyloid protein are a classic pathologic feature of AD and are associated with neuronal degeneration. Recent studies have led to development of the so-called inside-out hypothesis stating that extracellular amyloid plaques are the result of lysis of amyloid-burdened neurons. α7 nAChRs bind Aβ42 (the predominant beta-amyloid peptide species in amyloid plaques) with very high affinity,[92] and this interaction can have an antagonist effect on α7-receptor function.[93,94] The interaction of Aβ42 with α7 receptors is important for entry and accumulation of amyloid proteins in neurons, and is thought to be a key, early step in the pathogenesis of AD. Immunohistochemical analyses show the highest intracellular accumulation of Aβ42 in neurons expressing high levels of α7 receptors and that the receptor always colocalized with the peptide in the perikaryon of AD neurons.[91] Studies of cultured cells found that Aβ42 binding to α7 receptors and internalization and intracellular accumulation of Aβ42 were all

blocked by α-BTX.[95] Furthermore, the level of neuronal expression of α7 receptors is strongly correlated with the rate and extent of Aβ42 accumulations. Preventing the interaction between α7 receptor and Aβ42 has the potential to prevent intracellular accumulations of beta-amyloid protein and may have a positive effect on cognitive function and slow the progression of the neuronal degeneration underlying AD.[91] Thus, the α7 receptor is an important potential therapeutic target for treatment of AD.

Cholinergic Anti-Inflammatory Pathway

An interesting aspect of α7 receptor function in a non-neuronal system is its critical role in the cholinergic anti-inflammatory pathway.[13,96] Stimulation of the vagus nerve results in ACh release that reduces the release of proinflammatory cytokines. In vivo studies have demonstrated that nicotine administration attenuates the response to lipopolysaccharide and reduces the systemic inflammatory indicators associated with endotoxemia.[97] The α7 subunit is essential for inhibiting cytokine synthesis via the cholinergic anti-inflammatory pathway, because electrical stimulation of the vagus nerve inhibits secretion of tumor necrosis factor in wild-type mice but not in α7-deficient mice.[98] α-BTX binds to the surface of human and murine macrophages, indicating the presence of α7 nAChRs, and ACh reduces the release of proinflammatory cytokines in lipopolysaccharide-stimulated cultures of human macrophages. Physiologic or pharmacologic stimulation of α7 nAChRs on macrophages blocks the expression of tumor necrosis factor and the secretion of the high-mobility group box 1 (HMGB1) protein.[13] These results suggest that the α7 receptor may be an important therapeutic target for the prevention and treatment of the effects of inflammation and sepsis.

Pain

Early studies have shown that activation of the cholinergic system is antinoceptive in humans and laboratory animals.[99] Although many analgesic properties of nicotine are mediated by non-α7 receptors, α-BTX–sensitive α7 receptors may also play a role in pain modulation. Expression of these receptors was detected in both peripheral and central pain pathways. Using labeled α-BTX, mRNA for α7, and electrophysiology, α7 receptors were found in dorsal root ganglia and trigeminal ganglia neurons including nociceptive C fiber neurons (TRPV1 positive, capsaicin-sensitive).[57,59] Stimulation of the α7 receptors triggers the release of nitric oxide.[100] Although the physiologic role of C-fiber–induced nitric oxide release is unknown, nitric oxide can block voltage-gated calcium channels in bladder afferent neurons, causing an alteration in the excitability of these neurons.[101] α-BTX labeling was also shown in central brain areas involved in pain, including the substantia gelatinosa of the spinal cord (human[102]), thalamus (low levels of α7 rat[103]) or cortex (rat[104]) in several species.

The involvement of α7 receptors in pain modulation has been demonstrated in animal models of acute thermal, mechanical and inflammatory pain. Choline or CDP-choline (a drug used in the treatment of neurodegenerative disorders such as AD) administered intrathecally (IT), intraventricularly (ICV) or intravenously (IV) in mice subjected to acute thermal pain (hot plate paw withdrawal and tail flick tests), acute inflammatory pain (formalin test, acetic acid writhing test), or acute mechanical pain (paw pressure test), had antinociceptive properties that were blocked by α-BTX and MLA.[105-107]

α7 receptors in the brain are not only expressed in neurons but also in non-neuronal cells such as microglia, the primary immune cells in the brain.[108] Activation of α7 receptors in cultured microglia resulted in an α-BTX–sensitive decrease in the lipopolysaccharide-induced release of proinflammatory factors such as tumor necrosis factor-α.[108] This suggests that α7 receptors may be involved in a central cholinergic anti-inflammatory pathway similar to the one in the PNS.[13,96] Together, these studies indicate that α-BTX–sensitive receptors in the brain are potential targets for pain treatments.

On the other hand, an agent with α-BTX–like properties could potentially be useful in pain treatment, not because of its effect on nAChRs but because of the blockade of purinergic receptors. Adenosine triphosphate (ATP) is known to play a role in pain mechanisms. For example, release of ATP by bladder distension can activate afferent nerves and contribute to painful sensations.[109] In acutely dissociated dorsal root ganglion neurons, α-BTX inhibits purinergic receptors $P2X_3$

and $P2X_{2/3}$[110]; thus, α-BTX may have antinociceptive properties via different mechanisms in sensory neurons.

POTENTIAL CLINICAL APPLICATION OF DRUGS THAT TARGET nAChRs: TREATMENT OF LOWER URINARY TRACT DYSFUNCTION

Nicotinic cholinergic transmission in the CNS and PNS is essential for the neural control of all striated and visceral smooth muscle, as well as the regulation of some endocrine and exocrine glands. Thus, drugs that target nAChRs receptors have the potential for widespread clinical use. To illustrate the potential impact on organ function of pharmacotherapy directed at nAChRs, this section focuses on the treatment of neurogenic disorders of the lower urinary tract.

The ability of the lower urinary tract to store and periodically release urine is dependent upon neural circuitry in the brain and spinal cord that coordinates the activity of two functional units: (1) a reservoir, the urinary bladder, and (2) an outlet, consisting of bladder neck, urethra, and striated muscles of the urethral sphincter.[111] During urine storage, the bladder is quiescent and the urethra is tonically active; whereas during voiding, the pattern of activity is reversed. The bladder and urethral smooth muscle are controlled by autonomic nerves; whereas the urethral striated muscle is controlled by somatic motor nerves.

In rats, intravenous administration of α-BTX selectively blocks nicotinic transmission in the urethral sphincter, lowering urethral outlet resistance, but does not affect nicotinic ganglionic transmission in the autonomic pathways to the bladder and urethra.[112] Thus, bladder contractions and voiding are not affected by the toxin. On the other hand, ganglionic transmission, which is mediated by α3-type nAChRs, can be blocked by drugs (hexamethonium or mecamylamine) that selectively target these receptors. These drugs can block bladder activity without affecting urethral sphincter function.

Neurogenic lower urinary tract dysfunction that occurs after spinal cord injury consists of two deficits: (1) bladder hyperreflexia, resulting in failure to store urine, and (2) spasticity of the urethral sphincter (detrusor-sphincter-dys-synergia, DSD),[111] causing decreased voiding efficiency and urinary retention. DSD, which occurs when the bladder and external urethral sphincter contract simultaneously, can cause bladder infections and backflow of urine into ureters, and can lead to kidney failure. In chronic spinal cord–injured rats with DSD, systemic treatment with α-BTX suppresses urethral sphincter activity and improves voiding by blocking postjunctional nAChRs.[113] Local injection into the urethral sphincter of botulinum toxin, a toxin that acts presynaptically to suppress ACh release, has also been used in spinal cord–injured patients to block DSD and improve voiding.[114] α-BTX has not been used clinically to treat DSD because of its shorter duration of action.

nAChRs are also present in the afferent pathways controlling bladder function. Intravesical application of low concentrations of nicotine (50 nM–1 µM) to the luminal surface of the bladder suppressed the frequency of voiding.[115] This effect was blocked by pretreatment with 10 µM MLA, suggesting that it is mediated by α7 nAChRs. It has been proposed that this effect of nicotine is mediated by an action on urothelial cells that, in turn, release inhibitory substances such as nitric oxide that suppress afferent nerve activity. mRNA for the α7 subunit has been detected in cultured rat urothelial cells as well as in rat urothelial tissue.[114] Nicotine can release nitric oxide from cultured urothelial cells.[116]

Intravesical administration of high nicotine concentrations (1–10 mM) facilitated the micturition reflex, significantly increasing the frequency of voiding.[117] This effect was prevented by treatment with an α3 receptor antagonist (hexamethonium) and by capsaicin pretreatment, suggesting that the excitatory effect of nicotine was mediated by activation of C-fiber afferent nerves underlying the urothelium. α3 as well as β subunits necessary to form heteromeric receptors have been identified in afferent neurons as well as in urothelial tissue. Patch-clamp recordings from L6-S1 capsaicin-sensitive bladder afferent neurons revealed α3-mecamylamine–sensitive, nicotine-induced inward currents.[117] Thus, high concentrations of nicotine may affect sensory pathways in the bladder via a direct action on C-fiber bladder afferent nerves or by an indirect action through the release of neurotransmitters from the urothelium. Urothelial cells can synthesize ACh and mechanical or chemical stimulation of urothelial cells can release ACh.[118] Thus endogenous ACh may function as a neurotransmitter that acts on α7 and α3 receptor subtypes in the region of the urothelium to modulate afferent nerve excitability. Modulation of these receptors with drugs may be useful in controlling bladder dysfunction.

Cholinergic synapses in the CNS also appear to be involved in the neural control of the bladder. Intracerebroventricular administration of low does of epibatidine, an α3 receptor agonist, inhibited reflex bladder activity in the rat, whereas high doses facilitated bladder activity.[119] This effect was blocked by an α3 receptor antagonist, chlorisondamine. On the other hand, intrathecal injection of nicotine resulted in bladder overactivity (increased voiding frequency), whereas intracerebroventricular injection of nicotine inhibited bladder activity (decreased voiding frequency).[117] These effects were blocked by administration of the α3 receptor antagonist mecamylamine. Thus, activation of nAChRs at different levels of the neuraxis can alter lower urinary tract function. This raises the possibility that drugs might be developed to selectively target certain subtypes of nAChRs and be useful in treating urine storage and voiding dysfunctions.

References

1. Chang CC. Looking back on the discovery of a-bungarotoxin. *J Biomed Sci*. 1999;6:368-375.
2. Chang CC, Lee CY. Electrophysiological study of neuromuscular blocking action of cobra neurotoxin. *Br J Pharmacol Chemother*. 1966;28:172-181.
3. Nirthanan S, Gwee MC. Three-finger alpha-neurotoxins and the nicotinic acetylcholine receptor, forty years on. *J Pharmacol Sci*. 2004;94:1-17.
4. Chiappinelli VA. Kappa-neurotoxins and alpha-neurotoxins: effects on neuronal nicotinic acetylcholine receptors. In: Harvey AL, ed. *Snake toxins*. New York: Pergamon Press, 1991:223-258.
5. Love RA, Stroud RM. The crystal structure of alpha-bungarotoxin at 2.5 A resolution: relation to solution structure and binding to acetylcholine receptor. *Protein Eng*. 1986;1:37-46.
6. Dellisanti CD, Yao Y, Stroud JC, Wang ZZ, Chen L. Crystal structure of the extracellular domain of nAChR alpha1 bound to alpha-bungarotoxin at 1.94 A resolution. *Nat Neurosci*. 2007;10:953-962.
7. Scarselli M, Spiga O, Ciutti A, Bernini A, Bracci L, Lelli B, et al. NMR structure of alpha-bungarotoxin free and bound to a mimotope of the nicotinic acetylcholine receptor. *Biochemistry*. 2002;41:1457-1463.
8. Endo T, Tamiya N. Structure-function relationships of postsynaptic neurotoxins from snake venoms. In: Harvey AL, ed. *Snake Toxins*. New York: Pergamon Press, 1991:165-222.
9. Chen YH, Tai JC, Huang WJ, Lai MZ, Hung MC, Lai MD, et al. Role of aromatic residues in the structure-function relationship of alpha-bungarotoxin. *Biochemistry*. 1982;21:2592-2600.
10. Endo T, Oya M, Tamiya N, Hayashi K. Role of C-terminal tail of long neurotoxins from snake

venoms in molecular conformation and acetylcholine receptor binding: proton nuclear magnetic resonance and competition binding studies. *Biochemistry.* 1987;26:4592-4598.

11. Wu SH, Chen CJ, Tseng MJ, Wang KT. The modification of alpha-bungarotoxin by digestion with trypsin. *Arch Biochem Biophys.* 1983;227:111-117.

12. Zeng H, Moise L, Grant MA, Hawrot E. The solution structure of the complex formed between alpha-bungarotoxin and an 18-mer cognate peptide derived from the alpha 1 subunit of the nicotinic acetylcholine receptor from *Torpedo californica. J Biol Chem.* 2001;276:22930-22940.

13. Kalamida D, Poulas K, Avramopoulou V, Fostieri E, Lagoumintzis G, Lazaridis K, et al. Muscle and neuronal nicotinic acetylcholine receptors. Structure, function and pathogenicity. *FEBS J.* 2007;274:3799-3845.

14. Keesey J. How electric fish became sources of acetylcholine receptor. *J Hist Neurosci.* 2005;14:149-164.

15. Changeux JP, Kasai M, Lee CY. Use of a snake venom toxin to characterize the cholinergic receptor protein. *Proc Natl Acad Sci U S A.* 1970;67:1241-1247.

16. Miledi R, Molinoff P, Potter LT. Isolation of the cholinergic receptor protein of Torpedo electric tissue. *Nature.* 1971;229:554-557.

17. Dani JA, Bertrand D. Nicotinic acetylcholine receptors and nicotinic cholinergic mechanisms of the central nervous system. *Annu Rev Pharmacol Toxicol.* 2007;47:699-729.

18. Jensen AA, Frolund B, Liljefors T, Krogsgaard-Larsen P. Neuronal nicotinic acetylcholine receptors: structural revelations, target identifications, and therapeutic inspirations. *J Med Chem.* 2005;48:4705-4745.

19. Yu CR, Role LW. Functional contribution of the alpha5 subunit to neuronal nicotinic channels expressed by chick sympathetic ganglion neurones. *J Physiol.* 1998;509:667-681.

20. Gotti C, Clementi F. Neuronal nicotinic receptors: from structure to pathology. *Prog Neurobiol.* 2004;74:363-396.

21. Wilson PT, Lentz TL, Hawrot E. Determination of the primary amino acid sequence specifying the alpha-bungarotoxin binding site on the alpha subunit of the acetylcholine receptor from Torpedo californica. *Proc Natl Acad Sci U S A.* 1985;82:8790-8794.

22. Levandoski MM, Lin Y, Moise L, McLaughlin JT, Cooper E, Hawrot E. Chimeric analysis of a neuronal nicotinic acetylcholine receptor reveals amino acids conferring sensitivity to alpha-bungarotoxin. *J Biol Chem.* 1999;274:26113-26119.

23. Galzi JL, Bertrand D, Devillers-Thiery A, Revah F, Bertrand S, Changeux JP. Functional significance of aromatic amino acids from three peptide loops of the alpha 7 neuronal nicotinic receptor site investigated by site-directed mutagenesis. *FEBS J.* 1991;294:198-202.

24. Criado M, Mulet J, Bernal JA, Gerber S, Sala S, Sala F. Mutations of a conserved lysine residue in the N-terminal domain of alpha7 nicotinic receptors affect gating and binding of nicotinic agonists. *Mol Pharmacol.* 2005;68:1669-1677.

25. Schmidt J. Drug binding properties of an alpha-bungarotoxin-binding component from rat brain. *Mol Pharmacol.* 1977;13:283-290.

26. Mazurov A, Hauser T, Miller CH. Selective alpha7 nicotinic acetylcholine receptor ligands. *Curr Med Chem.* 2006;13:1567-1584.

27. Alkondon M, Albuquerque EX. Diversity of nicotinic acetylcholine receptors in rat hippocampal neurons. I. Pharmacological and functional evidence for distinct structural subtypes. *J Pharmacol Expl Ther.* 1993;265:1455-1473.

28. Revah F, Bertrand D, Galzi JL, Devillers-Thiery A, Mulle C, Hussy N, et al. Mutations in the channel domain alter desensitization of a neuronal nicotinic receptor. *Nature.* 1991;353:846-849.

29. Charpantier E, Wiesner A, Huh KH, Ogier R, Hoda JC, Allaman G, et al. Alpha7 neuronal nicotinic acetylcholine receptors are negatively regulated by tyrosine phosphorylation and Src-family kinases. *J Neurosci.* 2005;25:9836-49.

30. Kularatne SA. Common krait (*Bungarus caeruleus*) bite in Anuradhapura, Sri Lanka: a prospective clinical study, 1996-98. *Postgrad Med J.* 2002;78:276-280.

31. Singh G, Pannu HS, Chawla PS, Malhotra S. Neuromuscular transmission failure due to common krait (*Bungarus caeruleus*) envenomation. *Muscle Nerve.* 1999;22:1637-1643.

32. Chen IL, Lee CY. Ultrastructural changes in the motor nerve terminals caused by beta-bungarotoxin. *Virchows Arch.* 1970;6:318-325.

33. Dixon RW, Harris JB. Myotoxic activity of the toxic phospholipase, notexin, from the venom of the Australian tiger snake. *J Neuropathol Exp Neurol.* 1996;55:1230-1237.

34. Prasarnpun S, Walsh J, Harris JB. Beta-bungarotoxin-induced depletion of synaptic vesicles at the mammalian neuromuscular junction. *Neuropharmacology.* 2004;47:304-314.

35. Prasarnpun S, Walsh J, Awad SS, Harris JB. Envenoming bites by kraits: the biological basis of treatment-resistant neuromuscular paralysis. *Brain.* 2005;128:2987-2996.

36. Connolly S, Trevett AJ, Nwokolo NC, Lalloo DG, Naraqi S, Mantle D, et al. Neuromuscular effects of Papuan Taipan snake venom. *Ann Neurol.* 1995;38:916-920.

37. Hodgson WC, Wickramaratna JC. *In vitro* neuromuscular activity of snake venoms. *Clin Exp Pharmacol Physiol.* 2002;29:807-814.

38. Shapira M, Zhai RG, Dresbach T, Bresler T, Torres VI, Gundelfinger ED, et al. Unitary assembly of presynaptic active zones from Piccolo-Bassoon transport vesicles. *Neuron.* 2003;38:237-252.

39. Kasher R, Balass M, Scherf T, Fridkin M, Fuchs S, Katchalski-Katzir E. Design and synthesis of peptides that bind alpha-bungarotoxin with high affinity. *Chem Biol.* 2001;8:147-155.

40. Katchalski-Katzir E, Kasher R, Balass M, Scherf T, Harel M, Fridkin M, et al. Design and synthesis of peptides that bind alpha-bungarotoxin with high affinity and mimic the three-dimensional structure of the binding-site of acetylcholine receptor. *Biophys Chem.* 2003;100:293-305.

41. Salpeter MM, Eldefrawi ME. Sizes of endplate compartments, densities or acetylcholine receptor and other quantitative aspects of neuromuscular transmission. *J Histochem Cytochem.* 1973;21:769-778.

42. Fertuck HC, Salpeter MM. Localization of acetylcholine receptor by 125I-labeled a-bungarotoxin binding at mouse motor endplates. *Proc Natl Acad Sci U S A.* 1974;71:1376-1378.

43. Balice-Gordon RJ, Lichtman JW. *In vivo* visualization of the growth of pre- and postsynaptic elements of neuromuscular junctions in the mouse. *J Neurosci.* 1990;10:894-908.

44. Bambrick L, Gordon T. Neurotoxins in the study of neural regulation of membrane proteins in skeletal muscle. *J Pharmacol Toxicol Methods.* 1994;32:129-138.

45. Miledi R. The acetylcholine sensitivity of frog muscle fibres after complete or partial devervation. *J Physiol.* 1960;151:1-23.

46. Fambrough DM. Control of acetylcholine receptors in skeletal muscle. *Physiol Rev.* 1979;59:165-227.

47. Pestronk A, Drachman D, Griffin JW. Effect of botulinum toxin on trophic regulation of acetylcholine receptors. *Nature.* 1976;264:787-9.

48. Pestronk A, Drachman DB, Stanley EF, Price DL, Griffin JW. Cholinergic transmission regulates extrajunctional acetylcholine receptors. *Exp Neurol.* 1980;70:690-696.

49. Sanes JR, Lichtman JW. Induction, assembly, maturation and maintenance of a postsynaptic apparatus. *Nat Rev Neurosci.* 2001;2:791-805.

50. Salpeter MM, Loring RH. Nicotinic acetylcholine receptors in vertebrate muscle: properties, distribution and neural control. *Prog Neurobiol.* 1985;25:297-325.

51. Bowe MA, Fallon JR. The role of agrin in synapse formation. *Annu Rev Neurosci.* 1995;18:443-462.

52. McMahan UJ. The agrin hypothesis. *Cold Spring Harb Symp Quant Biol.* 1990;50:407-418.

53. Akaaboune M, Culican SM, Turney SG, Lichtman JW. Rapid and reversible effects of activity on acetylcholine receptor density at the neuromuscular junction *in vivo*. *Science.* 1999;286:503-507.

54. Conti-Fine BM, Milani M, Kaminski HJ. Myasthenia gravis: past, present, and future. *J Clin Invest.* 2006;116:2843-2854.

55. Walker MB. Case showing the effect of prostigmin on myasthenia gravis. *Proc R Soc Med.* 1935;28:759-761.

56. Chang KT, Berg DK. Nicotinic acetylcholine receptors containing a7 subunits are required for reliable synaptic transmission *in situ*. *J Neurosci.* 1999;19:3701-3710.

57. Genzen JR, Van Cleve W, McGehee DS. Dorsal root ganglion neurons express multiple nicotinic acetylcholine receptor subtypes. *J Neurophysiol.* 2001;86:1773-1782.

58. MacDermott AB, Role LW, Siegelbaum SA. Presynaptic ionotropic receptors and the control of transmitter release. *Annu Rev Neurosci.* 1999;22:443-485.

59. Rau KK, Johnson RD, Cooper BY. Nicotinic AChR in subclassified capsaicin-sensitive and -insensitive nociceptors of the rat DRG. *J Neurophysiol.* 2005;93:1358-1371.

60. Sargent PB. The diversity of neuronal nicotinic acetylcholine receptors. *Annu Rev Neurosci.* 1993;16:403-443.

61. Si ML, Lee JF. Pb^{2+} inhibition of sympathetic a7-nicotinic acetylcholine receptor-mediated nitrergic neurogenic dilation in porcine basilar arteries. *J Pharmacol Exp Ther.* 2003;305:1124-1131.

62. Berg DK, Conroy WG. Nicotinic a7 receptors: synaptic options and downstream signaling in neurons. *J Neurobiol.* 2002;53:512-523.

63. Loring RH, Zigmond RE. Characterization of neuronal nicotinic receptors by snake venom neurotoxins. *Trends Neurosci.* 1988;11:73-78.

64. Shoop RD, Martone ME, Yamada N, Ellisman MH, Berg DK. Neuronal acetylcholine receptors with a7 subunits are concentrated on somatic spines for synaptic signaling in embryonic chick ciliary ganglia. *J Neurosci.* 1999;19:692-704.

65. Loring RH, Chiappinelli VA, Zigmond RE, Cohen JB. Characterization of a snake venom neurotoxin which blocks nicotinic transmission in the avian ciliary ganglion. *Neuroscience.* 1984;11:989-999.

66. Vijayaraghavan S, Pugh PC, Zhang ZW, Rathouz MM, Berg DK. Nicotinic receptors that bind alpha-bungarotoxin on neurons raise intracellular free Ca^{2+}. *Neuron.* 1992;8:353-362.

67. Gahring LC, Rogers SW. Neuronal nicotinic acetylcholine receptor expression and function on nonneuronal cells. *AAPS J.* 2006;7:E885-E894.

68. Chernyavsky AI, Arredondo J, Marubio LM, Grando SA. Differential regulation of keratinocyte chemokinesis and chemotaxis through distinct nicotinic receptor subtypes. *J Cell Sci.* 2004;117:5665-5679.

69. Li XW, Wang H. Non-neuronal nicotinic alpha 7 receptor, a new endothelial target for revascularization. *Life Sci.* 2006;78:1863-1870.

70. Hunt SP, Schmidt J. The electron microscopic autoradiographic localization of alpha-bungarotoxin binding sites within the central nervous system of the rat. *Brain Res.* 1978;142:152-159.

71. Orr-Urtreger A, Goldner FM, Saeki M, Lorenzo I, Goldberg L, De Biasi M, et al. Mice deficient in the alpha7 neuronal nicotinic acetylcholine receptor lack alpha-bungarotoxin binding sites and hippocampal fast nicotinic currents. *J Neurosci.* 1997;17:9165-9171.

72. Gray R, Rajan AS, Radcliffe KA, Yakehiro M, Dani JA. Hippocampal synaptic transmission enhanced by low concentrations of nicotine. *Nature.* 1996;383:713-716.

73. Wang BW, Liao WN, Chang CT, Wang SJ. Facilitation of glutamate release by nicotine involves the activation of a Ca^{2+}/calmodulin signaling pathway in rat prefrontal cortex nerve terminals. *Synapse.* 2006;59:491-501.

74. Metherate R. Nicotinic acetylcholine receptors in sensory cortex. *Learn Mem.* 2004;11:50-59.

75. Katz LC, Shatz CJ. Synaptic activity and the construction of cortical circuits. *Science.* 1996;274:1133-1138.

76. Morley BJ. Nicotinic cholinergic intercellular communication: implications for the developing auditory system. *Hear Res.* 2005;206:74-88.

77. Pugh PC, Berg DK. Neuronal acetylcholine receptors that bind alpha-bungarotoxin mediate neurite retraction in a calcium-dependent manner. *J Neurosci.* 1994;14:889-896.

78. Chan J, Quik M. A role for the nicotinic alpha-bungarotoxin receptor in neurite outgrowth in PC12 cells. *Neuroscience.* 1993;56:441-451.

79. Messi ML, Renganathan M, Grigorenko E, Delbono O. Activation of alpha7 nicotinic acetylcholine receptor promotes survival of spinal cord motoneurons. *FEBS Lett.* 1997;411:32-38.

80. Levin ED. Nicotinic receptor subtypes and cognitive function. *J Neurobiol.* 2002;53:633-640.

81. Laroche S, Davis S, Jay TM. Plasticity at hippocampal to prefrontal cortex synapses: dual roles in working memory and consolidation. *Hippocampus.* 2000;10:438-446.

82. Hyman SE, Malenka RC, Nestler EJ. Neural mechanisms of addiction: the role of reward-related learning and memory. *Annu Rev Neurosci.* 2006;29:565-598.

83. Blaha CD, Allen LF, Das S, Inglis WL, Latimer MP, Vincent SR, et al. Modulation of dopamine efflux in the nucleus accumbens after cholinergic stimulation of the ventral tegmental area in intact, pedunculopontine tegmental nucleus-lesioned, and laterodorsal tegmental nucleus-lesioned rats. *J Neurosci.* 1996;16:714-722.

84. Fagen ZM, Mansvelder HD, Keath JR, McGehee DS. Short- and long-term modulation of synaptic inputs to brain reward areas by nicotine. *Ann N Y Acad Sci.* 2003;1003:185-195.

85. Solinas M, Scherma M, Fattore L, Stroik J, Wertheim C, Tanda G, et al. Nicotinic alpha 7 receptors as a new target for treatment of cannabis abuse. *J Neurosci.* 2007;27:5615-5620.

86. Martin LF, Kem WR, Freedman R. Alpha-7 nicotinic receptor agonists: potential new candidates for the treatment of schizophrenia. *Psychopharmacology.* 2004;174:54-64.

87. Stevens KE, Kem WR, Mahnir VM, Freedman R. Selective alpha7-nicotinic agonists normalize inhibition of auditory response in DBA mice. *Psychopharmacology* (Berl). 1998;136:320-327.

88. Adler LE, Olincy A, Waldo M, Harris JG, Griffith J, Stevens K, et al. Schizophrenia, sensory gating, and nicotinic receptors. *Schizophr Bull.* 1998;24:189-202.

89. Freedman R, Coon H, Myles-Worsley M, Orr-Urtreger A, Olincy A, Davis A, et al. Linkage of a neurophysiological deficit in schizophrenia to a chromosome 15 locus. *Proc Natl Acad Sci U S A.* 1997;94:587-592.

90. Kitagawa H, Takenouchi T, Azuma R, Wesnes KA, Kramer WG, Clody DE, et al. Safety, pharmacokinetics, and effects on cognitive function of multiple doses of GTS-21 in healthy, male volunteers. *Neuropsychopharmacology.* 2003;28:542-551.

91. D'Andrea MR, Nagele RG. Targeting the alpha 7 nicotinic acetylcholine receptor to reduce amyloid accumulation in Alzheimer's disease pyramidal neurons. *Curr Pharm Des.* 2006;12:677-684.

92. Wang HY, Lee DH, D'Andrea MR, Peterson PA, Shank RP, Reitz AB. Beta-amyloid(1-42) binds to alpha7 nicotinic acetylcholine receptor with high affinity. Implications for Alzheimer's disease pathology. *J Biol Chem.* 2000;275:5626-5632.

93. Liu Q, Kawai H, Berg DK. Beta-amyloid peptide blocks the response of alpha 7-containing nicotinic receptors on hippocampal neurons. *Proc Natl Acad Sci U S A.* 2001;98:4734-4739.

94. Pettit DL, Shao Z, Yakel JL. Beta-amyloid(1-42) peptide directly modulates nicotinic receptors in the rat hippocampal slice. *J Neurosci.* 2001;21:RC120.

95. Nagele RG, D'Andrea MR, Anderson WJ, Wang HY. Intracellular accumulation of beta-amyloid(1-42) in neurons is facilitated by the alpha 7 nicotinic acetylcholine receptor in Alzheimer's disease. *Neuroscience.* 2002;110:199-211.

96. Ulloa L. The vagus nerve and the nicotinic anti-inflammatory pathway. *Nat Rev Drug Discov.* 2005;4:673-684.

97. Wittebole X, Hahm S, Coyle SM, Kuman A, Calvano SE, Lowry SF. Nicotine exposure alters *in vivo* human responses to endotoxin. *Clin Exp Immunol.* 2007;147:28-34.

98. Wang H, Yu M, Ochani M, Amella CA, Tanovic M, Susarla S, et al. Nicotinic acetylcholine receptor a7 subunit is an essential regulator of inflammation. *Nature.* 2003;421:384-388.

99. Flores CM. The promise and pitfalls of a nicotinic cholinergic approach to pain management. *Pain.* 2000;88:1-6.

100. Haberberger RV, Henrich M, Lips KS, Kummer W. Nicotinic receptor alpha 7-subunits are coupled to the stimulation of nitric oxide synthase in rat dorsal root ganglion neurons. *Histochem Cell Biol.* 2003;120:173-181.

101. Yoshimura N, Seki S, de Groat WC. Nitric oxide modulates Ca(2+) channels in dorsal root ganglion neurons innervating rat urinary bladder. *J Neurophysiol.* 2001;86:304-311.

102. Gillberg PG, Aquilonius SM. Cholinergic, opioid and glycine receptor binding sites localized in human spinal cord by *in vitro* autoradiography. Changes in amyotrophic lateral sclerosis. *Acta Neurol Scand.* 1985;72:299-306.

103. Ryan RE, Loiacono RE. Nicotinic receptor subunit mRNA in the thalamus of the rat: relevance to schizophrenia? *Neuroreport.* 2000;11:3693-3698.

104. Seguela P, Wadiche J, Dineley-Miller K, Dani JA, Patrick JW. Molecular cloning, functional properties, and distribution of rat brain alpha 7: a nicotinic cation channel highly permeable to calcium. *J Neurosci.* 1993;13:596-604.

105. Damaj MI, Meyer EM, Martin BR. The antinociceptive effects of alpha7 nicotinic agonists in an acute pain model. *Neuropharmacology.* 2000;39:2785-2791.

106. Hamurtekin E, Gurun MS. The antinociceptive effects of centrally administered CDP-choline on acute pain models in rats: the involvement of cholinergic system. *Brain Res.* 2006;1117:92-100.

107. Wang Y, Su DM, Wang RH, Liu Y, Wang H. Antinociceptive effects of choline against acute and inflammatory pain. *Neuroscience.* 2005;132:49-56.

108. Shytle RD, Mori T, Townsend K, Vendrame M, Sun N, Zeng J, et al. Cholinergic modulation of microglial activation by alpha 7 nicotinic receptors. *J Neurochem.* 2004;89:337-343.

109. Ruggieri MR, Sr. Mechanisms of disease: role of purinergic signaling in the pathophysiology of bladder dysfunction. *Nat Clin Pract Urol.* 2006;3:206-215.

110. Lalo U, Pankratov Y, Krishtal O, North RA. Methyllycaconitine, alpha-bungarotoxin and (+)-tubocurarine block fast ATP-gated currents in rat dorsal root ganglion cells. *Br J Pharmacol.* 2004;142:1227-1232.

111. Morrison J, Birder LA, Craggs M, de Groat WC, Downie J, Drake M, et al. Neural control. In: Abrams L, Cardozo L, Khoury S, Wein A, eds. *Incontinence.* Paris: Health Publications, Ltd; 2005:363-422.

112. Kakizaki H, de Groat WC. Reorganization of somatourethral reflexes following spinal cord injury in the rat. *J Urol.* 1997;158:1562-1567.

113. Yoshiyama M, deGroat WC, Fraser MO. Influences of external urethral sphincter relaxation induced by alpha-bungarotoxin, a neuromuscular junction blocking agent, on voiding dysfunction in the rat with spinal cord injury. *J Urol.* 2000;55:956-960.

114. Schurch B, Hauri D, Rodic B, Curt A, Meyer M, Rossier AB. Botulinum-A toxin as a treatment of detrusor-sphincter dyssynergia: a prospective study in 24 spinal cord injury patients. *J Urol.* 1996;155:1023-1029.

115. Beckel JM, Kanai A, Lee SJ, de Groat WC, Birder LA. Expression of functional nicotinic acetylcholine

receptors in rat urinary bladder epithelial cells. *Am J Physiol Renal Physiol.* 2006;290:F103-110.

116. Birder LA, Truschel S, Kiss S, Apodaca G, Dineley K, de Groat WC, et al. Nicotine Evokes Nitric Oxide Release from Urinary Bladder Epithelium. The 10th Neuropharmacology Conference, 2000.

117. Masuda H, Hayashi Y, Chancellor MB, Kihara K, de Groat WC, de Miguel F, et al. Roles of peripheral and central nicotinic receptors in the micturition reflex in rats. *J Urol.* 2006;176:374-379.

118. Hanna-Mitchell AT, Beckel JM, Barbadora S, Kanai AJ, de Groat WC, Birder LA. Non-neuronal acetylcholine and urinary bladder urothelium. *Life Sci.* 2007;80:2298-2302.

119. Lee SJ, Nakamura Y, de Groat WC. Effect of (+/-)-epibatidine, a nicotinic agonist, on the central pathways controlling voiding function in the rat. *Am J Physiol Regul Integr Comp Physiol.* 2003;285:R84-R90.

Biology and Pharmacology of Conotoxins

36

Russell W. Teichert, Elsie C. Jimenez, and Baldomero M. Olivera

INTRODUCTION

Over the course of evolution, the approximately 700 living species of predatory marine cone snails (genus *Conus*) (Fig. 36-1) have generated in their venoms a vast array of peptide toxins, known colloquially as conotoxins (alternatively, conopeptides or *Conus* peptides). Cone snails occupy diverse marine habitats in tropical and subtropical oceans globally, ranging from shallow water coral reefs to deep water habitats. As a consequence of occupying an exclusive ecologic niche, each *Conus* species appears to have evolved its own unique set of venom peptides tailored to the combination of prey, predators, and competitors that the species interacts with. Even very closely related species have different peptides in their venoms. Because every species of cone snail produces 100 to 200 unique peptide toxins in its venom, there are estimated to be more than 100,000 unique peptide toxins distributed across the approximately 700 species of cones.[1-3]

The vast structural and functional diversity of conopeptides has arisen via several mechanisms. One source of conopeptide diversity is the different gene superfamilies that encode conopeptides (Table 36-1). Within a gene superfamily, conopeptides typically share a single structural scaffold, most often determined by a common framework of disulfide bonds. Most conotoxins are disulfide-rich peptides, which fold in three-dimensional conformations required for their high affinity and specificity for their respective targets. Relatively few gene superfamilies encode the great majority of conopeptides; thus, cone snails have used relatively few structural scaffolds to achieve extensive functional diversity. Although conopeptides in a superfamily are genetically and structurally related, the cone snails generate diversity by mechanisms that include accelerated evolution (e.g., rapid divergence in amino acid sequence), numerous post-translational modifications, and (rarely) changing the disulfide-bonding framework of an existing peptide family.[2,4-6]

Over the past two decades, numerous conopeptide families have been characterized, demonstrating that the diversity of their molecular targets parallels the diversity of the conopeptides themselves.[6] The biologic mechanisms that have altered conopeptides, and the evolutionary forces that have selected for comparative advantages in predation, defense, and competitive interactions, collectively have optimized many conopeptides for high affinity and specificity for particular targets, often subtypes of receptors or ion channels in the nervous system. Their targets include many subtypes of voltage-gated ion channels (Table 36-2), ligand-gated ion channels (Table 36-3), and G protein–coupled receptors (Table 36-4); many of these targets are described in this chapter. Their unique

Dr. Teichert is disclosing that he is currently employed by Vertex Pharmaceuticals, San Diego, CA. His entire contribution to this chapter was completed while he was previously employed as a Research Assistant Professor, Department of Biology, University of Utah. Dr. Jimenez is disclosing that she holds US patents on conopeptides, such as contryphan peptides, bromotryptophan conopeptides, conantokins, and I-superfamily conotoxins. Contryphan is currently marketed as a research biochemical by Bachem, a biotechnology company with headquarters in Bubendorf, Switzerland, and affiliates in Europe and the United States. Dr. Olivera does not report any conflicts of interest.

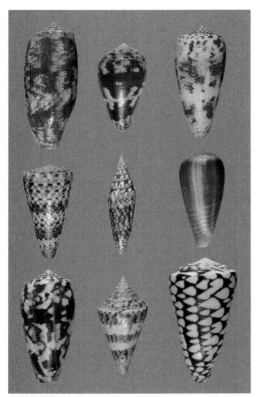

FIGURE 36-1. Shells of some cone snails (genus *Conus*) that produce pharmacologically active venom peptides. The venoms of most *Conus* species shown are well characterized and have provided peptides of biomedical interest with therapeutic potential. Two of the species, *Conus milneedwardsi*, the Glory of India cone and *Conus delesserti*, Delessert's cone (center middle row and center bottom row, respectively) are virtually unexplored; these represent the significant number of cone-snail species with unexplored venoms, a frontier for new conopeptide discovery. The species shown are, left to right, **top row:** *Conus geographus*, the geography cone; *Conus purpurascens*, the purple cone; *Conus magus*, the magician's cone. **Middle row,** *Conus imperialis*, the imperial cone; *Conus milneedwardsi*; *Conus radiatus*, the radial cone. **Bottom row,** *Conus striatus*, the striated cone; *Conus delesserti*; *Conus marmoreus*, the marble cone. Most species shown are fish hunting except for *Conus imperialis* and *Conus delesserti*, which prey on worms, and *Conus marmoreus* and *Conus milneedwardsi*, which are snail hunters.

specificity makes conopeptides increasingly important as research tools for defining the physiologic roles of closely related subtypes of receptors and ion channels, and for various clinical applications, including direct application as therapeutic drugs. In this chapter, we systematically review the structural and functional diversity of conopeptides, with a discussion of their pharmacologic selectivity and utility.

BIOLOGY AND ECOLOGY OF CONE SNAILS: SOURCE OF PEPTIDE DIVERSITY

The cone snails comprise one of the largest genera (*Conus*) of marine animals.[7] Cone snails are divided into three groups, based on their prey. The largest group includes the vermivorous (worm-hunting) species that feed on polychaete, hemichordate, and echiuroid worms. The second class comprises the molluscivorous (snail-hunting) species that hunt other mollusks. A notable group consists of the piscivorous (fish-hunting) cone snails; these have venoms that very rapidly immobilize fish.[1,8,9] The different predatory specializations of cone snails provide one rationale for the diversity of peptides found in their venoms.

As mentioned earlier, different *Conus* species have divergent biotic interactions leading to the rapid divergence of conopeptides between *Conus* species. Cone snails particularly thrive in tropical marine habitats; these contain the most diverse array of *Conus* species. In addition to the predatory specializations cited earlier, the incredibly complex web of biologic interactions (e.g., defense and competition with myriad species) in tropical marine environments provides another rationale for the unique and divergent spectrum of conopeptides evolved by each *Conus* species.[2]

Venom is the major weapon used by cone snails for prey capture, defense, and deterrence of competitors. Because these predatory snails are not notable for their speed or mechanical weaponry, they have evolved rapidly acting, potent venoms. Targeting various ion channels using combinations of conotoxins is a sensible strategy; the rich molecular diversity of potential targets and the ability to interfere with the rapid signaling of ion channels provide an additional rationale for the molecular complexity of peptides in cone snail venoms.[1] As a consequence of all the factors cited earlier, *Conus* venoms have become a discovery engine for ligands with subtype selectivity for many classes and families of receptors and ion channels.

SUPERFAMILIES OF CONOPEPTIDES

An overview of the superfamilies of conopeptides is shown in Table 36-1. Two broad

TABLE 36-1 Conopeptide Gene Superfamilies

Superfamily	Family	Cys Pattern	Cys Pattern Class	Molecular Target
Disulfide-Rich Peptides				
A	α	CC-C-C	I/II	nAChR
A	αA	CC-C-C-C-C	IV	nAChR
A	κA	CC-C-C-C-C	IV	K^+ or Na^+ channel
I_1	ι	C-C-CC-CC-C-C	XI	Na^+ channel
I_2		C-C-CC-CC-C-C	XI	K^+ channel
J	κJ	C-C-C-C	XIV	K^+ channel
M	μ	CC-C-C-CC	III	Na^+ channel
M	ψ	CC-C-C-CC	III	nAChR
M	κM	CC-C-C-CC	III	K^+ channel
O	δ	C-C-CC-C-C	VI/VII	Na^+ channel
O	μO	C-C-CC-C-C	VI/VII	Na^+ channel
O	κ	C-C-CC-C-C	VI/VII	K^+ channel
O	ω	C-C-CC-C-C	VI/VII	Ca^{2+} channel
P		C-C-C-C-C-C	IX	
S	σ	C-C-C-C-C-C-C-C-C-C	VIII	5-HT_3 Receptor
S	αS	C-C-C-C-C-C-C-C-C-C	VIII	nAChR
T	χ	CC-CPC	I/II	NE Transporter
T		CC-CC	V	
Non–Disulfide-Rich Peptides and Polypeptides				
	Conantokin	NA	NA	NMDA Receptor
	Conorfamide	NA	NA	Rifamide Receptor
C	Contulakin	NA	NA	Neurotensin Receptor
C	αC	C-C	X	nAChR
	Conopressin	C-C		Vasopressin Receptor
	Contryphan	C-C		Ca^{2+} channel
	Conkunitzins	C-C-C-C		K^+ channel

NA, not applicable; nAChR, nicotinic acetylcholine receptor; NMDA, N-methyl-D-aspartate, NE, norepinephrine; 5-HT, 5-hydroxytryptamine (serotonin). Blanks in the table are either undefined or unknown.

Many references for each peptide family are provided in the text and in the subsequent tables in this chapter. For each Cys pattern, the dash represents a variable number of amino acids between Cys residues. Cys pattern class is utilized as a naming convention, e.g. μ-conotoxin GIIIA has a class III Cys pattern (CC-C-C-CC) and thus has "III" in its name. Conkunitzins are not considered disulfide rich because each polypeptide is approximately 60 AA in length.

divisions of venom components are shown: disulfide-rich and non–disulfide-rich conopeptides. In most of the disulfide-rich conotoxins, cysteine residues occur at an unusually high frequency. However, the arrangement of cysteine residues is limited to relatively few patterns; in general, each pattern corresponds to a specific disulfide-bonding framework. Furthermore, the cysteine pattern is indicative of the gene superfamily that encodes the conopeptide and, in some cases, can be indicative of the pharmacologic target.[6]

Despite the incredible diversity among conotoxins, they are encoded by relatively few gene superfamilies. Characterization of cDNA clones from venom ducts has established that conopeptides are initially translated as prepropeptide precursors.[10] The organization of conopeptide precursors consists of a typical signal sequence (the "pre" region) at the N-terminal end, followed by an intervening "pro" region, and the mature toxin region at the C-terminal end of the open reading frame. Proteolytic cleavage of the precursor to form the functional

TABLE 36-2 Some Conopeptides Targeted to Voltage-Gated Ion Channels

Peptide	Amino Acid Sequence	Target (Specificity)	Reference
μ-GIIIA	RDCCTOOKKCKDRQCKOQRCCA*	Na$^+$ channel (Na$_V$1.4)	26-29
μ-GIIIB	RDCCTOORKCKDRRCKOMKCCA*	Na$^+$ channel (Na$_V$1.4)	26, 27
μ-PIIIA	ZRLCCGFOKSCRSRQCKOHRCC*	Na$^+$ channel (Na$_V$1.4)	33
μ-SmIIIA	ZRCCNGRRGCSSRWCRDHSRCC*	Na$^+$ channel (TTX-R)#	35
μO-MrVIA	ACRKKWEYCIVPIIGFIYCCPGLICGPFVCV	Na$^+$ channel	39
μO-MrVIB	ACSKKWEYCIVPILGFVYCCPGLICGPFVCV	Na$^+$ channel (Na$_V$1.8)	39, 42
ι-RXIA	GOSFCKADEKOCEYHADCCNCCLSG ICAOSTNWILPGCSTSSFFKI	Na$^+$ channel	44, 45
δ-PVIA	EACYAOGTFCGIKOGLCC$\overline{\text{S}}$EFCLPGVCFG	Na$^+$ channel	47
δ-TxVIA	WCKQSGEMCNLLDQNCCDGYCIVLVCT	Na$^+$ channel	46
δ-GmVIA	VKPCRKEGQLCDPIFQNCCRGWNCVLFCV	Na$^+$ channel	49
κ-PVIIA	CRIONQKCFQHLDDCCSRKCNRFNKCV	K$^+$ channel (K$_V$1.X)	51
κM-RIIIK	LOSCCSLNLRLCOVOACKRNOCCT*	K$^+$ channel (K$_V$1.2)	53, 54
Conkunitzin-S1	KDRPSLCDLPADSGSGTKAEKRIYYNSARKQ CLRFDYTGQQGGNENNFRRTYDCQRTCLYT	K$^+$ channel (K$_V$1.X)	55
κA-SIVA	ZKSLVP$VITTCCGYDOGTMCOOCRCTNSC*	K$^+$ or Na$^+$ channel	73
p114a (κJ-PIXIVA)	FPRPRICNLACRAGIGHKYPFCHCR*	K$^+$ channel (K$_V$1.6) and nAChRs	72
ω-GVIA	CKSOGSSCSOTSYNCCRSCNOYTKRCY*	Ca^{2+} channel (N-type)	57, 58
ω-MVIIA	CKGKGAKCSRLMYDCCTGSCRSGKC*	Ca^{2+} channel (N-type)	59, 60
ω-MVIIC	CKGKGAPCRKTMYDCCSGSCGRRGKC*	Ca^{2+} channel (P/	59, 60, 65
ω-CVID	CKSKGAKCSKLMYDCCSGSCSGTVGRC*	Q-type)	66
ω-TxVII†	CKQADEPCDVFSLDCCTGICLGVCMW	Ca^{2+} channel (N-type) Ca^{2+} channel (L-type)	77
Glacontryphan	NγSγCPWHPWC*	Ca^{2+} channel (L-type)	77
Am 975; Cont-P	GCOWD$\overline{\text{P}}$WC*	Ca^{2+} channel	78

O, 4-trans-hydroxyproline; Cont, contryphan; Z, pyroglutamate; $, O-glycosylated serine residue; TTX-R, tetrodotoxin resistant sodium current; γ, γ-carboxyglutamate; F, D-phenylalanine; W, D-tryptophan; *, amidated C-terminus; †, molluscan L-type calcium channel; #, TTX resistant in amphibians only. The peptide previously designated p114a is designated here as κJ-PIXIVA, the defining member of the κJ-family.

(mature) toxin is an obligatory step in the maturation of all conopeptides.

A comparison of homologous cDNA sequences from different *Conus* species reveals a striking pattern; peptides with similar arrangements of cysteine residues in the primary sequence of the mature toxin share a highly conserved signal sequence. These features define members of a conopeptide gene superfamily. These gene superfamilies have diverged structurally and functionally to produce the majority of the more than 100,000 different conopeptides found in the venoms of cone snails.[1-3] A variety of mechanisms that lead to the conservation of the signal sequences juxtaposed with the hyperdivergence in the mature toxin region have been proposed.[5,10-13] In addition, the occurrence of a variety of post-translational modifications contributes to the molecular diversity of conopeptides.[14,15]

One insight into the mechanism of post-translational modification of conopeptides has been obtained from studies of the γ-carboxylation of glutamate to the nonstandard amino acid γ-carboxyglutamate.[16,17] The post-translational modification enzyme γ-glutamyl carboxylase has been found in *Conus* venom ducts. Its gene was subsequently cloned and expressed. The *Conus* enzyme is highly homologous to the mammalian enzyme.[18-20] It recognizes a sequence in the pro region of the precursor peptide, where that signal engages and initiates the enzyme to modify specific amino acid residues in the mature toxin region. The pro region of the conopeptide precursor provides potential anchor-binding sites for the γ-glutamyl carboxylase.[21]

General Physiology and Pharmacology of Conopeptides

A pharmacologic insight into the mode of action of conopeptides is that cone snails

TABLE 36-3 Some Conopeptides Targeted to Ligand-Gated Ion Channels

Peptide	Amino Acid Sequence	Target (Specificity)	Reference
α-Iml	GCCSDPRCAWRC*	nAChR (α7)	82
α-MII	GCCSNPVCHLEHSNLC*	nAChR (α3β2; α6βX)	4, 89
α-RgIA	GCCSDPRCRYRCR	nAChR (α9α10)	86, 87
αA-EIVA	GCCGPYONAACHOCGCKVGROOYCDRO SGG*	nAChR (α/δ, α/γ interfaces)	93
αA-OIVA	CCGVONAACHOCVCKNTC*	nAChR (α/γ interface)	91, 92
αS-RVIIIA	KCNFDKCKGTGVYNCGγSCSCγGLHSCRC TYNIGSMKSGCACICTYY	nAChR (nonspecific)	94
αC-PrXA	TYGIYDAKPOFSCAGLRGGCVLPONLROK FKE*	nAChR (α/δ interface)	95
φ-PIIIE	HOOCCLYGKCRRYOGCSSASCCQR*	nAChR (muscle-noncompetitive)	96, 97
σ-GVIIIA	GCTRTCGGOKCTGTCTCTNSSKCGCRYN VHPSGUGCGCACS*	5-HT₃ Receptor	100
Conantokin-G	GEγγLQγNQγLIRγKSN*	NMDAR (NR2B)	17, 101
Conantokin-T	GEγγYQKMLγNLRγAEVKKNA*	NMDAR	102
Conantokin-L	GEγγVAKMAAγLARγDAVN*	NMDAR	103

O, 4 trans-hydroxyproline; γ, γ-carboxyglutamate; U, 6-bromotryptophan; *, C-terminal amidation; nAChR, nicotinic acetylcholine receptor; 5-HT, 5-hydroxytryptamine (serotonin); NMDAR, N-methyl-D-aspartate receptor.

employ sophisticated combinations of peptide ligands with divergent specificities to elicit a variety of physiologic responses that are critical to predation, defense, and competitive interactions. To efficiently inflict the physiologic effect on the prey, predator. or competitor, multiple conopeptides act together in a synergistic manner to affect the targeted animal. There are similarities between the evolution of conopeptides and modern pharmacologic practices. The hypermutation that

occurs in conopeptide-encoding regions accompanying cone snail speciation is the evolutionary equivalent of a combinatorial library strategy for drug development. Post-translational modifications of conopeptides achieve the same goals as the medicinal chemistry done after an initial lead candidate for drug development is identified.[1,6]

To better understand the diversity of conopeptides within a single venom, we have conceptually grouped conopeptides acting

TABLE 36-4 Miscellaneous Constituents of *Conus* Venoms

Peptide	Amino Acid Sequence	Target/Function	Reference
Conopressin-G	CFIRNCPLG*	Vasopressin receptor	115
Contulakin-G	ZSEEGGSNATKKPYIL	Neurotensin receptor	116
ρ-TIA	FNWRCCLIPĀCRRNHKKFC*	α₁-Adrenergic receptor	117
mr5a; χ-MrIA	NGVCCGYKLCHOC	Norepinephrine transporter	117-119
tx5a; TxIX	γCCγDGWCCTAAO	Reduces Ca²⁺ flux	120, 121
μ-PnIVA	CCKYGW̲T̄CLL̲GCSPCGC	Na⁺ channel-molluscan	122
γ-PnVIIA	DCTSWFGRCTVNSγCCSNSCDQTYCγLYAFOS	Pacemaker channel-molluscan	123
Conorfamide	GPMGWVPVFYRF*	RFamide R; Na⁺ channel	124
Contryphan-Vn	GDCPWKPWC*	Ca²⁺-dependent K⁺ channel	79
Bromosleeper	UATIDγCγγTCNVTFKTCCGOOGDWQCVγACPV	Unknown target	125
Light sleeper r7a	UFGHγγCTYULGPCγVDDTCCSASCγSKFCGLU	Unknown target	126
Spasmodic-Tx	GCNNSCQγHSDCγSHCICTFRGCGAVN*	Unknown target	127

Z, pyroglutamate; O, 4-*trans*-hydroxyproline; γ, γ-carboxyglutamate; T̲, O-glycosylated threonine; W̲, D-tryptophan; U, 6-bromotryptophan; *, C-terminal amidation.

concertedly to bring about a particular physiologic effect and refer to such groups as "toxin cabals."[1,22] The characterization of conotoxins from the venom of the fish-hunting species *Conus purpurascens* defined the presence of two different toxin cabals with distinct effects.[9] The "lightning-strike cabal" causes immediate immobilization of the injected prey; components of the lightning-strike cabal include peptides that delay inactivation of voltage-gated Na^+ channels, reduce the threshold for Na^+ channel activation, and block K^+ channels (see the section entitled Conotoxins Targeted to Voltage-Gated Ion Channels). This mixture synergistically leads to the massive depolarization of axons in the immediate vicinity of the venom injection site, causing an effect similar to electrocution of the fish. Thus, the characteristic tetanic state elicited by the peptides of the lightning-strike cabal are evident immediately after venom injection. A second group of venom peptides, the "motor cabal," causes complete inhibition of neuromuscular transmission. This is accomplished more slowly; components of the motor cabal are conotoxins that act at sites that are remote from the venom injection site, for example, at neuromuscular junctions. Because transport of the peptides to the target sites is required before the desired physiologic effects are completed, the effects of the motor cabal are observed after those of the lightning-strike cabal. The motor cabal, which is found in all fish-hunting *Conus* venoms studied so far, can include peptides that inhibit the presynaptic Ca^{2+} channels that control neurotransmitter release, the postsynaptic nicotinic acetylcholine receptors (nAChRs), and the Na^+ channels that trigger the muscle action potential (see the sections entitled Contoxins Targeted to Voltage-Gated Ion Channels and Conopeptides Targeted to Ligand-Gated Ion Channels).

There is evidence that different fish-hunting *Conus* species may have a divergent array of toxin cabals for prey capture.[2] In part, this divergence can be correlated with different behavioral strategies for capturing fish. The combination of lightning-strike and motor cabals is found in the venoms of *Conus* species that extend their proboscis to initially approach and then harpoon the fish prey. Some species use an alternative strategy for capturing fish; such cone snails can greatly distend their "false mouths," effectively using them as a net. These cone snails engulf the fish with the false mouth before they inject venom. Thus the venom of fish-hunting *Conus geographus* appears to have peptides whose function is to deaden the sensory circuitry of the prey; these have been referred to as the "nirvana cabal."[1,6,22] It has been proposed that conopeptide antagonists of a serotonin-gated ion channel (5-HT_3) and the N-methyl-D-aspartate (NMDA) class of ionotropic glutamate receptors (see the section entitled Conopeptides Targeted to Ligand-Gated Ion Channels), together with a neurotensin receptor agonist (see the section entitled Other Biologically Active Constituents of *Conus* Venoms), can elicit a sedated state, making prey capture using the net strategy more facile.

The combination drug strategy employed by cone snails provides an additional rationale for the complexity of *Conus* venoms, as well as for the notable pharmacologic diversity of conopeptides. Different toxin cabals may include peptides that act on the same general class of targets but through different mechanisms and kinetics. The radiation of cone snails has given rise to many venom peptides that synergistically target distinct ion channel subtypes to achieve a particular physiologic result. Thus, different conopeptides may be effective constituents of different cabals, acting within different time frames, without causing any functional cross-interference.

OVERVIEW OF MAIN TARGETS OF CONUS PEPTIDES: VOLTAGE-GATED AND LIGAND-GATED ION CHANNELS

Voltage-gated ion channels are targets of toxins from various organisms. In the following sections, we describe the properties of conotoxins interacting with the pore-forming α-subunit of Na^+, K^+, and Ca^{2+} channels.[23] Voltage-activated Na^+ channels are key molecules for generating action potentials in electrically excitable cells. They have been divided into two pharmacologic classes, based on their sensitivity to tetrodotoxin (TTX), the classic blocker of Na^+ currents; thus, there are TTX-sensitive and TTX-insensitive Na^+ channels. The interaction site of TTX with the channel protein is designated site I; it is proposed to be at the extracellular end of the ion channel pore. In addition, up to five ligand-binding sites on the channel protein have been distinguished.[24] Most ligands that target these other sites cause a net increase in

Na$^+$ currents either by shifting the current-voltage relationship or by blocking the fast inactivation of the channels. Molecular isoforms of Na$^+$ channels are designated as Na$_V$1.x, where x is 1, 2, 3, and so on.

Potassium channels are important in the repolarization phase of action potentials, in setting the resting membrane potential, and in bursting activity; they have a wide diversity of specialized functions in various cell types.[23] In line with this broad spectrum of different physiologic roles, about 100 genes encoding different K$^+$ channels have been identified, and several families of voltage-gated K$^+$ channels (K$_V$1.x, K$_V$2.x, where x is 1, 2, and so on) are known.

Calcium signaling is involved in a great variety of different physiologic processes including neurotransmitter release. Voltage-gated Ca^{2+} channels, which mediate the Ca^{2+} influx in response to depolarization, are heteromeric protein complexes with four or five different subunits. The observed physiologic and pharmacologic diversity of Ca^{2+} channels is mainly due to the properties of the pore-forming α_1-subunits. Based on their different physiologic and pharmacologic properties, voltage-gated Ca^{2+} channels were initially classified into L-, N-, P-, Q-, R-, and T-type channels. A standardized, more genetically derived nomenclature is now generally used for Ca^{2+} channels, based on the system originally developed for K$^+$ channels. In this nomenclature, the Ca$_V$1 family includes the channels that mediate L-type Ca^{2+} currents; the Ca$_V$2 family comprises those that mediate N-, P/Q-, and R-type Ca^{2+} currents; and the Ca$_V$3 family includes those that mediate T-type Ca^{2+} currents.

Ligand-gated ion channels mediate fast synaptic transmission (for an overview, see reference 25); there are several groups. One includes those that are activated by acetylcholine, serotonin, gamma-aminobutyric acid (GABA), or glycine; these belong to the Cys-loop receptor superfamily. Aside from their ligand specificity, these channels may differ in their selectivity for permeant ions. The functional channel complexes are comprised of five subunits, with each subunit containing four transmembrane helices. The other gene superfamily of ligand-gated ion channels comprises the ionotropic glutamate receptors, usually classified into NMDA and kainate/AMPA receptors. A third family of ligand-gated ion channels includes the adenosine triphosphate (ATP) receptors. The nicotinic acetylcholine receptors (nAChRs) and NMDA receptors, which are important targets of *Conus* peptides, are discussed briefly below.

Most vertebrate nAChRs are heteromeric pentamers. Most subtypes consist of two α-subunits and three non–α-subunits. One group of nAChRs (α7, α9, α10) can be assembled exclusively from α-subunits. There are generally two to four different types of subunits comprising native functional heteromeric nAChR complexes. The acetylcholine binding sites (also the binding site for other agonists) are generally located at interfaces between α- and non–α-subunits. Two acetylcholine molecules must bind before gating of the ion channel from a closed to an open state can occur.

Glutamate receptors are believed to be tetramers, and in the NMDA subclass, the functional native receptors consist of two types of subunits, NR1 and NR2. Only one gene has been found to encode NR1 subunits, but eight different splice variants of NR1 have been identified in mammals. In contrast, the four NR2 subunits, NR2A, NR2B, NR2C, and NR2D, are encoded by different genes. These ligand-gated ion channels are gated by two coagonists: glutamate, which binds the NR2 subunit, and glycine, which binds the NR1 subunit. NMDA receptors are normally blocked by Mg^{2+}, which binds in the pore region and must be removed by membrane depolarization in order for the co-agonists to elicit currents.

In the following sections, we review the major conopeptide families and their molecular targets. One section summarizes conopeptides targeted to voltage-gated ion channels (see Table 36-2), whereas the following section summarizes conopeptides targeted to ligand-gated ion channels (see Table 36-3).

CONOTOXINS TARGETED TO VOLTAGE-GATED ION CHANNELS

Four different conopeptide families are known to target voltage-gated Na$^+$ channels; each has a distinct mechanism of action. As described later, the μ-conotoxins are Na$^+$-channel blockers; the μO-conotoxins inhibit Na$^+$-channel activation; the ι-conotoxins reduce the threshold for activation of voltage-activated Na$^+$ channels; and the δ-conotoxins delay or inhibit fast Na$^+$-channel inactivation. Several conopeptide families have been shown to target K$^+$

channels. A remarkable difference between peptides that target K^+ channels and those that target Na^+ channels is that the Na^+ channel-targeted conopeptide families appear to be widely conserved over a broad range of *Conus* species. In contrast, genetically and structurally divergent conopeptide families that target K^+ channels have evolved in different clades of *Conus* species. The venoms of fish-hunting *Conus* have multiple ω-conotoxin isoforms that may differ in their selectivity for different Ca^{2+} channel subtypes.

μ-Conotoxins: Sodium Channel Blockers

The μ-conotoxins, which have six cysteine residues forming three disulfide bonds, belong to the M-superfamily. The first μ-conotoxins were isolated from the venom of *Conus geographus*.[26,27] The μ-conotoxin GIIIA (μ-GIIIA) is known to specifically block skeletal muscle Na^+ channels ($Na_V1.4$)[28,29]; it interacts with the pore region of the ion channel and competes with TTX for binding to site I. In μ-GIIIA, Arg-13 likely occludes the pore; this residue seems to act as a steric and electrostatic barrier.[30-32] The μ-conotoxin PIIIA (μ-PIIIA) from *Conus purpurascens* venom also contains an Arg residue (Arg-14), shown to be a major determinant for binding to site I.[33] In amphibian systems, μ-PIIIA, but not μ-GIIIA, irreversibly blocks muscle Na^+ channels. Using cloned mammalian Na^+ channels, μ-PIIIA is not as highly specific for $Na_V1.4$ as μ-GIIIA; although μ-PIIIA has higher affinity for $Na_V1.4$ skeletal muscle Na^+ channels, it also blocks neuronal $Na_V1.2$ channels with affinity in the submicromolar range.[33] The peptide μ-conotoxin SmIIIA (μ-SmIIIA), from fish-hunting *Conus stercusmuscarum*, has several unique features.[34,35] In voltage-clamped dissociated neurons from frog sympathetic and dorsal root ganglia, μ-SmIIIA inhibited most TTX-resistant Na^+ current irreversibly but had no effect on the TTX-sensitive Na^+ currents. The TTX-resistant Na^+ channel blockers, μ-conotoxins SIIIA and KIIIA (μ-SIIIA and μ-KIIIA), from the fish-hunting *Conus striatus* and *Conus kinoshitai* inhibit TTX-resistant Na^+ currents in neurons of frog sympathetic and dorsal root ganglia but weakly inhibit action potentials in frog skeletal muscle, which are mediated by TTX-sensitive sodium channels.[36] μ-KIIIA was recently shown to irreversibly block the mammalian neuronal sodium channel $Na_V1.2$.[37] Both μ-KIIIA and μ-SIIIA exhibit potent analgesic activity in animal models of pain.[37,38] As more μ-conotoxins are discovered and characterized, it is likely that this peptide family will yield ligands selective for neuronal subtypes of mammalian sodium channels.

μO-Conotoxins: Inhibitors of Sodium Channel Activation

The μO-conotoxins, which are hydrophobic peptides with six cysteine residues forming three disulfide bonds, belong to the O-superfamily. Two closely related peptides, μO-conotoxin MrVIA (μO-MrVIA) and μO-conotoxin MrVIB (μO-MrVIB), were isolated from the venom of the snail-hunting *Conus marmoreus*.[39] μO-MrVIA appears to block both TTX-sensitive and TTX-insensitive Na^+ channels; it blocks $Na_V1.2$ channels expressed in *Xenopus* oocytes in the nanomolar range, as well as Na^+ currents recorded from hippocampal pyramidal neurons in culture.[40] Unlike μ-conotoxins, μO-conotoxins did not compete for binding with saxitoxin (STX), indicating that these peptides do not interact with site I and, therefore, act through a different mechanism. Recent work demonstrated that μ-MrVIA interacts with domain III of the alpha subunit of sodium channels.[41] μO-MrVIB potently inhibited the rat $Na_V1.8$ sodium channel and had potent and long-lasting local analgesic effects when tested in pain assays in rats.[42,43] Moreover, μO-MrVIB was shown to block the propagation of action potentials in A- and C-fibers in sciatic nerve and skeletal muscle in rat preparations.[42]

ι-Conotoxins: Enhancers of Sodium Channel Activation

The ι-conotoxins characteristically have eight cysteine residues forming four disulfide bonds, and are notable for the very unusual presence of a D-amino acid in their sequence. These peptides belong to a branch of the I-superfamily designated the I_1-superfamily. Unlike any of the other Na^+ channel-targeted conotoxins, the ι-conotoxins reduce the threshold for activation of voltage-activated Na^+ channels. Consequently, these peptides are part of the lightning-strike cabal, similar to δ-conotoxins, but through a distinct mechanism of action. The ι-conotoxins have a disulfide framework that is notably distinct from other *Conus* peptides targeted to voltage-gated ion channels.[44,45]

δ-Conotoxins: Inhibitors of Sodium Channel Inactivation

The δ-conotoxins are unusually hydrophobic peptides that belong to the O-conotoxin superfamily; they share a common arrangement of Cys residues with the ω-conotoxins, which block Ca^{2+} channels (see the section entitled ω-Conotoxins: Calcium Channel Blockers), and resemble the μO-conotoxins in their hydrophobic character (see the section entitled μO-Conotoxins: Inhibitors of Sodium Channel Activation). The δ-conotoxin TxVIA (δ-TxVIA) from the snail-hunting *Conus textile* (originally called the "King Kong" peptide because it caused a dominant behavior upon injection into lobster)[46] was shown to prolong Na^+ currents in molluscan neuronal membranes. The δ-conotoxin PVIA (δ-PVIA) from the venom of *Conus purpurascens* elicited specific muscle contractions in fish, resulting in a characteristic extension of the mouth, which was termed the "lockjaw syndrome"[47]; In contrast to μ- and μO-conotoxins, which are part of the motor cabal, δ-conotoxin are constituents of the lightning-strike cabal in the venom. The excitatory effects of δ-PVIA are synergistic with the K^+ channel-blocking peptide κ-conotoxin PVIIA (κ-PVIIA) (see the section entitled κ-, κM-Conotoxins and Conkunitzins: Potassium Channel Blockers), resulting in the almost immediate immobilization of the fish prey. δ-PVIA inhibits fast inactivation of $Na_V1.2$-mediated currents expressed in the *Xenopus* expression system, as well as Na^+ currents recorded from hippocampal neurons in culture.[9] Like δ-PVIA, δ-conotoxin SVIE (δ-SVIE) caused a delayed inactivation of Na+ current in frog sympathetic neurons.[48] The δ-conotoxin GmVIA (δ-GmVIA) isolated from the snail-hunting *Conus gloriamaris* caused action potential broadening in *Aplysia* neurons[49,50]; this peptide has micromolar affinity for $Na_V1.2$ and $Na_V1.4$ but does not affect $Na_V1.6$-mediated Na^+ currents.

κ-, κM-Conotoxins and Conkunitzins: Potassium Channel Blockers

The κ-conotoxins, which have six cysteines forming three disulfide bonds, are members of the O-superfamily. As mentioned earlier, κ-PVIIA, isolated from *Conus purpurascens*, was the first conotoxin shown to target voltage-gated K^+ channels.[9,51] The K^+ channel inhibition of κ-PVIIA is physiologically significant for prey capture; this activity is synergistic with δ-PVIA, leading to massive hyperexcitation of the targeted prey, resulting in an almost instant tetanic paralysis.[9] Using the *Xenopus* expression system, it was demonstrated that this peptide inhibited the *Shaker* K^+ channel cloned from *Drosophila*.[51] κ-PVIIA was shown to differentiate between splice variants of the *Shaker* K^+ channel homolog from lobster, indicating its subtype selectivity.[52]

The κM-conotoxins, which share a common Cys pattern with the μ-conotoxins, belong to the M-superfamily. The first characterized peptide belonging to this family, κM-conotoxin RIIIK (κM-RIIIK), was cloned from the venom duct of the fish-hunting *Conus radiatus*. κM-RIIIK blocks *Shaker* K^+ channels and TSha1, a *Shaker* homolog K^+ channel from trout, with high affinity.[53] It was shown that κM-RIIIK blocked the human $K_V1.2$ K^+ channel without any significant effect on $K_V1.5$- and $K_V1.6$-mediated currents.[54]

The conkunitzins are polypeptides, approximately 60 AA in length with four to six Cys residues, that belong to a new *Conus* peptide superfamily. Members of the conkunitzin family were recently extracted from the venom of *Conus striatus* and identified as inhibitors of *Shaker* potassium channels. These conopeptides share a motif, known as a Kunitz domain, that is found in various proteins, including protease inhibitors and snake toxins targeted to potassium channels.[55,56]

Notably, κ-conotoxins, κM-conotoxins, and conkunitzins are channel blockers targeted to the K_V1 subfamily of voltage-gated potassium channels. However, they are structurally different and are encoded by different gene superfamilies. Significantly, each of these conopeptide families appears to have evolved independently within different clades of fish-hunting cone snails to achieve the same physiologic end point.[55]

ω-Conotoxins: Calcium Channel Blockers

The ω-conotoxins have six cysteine residues and belong to the O-superfamily, along with the ω-, δ- and μO-conotoxins. The ω-conotoxin GVIA (ω-GVIA) (also designated ω-CgTX in the neuroscience literature) isolated from *Conus geographus*[57] is widely used as a pharmacologic tool, mainly to inhibit synaptic transmission; it is specific for N-type Ca^{2+} channels.[58] In *Conus magus* venom, multiple ω-conotoxin isoforms were found: ω-conotoxin MVIIA (ω-MVIIA), which is highly specific for N-type Ca^{2+} channels ($Ca_V2.2$), and ω-conotoxin MVIIC (ω-MVIIC), which selectively targets the P/Q channels ($Ca_V2.1$).[59,60] A characteristic feature of ω conotoxins is their high content of basic amino acid residues that have an essential role in the inhibition of Ca^{2+} channels.[61] In addition to the positive charges, it is known that a tyrosine residue (Tyr-13 in ω-MVIIA and ω-MVIIC) is important for the binding to $Ca_V2.2$ and $Ca_V2.1$ channels.[62-64] The ω-conotoxin CVID (ω-CVID) from *Conus catus* was shown to target an N-type Ca^{2+} channel in preganglionic nerve terminals.[65] Another peptide, ω-conotoxin TxVII (ω-TxVII), targets the molluscan L-type Ca^{2+} channels.[66] Several ω-conotoxins have been identified and functionally characterized; since this field has previously been reviewed comprehensively (for overviews, see references 67-69), the reader is referred to the earlier literature on ω-conotoxins.

OTHER *CONUS* PEPTIDES REPORTED TO TARGET VOLTAGE-GATED ION CHANNELS

I_2-Superfamily Conotoxins

As stated earlier, the ι-conotoxins belong to the I_1-superfamily. The genetically distant I_2-superfamily (which has the same Cys pattern as the I_1-superfamily) includes peptides that purportedly target potassium channels. A peptide designated κ-BtX has been reported to upmodulate the Ca^{2+}- and voltage-sensitive BK currents measured from rat adrenal chromaffin cells without any effect on other voltage-gated channels.[70] In contrast, another member of the I_2-superfamily designated VcTx was shown to inhibit vertebrate $K_V1.1$ and $K_V1.3$ subtypes but not $K_V1.2$.[71] This situation may parallel the related μO- and δ-conotoxins that target sodium channels (see the sections entitled μO-Conotoxins: Inhibitors of Sodium Channel Activation and δ-Conotoxins: Inhibitors of

Sodium Channel Inactivation), but one enhances and the other inhibits channel conductance.

J-Superfamily Conotoxins

A recently characterized conopeptide with four cysteines, designated pl14a, defines a new conopeptide superfamily (J-superfamily). This peptide inhibited the $K_V1.6$ subtype of voltage-gated ion channel with micromolar affinity. Surprisingly, it also inhibited some nAChR subtypes with micromolar affinity. This was the first conopeptide characterized to date that has demonstrated inhibition of both a voltage-gated and ligand-gated ion channel.[72] For its inhibition of $K_V1.6$, pl14a is considered the defining member of the κJ-conotoxin family.

Glycosylated A-Superfamily Conotoxins

The first peptide of the group was identified from the venom of the fish-hunting *Conus striatus*.[73] The peptide, originally designated κA-conotoxin SIVA (κA-SIVA), contains an O-glycosylated serine, which was the first evidence for O-glycosylation as a post-translational modification in a biologically active conotoxin. The arrangement of the six Cys residues in κA-SIVA is similar to the pharmacologically distinct αA-conotoxins. Although the peptide is clearly an excitotoxin, there is not yet definitive evidence for its molecular target. Electrophysiologic assays suggested that κA-SIVA blocks K^+ channels. However, it has also been suggested that a homologous peptide designated CcTx from *Conus consors*, which has the same cysteine scaffold as κA-SIVA, activates neuronal voltage-gated Na^+ channels at a resting membrane potential.[74] Thus, it is likely that the glycosylated A-superfamily conotoxins target voltage-gated ion channels, but the basic mechanism that underlies their potent biologic activity needs to be clarified.

Contryphans

The contryphans contain a single disulfide bond and belong to an undesignated conopeptide superfamily. These peptides contain a post-translationally modified D-amino acid (D-tryptophan or D-leucine). The first contryphan isolated from *Conus radiatus* elicited "stiff tail" syndrome when administered intracranially to mice[75]; Leu-contryphan from *Conus purpurascens* caused body tremor and excessive mucous secretion in fish.[76] Electrophysiologic assays using mouse pancreatic B-cells suggested that glacontryphan-M from *Conus marmoreus* targeted the L-type Ca^{2+} channel.[77] Using dorsal root ganglion neurons, contryphans Am 975 and Lo959 from the snail-hunting *Conus amadis* and the worm-hunting *Conus loroisii*, respectively, were reported to affect high voltage-activated Ca^{2+} channels; whereas Am975 caused inhibition, Lo959 resulted in an increase in Ca^{2+} current.[78] The two peptides with eight amino acid residues differ in only a single hydroxyl group (4-*trans*-hydroxyproline in Am975 and proline in Lo959 at position three). Contryphan-Vn has been reported to modulate Ca^{2+} activated K^+ channels.[79] However, the precise molecular targets have not been defined.

CONOPEPTIDES TARGETED TO LIGAND-GATED ION CHANNELS

Conopeptides that target ligand-gated ion channels include those that antagonize nAChRs, the $5-HT_3$ serotonin-gated ion channel, and the NMDA class of ionotropic glutamate receptors. The most extensively characterized groups of conopeptides targeted to ligand-gated ion channels are the nAChR antagonists. The most widely distributed of the nAChR-antagonist conopeptides are the α-conotoxins.

α-Conotoxins: A Widely Distributed Family of Competitive nAChR Antagonists

The α-conotoxins, which have two disulfide bonds, belong to the A-Superfamily. This widely distributed family of venom peptides can be classified into subfamilies based on the sequence motif: $-CCX_mCX_nC-$. The major subfamilies are the α3/5-conotoxins (m=3, n=5), α4/3-conotoxins (m-4, n=3), and α4/7-conotoxins (m=4, n=7). The first members of the α-conotoxin family to be characterized were members of the α3/5-conotoxin subfamily,[80] which are found in many fish-hunting *Conus* venoms; these paralyze prey by competitive

antagonism of the neuromuscular nAChR. When tested on mammalian nAChRs, many α3/5-conotoxins appear to be highly specific for only one of the two acetylcholine-binding sites. α-Conotoxin MI (α-MI) has approximately 10,000-fold higher affinity for the binding site at the α1/δ-interface than the α1/γ-interface.[81]

The best studied of the α4/3-conotoxin subfamily are α-conotoxins ImI and ImII (α-ImI and α-ImII) from the worm-hunting *Conus imperialis* (see Fig. 36-1); both α-ImI and α-ImII inhibit homomeric nicotinic receptors composed exclusively of α7-subunits. α-ImII is almost identical in sequence to α-ImI (in nine out of 12 amino acids) and thus was expected to target the same α7-subtype as does α-ImI. Surprisingly, α-ImII did not act at the competitive ligand site that is the high-affinity target of both α-bungarotoxin and α-ImI.[82,83] It was shown that proline-5 in α-ImI was required for targeting these peptides to the competitive ligand site; α-ImII lacks this proline residue at this locus. It is worth noting that most α-conotoxins have the proline residue critical for competitive antagonism in α-ImI; the small minority of α-conotoxins (such as α-ImII) that lack this highly conserved proline residue are potential candidates for acting through a different site. The structure of α-ImI bound to the acetylcholine binding protein has been determined.[84,85] A recently characterized α4/3-conotoxin, α-conotoxin RgIA (α-RgIA), proved to be a specific antagonist of the α9α10 subtype of neuronal nAChR; the peptide exhibits analgesic effects in rat nerve pain models.[86,87]

The largest and most widely distributed subfamily of the α-conotoxins is the α4/7-conotoxin subfamily. The targets of individual members of this subfamily comprise every class of nAChR, including the muscle subtype (e.g., α-conotoxin EI [α-EI]), homomeric nAChR subtypes such as α7 (e.g., α-conotoxin PnIB [α-PnIB]), and heteromeric neuronal nAChR subtypes (e.g., α-conotoxins MII and AuIB [α-MII and α-AuIB]). Very few amino acid substitutions in α4/7-conotoxins can apparently cause a shift in targeting specificity and affinity. For instance, α-conotoxin PnIA (α-PnIA) and α-PnIB from the venom of *Conus pennaceus* differ in sequence by only two amino acids, but one preferentially targets the α7 nAChR subtype, whereas the other targets the α3β2 nAChR subtype.[88]

One proposed mechanism for the high subtype selectivity of α-conotoxins is known as the Janus ligand hypothesis; α-conotoxins have two pharmacophores for two distinct recognition sites on the receptor complex.[1,4] In this way, α-conotoxin can be specific for an interface between two particular nAChR subunits. The experimental data supporting the Janus ligand hypothesis comes from studies with α-conotoxin MII (α-MII) and its interaction between a high-affinity target nAChR subtype, the α3β2-receptor, and another subtype, the α3β4-receptor, for which the peptide has much lower affinity.[89]

αA-, αS-, and αC-Conotoxins: Competitive nAChR Antagonists with Limited Distribution

The αA-conotoxin family belongs to the A-superfamily; however, these peptides have three disulfide bonds rather than the two disulfide–bond framework of the α-conotoxins, the most widely distributed members of the A-superfamily. αA-Conotoxin PIVA (αA-PIVA), from *Conus purpurascens*, is a competitive nAChR antagonist.[90] Although αA-conotoxin OIVA (αA-OIVA), from *Conus obscurus*, is also a competitive nAChR antagonist, these peptides differ in their disulfide-bonding framework, although they are similar in their paralytic effects on fish and their antagonism of the neuromuscular nAChR.[91] Thus the αA-conotoxin family can be subdivided into two subfamilies: one group includes αA-PIVA and the other group includes αA-OIVA; they are designated as the αA$_L$- (e.g., αA-PIVA) and the αA$_S$-subfamilies (e.g., αA-OIVA), respectively[92]: the αA$_L$ peptides are longer than the αA$_S$ peptides. The known αA$_L$ peptides are inhibitors of both the mammalian fetal and adult muscle nAChRs that compete with acetylcholine for binding at both α/δ and α/γ interfaces of the nAChR.[93] The αA$_S$ peptides are selective antagonists of the fetal subtype that compete with acetylcholine for binding at the α/γ interface only.[92]

Although most nAChR antagonists in *Conus* venom appear to be from the A-superfamily (α- and αA-conotoxins), recently peptides from two other conopeptide superfamilies were characterized that target the nAChR; these are known as αS-conotoxins from the S-superfamily with five disulfide bonds[94] and the αC-conotoxins from the C-superfamily with a single disulfide bond.[95] The αS-conotoxin RVIIIA (αS-RVIIIA) isolated from *Conus radiatus* broadly targets neuromuscular and neuronal nAChRs.[94] In contrast, αC-conotoxin PrXA

(αC-PrXA) specifically blocks the muscle subtype of nAChR; it competes with α-bungarotoxin for binding at the α/γ and α/δ subunit interfaces of the nAChR, with higher affinity for the α/δ subunit interface.[95]

ψ-Conotoxins: Noncompetitive nAChR Antagonists

Unlike most other conopeptide nAChR antagonists, the ψ-conotoxins are noncompetitive antagonists of the muscle subtype of nicotinic receptors; these include ψ-conotoxins PIIIE and PIIIF (ψ-PIIIE, and ψ-PIIIF). NMR structures have been determined for these peptides.[96-98] The ψ-conotoxins were originally believed to be restricted to a single clade of fish-hunting cone snails in the Eastern Pacific and the Caribbean. However, they have recently been found in Indo-Pacific fish-hunting cone snails as well.[99] Structurally, the ψ-conotoxins are most closely related to the μ-conotoxins that are Na$^+$ channel blockers, and the κM-conotoxins that block K$^+$ channels. Although ψ-, μ- and κM-conotoxins affect different targets, they may effectively act by plugging the ion permeation pathway.

σ-Conotoxin: Serotonin-Gated Ion Channel Receptor Antagonist

An unusual conopeptide containing 6-bromo-tryptophan and 10 cysteine residues, designated σ-conotoxin GVIIIA (σ-GVIIIA), was isolated from *Conus geographus* and shown to be a competitive antagonist of the 5-HT$_3$ serotonin-gated ion channel.[100] So far, this is the only peptidic toxin known to target this receptor. Many other peptides belong to the same gene superfamily (S-superfamily) as σ−GVIIIA, but because of their sequence divergence, they appear unlikely to target the 5-HT$_3$ receptor. As mentioned earlier, αS-RVIIIA, which also belongs to the S-superfamily, targets nAChRs.[94]

CONANTOKINS: N-METHYL-D-ASPARTATE RECEPTOR ANTAGONISTS

The conantokins (originally called "sleeper peptides") were first discovered because of their ability to induce sleep in young mice and hyperactivity in older mice.[17,101] They are antagonists of NMDA receptors; these peptides are biochemically distinctive in their high content of γ-carboxyglutamate, while cysteine residues are generally absent.[17,102,103] Biochemical characterization of conantokin-G (con-G) revealed five γ-carboxyglutamate (Gla) residues. Because of the absence of disulfide bonds in this peptide, it is the Gla residues that provide the structural framework to form an α-helical conformation.[104-107]

The first evidence suggesting that conantokins inhibited NMDA receptors was obtained using a neonatal rat cerebellum preparation; con-G blocked the rise in cyclic guanosine monophosphate levels induced by the addition of NMDA.[108] It was shown that the peptide was a competitive antagonist of the glutamate binding site.[109-111] It has been established that the glutamate binding site is located on the extracellular domains of NR2 subunits,[112] whereas the homologous positions in the NR1 subunit interact with glycine, the coagonist for NMDA receptors. Two studies suggested that con-G is a selective antagonist of NMDA receptors containing an NR2B subunit[109,113]; however, this strong selectivity for the NR2B subunit was not observed in a third study.[111]

Other conantokins have been characterized from various fish-hunting *Conus* species: conantokin-T (con-T),[102] conantokin-L (con-L),[103] and conantokin-R (con-R).[114] In contrast to con-G, these peptides do not appear to discriminate between NR2B- and NR2A-containing complexes[111,113,114]; however, con-R showed NMDA receptor subtype selectivity because the peptide did not inhibit NR2D-containing receptor complexes.[114] With the Frings audiogenic seizure mouse model, con-R proved to be an antagonist of NMDA receptors, with potent anticonvulsant activity and relatively low toxicity.[114] Although con-L has a sequence that is almost identical to that of con-R near the N-terminus, and is as potent as conantokin-R in blocking NMDA receptors in vitro, it has much lower anticonvulsant potency in vivo compared with con-R.[103]

OTHER BIOLOGICALLY ACTIVE CONSTITUENTS OF *CONUS* VENOMS

In previous sections, we focused on *Conus* peptides that target either voltage-gated or ligand-gated ion channels. In this section, we briefly summarize other conopeptides that do not belong to the categories reviewed earlier (see Table 36-4). One group of conopeptides have been shown to target G protein–coupled receptors: conopressin-G, an agonist of the vasopressin receptor,[115] and contulakin-G, which is an agonist of the neurotensin receptor.[116] These two conopeptides have sequence similarity to the mammalian neuropeptides that are the endogenous agonists of these receptors. The ρ-conotoxin TIA (ρ-TIA), which has been shown to target the α_1-adrenergic receptor, is a G protein–coupled receptor antagonist.[117] The χ-conotoxins, including χ-conotoxin MrIA (χ-MrIA) (also called mr5a), target the norepinephrine transporter.[117-119] Peptide tx5a (also termed ε-TxIX) likely targets either a G protein–coupled receptor or an ion channel.[120,121]

Several conopeptides were reported to have an ion channel target but do not fall under any of the families as presently defined; these include μ–PnIVA and γ-conotoxin PnVIIA (γ-PnVIIA) from *Conus pennaceus*,[122,123] which target molluscan voltage-gated Na^+ channels and pacemaker channels, respectively. The conorfamide from the worm-hunting *Conus spurius* venom is possibly an agonist of FMRFamide-gated ion channels and a modulator of epithelial Na^+ channels in mammals.[124]

There are biologically active conopeptides whose targets have not been defined; these include the bromosleeper peptide,[125] the light sleeper peptide r7a,[126] and the spasmodic peptide.[127] In many cases, it has been difficult to determine the functions of the individual venom constituents. The constituents that are biochemically and structurally unrelated may have convergent physiologic roles. Often, it is the synergy between multiple conotoxins that makes *Conus* venoms rapidly acting, potent, and effective neuropharmacologic concoctions.

THERAPEUTIC APPLICATIONS OF CONOTOXINS

The increasing interest in conotoxins arises in part from their clinical potential. In addition to their widespread use as tools for neurobiologists, several conopeptides are being developed for therapeutic applications. Notably, six different conopeptides have reached human clinical trials for pain, with five distinct mechanisms of action (Table 36-5).[3,128-130]

TABLE 36-5 Conopeptides That Have Reached Human Clinical Trials as Therapeutic Drugs

Peptide	Amino Acid Sequence	Target	Reference
ω-MVIIA	CKGKGAKCSRLMYDCCTGSCRSGKC*	Ca^{2+} channel (N-type)	59, 60
ω-CVID	CKSKGAKCSKLMYDCCSGSCSGTVGRC*	Ca^{2+} channel (N-type)	65
Conantokin-G	GEγγLQγNQγLIRγKSN*	NMDAR (NR2B)	17, 101
Contulakin-G	ZSEEGGSNATKKPYIL	Neurotensin receptor	116
α-Vc1.1	GCCSDPRCNYDHPEIC*	nAChR (α9α10)	87, 139
χ-MrIA	NGVCCGYKLCHOC	Norepinephrine transporter	140

Z, pyroglutamate; nAChR, nicotinic acetylcholine receptor; NMDAR, N-methyl-D-aspartate receptor, O, 4-*trans*-hydroxyproline; γ, γ-carboxyglutamate; T, O-glycosylated threonine; *, C-terminal amidation. All of these peptides advanced to human clinical trials as drugs for pain. Conantokin-G also advanced to clinical trials as a drug for epilepsy. A derivative of χ-MrIA, rather than the native peptide, advanced to human clinical trials.

In December, 2004, the United States Food and Drug Administration approved ω-conotoxin MVIIA (ω-MVIIA) as a drug, which is called Prialt (Ziconitide, Elan Corporation), for the treatment of intractable chronic pain. This peptide is a specific inhibitor of the N-type calcium channel, Ca$_V$2.2. A related peptide, ω-conotoxin CVID (ω-CVID), is now being developed as a drug (AM336, Zenyth Therapeutics, formerly Amrad) for intractable pain. In the mammalian spinal cord, the synapses with incoming C-fibers that propagate nociceptive signals are particularly sensitive to inhibition of Ca$_V$2.2 by these ω-conotoxins.[129-133]

In addition to the N-type calcium channel antagonists, conopeptides with diverse mechanisms of action are in development as analgesic drugs. Conantokin-G targets NMDA receptors; it is a potent anticonvulsant and analgesic, and has reached human clinical trials as a drug (CGX-1007, Cognetix) for both epilepsy and pain.[134] Moreover, it has been shown to be neuroprotective in rat models of ischemia.[135,136] Contulakin-G, which appears to be a neurotensin receptor agonist has advanced to Phase I clinical trials as an analgesic drug (CGX-1160, Cognetix).[73,116] The α9α10 nAChR antagonist, α-conotoxin Vc1.1 (α-Vc1.1), has reached Phase II clinical trials for pain (ACV-1, Metabolic Pharmaceuticals).[137-139] Finally, a derivative of χ-conotoxin Mr1A (χ-Mr1A), which inhibits norepinephrine uptake, has advanced to Phase I clinical trails as an analgesic drug (Xen2174, Xenome).[140] Although the analgesic properties of conopeptides have been investigated extensively, there are many additional potential clinical applications. As just one exmple, κ-PVIIA (CGX-1051, Cognetix, Inc.) has demonstrated

cardioprotection for myocardial ischemia and reperfusion injury.[141,142]

From many perspectives, conopeptides have proven to be valuable and interesting. The applications in neuroscience research and the emerging clinical applications decisively validate their utility. In addition, both basic and applied science have advanced significantly from the valuable insights gained by studying the biology of cone snails, and the vast array of unique pharmacologic agents that have evolved to enable the cone snails to thrive in their complex environments.

ACKNOWLEDGMENT

The research was supported by National Institute of General Medical Sciences Grant GM-48677. We thank Maren Watkins for her help in preparing this review.

References

1. Olivera BM. E.E. Just Lecture, 1996. Conus venom peptides, receptor and ion channel targets, and drug design: 50 million years of neuropharmacology. *Mol Biol Cell.* 1997;8:2101-2109.
2. Olivera BM. Conus venom peptides: reflections from the biology of clades and species. *Annu Rev Ecol Syst.* 2002;33:25-47.
3. Olivera BM. Conus peptides: biodiversity-based discovery and exogenomics. *J Biol Chem.* 2006;281:31173-31177.
4. Olivera BM, Imperial JS, Bulaj G. Cone snails and conotoxins: evolving sophisticated neuropharmacology. In: Menez A, ed. *Perspectives in Molecular Toxinology,* West Sussex, England: John Wiley and Sons Ltd.; 2002:143-158.
5. Olivera BM, Walker C, Cartier GE, Hooper D, Santos AD, Schoenfeld R, et al. Speciation of cone snails and interspecific hyperdivergence of their venom peptides.

Potential evolutionary significance of introns. *Ann N Y Acad Sci.* 1999;870:223-237.

6. Terlau H, Olivera BM. Conus venoms: a rich source of ion channel-targeted peptides. *Physiol Rev.* 2004;84:41-68.

7. Röckel D, Korn W, Kohn AJ. *Manual of the Living Conidae.* Wiesbaden, Germany: Verlag Christa Hemmen; 1995.

8. Olivera BM, Gray WR, Zeikus R, McIntosh JM, Varga J, Rivier J, et al. Peptide neurotoxins from fish-hunting cone snails. *Science.* 1985;230:1338-1343.

9. Terlau H, Shon KJ, Grilley M, Stocker M, Stuhmer W, Olivera BM. Strategy for rapid immobilization of prey by a fish-hunting marine snail. *Nature.* 1996;381:148-151.

10. Woodward SR, Cruz LJ, Olivera BM, Hillyard DR. Constant and hypervariable regions in conotoxin propeptides. *Embo J.* 1990;9:1015-1020.

11. Conticello SG, Gilad Y, Avidan N, Ben-Asher E, Levy Z, Fainzilber M. Mechanisms for evolving hypervariability: the case of conopeptides. *Mol Biol Evol.* 2001;18:120-131.

12. Duda Jr TF, Palumbi SR. Molecular genetics of ecological diversification: duplication and rapid evolution of toxin genes of the venomous gastropod Conus. *Proc Natl Acad Sci U S A.* 1999;96:6820-6823.

13. Espiritu DJ, Watkins M, Dia-Monje V, Cartier GE, Cruz LJ, Olivera BM. Venomous cone snails: molecular phylogeny and the generation of toxin diversity. *Toxicon.* 2001;39:1899-1916.

14. Buczek O, Bulaj G, Olivera BM. Conotoxins and the posttranslational modification of secreted gene products. *Cell Mol Life Sci.* 2005;62:3067-3079.

15. Craig AG, Bandyopadhyay P, Olivera BM. Post-translationally modified neuropeptides from Conus venoms. *Eur J Biochem.* 1999;264:271-275.

16. Bandyopadhyay PK, Colledge CJ, Walker CS, Zhou LM, Hillyard DR, Olivera BM. Conantokin-G precursor and its role in γ-carboxylation by a vitamin K-dependent carboxylase from a Conus snail. *J Biol Chem.* 1998;273:5447-5450.

17. McIntosh JM, Olivera BM, Cruz LJ, Gray WR. γ-carboxyglutamate in a neuroactive toxin. *J Biol Chem.* 1984;259:14343-14346.

18. Bandyopadhyay PK, Garrett JE, Shetty RP, Keate T, Walker CS, Olivera BM. γ-Glutamyl carboxylation: An extracellular posttranslational modification that antedates the divergence of molluscs, arthropods, and chordates. *Proc Natl Acad Sci U S A.* 2002;99:1264-1269.

19. Czerwiec E, Begley GS, Bronstein M, Stenflo J, Taylor KL, Furie BC, et al. Expression and characterization of recombinant vitamin K-dependent γ-glutamyl carboxylase from an invertebrate, Conus textile. *Eur J Biochem.* 2002;269:6162-6172.

20. Stanley TB, Stafford DW, Olivera BM, Bandyopadhyay PK. Identification of a vitamin K-dependent carboxylase in the venom duct of a Conus snail. *FEBS Lett.* 1997;407:85-88.

21. Hooper D, Lirazan MB, Schoenfeld R, Cook B, Cruz LJ, Olivera BM, et al. Post-translational modifications: a two-dimensional strategy for molecular diversity of Conus peptides. In: Fields GB, Tam JP, Barany G, eds. *Peptides for the New Millennium: Proceedings of the Sixteenth American Peptide Symposium.* Dordrecht, The Netherlands: Kluwer Academic Publishers; 2000:727-729.

22. Olivera BM, Cruz L. Conotoxins, in retrospect. *Toxicon.* 2001;39:7-14.

23. Hille B. *Ion Channels of Excitable Membranes.* 3rd ed. Sunderland, MA: Sinauer Associates, Inc; 2001.

24. Catterall WA. Cellular and molecular biology of voltage-gated sodium channels. *Physiol. Rev.* 1992;72:S15-S48.

25. Kandel ER, Schwartz JH, Jessel TM. *Principles of Neural Science.* 4th ed, New York: McGraw-Hill; 2000.

26. Cruz LJ, Gray WR, Olivera BM, Zeikus RD, Kerr L, Yoshikami D, et al. Conus geographus toxins that discriminate between neuronal and muscle sodium channels. *J Biol Chem.* 1985;260:9280-9288.

27. Sato S, Nakamura H, Ohizumi Y, Kobayashi J, Hirata Y. The amino acid sequences of homologous hydroxyproline containing myotoxins from the marine snail Conus geographus venom. *FEBS Lett.* 1983;155:277-280.

28. Becker S, Prusak-Sochaczewski E, Zamponi G, Beck-Sickinger AG, Gordon RD, French RJ. Action of derivatives of mu-conotoxin GIIIA on sodium channels. Single amino acid substitutions in the toxin separately affect association and dissociation rates. *Biochemistry.* 1992;31:8229-8238.

29. Gray WR, Olivera BM, Cruz LJ. Peptide toxins from venomous Conus snails. *Annu Rev Biochem.* 1988;57:665-700.

30. Dudley Jr SC, Todt H, Lipkind G, Fozzard HA. A mu-conotoxin-insensitive Na+ channel mutant: possible localization of a binding site at the outer vestibule. *Biophys J.* 1995;69:1657-1665.

31. French RJ, Prusak-Sochaczewski E, Zamponi GW, Becker S, Kularatna AS, Horn R. Interactions between a pore-blocking peptide and the voltage-sensor of the sodium channel: an electrostatic approach to channel geometry. *Neuron.* 1996;16:407-413.

32. Hui K, Lipkind G, Fozzard HA, French RJ. Electrostatic and steric contributions to block of the skeletal muscle sodium channel by mu-conotoxin. *J Gen Physiol.* 2002;119:45-54.

33. Shon KJ, Olivera BM, Watkins M, Jacobsen RB, Gray WR, Floresca CZ, et al. mu-Conotoxin PIIIA, a new peptide for discriminating among tetrodotoxin-sensitive Na channel subtypes. *J Neurosci.* 1998;18:4473-4481.

34. Keiser DW, West PJ, Lee EF, Yoshikami D, Olivera BM, Bulaj G, et al. Structural basis for tetrodotoxin-resistant sodium channel binding by mu-conotoxin SmIIIA. *J Biol Chem.* 2003;278:46805-46813.

35. West PJ, Bulaj G, Garrett JE, Olivera BM, Yoshikami D. mu-conotoxin SmIIIA, a potent inhibitor of tetrodotoxin-resistant sodium channels in amphibian sympathetic and sensory neurons. *Biochemistry.* 2002;41:15388-15393.

36. Bulaj G, West PJ, Garrett JE, Watkins M, Zhang MM, Norton RS, et al. Novel conotoxins from Conus striatus and Conus kinoshitai selectively block TTX-resistant sodium channels. *Biochemistry.* 2005;44:7259-7265.

37. Zhang MM, Green BR, Catlin P, Fiedler B, Azam L, Chadwick A, et al. Structure/function characterization of mu-conotoxin KIIIA, an analgesic, nearly irreversible blocker of neuronal mammalian sodium channels. *J Biol Chem.* 2007;282:30699-39706.

38. Green BR, Catlin P, Zhang MM, Fiedler B, Bayudan W, Morrison A, et al. Conotoxins containing nonnatural backbone spacers: cladistic-based design, chemical synthesis, and improved analgesic activity. *Chem Biol.* 2007;14:399-407.

39. McIntosh JM, Hasson A, Spira ME, Gray WR, Li W, Marsh M, et al. A new family of conotoxins that

blocks voltage-gated sodium channels. *J Biol Chem.* 1995;270:16796-16802.

40. Terlau H, Stocker M, Shon KJ, McIntosh JM, Olivera BM. μO-conotoxin MrVIA inhibits mammalian sodium channels, but not through site I. *J Neurophysiol.* 1996;76:1423-1429.

41. Zorn S, Leipold E, Hansen A, Bulaj G, Olivera BM, Terlau H, et al. The μO-conotoxin MrVIA inhibits voltage-gated sodium channels by associating with domain-3. *FEBS Lett.* 2006;580:1360-1364.

42. Bulaj G, Zhang MM, Green BR, Fiedler B, Layer RT, Wei S, et al. Synthetic μO-conotoxin MrVIB blocks TTX-resistant sodium channel NaV1.8 and has a long-lasting analgesic activity. *Biochemistry.* 2006;45:7404-7414.

43. Ekberg J, Jayamanne A, Vaughan CW, Aslan S, Thomas L, Mould J, et al. μO-conotoxin MrVIB selectively blocks NaV1.8 sensory neuron specific sodium channels and chronic pain behavior without motor deficits. *Proc Natl Acad Sci U S A.* 2006;103:17030-17035.

44. Buczek O, Wei D, Babon JJ, Yang X, Fiedler B, Yoshikami D, et al. Structure and sodium channel activity of an excitatory I(1)-superfamily conotoxin. *Biochemistry.* 2007;46:9929-9940.

45. Buczek O, Yoshikami D, Watkins M, Bulaj G, Jimenez EC, Olivera BM. Characterization of D-amino-acid-containing excitatory conotoxins and redefinition of the I-conotoxin superfamily. *FEBS J.* 2005;272:4178-4188.

46. Hillyard DR, Olivera BM, Woodward S, Corpuz GP, Gray WR, Ramilo CA, et al. A molluscivorous Conus toxin: conserved frameworks in conotoxins. *Biochemistry.* 1989;28:358-361.

47. Shon KJ, Grilley MM, Marsh M, Yoshikami D, Hall AR, Kurz B, et al. Purification, characterization, synthesis, and cloning of the lockjaw peptide from Conus purpurascens venom. *Biochemistry.* 1995;34:4913-4918.

48. West PJ, Bulaj G, Yoshikami D. Effects of delta-conotoxins PVIA and SVIE on sodium channels in the amphibian sympathetic nervous system. *J Neurophysiol.* 2005;94:3916-3924.

49. Hasson A, Shon KJ, Olivera BM, Spira ME. Alterations of voltage-activated sodium current by a novel conotoxin from the venom of Conus gloriamaris. *J Neurophysiol.* 1995;73:1295-1301.

50. Shon KJ, Hasson A, Spira ME, Cruz LJ, Gray WR, Olivera BM. δ-conotoxin GmVIA, a novel peptide from the venom of Conus gloriamaris. *Biochemistry.* 1994;33:11420-11425.

51. Shon KJ, Stocker M, Terlau H, Stuhmer W, Jacobsen R, Walker C, et al. κ-Conotoxin PVIIA is a peptide inhibiting the shaker K+ channel. *J Biol Chem.* 1998;273:33-38.

52. Kim M, Baro DJ, Lanning CC, Doshi M, Farnham J, Moskowitz HS, et al. Alternative splicing in the pore-forming region of shaker potassium channels. *J Neurosci.* 1997;17:8213-8224.

53. Ferber M, Sporning A, Jeserich G, DeLaCruz R, Watkins M, Olivera BM, et al. A novel conus peptide ligand for K+ channels. *J Biol Chem.* 2003;278:2177-2183.

54. Ferber M, Al-Sabi A, Stocker M, Olivera BM, Terlau H. Identification of a mammalian target of κM-conotoxin RIIIK. *Toxicon.* 2004;43:915-921.

55. Imperial JS, Silverton N, Olivera BM, Bandyopadhyay PK, Sporning A, Ferber M, et al. Using chemistry to reconstruct evolution: On the origins of fish-hunting is venomous cone snails. *Proc Am Philos Soc.* 2007;151:185-200.

56. Pritchard L, Dufton MJ. Evolutionary trace analysis of the Kunitz/BPTI family of proteins: functional divergence may have been based on conformational adjustment. *J Mol Biol.* 1999;285:1589-1607.

57. Olivera BM, McIntosh JM, Cruz LJ, Luque FA, Gray WR. Purification and sequence of a presynaptic peptide toxin from Conus geographus venom. *Biochemistry.* 1984;23:5087-5090.

58. Reynolds IJ, Wagner JA, Snyder SH, Thayer SA, Olivera BM, Miller RJ. Brain voltage-sensitive calcium channel subtypes differentiated by ω-conotoxin fraction GVIA. *Proc Natl Acad Sci U S A.* 1986;83:8804-8807.

59. Hillyard DR, Monje VD, Mintz IM, Bean BP, Nadasdi L, Ramachandran J, et al. A new Conus peptide ligand for mammalian presynaptic Ca2+ channels. *Neuron.* 1992;9:69-77.

60. Olivera BM, Cruz LJ, de Santos V, LeCheminant GW, Griffin D, Zeikus R, et al. Neuronal calcium channel antagonists. Discrimination between calcium channel subtypes using omega-conotoxin from Conus magus venom. *Biochemistry.* 1987;26:2086-2090.

61. Nadasdi L, Yamashiro D, Chung D, Tarczy-Hornoch K, Adriaenssens P, Ramachandran J. Structure-activity analysis of a Conus peptide blocker of N-type neuronal calcium channel. *Biochemistry.* 1995;34:8076-8081.

62. Kim JI, Takahashi M, Ogura A, Kohno T, Kudo Y, Sato K. Hydroxyl group of Tyr13 is essential for the activity of ω-conotoxin GVIA, a peptide toxin for N-type calcium channel. *J Biol Chem.* 1994;273:23876-23878.

63. Lew MJ, Flinn JP, Pallaghy PK, Murphy R, Whorlow SL, Wright CE, et al. Structure-function relationships of ω-conotoxin GVIA. Synthesis, structure, calcium channel binding, and functional assay of alanine-substituted analogs. *J Biol Chem.* 1997;272:12014-12023.

64. Nielsen KJ, Adams DA, Alewood PF, Lewis RJ, Thomas L, Schroeder T, et al. Effects of chirality at Tyr13 on the structure-activity relationships of ω-conotoxins from Conus magus. *Biochemistry.* 1999;38:6741-6751.

65. Adams DJ, Smith AB, Schroeder CI, Yasuda T, Lewis RJ. Omega-conotoxin CVID inhibits a pharmacologically distinct voltage-sensitive calcium channel associated with transmitter release from preganglionic nerve terminals. *J Biol Chem.* 2003;278:4057-4062.

66. Fainzilber M, Lodder JC, van der Schors RC, Li KW, Yu Z, Burlingame AL, et al. A novel hydrophobic ω-conotoxin blocks molluscan dihydropyridine-sensitive calcium channels. *Biochemistry.* 1996;35:8748-8752.

67. Dunlap K, Luebke JI, Turner TJ. Exocytotic Ca2+ channels in mammalian central neurons. *Trends Neurosci.* 1995;18:89-98.

68. McIntosh JM, Olivera BM, Cruz LJ. Conus peptides as probes for ion channels. *Methods Enzymol.* 1999;294:605-624.

69. Olivera BM, Miljanich GP, Ramachandran J, Adams ME. Calcium channel diversity and neurotransmitter release: the ω-conotoxins and omega-agatoxins. *Annu Rev Biochem.* 1994;63:823-867.

70. Fan C-X, Chen X-K, Zhang C, Wang L-X, Duan KL, He LL, et al. A novel conotoxin from Conus betulinus, κ-BtX, unique in cysteine pattern and in function is a specific BK channel modulator. *J Biol Chem.* 2003;278:12624-12633.

71. Kauferstein S, Huys I, Lamthanh H, Stöcklin R, Sotto F, Menez A, et al. A novel conotoxin inhibiting vertebrate voltage-sensitive potassium channels. *Toxicon.* 2003;42:43-52.

72. Imperial JS, Bansal PS, Alewood PF, Daly NL, Craik DJ, Sporning A, et al. A novel conotoxin inhibitor of Kv1.6 channel and nAChR subtypes defines a new superfamily of conotoxins. *Biochemistry*. 2006;45: 8331-8340.

73. Craig AG, Zafaralla G, Cruz LJ, Santos AD, Hillyard DR, Dykert J, et al. An O-glycosylated neuroexcitatory Conus peptide. *Biochemistry*. 1998;37:16019-16025.

74. Le Gall F, Favreau P, Benoit E, Mattei C, Bouet F, Menou J-L, et al. A new conotoxin isolated from Conus consors venom acting selectively on axons and motor nerve terminals through a Na+-dependent mechanism. *Eur J Neurosci*. 1999;11:3134-3142.

75. Jimenez EC, Olivera BM, Gray WR, Cruz LJ. Contryphan is a D-tryptophan-containing Conus peptide. *J Biol Chem*. 1996;271:28002-28005.

76. Jacobsen RB, Jimenez EC, De la Cruz RG, Gray WR, Cruz LJ, Olivera BM. A novel D-leucine-containing Conus peptide: diverse conformational dynamics in the contryphan family. *J Pept Res*. 1999;54:93-99.

77. Hansson K, Ma X, Eliasson L, Czerwiec E, Furie B, Furie BC, et al. The first Gla-containing contryphan: a selective L-type calcium ion channel blocker isolated from the venom of Conus marmoreus. *J Biol Chem*. 2004;279:32453-32463.

78. Sabareesh V, Gowd KH, Ramasamy P, Sudarslal S, Krishnan KS, Sikdar SK, et al. Characterization of contryphans from Conus loroisii and Conus amadis that target calcium channels. *Peptides*. 2006;27:2647-2654.

79. Massilia GR, Eliseo T, Grolleau F, Lapied B, Barbier J, et al. Contryphan-Vn: a modulator of Ca2+-dependent K+ channels. *Biochem Biophys Res Commun*. 2003;303: 238-246.

80. McIntosh JM, Santos AD, Olivera BM. Conus peptides targeted to specific nicotinic acetylcholine receptor subtypes. *Annu Rev Biochem*. 1999;68:59-88.

81. Sine SM, Kreienkamp H-J, Bren N, Maeda R, Taylor P. Molecular dissection of subunit interfaces in the acetylcholine receptor: identification of determinants of α-conotoxin MI selectivity. *Neuron*. 1995;15:205-211.

82. Ellison M, McIntosh JM, Olivera BM. α-conotoxins ImI and ImII. Similar α7 nicotinic receptor antagonists act at different sites. *J Biol Chem*. 2003;278:757-764.

83. McIntosh JM, Yoshikami D, Mahe E, Nielsen DB, Rivier JE, Gray WR, et al. A nicotinic acetylcholine receptor ligand of unique specificity, α-conotoxin ImI. *J Biol Chem*. 1994;269:16733-16799.

84. Hansen SB, Sulzenbacher G, Huxford T, Marchot P, Taylor P, Bourne Y. Structures of Aplysia AChBP complexes with nicotinic agonists and antagonists reveal distinctive binding interfaces and conformations. *EMBO J*. 2005;24:3635-3646.

85. Ulens C, Hogg RC, Celie PH, Bertrand D, Tsetlin V, Smit AB, et al. Structural determinants of selective alpha-conotoxin binding to a nicotinic acetylcholine receptor homolog AChBP. *Proc Natl Acad Sci U S A*. 2006;103:3615-3620.

86. Ellison M, Haberlandt C, Gomez-Casati ME, Watkins M, Elgoyhen AB, McIntosh JM, et al. Alpha-RgIA: a novel conotoxin that specifically and potently blocks the alpha9alpha10 nAChR. *Biochemistry*. 2006;45:1511-1517.

87. Vincler M, Wittenauer S, Parker R, Ellison M, Olivera BM, McIntosh JM. Molecular mechanism for analgesia involving specific antagonism of α9α10 nicotinic acetylcholine receptors. *Proc Natl Acad Sci U S A*. 2006;103:17880-17884.

88. Luo S, Nguyen TA, Cartier GE, Olivera BM, Yoshikami D, McIntosh JM. Single-residue alteration in alpha-conotoxin PnIA switches its nAChR subtype selectivity. *Biochemistry*. 1999;38:14542-14548.

89. Cartier GE, Yoshikami D, Gray WR, Luo S, Olivera BM, McIntosh JM. A new α-conotoxin which targets α3β2 nicotinic acetylcholine receptors. *J Biol Chem*. 1996;271:7522-7528.

90. Hopkins C, Grilley M, Miller C, Shon KJ, Cruz LJ, Gray WR, et al. A new family of Conus peptides targeted to the nicotinic acetylcholine receptor. *J Biol Chem*. 1995;270:22361-22367.

91. Teichert RW, Rivier J, Dykert J, Cervini L, Gulyas J, Bulaj G, et al. αA-Conotoxin OIVA defines a new αA-conotoxin subfamily of nicotinic acetylcholine receptor inhibitors. *Toxicon*. 2004;44:207-214.

92. Teichert RW, Lopez-Vera E, Gulyas J, Watkins M, Rivier J, Olivera BM. Definition and characterization of the short αA-conotoxins: a single residue determines dissociation kinetics from the fetal muscle nicotinic acetylcholine receptor. *Biochemistry*. 2006;45:1304-1312.

93. Jacobsen R, Yoshikami D, Ellison M, Martinez J, Gray WR, Cartier GE, et al. Differential targeting of nicotinic acetylcholine receptors by novel alphaA-conotoxins. *J Biol Chem*. 1997;272:22531-22537.

94. Teichert RW, Jimenez EC, Olivera BM. αS-conotoxin RVIIIA: a structurally unique conotoxin that broadly targets nicotinic acetylcholine receptors. *Biochemistry*. 2005;44:7897-7902.

95. Jimenez EC, Olivera BM, Teichert RW. αC-Conotoxin PrXA: a new family of nicotinic acetylcholine receptor antagonists. *Biochemistry*. 2007;46:8717-8724.

96. Mitchell SS, Shon KJ, Foster MP, Davis DR, Olivera BM, Ireland CM. Three-dimensional solution structure of conotoxin ψ-PIIIE, an acetylcholine gated ion channel antagonist. *Biochemistry*. 1998;37:1215-1220.

97. Shon KJ, Grilley M, Jacobsen R, Cartier GE, Hopkins C, Gray WR, et al. A noncompetitive peptide inhibitor of the nicotinic acetylcholine receptor from Conus purpurascens venom. *Biochemistry*. 1997;36:9581-9587.

98. Van Wagoner RM, Jacobsen RB, Olivera BM, Ireland CM. Characterization and three-dimensional structure determination of ψ-conotoxin PIIIF, a novel noncompetitive antagonist of nicotinic acetylcholine receptors. *Biochemistry*. 2003;42:6353-6362.

99. Lluisma AO, Lopez-Vera E, Bulaj G, Watkins M, Olivera BM. Characterization of a novel psi-conotoxin from Conus parius Reeve. *Toxicon*. 2008;51:174-180.

100. England LJ, Imperial J, Jacobsen R, Craig AG, Gulyas J, Akhtar M, et al. Inactivation of a serotonin-gated ion channel by a polypeptide toxin from marine snails. *Science*. 1998;281:575-578.

101. Olivera BM, McIntosh JM, Clark C, Middlemas D, Gray WR, Cruz LJ. A sleep-inducing peptide from Conus geographus venom. *Toxicon*. 1985;23:277-282.

102. Haack JA, Rivier J, Parks TN, Mena EE, Cruz LJ, Olivera BM. Conantokin-T. A γ-carboxyglutamate containing peptide with N-methyl-d-aspartate antagonist activity. *J Biol Chem*. 1990;265:6025-6029.

103. Jimenez EC, Donevan S, Walker C, Zhou LM, Nielsen J, Cruz LJ, et al. Conantokin-L, a new NMDA receptor antagonist: determinants for anticonvulsant potency. *Epilepsy Res*. 2002;51:73-80.

104. Chen Z, Blandl T, Prorok M, Warder SE, Li L, Zhu Y, et al. Conformational changes in conantokin-G induced upon binding of calcium and magnesium as revealed by NMR structural analysis. *J Biol Chem*. 1998;273:16248-16258.

105. Myers RA, McIntosh JM, Imperial J, Williams RW, Oas T, Haack JA, et al. Peptides from Conus venoms which which affect Ca++ entry into neurons. *J Toxin Toxin Rev.* 1990;9:179-202.

106. Rigby AC, Baleja JD, Furie BC, Furie B. Three-dimensional structure of a γ-carboxyglutamic acid-containing conotoxin, conantokin-G, from the marine snail Conus geographus. The metal-free conformer. *Biochemistry.* 1997;36:6906-6914.

107. Skjaebaek N, Nielsen KJ, Lewis RJ, Alewood P, Craik DJ. Determination of the solution structures of con-antokin-G and conantokin-T by CD and NMR spectroscopy. *J Biol Chem.* 1997;272:2291-2299.

108. Mena EE, Gullak MF, Pagnozzi MJ, Richter KE, Rivier J, Cruz LJ, et al. Conantokin-G: a novel peptide antagonist to the N-methyl-D-aspartic acid (NMDA) receptor. *Neurosci Lett.* 1990;118:241-244.

109. Donevan SD, McCabe RT. Conantokin-G is an NR2B-selective competitive antagonist of N-methyl-D-aspartate receptors. *Mol Pharmacol.* 2000;58:614-623.

110. Hammerland LG, Olivera BM, Yoshikami D. Conantokin-G selectively inhibits N-methyl-D-aspartate-induced currents in Xenopus oocytes injected with mouse brain mRNA. *Eur J Pharmacol.* 1992;226:239-244.

111. Wittekindt B, Malany S, Schemm R, Otvos L, Maccecchini ML, Laube B, et al. Point mutations identify the glutamate binding pocket of the N-methyl-D-aspartate receptor as a major site conantokin-G inhibition. *Neuropharmacology.* 2001;41:753-761.

112. Laube B, Hirai H, Sturgess M, Betz H, Kuhse J. Molecular determinants of agonist discrimination by NMDA receptor subunits: analysis of the gluta-mate binding site on the NR2B subunit. *Neuron.* 1997;18:493-503.

113. Klein RC, Prorok M, Galdzicki Z, Castellino FJ. The amino acid residue at sequence position 5 in the con-antokin peptides partially governs subunit-selective antagonism of recombinant N-methyl-D-aspartate receptors. *J Biol Chem.* 2001;276:26860-26867.

114. White HS, McCabe RT, Armstrong H, Donevan SD, Cruz LJ, Abogadie FC, et al. In vitro and in vivo characterization of conantokin-R, a selective NMDA receptor antagonist isolated from the venom of the fish-hunting snail Conus radiatus. *J Pharmacol Exp Ther.* 2000;292:425-432.

115. Cruz LJ, Johnson DS, Olivera BM. Characterization of the ω-conotoxin target. Evidence for tissue-specific heterogeneity in calcium channel types. *Biochemistry.* 1987;26:820-824.

116. Craig AG, Norberg T, Griffin D, Hoeger C, Akhtar M, Schmidt K, et al. Contulakin-G, an O-glycosylated invertebrate neurotensin. *J Biol Chem.* 1999;274:13752-13759.

117. Sharpe IA, Gehrmann J, Loughnan ML, Thomas L, Adams DA, Atkins A, et al. Two new classes of con-opeptides inhibit the α1-adrenoceptor and noradren-aline transporter. *Nat Neurosci.* 2001;4:902-907.

118. Balaji RA, Ohtake A, Sato K, Gopalakrishnakone P, Kini RM, Seow KT, et al. Lambda-conotoxins, a new family of conotoxins with unique disulfide pattern and protein folding. Isolation and characterization from the venom of Conus marmoreus. *J Biol Chem.* 2000;275:39516-39522.

119. McIntosh JM, Corpuz GO, Layer RT, Garrett JE, Wagstaff JD, Bulaj G, et al. Isolation and characterization of a novel Conus peptide with apparent antino-ciceptive activity. *J Biol Chem.* 2000;275:32391-32397.

120. Rigby AC, Lucas-Meunier E, Kalume DE, Czerwiec E, Hambe B, Dahlqvist I, et al. A conotoxin from Conus textile with unusual posttranslational modifications reduces presynaptic Ca2+ influx. *Proc Natl Acad Sci U S A.* 1999;96:5758-5763.

121. Walker CS, Steel D, Jacobsen RB, Lirazan MB, Cruz LJ, Hooper D, et al. The T-superfamily of conotoxins. *J Biol Chem.* 1999;274:30664-30671.

122. Fainzilber M, Nakamura T, Gaathon A, Lodder JC, Kits KS, Burlingame AL, et al. A new cysteine frame-work in sodium channel blocking conotoxins. *Biochemistry.* 1995;34:8649-8656.

123. Fainzilber M, Nakamura T, Lodder JC, Zlotkin E, Kits KS, Burlingame AL. γ-Conotoxin PnVIIA, a γ-carbox-yglutamate-containing peptide agonist of neuronal pacemaker cation currents. *Biochemistry.* 1998;37:1470-1477.

124. Maillo M, Aguilar MB, Lopez-Vera E, Craig AG, Bulaj G, Olivera BM, et al. Conorfamide, a Conus venom peptide belonging to the RFamide family of neuro-peptides. *Toxicon.* 2002;40:401-407.

125. Craig AG, Jimenez EC, Dykert J, Nielsen DB, Gulyas J, Abogadie FC, et al. A novel post-translational modi-fication involving bromination of tryptophan. Identification of the residue, L-6-bromotryptophan, in peptides from Conus imperialis and Conus radia-tus venom. *J Biol Chem.* 1997;272:4689-4698.

126. Jimenez EC, Watkins M, Olivera BM. Multiple 6-bro-motryptophan residues in a sleep-inducing peptide. *Biochemistry.* 2004;43:12343-12348.

127. Lirazan MB, Hooper D, Corpuz GP, Ramilo CA, Bandyopadhyay P, Cruz LJ, et al. The spasmodic pep-tide defines a new conotoxin superfamily. *Biochemistry.* 2000;39:1583-1588.

128. Jones RM, Bulaj G. Conotoxins—new vistas for pep-tide therapeutics. *Curr Pharm Des.* 2000;6:1249-1255.

129. Miljanich GP. Venom peptides as human pharmaceu-ticals. *Science & Medicine* 1997;Sept/Oct:6-15.

130. Olivera BM. ω-Conotoxin MVIIA: from marine snail venom to analgesic drug. In: Fusetani N, ed. *Drugs from the Sea.* Basel: Karger; 2000:75-85.

131. Lewis RJ, Nielsen KJ, Craik DJ, Loughnan ML, Adams DA, Sharpe IA, et al. Novel ω-conotoxins from Conus catus discriminate among neuronal calcium channel subtypes. *J Biol Chem.* 2000;275:35335-35344.

132. Scott DA, Wright CE, Angus JA. Actions of intrathecal omega-conotoxins CVID, GVIA, MVIIA, and mor-phine in acute and neuropathic pain in the rat. *Eur J Pharmacol.* 2002;451:279-286.

133. Smith MT, Cabot PJ, Ross FB, Robertson AD, Lewis RJ. The novel N-type calcium channel blocker, AM336, produces potent dose-dependent antinoci-ception after intrathecal dosing in rats and inhibits substance P release in rat spinal cord slices. *Pain.* 2002;96:119-127.

134. Malmberg AB, Gilbert H, McCabe RT, Basbaum AI. Powerful antinociceptive effects of the cone snail venom-derived subtype selective NMDA receptor antagonists conantokins G and T. *Pain.* 2003;101:101-116.

135. Williams AJ, Dave JR, Phillips JB, Lin Y, McCabe RT, Tortella FC. Neuroprotective efficacy and therapeutic window of the high-affinity N-methyl-D-aspartate antagonist conantokin-G: in vitro (primary cerebellar neurons) and in vivo (rat model of transient focal brain ischemia) studies. *J Pharmacol Exp Ther.* 2000;294:378-386.

136. Williams AJ, Ling G, McCabe RT, Tortella FC. Intrathecal CGX-1007 is neuroprotective in a rat

model of focal cerebral ischemia. *NeuroReport*. 2002;13:821-824.

137. Livett BG, Sandall DW, Keays D, Down J, Gayler KR, Satkunanathan N, et al. Therapeutic applications of conotoxins that target the neuronal nicotinic acetylcholine receptor. *Toxicon*. 2006;48:810-829.

138. Sandall DW, Satkunanathan N, Keays DA, Polidano MA, Liping X, Pham V, et al. A novel alpha-conotoxin identified by gene sequencing is active in suppressing the vascular response to selective stimulation of sensory nerves in vivo. *Biochemistry*. 2003;42:6904-6911.

139. Satkunanathan N, Livett B, Gayler K, Sandall D, Down J, Khalil Z. Alpha-conotoxin Vc1.1 alleviates neuropathic pain and accelerates functional recovery of injured neurones. *Brain Res*. 2005;1059:149-158.

140. Nielsen CK, Lewis RJ, Alewood D, Drinkwater R, Palant E, Patterson M, et al. Anti-allodynic efficacy of the chi-conopeptide, Xen2174, in rats with neuropathic pain. *Pain*. 2005;118:112-124.

141. Lubbers NL, Campbell TJ, Polakowski JS, Bulaj G, Layer RT, Moore J, et al. Postischemic administration of CGX-1051, a peptide from cone snail venom, reduces infarct size in both rat and dog models of myocardial ischemia and reperfusion. *J Cardiovasc Pharmacol*. 2005;46:141-146.

142. Zhang SJ, Yang XM, Liu GS, Cohen MV, Pemberton K, Downey JM. CGX-1051, a peptide from Conus snail venom, attenuates infarction in rabbit hearts when administered at reperfusion. *J Cardiovasc Pharmacol*. 2003;42:764-771.

Therapeutic 37 Applications of Conotoxins

Michael F. Saulino

INTRODUCTION

The primary biologic activity of conotoxins occurs through interactions with specific ion channels. Most commonly, these peptides modulate voltage-gated channels and inhibit the entrance of Na^+, K^+, and Ca^{2+} ions into cells. Conotoxins are among estimated 100,000 small, disulfide-rich peptide venoms produced by predatory cone snails (genus *Conus*). The remarkable diversity of pharmacologic structure, function, and utility has been recently reviewed.[1] The typical physiologic role of voltage-gated ion channels is the production, modulation, and transduction of the electrical signals. Thus, the potential clinical utility of these agents would be alteration of biologic processes that depend upon electrical signaling. Human disease states that have been explored as conotoxin targets include pain, stroke, brain injury, mental illness, addiction, and epilepsy.

At present, only a single conotoxin has received approval from the U.S. Food and Drug Adminstration (FDA) for therapeutic use. Ziconotide, a synthetic form of conotoxin MVIIa, is marketed by Élan pharmaceuticals under the name Prialt.[2] This compound was originally isolated from the venom of the cone snail *Conus magus*. This drug was also known as SNX-111 when it was an investigational pharmaceutical by Neurex Corporation. The indication for this agent is severe chronic pain in patients for whom intrathecal therapy is warranted, and who are intolerant of or refractory to other treatments, such as systemic analgesics, adjunctive therapies, or intrathecal morphine.[3] The majority of this chapter will focus on the use of the medication with a smaller discussion reserved for conotoxins in clinical development.

Ziconotide is a 25 amino acid peptide that blocks a neural specific calcium channel on small myelinated and unmyelinated nociceptive afferents that are primarily localized in the superficial Rexed laminae (I and II).[4] The analgesic effect of ziconotide is produced when this channel blockade results in diminishing neurotransmitter release from these primary nociceptive afferents. Thus, the transmission of the pain signal never crosses the synaptic cleft from the primary afferents to the second-order neurons.

One of the clinical challenges with ziconotide use is need for chronic spinal exposure of the agent in order to achieve therapeutic efficacy. Oral intake of ziconotide results in rapid breakdown into inactive peptides. Vascular exposure of ziconotide produces hypotension in rats and humans, probably due to cross-reactivity to vascular calcium channels. Intravenous administration of ziconotide was also found to be neuroprotective in brain ischemia models which lead to the some early investigations for this agent in acute stroke and head injury.[5] Epidural administration of this agent did not result in consistent therapeutic efficacy. Thus, ziconotide is indicated for use only via an intrathecal delivery system. This agent has been formally evaluated with both temporary (CADD-Micro ambulatory infusion pump, Smiths Medical MD, Inc., St. Paul, MN) and permanent (SynchroMed EL and SynchroMed II Infusion System, Medtronic Inc., Minneapolis, MN) intrathecal pumps.[5]

Dr. Saulino is disclosing that he is a member of the speaker's bureau for Medtronic Intrathecal Baclofen and Élan Pharmaceuticals Intrathecal Ziconotide.

Ziconotide's role in chronic pain management is evolving. This agent is entirely different from all other medications that are routinely used for intrathecal therapy. While several agents are commonly used,[6,7] only three agents currently have FDA approval for intrathecal use: baclofen, morphine and ziconotide. Baclofen, a GABA-B agonist, is the mainstay of intrathecal therapy for spasticity and has FDA approval for spasticity of both cerebral and spinal origin. Morphine, considered by many clinicians to be the first-line agent for intrathecal pain management, has been approved by the FDA for clinical use for more than decades. Intraspinal opiates, such as morphine and hydromorphone, are thought to exert their therapeutic effect presynaptically by inhibiting calcium ion influx and postsynaptically by increasing potassium flux.[8] Other commonly used agents for chronic intraspinal infusion include bupivacaine and clonidine. Treatment algorithms for use of these agents, both in monotherapy and combination therapy, are far from standardized. The highest level of evidence-based decision making for intrathecal pain therapy is consensus statements of experienced clinicians. When the last consensus statement was produced in 2004, ziconotide was still an investigational agent. Accordingly, ziconotide was not placed within the treatment algorithm.[6] In January 2007, a consensus of experts again convened to review the current medical literature and put forth updated guidelines for intrathecal pain therapy. The 2007 consensus guidelines have recently been published with ziconotide monotherapy being put forth as a first-line agent with combination therapy of ziconotide and other agents attaining secondary indications.[9]

There are two major clinical trials that support a positive therapeutic effect of intrathecal ziconotide. Staats and colleagues[11] explored the use of this agent in 111 patients with pain associated with cancer or acquired immunodeficiency syndrome (AIDS) in a randomized, controlled, double-blinded trial. The pain diagnoses included in this trial were variable for both cancer-related pain (neuropathy, postherpetic neuralgia, pathologic fractures and complications of radiation therapy) and AIDS-related (peripheral neuropathy, Kaposi sarcoma and postherpetic neuralgia) pain syndromes. The study population is notable for a relatively high percentage of neuropathic pain, which is considered relatively challenging to treat with intrathecal therapy. Patients were required to either have a permanent SynchroMed intrathecal infusion system implanted or have a temporary external intrathecal infusion system. Individuals who were treated with ziconotide started at either 0.1 µg per hour or 0.4 µg per hour. Patients had to rate their pain at least 50 mm of 100 mm line on a Visual Analog Score of Pain Intensity (VASPI). Dosing adjustments occurred every 12 to 24 hours based on the appearance of either adverse effects or pain relief. Intrathecal ziconotide exposure continued for up to 2 weeks. Patients were allowed to adjust their systemic pain regimens as needed but could not use any other intrathecal agent.

At the conclusion of the trial, the mean VASPI improved 53% for the ziconotide-treated group compared with 19% for the placebo group. Positive responders, defined as a 30% improvement in VASPI compared with baseline, was achieved in 50% of the active treatment group and in 17.5% in the placebo-treated group. Moderate to complete pain relief as measured by the Category Pain Relief Scale (CPRS) was achieved in 52.9% of ziconotide-treated patients compared with 17.5% of placebo-treated patients. Oral opioid consumption decreased 9.9% in the ziconotide-treated group, whereas the placebo-treated group increased oral opioid consumption by 5.1%. Following the rapid titration phase of this study, patients treated with ziconotide were permitted to enter an extension maintenance phase, and placebo-treated patients were allowed to cross over to ziconotide therapy. All of the patients who continued ziconotide therapy maintained therapeutic efficacy, resulting in a 69.2% decrement in VASPI scores. Pain relief continued without dose escalation, which suggests that tolerance does not occur with this agent. Initial placebo patients experienced a 45% decrement in VASPI at the conclusion of the crossover phase. The positive therapeutic effect of ziconotide in this trial was statistically significant for both starting-dose subgroups (< 0.1 µg/h and > 0.1 µg/h) as well as for either disease subgroups (those with cancer or AIDS). No statistical significance in pain relief was seen with respect to age, gender or prior intrathecal therapy.

The adverse event profile for ziconotide therapy during this trial was significant. Seventy-one patients were initially assigned to receive ziconotide. Twenty-seven of these 71 individuals (38%) discontinued ziconotide therapy, in which 12 were discontinued due to adverse events (17%). The dropout rate for the placebo group was less compared with the active treatment group. Nine of the 40 subjects who were assigned to the placebo group dropped (22%), out of which 4 (10%) dropped out due to adverse events. During the titration phase, 22 of 72 patients (30.6%) exposed to ziconotide experienced a total of 31 serious adverse effects. In the opinion of the investigators, 14 of these 31 events were considered related to ziconotide treatment. All of these serious adverse events involved the nervous system with confusion, somnolence, and urinary retention being reported most commonly. Other common but less serious adverse events included dizziness, vomiting, postural hypotension, and fever. An interesting observation on these adverse events was that the appearance of adverse events occurred 2 to 3 days following a dosing adjustment. The central nervous system adverse events had a median time to resolution of 4 days (range 0 to 58 days) following a dosing decrement. These time lags supports the concept that ziconotide must penetrate neural tissue to exert an effect. A total of 15 patients died during or immediately after the study period. Death rates were not significantly different between the ziconotide- and placebo-treated groups. Twelve of the 15 deaths were due to the incident neoplasm. There were no reports of anaphylaxis or hypersensitivity to ziconotide.[11]

The other major controlled trial that explored the therapeutic benefit of ziconotide was performed Rauck and colleagues.[12] This study reported on 220 patients with nonmalignant pain who were randomized to receive either ziconotide (112 subjects) or placebo (108 subjects). Similarly, the pain diagnoses were variable, but a high percentage of neuropathic pain patents were again enrolled (76% for the ziconotide group and 71% for the placebo group). In this study, patients were required to have an implanted SynchroMed infusion system before enrollment in the trial. Subjects were weaned from prior intrathecal medications before being exposed to ziconotide. Patients were required to have a VASPI score of greater than 50 mm at the conclusion of intrathecal weaning and to have a stabilized systemic analgesic regimen. The starting dose of ziconotide was 0.1 µg/h. The titration phase of this trial lasted for 3 weeks, during which dosing adjustments upward of 0.05 or 0.1 µg/h were performed until patients attained analgesia or reported intolerable side effects. At least 24 hours was required between each dosing increase, but downward adjustments were allowed at any time point to improve tolerability. Again, patients were allowed to adjust systemic medications as needed but could not use any intrathecal agent other than ziconotide.

During this trial, the primary outcome measure was improvement in VASPI scores. At the conclusion of the 3 weeks of titration, ziconotide-treated subjects demonstrated a statistically significant improvement in their VAPSI scores (14.7%) compared with placebo-treated subjects (7.2%). The onset of pain relief was observed among ziconotide-treated patients as early as Week 1, with a mean percent improvement on the VASPI of 16.6%, compared with a mean percent improvement of 5.0% among the placebo-treated patients. At Week 2, the mean percent improvement in VASPI scores for the ziconotide-treated group (13.8%) was greater than that for the placebo-treated group (8.2%), but this difference was not statistically significant. Another measure of treatment response was the portion of subjects who demonstrated at least a 30% improvement in VASPI score. For this outcome measure, there was no significant difference between the ziconotide-treated group (16.1%) and the placebo-treated group (12.0%). On the clinician's global impression (CGI) satisfaction scale, 28.4% of ziconotide-treated patients reported "a lot" or "complete" satisfaction compared with 12.1% of placebo-treated subjects. On the CGI Overall Pain Control measure, 11.9% of ziconotide-treated subjects reported "very good" or "excellent" pain control at study termination, compared with 0.9% of placebo-treated patients. Both of these CGI measures were statistically significant. The change in the Global McGill Pain Relief total score was significantly reduced in the ziconotide group compared with that of the placebo group. The Categorical Pain Relief Scale (CPRS) at study termination showed a trend in favor of ziconotide, but the difference did not reach statistical significance. With regard to oral opiate consumption, there was a 23.7% mean decrease in weekly opioid use (in morphine equivalents) from pretreatment stabilization to Week 3 for the ziconotide-treated group compared with a 17.3% decrease in the placebo group. Similarly, this result demonstrated a trend that did not achieve statistical significance.

The adverse event profile observed during this trial was also considerable, with the majority of subjects in both treatment arms experiencing side effects (92.9% of ziconotide subjects and 82.4% of placebo subjects). The severity of adverse events reported was primarily mild or moderate (ziconotide, 83.6%; placebo, 83.8%). The spectrum of adverse effects in this trial was similar to that of the cancer/AIDS trial. The side effects that occur with statistically greater frequency in the ziconotide group included dizziness (47.3% versus 13.0%), confusion (17.9% versus 4.6%), ataxia (16.1% versus 1.9%), abnormal gait (15.2% versus 1.9%) and memory impairment (11.6% versus 0.9%). The incidence of serious adverse event was similar for both the ziconotide-treated and placebo-treated groups (11.6% versus 9.3%). There were no reported deaths during this trial, which supports the hypothesis that the deaths noted in the earlier trial were due to the disease processes and were not directly related to ziconotide treatment. The onset and resolution of adverse effects were delayed in a fashion similar to that of the Staats study. The median time to onset for the most commonly reported ziconotide-related side effects (dizziness, nausea, confusion, ataxia, and asthenia) ranged from 3.0 to 9.5 days. The median time to resolution for most of these adverse events was within 1 to 2 weeks of drug discontinuation.[12]

As a result of the above-mentioned factors as well as other trials with ziconotide, this agent was approved by the FDA in December 2004. This event represents the first intrathecal agent for pain control that has successfully passed the high standards of the approval process. Morphine was approved more than a decade ago, but it was "grandfathered" in the FDA. Intrathecal baclofen is an FDA-approved intervention for spasticity. It is estimated that more than 1500 patients over 12 years have been exposed to ziconotide. During this exposure, there have been no permanent sequelae that have been unequivocally linked to the drug. Also, no withdrawal or abstinence syndrome following sudden cessation of drug delivery has been reported with this agent. This feature is distinctly different from intrathecal opiates, which can have a profound withdrawal syndrome.

One important observation during the clinical trials as well as after approval surveillance is that the incidence of ziconotide-related side effects corresponds not only to total daily dose but the titration rate at which a particular dose is achieved. Figure 37-1 demonstrates the adverse event profile during two early ziconotide clinical trials. The majority of side effects demonstrated an increased incidence during the "fast" trial (mean daily dose of 36 µg per day achieved in 5–6 days) compared to the "slow" trial (mean daily 7.2 µg per day achieved in 28 days). The current package insert describes a titration schedule as follows: starting dose of no more than 2.4 µg/day, upward titration by up to 2.4 µg/day at intervals of no more than 2 to 3 times per week, up to a recommended maximum of 19.2 µg/d (0.8 µg/h) by Day 21. Even this titration schedule, which is slower than the initial clinical trials, has been considered excessively rapid by experienced clinicians. One small group of experts has put forth the following titration recommendations: starting dosage of 0.5 µg/d, with increases of no more often than weekly.[13]

Another challenge with the use of ziconotide is the issue of stability. In contrast to opiates and other commonly used intrathecal agents, which have acceptable stability profiles,[14] ziconotide is susceptible to breakdown at a rate that is clinically significant. All patients with implanted intrathecal delivery systems require

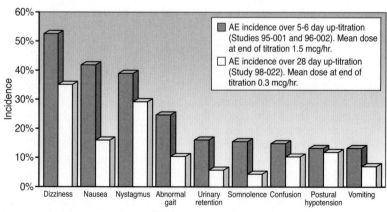

FIGURE 37-1. Comparison of adverse event (AE) profile during two different intrathecal ziconotide titration schedules.

refill of the pump reservoir to maintain a constant delivery of medication. Typically, refill intervals are between 2 and 6 months.[10] The phyical stability of the ziconotide molecule can potentially interfere with refill frequency. Ziconotide degradation occurs primarily through oxidation to the methionine sulfoxide form of the drug. The breakdown products of ziconotide are both nontoxic and inactive. Two accelerants of the oxidation process are (1) heat and (2) the presence of dissolved oxygen in a solution. For these two reasons, ziconotide is stored in a refrigerator and is package in a methionine buffer. Using these strategies, ziconotide should be capable of maintaining acceptable stability for clinical use. Undiluted ziconotide solutions maintain greater than 90% stability for approximately 84 days.[15]

An increasing concern with long-term infusion of intrathecal agents is the development of inflammatory, noninfectious mass at the tip of the intrathecal cathter. Although the exact pathophysiology of these masses is unknown, there are several causally linked factors including the medication infused, catheter position, low cerebrospinal fluid volume, and the dose and concentration of the infused drug. Granuloma development is the most serious adverse effect associated with intrathecal pain therapy, with some clinicians considering this issue the most significantly barrier to patient access.[9] To date, no granulomas have ever been detected in patients exposed to intrathecal ziconotide. Although this may represent a therapeutic advantage of this agent, it is important to acknowledge that the relatively low prevalence of ziconotide use and the rarity of granuloma development preclude a definite statement that use of this agent is not associated with granuloma development.

Many patients are exposed to ziconotide by converting the agents in their current intrathecal pump as opposed to having ziconotide as their initial intrathecal agent. If a patient has intrathecal opiates in his or her pump and a decision is made to attempt intrathecal ziconotide therapy, then weaning from the opiates should occur. Weaning of patients from intrathecal opioid therapy can be challenging. Many clinicians mistakenly adhere strictly to the belief that any decrease in the intrathecal opioid dose should be replaced with equianalgesic doses of systemic opioids. Various equianalgesic oral to intrathecal dosing ratios have been suggested, ranging from 12:1 to 300:1.[16] These equianalgesic doses are typically inappropriate for weaning from chronic intrathecal

opioid therapy, and patients can be weaned without strict adherence to equianalgesic conversion ratios. Patients may experience opioid withdrawal during the weaning process. Signs and symptoms may include lacrimation, rhinorrhea, yawning, insomnia, restlessness, mydriasis, nausea, vomiting, diarrhea, piloerection, abdominal cramps, anxiety, agitation, muscle twitching, diaphoresis, palpitations, flu-like symptoms, hypertonia, and increased pain.[17] During some of the ziconotide trials described earlier, intrathecal opiates weaning periods varied from 2 to 8 weeks. A descriptive method for intrathecal opiate weaning has recently been published.[18]

CONCLUSION

Although the majority of investigation into the use of ziconotide that occurred before FDA approval examined the use of this agent as monotherapy, the most commonly used strategy since the release of this agent is ziconotide in combination with other medications. The current estimate is that ziconotide monotherapy represents only 20% to 25% of ziconotide use in the United States. A variety of agents have been attempted in combination with ziconotide, including morphine, hydromorphone, fentanyl, bupivacaine, clonidine, and baclofen. The utility of this approach to chronic pain is presently guided by clinical experience and will likely continue to evolve. Because intrathecal ziconotide and other intrathecal agents have different mechanisms of action, it is possible that combination therapy could result in a synergistic effect. Additionally, multiple pain syndromes could be present in one patient with differential responsiveness observed to each syndrome.[19] Although combination ziconotide therapy does not appear to produce any additive risk, the issues of stability makes this approach somewhat daunting. As noted earlier, ziconotide has a degradation profile when used in isolation. This process is accelerated in the presence of additional agents and would appear to a concentration-dependent phenomenon of the non-ziconotide agent.[15,20] Despite this complexity, it would appear that most practioners favor this approach.

Several other conotoxins are in various stages of development for therapeutic utility. A summary of these agents are presented in Table 37-1. All of these agents are small peptides and thus may require the same

TABLE 37-1 Conotoxins Under Investigation for Clinical Human Use

Toxin	Class	Species	Proposed indication
Vc1.1 (ACV1)	α	*C. victoria*	Neuropathic pain
CVID (AM336)	ω	*C. canus*	Neuropathic pain
MrIA/B (Xen2174)	χ	*C. marmoreus*	Cancer pain
Contulakin-G (CGX-1160)	Contulakin	*C. geographus*	Chronic pain
Conantokin-G (CGX-1007)	Conantokin	*C. geographus*	Epilepsy

challeneges of intrathecal delivery and stability that face ziconotide.[5] Despite the challenges associated with the clinical use of conotoxins, this class of neurotoxins can have a profound effect on clinical medicine. As demonstrated by the 2007 PolyAnalgesic Consensus conference, ziconotide has changed the face of intrathecal drug delivery for chronic pain mamagment. With continued research efforts, these other contoxins can have a similar impact.

References

1. Olivera BM, Teichert RW. Diversity of the neurotoxic Conus peptides: a model for concerted pharmacological discovery. *Mol Interv.* 2007;7:251-260.
2. Élan Pharmaceuticals. Prialt package insert. San Diego, CA, 2007.
3. Thompson JC, Dunbar E, Laye RR. Treatment challenges and complications with ziconotide monotherapy in established pump patients. *Pain Physician.* 2006;9:147-152.
4. Kristipati R, Nádasdi L, Tarczy-Hornoch K, Lau K, Miljanich GP, Ramachandran J, et al. Characterization of the binding of omega-conopeptides to different classes of non-L-type neuronal calcium channels. *Mol Cell Neurosci.* 1994;5:219-228.
5. Wang C, Chi C. Conus peptides—a rich pharmaceutical treasure. *Acta Biochim Biophys Sin.* 2004;36:713-723.
6. Hassenbusch S, Portenoy R, Cousins M, Buchser E, Deer TR, Du Pen SL, et al. Polyanalegesic Consensus Conference 2003: an update on the management of pain by intraspinal drug delivery—report of an expert panel. *J Pain Symptom Manage.* 2004;27:540-563.
7. Ivanhoe C, Tilton A, Francisco G. Intrathecal baclofen therapy for spastic hypertonia. *Phys Med Rehab Clins N Am.* 2001;12:923-929.
8. Pirec V, Laurito C, Lu Y, Yeomans D. The combined effects of N-type calcium channel blockers and morphine on A delta versus C fiber mediated nociception. *Anesth Anal.* 2001;92:239-243.
9. Deer T, Krames E, Hassenbusch S, Burton A, Caraway D, Dupen S, et al. Polyanalgesic Consensus Conference 2007: Recommendations for the Management of Pain by Intrathecal (Intraspinal) Drug Delivery: Report of an expert panel. *Neuromodulation.* 2007;10:300-328.
10. Staats P, Whitworth M, Barakat M, Anderson W, Lilienfeld S. The use of implanted programmable infusion pumps in the management of nonmalignant, chronic low-back pain. *Neuromodulation.* 2007;10:376-380.
11. Staats P, Yearwood T, Charapata S, Presley R, Wallace M, Bryce D, et al. Intrathecal ziconotide in the treatment of refractory pain in patients with cancer or AIDS: A randomized clinical trial. *JAMA.* 2004;291:63-70.
12. Rauck R, Wallace M, Leong M, MineHart M, Webster L, Charapata S, et al. A randomized, double-blind, placebo-controlled study of intrathecal ziconotide in adults with severe chronic pain. *J Pain Symptom Manage.* 2006;31:393-406.
13. Fisher R, Hassenbusch S, Krames E, Leong M, Minehart M, Prager J, et al. A consensus statement regarding the present suggested titration for Prialt (Ziconotide). *Neuromodulation.* 2005;8:153-154.
14. Trissel L, Xu Q, Pharm L. Physical and chemical stability. *Int J Pharm Compound.* 2002;6:74-76.
15. Shields D, Montenegro R. Chemical stability of ziconotide-clonidine hydrochloride admixtures with and without morphine during simulated intrathecal administration. *Neuromodulation.* 2007;(suppl 1):1-121.
16. Sylvester R, Lindsay S, Schauer C. The conversion challenge: from intrathecal to oral morphine. *Am J Hosp Palliat Care.* 2004;18:143-147.
17. Olmedo R, Hoffman R. Withdrawal syndromes. *Emerg Med Clin North Am.* 2000;18:273-288.
18. Caraway D, Saulino M, Fisher R, Rosenblum S. Intrathecal therapy trials with ziconotide. *Pract Pain Manage.* 2008;8:53-56.
19. Saulino M. Successful reduction of neuropathic pain associated with spinal cord injury via of a combination of intrathecal hydromorphone and ziconotide: a case report. *Spinal Cord.* 2007;45:749-752.
20. Shields D, Montenegro B, Ragusa M. Chemical stability of admixtures combining ziconotide with morphine and hydromorphone during simulated intrathecal administration. *Neuromodulation.* 2005;8:257-263.

Spider and Wasp Neurotoxins

38

Wagner Ferreira dos Santos

INTRODUCTION

In an experimental model for glaucoma in which rat retinas are subject to ischemia followed by reperfusion, PbTx1.2.3., purified from *Parawixia bistriata* spider venom (Brazilian "cerrado" spider), protected neurons from excitotoxic death in both outer and inner nuclear layers, and ganglion cell layers.[1] The venom of spider *Macrothele raveni* (Chinese spider) can inhibit cell proliferation and DNA synthesis of BEL-7402 cells in human hepatocellular carcinoma, probably through inducing cell apoptosis, downregulating C-myc, and arresting cell cycle progression.[2] These were the conclusions of studies in just two instances, about the therapeutic applications and many possibilities in the vast unexplored field of venoms research.

Venomous animals have evolved a flurry of toxins, for prey capture and defense. These toxins target a wide variety of pharmacologic sites, making them an invaluable source of ligands for studying the properties of these targets in different experimental paradigms. Among the many venomous animals of different phyla, spiders and wasps should be recognized because they are useful sources of polypeptides, acylpolyamines, alkaloids, sulfated nucleosides, cinines, mastoparans, among other types of molecules that function as neurotoxins. These molecules have proved to be extremely useful tools for the understanding of synaptic transmission events, and they have contributed to the design of novel drug models for treatment of acute and chronic neurologic disorders and pain.[3] Some invertebrate neurotoxins are described in Figure 38-1.

A general example is the number of peptides of venomous animals that have been used in vivo for proof-of-concept studies, with several having undergone preclinical or clinical development for the treatment of pain, diabetes, multiple sclerosis, and cardiovascular diseases.[4]

Wasps are grouped into the class of the insects, being extraordinarily prevalent and widespread over the Earth because their adaptability and variety have assured their continuous existence. They have been surviving for the last 300 million years, mainly due to their wings, exoskeleton, adaptability to different niches, chemical communications, capacity for metamorphosis, and production of toxins.[5] For the wasp venoms, the main focus is directed to the medical area, because their venoms are cocktails of harmful compounds, mainly enzymes, which generally trigger inflammatory responses after sting.

The spiders had evolved from ancestors during the Devonian period. The oldest spider fossil is the *Attercopus fimbriunguis*, of the medium Devonian (380–374 million years ago), that was found in the Gilboa farm, in the state of New York.[6] Two species of spiders with orb-weaver are known from the beginning of the Cretaceo in Spain.[7] Also, an orb made by a spider of the genus Arancoidea was found in amber in Sant Just, Spain and was dated of 110 million years ago, in the beginning of the Cretaceo.[7]

In evolutionary terms, spiders (class: Aracnida; order: Araneae) are the most successful predatory invertebrates and they maintain by far the largest pool of toxic peptides, besides other compounds. There are approximately 38,000 described species,[6] with an even greater number waiting characterization.[7] Sollod and colleagues[8] estimate that of approximately 50 peptides per venom obtained from mass spectrometric analysis of 55 tarantula venoms and a conservative species count of 80,000, there should be an amount of 4 million spider venom polypeptides.

Dr. dos Santos does not report any conflicts of interest.

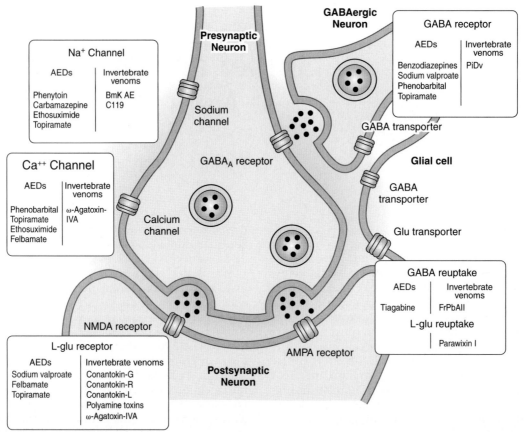

FIGURE 38-1. Molecular targets of antiepileptic drugs (AEDs), and invertebrate venoms and neurotoxins.[3] Models of action include the Na$^+$ and Ca^{2+} channels blockade; of inhibitory neurotransmission, such as GABAreceptor agonists and neuronal and astrocytic GABA transporter inhibitors, and inhibition excitatory neurotransmission through the antagonism of N-methyl-D-aspartate, AMPA and kainate receptors. "Agatoxins," *Agelenopsis aperta* toxins; "Conantokins," *Conus sp.* toxins; BmKAE, *Buthus martensi* Karsch antiepileptic pepitide; C119, *Centruroides limpidus* toxin; FrPbAll, *Parawixia bistriata* GABA neurotoxin; Parawixin1, *Parawixia bistriata* glutamate neurotoxin; PiDv, *Polybia ignobilis* venom.

In this chapter, I summarize and compile several biochemical and pharmacologic aspects and therapeutic applications of spider and wasp neurotoxins (Table 38-1).

TOXINS ACTING ON NA$^+$ CHANNELS

Voltage-gated Na$^+$ channels are present in most excitable cell membranes, and are responsible for the generation and propagation of action potentials in these cells. They represent transmembrane proteins composed of a major α-subunit of approximately 260 kDa, sufficient for functional expression, and of at least three different auxiliary β-subunits of 30 to 40 kDa, which modify the kinetics and voltage dependence of channel gating.[9,10] A number of toxins and chemicals that block or modulate the function of voltage-gated Na$^+$ channels have been discovered; some of which are presently being used as chemical tools to study these channels.

Some spider toxins acting on Na$^+$ channels, like δ-atracotoxin, δ-palutoxin, and pompilidotoxins, bind at site 3, which involves the extracellular loops IS5-S6, IVS3-S4, and IVS5-S6 of the ionic channel.[11] Most of the studies in spider toxins interfering with Na$^+$ channels deal with molecules purified from *Agelenopsis aperta*, *Phoneutria nigriventer*, *Atrax robustus*, and *Hadronyche versuta*.

Spider Venoms

A. aperta (Agelenidae; American funnel-web) spider venom is a rich source of toxins acting

TABLE 38-1 Neurotoxins from Invertebrates and Biologic Activities

Animal	Neurotoxin	Na⁺ Channel	Ca²⁺ Channel	Inhibitory Transmission	Excitatory Transmission	K⁺ Channels	Cl⁻ Channels	Observation
Spider								
P. bistriata	FrPbAII							Pain control
	Parawixin1			Increase				
N. clavata	Jorotoxin-3				Diminish			
S. raptoria	SrTxl.3				Diminish			
A. lobata	Argiotoxin$_{636}$				Diminish		Inhibit Ca²⁺-activated Cl⁻ currents	
	Argiotoxin$_{636}$/argiopine					Inhibit current Kir2.1		
Argiope sp.	aFTX3.3	Inhibits currents			Diminish		Inhibit Ca²⁺-activated Cl⁻ currents	
	AG2							
	ω-Aga-IVA		Diminish (P/Q)					Pain control
	ω-Agala-IC		Block L					
A. aperta	μ-Agal-VII	TTX sensitive			Diminish		Inhibit Ca²⁺-activated Cl⁻ currents	
	FTX3.3 (synthetic toxin)							
	PhTx3, 3-3 and 3-4		P/Q type					
	PhTx3, 3-2 and 3-5		L type					
P. nigriventer	PhTx2 and 2-6							
	Tx3-1		Inhibit activation					
H. versuta	PaTx 1 and 2					Inhibit current A-type Kv4.2 and 4.4 channels		
G. spatulata	ω-grammatoxin SIA					Inhibit current		
Wasp								
P. trangulum	Philanthotoxin-343				Diminish			Pain control
	Philanthotoxin-433				Diminish			Pain control
P. occidentalis	Th6-BK							
	Venom			Increase				
P. ignobilis	Venom				Diminish			

on Na+ channels.[12,13] This spider possesses μ-agatoxins I to IV, which belong to a family of six 36- to 37-residue peptides containing four disulfide bridges that present high-sequence homology to Curtatoxins from the related Agelenid spider *Hololena curta*.[14] They cause convulsive irreversible paralysis and repetitive firing in presynaptic terminals of *Musca domestica*. This action is correlated with repetitive firing in the terminal branches of insect motor axons, resulting in a significant increase in spontaneous neurotransmitter release in the fly.[15] This massive release of neurotransmitters occurs due to the increase of Na+ influx through tetrodotoxin-sensitive channels, shifting the activation curve to more negative potentials.[16] However, μ-agatoxins also slow Na_v channel inactivation in insect motoneurons from budworm *Heliothis virescens* an action shared by δ-PaluIT toxins, isolated from *Paracoelotes luctuosus* spider venom with which they shared considerable sequence homology.[13]

Several specific insect neurotoxins are still awaiting the identification of their mode of action and thus their target sites, since the methods of the bioassay used are nonspecific. These include acute oxicity testing systemic injection or isolated organ bath screening, for example, Lasiotoxins 1 and 2 (LpTx1, 2) isolated from *Lasiodora parahybana* (Brazilian rosean tarantula), *Euripelma toxins* (EsTx1, 2), Covalitoxin II from *Coremiocnemis validus* (Singapura tarantula), and Atracotoxin-Hvf17 from *H. versuta*. A family of 56- to 61-residue potent insecticidal peptides, named DTX9.2, 10, and 11 have been isolated from the venom of the North American primitive weaving spider *Diguetia canities* (Araneomorphae, Diguetidae). These neurotoxins cause progressive spastic paralysis in tabacco budworm larvae, with no effects on mice following intraperitoneal (IP) or intracerebroventricular (ICV) injections. On the other hand, lepidopteron larvae presented 50% paralytic doses (PD_{50}) ranging from 0.38 to 3.18 nmol/g, perhaps being among the most potent insecticidal compounds yet described from arthropod venoms. However, binding studies demonstrated only a partial inhibition of ^{125}I-AahIT binding to site 3 at Na+ channels of housefly head membranes. In neurophysiologic experiments, DTX9.2 elevated spikes discharges in sensory nerves at neuromuscular junction and also caused a depolarization of the membrane potential in cockroach giant axons.[17] The gene encoding DTX9.2 was isolated and characterized.[18]

A variety of noninsecticidal spider toxins are proving to be useful in the study of molecular differences in Na_v channel subtypes such as; ceratotoxins (CcoTx1, CcoTx2, and CcoTx3) from Latin American *Phrixotrichus cornuatus*, and phrixotoxin 3 (PaurTx3) from *P. auratus*. These neurotoxins block ion conductance and shift the voltage-dependence of activation towards more positive values, without affecting inactivation of these channels. A single amino acid mutation in ceratotoxin from Tyr^{32} 2 to Asp^{32} in ceratotoxin 1 completely blocks actions on the Na_v1.3 channel subtype. The specific site of action of these toxins on the Na_v channel remains speculative, but probably is associated with site 4.[13] The pharmacological profiles of these new toxins were characterized by electrophysiological measurements on six cloned voltage-gated sodium channel subtypes expressed in *Xenopus laevis* oocytes (Na(v)1.1/beta(1), Na(v)1.2/beta(1), Na(v)1.3/beta(1), Na(v)1.4/beta(1), Na(v)1.5/beta(1), and Na(v)1.8/beta(1)). In general, these novel toxins modulate voltage-gated sodium channels with properties similar to those of typical gating-modifier toxins, both by causing a depolarizing shift in gating kinetics and blocking the inward component of the sodium current.[19]

Futhermore, pore blocking toxins that are potential ligands site-1 of Na_v channels have been isolated from spider venoms. They are part of this group a family of 33-35 residue toxins with three disulfides known as the hainantoxins and huwentoxins, which were isolated from *Ornithoctus spp* (Chinese bird spider) (formerly Selenocosmia genera). Dorsal root ganglion cells with diameters of 20-40 μm were selected to study Na+ channels, for larger dorsal root ganglion cells from older animals tend to express fast tetrodotoxin-sensitive Na+ currents while smaller ones (<10 μm) tend to express slow tetrodotoxin-resistant Na+ currents. Completely inhibited the inactivation Na+ currents induced by BMK-I from *Buthus martensi* scorpion. The Na+ current reductions caused by hanantoxin-III and hanantoxin-IV were concentration-dependent with the IC_{50} value of 1.1 and 44.6 nM, respectively. Also, hanantoxin-III and hainantoxin-IV affected the mammalian neural Na+ channels in this paradigm through a mechanism quite different from other spider toxins targeting the neural receptor site 3, such as delta-aractoxins and μ-agatoxins.[20] Therefore, the two hanantoxins will **be useful tools** to discriminate different Na+ channel subtypes and disclose the structure-function relationship of Na$^+$ channels.

It is recognized that this group of polypeptides are the first family of spider toxins to selectively block Na$^+$ conductance via an interaction with site-1 of the Na$_v$ channel. However, competition binding studies with radionuclide-STX are necessary to confirm this interaction. Actions that differ from that of site-1 include the closing of the pore, or the modulation at a distant site, which allosterically leads to a conformational change in the channel protein resulting in a block of ion conductance. Nevertheless, HNTX-I represents the first insect-selective spider toxin interacting with either site-1 or a novel site on the Na$_v$ channel. Therefore, these peptides represent the first family of spider toxins to selectively block Na$^+$ conductance and, in the case of HNTX-I, the first insect-selective toxin to block the Na$_v$ channel.[20]

Jingzhaotoxin-I (JZTX-I) was purified from another Chinese tarantula *Chilobrachys jingzhao* venom that preferentially inhibits cardiac sodium channel inactivation and may define a new subclass of spider sodium channel toxins. In this study, the authors describe the contrast to other spider sodium channel toxins acting presynaptically rather than postsynaptically, because JZTX-I augmented frog end-plate potential amplitudes and caused an increase in both nerve mediated and unmediated muscle twitches. JZTX-I acted both presynaptically and postsynaptically, and facilitated neurotransmitter release by biasing the activities of Na$^+$ channels toward the open state. These actions are similar to those of *Leiurus quinquestriatus hebraeus* scorpion alpha-toxin Lqh II.[21]

From the venom of the Chilean "Roseantarantula" *Grammostola rosea*, a peptide named GrTx1 was described. GrTx1 has 29 amino-acid residues, compactly folded by three disulfide bridges with a molecular weight of 3697 Da. This peptide blocks Na$^+$ currents of neuroblastoma F-11 cells with an IC$_{50}$ of 2.8 ± 0.1 μM, up to a maximum of about 85% at 10 μM. Moreover, the right-shift (+20.1 ± 0.4 mV) of the fractional voltage-dependent conductance could also be compatible with a putative gating-modifier mechanism. Sequence analysis showed that GrTx1 is closely related to other spider toxins reported to affect various distinct ion channel functions.[22]

ProTx-II is a 30-amino acid peptide toxin from the venom of the Peruvian green velvet tarantula, *Thrixoplema pruriens*, that conforms to the inhibitory cystine knot motif and that modifies the activation kinetics of Na$^+$(v) and Ca^{2+}(v) but not K$^+$(v), channels. ProTx-II inhibits ion current by shifting the voltage dependence of activation to more depolarized potentials. Therefore, it differs from the classic site 4 toxins that shift voltage dependence of activation in the opposite direction.[23]

From the venom of the Brazilian Ctenid spider *Phoneutria nigriventer*, some neurotoxins that target sodium and calcium channels were purified. Peptides isolated from the toxic fraction PnTx1 of the venom of this *"armed" spider* produced reversible inhibition of recombinant Na$_v$1.2 interacting with specific sites of conotoxins.[24] Later, another toxin was isolated and the sequence analysis pointed to a molecular mass of 8600 Da and a C-terminally amidated glycine residue, apparently being identical to Toxin 1 (Tx1) isolated previously from this venom. Tx1 reversibly inhibited sodium currents in Chinese hamster ovary cells expressing recombinant sodium (Na(v)1.2) channels without affecting their fast biophysical properties.[25] Patch-clamp and binding data showed that *P. nigriventer* Tx1 is a novel, state-dependent sodium-channel blocker that binds to a site close to pharmacologic site 1, overlapping μ-conotoxin but not TTX binding sites.

CALCIUM CHANNEL TOXINS

Calcium channels are prevalent in many tissues throughout the body, being relevant to the nervous tissue where the entry of Ca^{2+} into nerve terminals plays a key role in cardiac, muscular, and neuronal functions. Spider venoms contain a diversity of polypeptide toxins acting on voltage-sensitive calcium channels (VSCCs). There are six different types of VSCCs: T-, L-, N-, P-, Q- and R-types. This criterion is based on their electrophysiologic properties and sensitivity to various activators-inhibitors and ions.[26]

The presence of Ca^{2+} channel blocking toxins in spiders were verified with the characterization of the venoms of three spiders: *A. aperta*, which produce an irreversible presynaptic block at the *Drosophila* neuromuscular junction; peptide toxins isolated from *Plecteurys tristes* spider (PLTXs I-III, MW 6 to 7 kDa) and one from *Hololena curta* (Hololena toxin, MW 16 kDA), whose activities were consistent with long-lasting specific block of presynaptic Ca^{2+} channels. Hololena toxin selectively blocked noninactivating Ca^{2+} current, whereas PLTX-II blocked band noninactivating Ca^{2+} currents in cultured *Drosophila* neurons.[27]

From *A. aperta* several toxins have been purified. Type I agatoxins (ω-AgaIA, IB and IC) are heterodimeric peptides of similar size with MW 7.5 kDa and five disulfide bonds. Studies demonstrated that ω-AgaIA potently blocks voltage-sensitive Ca^{2+} channels in insects, blocks neurotransmission at the frog neuromuscular junction, and suppresses high-threshold Ca^{2+} currents in rat dorsal root ganglion cells. Therefore, the toxin affects Ca^{2+} channels from both vertebrates and invertebrates with relative selectivity for L-type channels.

Type ω-AgaII (IIA and IIB, MW 10 kDa), which have homology of 43% at NH_2 terminal end with type IA toxins, also block presynaptically the insect neuromuscular transmission. Unlike, type I ω-agatoxins, type II ω-Aga inhibit the binding of ω-conotoxin GVIA from *Conus sp* in chick synaptosomes and potently block the potassium-stimulated Ca^{2+} entry; hence, their classification as N-type channel blockers. Low molecular weight (200 to 400 Da) fractions of *A. aperta* venom blocks P-type Ca^{2+} channels in guinea pig cerebellar Purkinje cells, in squid giant synapse, and in Xenopus oocytes injected with rat brain mRNA. The funnel-web spider toxin (FTX) isolated from *A. aperta* venom was identified as a polyamine.[28]

Hysterocrates gigas is an African spider from which several toxins were isolated, such as SNX-482, which is a selective peptide antagonist of R- and L-type VSCCs. Assays using chimeric channels combining structural features of R- (a1E) and L-type (a1C) calcium channel subunits showed that the presence of domains III and IV of the R-type current is a prerequisite for strong gating inhibition.[29]

The analysis of the venom of Brazilian "armed" *P. nigriventer* led to the isolation of several toxins. Large peptides such as ω-phonetoxin-IIA (ω-PnTxIIA) and PnTx3-6 blocked P/Q-type and N-type calcium currents almost irreversibly at 3 nM for ω-PnTxIIA, whereas R-type currents presented partial and readily reversible inhibition. Binding and displacement studies using ^{125}I-ω-PnTxIIA, showed that rat cerebral cortex synaptosomes displayed many kinds of binding sites. Radioactive type IIA was totally displayed by cold IIA at Ki=100 pM, and 25% by GVIA and 50% by MVIIC from the *Conus sp* snail.[29]

Another neurotoxin of *P. nigriventer* is PhTx3, which has a broad-spectrum calcium channel blocker that inhibits glutamate release, calcium uptake, and also glutamate uptake in synaptosomes. The effects of PhTx3 (1.0 μg/mL), ω-conotoxin GVIA (1.0 μmol/L) and ω-conotoxin MVIIC (100 nmol/L) were described on neuroprotection of hippocampal slices and SN56 cells subjected to ischemia by oxygen deprivation and low glucose insult. Confocal images of the CA1 region of rat hippocampal slices subjected to ischemia insult and treated with PhTx3 showed 18% dead cells. The SN56 cells derived from mouse septal cholinergic neurons under ischemia were protected from damage by PhTx3. Omega-conotoxin GVIA or ω-conotoxin MVIIC produced partial protection in the same paradigm.[30] Therefore, PhTx3 provided a new class of agents that targets multiple components in the in vitro model of brain ischemia.

Lambert-Eaton myasthenic syndrome (LEMS) is a neurologic autoimmune disease in which downregulation of VGCCs leads to reduced acetylcholine release from motoneuron terminals. Serological assays for LEMS autoantibodies by immunoprecipitation of calcium channels labeled with ^{125}I-ω-conotoxins are well established. However, an assay using the spider venom peptide ^{125}I-ω-Phonetoxin IIA (^{125}I-ω-PtxIIA) was developed. ^{125}I-ω-PtxIIA–labeled recombinant Cav2.1 and Cav2.2 channels and endogenous VGCCs in rat brain membranes. Autoantibodies that immunoprecipitate a ^{125}I-ωPtxIIA/channel complex were detected in 84% of patients with LEMS. Patients who were seropositive in the ^{125}I-ωPtxIIA assay corresponded precisely to the population that was positive for Cav2.1 or Cav2.2 antibodies detected using two different ω-conotoxins. Therefore, the ^{125}I-ω-PtxIIA assay detects a broader spectrum of autoantibody specificities than current ω-conotoxin–based assays.[31]

Another peptide named GsTxSIA was isolated from the Chilean theraposid *Gramostola spatula* venom. This peptide blocks N-, P-, and Q-type VSCCs. Aside from these actions on voltage-gated Ca^{2+} channels, it also binds to K^+ channels, although with much lower affinity. When the structures of HaTx1 and GsTxSIA were compared, a conserved motif containing a large hydrophobic pattern surrounded by positively charged residues were identified. It appeared to play an important role in the binding of the receptor site on the channel, probably located on or close to the voltage sensor. This also suggests a conserved binding domain relating to the voltage-sensing capability of ion channels of different ion selectivity as revealed by toxin binding.[29]

The peptide DW13.3 was isolated from the venom of the Filistatid spider *Filistata hibernalis*, which is commonly found throughout Florida and the southern region of the United States in human populated areas and causes a potent but transient block of native Ca^{2+} channels. This toxin has the highest affinity for P- and Q-type, following by N-, L- and R-type; without effect on T-type currents recorded from GH3 cells. Yet, DW13.3 elicited a block of both a1A in 60% and P-type in 76% currents from Purkinje cells.[32]

Segestria florentina is recognized as Tube web spider and originally a native of southern Europe as far as east Georgia. An example of neurotoxin purified from *S. florentina* venom is SNX-325 that a selective blocker of the N-type but not cardiac L-, P/Q, or R-type calcium channels. Similarly, huwentoxin-I and huwentoxin-X isolated from Chinese theraphosid *Selenocosmia huwena* venom inhibited N-type Ca^{2+} channels and had a weak effect on L-type Ca^{2+} channels.[33]

POTASSIUM CHANNEL TOXINS

The largest and most diverse family of ion channels comprises those selective for K^+, which plays a central role in regulating the membrane potential of cells and controls a wide variety of cellular processes throughout the body. These processes include: neurotransmitter release, insulin secretion, neuronal excitability, smooth muscle contraction, heart beat, and cell volume control.

From *Drosophila* shaker K^+ channel, many K^+ channels have been cloned. These studies have shown that K^+ channels are formed by coassembly of four subunits and are sometimes associated with auxiliary β subunits that can modify the gating properties of the heteromultimeric channel complex. With only a few exceptions, the molecular basis of cardiac K^+ currents have been defined. These channels can be grouped in many ways, for instance, by amino acid sequence homology. Another classification is based on biophysical properties of the currents determined by voltage-clamp methodology. Based on function, cardiac K^+ channels can be placed into one of four categories: transient outward, delayed rectifier, inward rectifier, and leak channels.[34]

More than 50 human genes encoding several K^+ channel subunits have been cloned during the past decade. Although the genes for many subunits have been cloned, there is still a substantial gap in the correlation between cloned Kv channels and native currents.[27,29]

Hanatoxins 1 and 2 from *G. spatulata* venom inhibit rat brain Shab- (Kv2.1) and Shal-related K^+ channels expressed in Xenopus sp oocytes, whereas Shaker-, Shaw-, and eag channels are relatively insensitive to this toxin. The Kv4 family of channels is also target by neurotoxins from two other spiders. Hetrapodatoxins (HpTx1-3), isolated from *Hetrapoda venatoria* venom, prolonged the action potential duration in rat ventricular myocytes by blocking the transient outward K^+ current (I_{to}).[35] The phrixotoxins (PaTxs) were isolated from Chilean *Theraphosid Phrixotrichus auratus* venom. These toxins specifically block Kv4.3 and Kv4.2 currents, with IC_{50} ranging from 5 nM to 70 nM, apparently by altering the gating properties of the channels. Also, PaTxs blocked cardiac I_{to} currents in isolated murine cardiomyocytes.[36]

From *Scodra griseipes* African spider venom the novel toxin SGTx1 was isolated, and it has been suggested that it acts partially and reversibly inhibiting both fast transient and delayed rectifier K^+ currents in rat cerebellar granule cells, similarly to hanatoxins. SGTx1 reversibly inhibited K^+ currents in oocytes expressing Kv2.1 channels. Moreover, generation of steady-state activation curves showed that, consistent with other gating modifiers, SGTx1 acted by shifting the activation of the channel to more depolarized voltages. When comparing the effects of SGTx1 and HaTx, differences in binding affinity and conformational homogeneity were revealed. These might result from different charge distributions at the binding surface and in the amino acid composition of the respective β-hairpin structures in the peptides.[37]

SGTx1 is thought to bind to the S3b-S4a region of the voltage sensor, and it is thought to alter the energetics of gating. However, there are experimental data for SGTx1, such as its interaction with lipid bilayer membranes, that remain to be characterized. An atomistic and coarse-grained molecular dynamics simulation to study the interaction of SGTx1 with a POPC and a 3:1 POPE/POPG lipid bilayer membrane was developed. It revealed the preferential partitioning of SGTx1 into the water/membrane interface of the bilayer, and also has been showed that electrostatic interactions between the charged residues of SGTx1 and the lipid head groups play an important role in stabilizing SGTx1 in a bilayer environment.[38]

Studies using whole-cell patch clamping on CH3 cells demonstrated that Tx3-1 from *P. nigriventer* venom inhibits A-type currents without affecting delayed rectifying, inward-rectifying and Ca^{2+}-sensitive K^+ currents or T- and L-type Ca^{2+} channels.[39]

Also, studies on the intra- and extracellular applications, of a well-known acyl-poliamine, argiotoxin-636 isolated from *Argiope lobata* venom, showed that it reduced the excitability of rat DRG neurons in part by inhibiting Na^+ channels, and in addition, dose-dependently inhibited voltage-activated K^+ channels, without affecting the voltage dependence of activation or steady-state inactivation. Lee and colleagues[40] analyzed the interactions between argiotoxin and the polyamine toxin philanthotoxin isolated from the venom of the solitary wasp *Philanthus triangulum*, on inward rectification in Kir2.1 using patch-clamping of *Xenopus* oocytes. These authors demonstrated that the high-affinity polyamine block is not consistent with direct open channel block, but instead involves polyamine binding to another region of the channel (intrinsic gate) to form a blocking complex that occludes the pore. This interaction defined a novel mechanism of ion channel closure.[40]

CHLORIDE CHANNEL TOXINS

Chloride channels are involved in many physiologic processes, such as cell volume control, transport across membranes, control of cellular excitability, as components of GABA receptors in both the vertebrate and invertebrate central nervous system, and acidification of intracellular organelles. Few neurotoxins of spider and wasp venoms affect these channel type.

An example is the neurotoxin sFTX3.3., isolated from *A. aperta* venom, which inhibited both voltage-activated Ca^{2+} currents and Ca^{2+}-activated Cl^- currents $[I_{Cl(Ca)}]$ in rat cultured dorsal root ganglion neurons, whereas synthetic analogue FTX and Arg_{636} inhibit $I_{Cl(Ca)}$ but not the Ca^{2+} currents.[27]

GLUTAMATE RECEPTOR AND TRANSPORTERS TOXINS

L-glutamate (L-Glu) is the main excitatory transmitter in the mammalian central nervous system and is also an important transmitter in the neuromuscular junction of invertebrates with both excitatory and inhibitory functions. The action of L-Glu is terminated by its removal from the synapse via high-affinity transporters (GluTs) located on both neurones and glial cells. Until now, five different types of GluTs have been described: EAAT1 to 5. There are several types of L-Glu receptors classified as ionotropic (iGluR) and metabotropic glutamate receptors (mGluR). The iGluRs are currently grouped into N-methyl-D-aspartate receptor (NMDA-R) and non-NMDA-R (AMPA, kainate and AP4) subtypes, being named after their sensitivity to selective agonists. The L-glutamate system is involved in nervous tissue development and embryology, learning, and memory. Many acute and chronic dysfunctions that affect the nervous system are related to glutamatergic system, such as epilepsy, trauma, amyotrophic lateral sclerosis (ALS), glaucoma, and so on. Drugs that modulate this system by blocking glutamatergic receptors or potentiating its uptake have been used to control many experimental diseases.

In the early 1980s, a neurotoxin named Joro spider toxin (JSTX), was isolated from *Nephila clavata* venom. This spider is a member of golden orb-weaver spider family, and can be found throughout Japan, China, and Korea, except Hokkaido island. Joro spider toxin irreversibly suppressed excitatory postsynaptic potentials (EPSP) and depolarization elicited by exogenous L-Glu, without affecting inhibitory postsynaptic potentials or depolarization due to aspartate on lobster neuromuscular junction. JSTX was also found to block glutamatergic synapses in mammalian brain. Several neurotoxins from the orb-weaver spider and solitary wasp were isolated, and the chemical structures of many of these have now been elucidated and they have been grouped into a family of closely related compounds, the acylpolyamines or simply polyamines.[41]

Another polyamine toxin has been identified from several venoms: *A. aperta* and *H. curta*, a trapdoor spider *H. theveniti*, and two tarantulas, *Herpactirella sp* and Desert blonde tarantula *Aphonopelma chalcodes* is common throughout the Southwestern United States, especially

Arizona, New Mexico, and Southern California. The α-agatoxins, purified from *A. aperta* venom, are selective and reversible, noncompetitive antagonists of NMDA-R in mammalian brain. Those polyamines from *H. theveniti* were paralytic to lepdopteram insect larvae. However, the studies are scarce and the mechanism of action was not investigated. In the chick nervous tissue, the venom from *H. curta* irreversibly blocked on-NMDA-R–mediated transmission. Further fractionation of this venom led to the neurotoxin of 5 to 10 kDa, 10 paralytic polyamines, and one insecticidal peptide, all of which are known as curtatoxins. Moreover, two polyamines (HO_{489} and HO_{505}) and one peptide previously described in the *A. aperta* venom (μ-AgaII) were characterized.[12,27,29]

PhTx4 isolated from *P. nigriventer* venom inhibited glutamate uptake in a dose-dependent manner on rat cerebrocortical synaptosomes. The IC_{50} value obtained was 2.35 ± 0.9 μg/mL, which is in the observed range reported for glutamate uptake blockers. Tx4-7, one of PhTx4 toxins, showed the strongest inhibitory activity ($50.3 \pm 0.69\%$).[42,43]

From the *Parawixia bistiata* Brazilian "cerrado" spider venom were isolated several neurotoxins that paralyze insects and have glutamatergic and GABAergic targets in neurons of mammals, too. The active fraction, named PbTx1.2.3. (now Parawixin-1), stimulated L-Glu uptake in cerebrocortical synaptosomes of rats without changing the K_M value, and did not effect GABA uptake. Subsequently experiments showed that the enhancement of L-glu uptake by this neurotoxin occurs when ionotropic L-glu receptors or voltage-gated sodium and calcium channels are completely inhibited or when GABA receptors and potassium channels are activated, indicating that the molecule may have a direct action on the transporters. In an experimental model for glaucoma in which rat retinas are subject to ischemia followed by reperfusion, Parawixin-1 protected neurons from excitotoxic death in both outer and inner nuclear layers, and ganglion cell layers.[1]

In GluTs after solubilization and reconstitution in liposomes and in transfected COS-7 cells, Parawixin1 promotes a direct and selective enhancement of L-Glu influx by the EAAT2 transporter subtype through a mechanism that does not alter the apparent affinities for the cosubstrates L-Glu or sodium. In liposomes, maximal enhancement by Parawixin-1 was observed when extracellular sodium and intracellular potassium concentrations was within

physiologic range. Moreover, the compound does not enhance the reverse transport of glutamate under ionic conditions that favor efflux, when extracellular potassium is elevated and the sodium gradient is reduced. Nor does it alter the exchange of glutamate in the absence of internal potassium. These observations suggest that Parawixin1 facilitates the reorientation of the potassium-bound transporter, the rate-limiting step in the transport cycle. This conclusion was further supported by experiments using EAAT2 transport mutant (E405D), which is defective in the potassium-dependent reorientation step,[44] and in this case, Parawixin1 does not stimulate L-Glu uptake.[44] These data demonstrated the potential role of this neurotoxin as a probe for the designing of therapeutic drugs to be used in pathologies that involve the hyperactivation of glutamatergic synapses, such as epilepsies and neurodegenerative diseases.

GABA RECEPTOR AND TRANSPORTERS TOXINS

The GABAergic neurotransmission has been implicated in the modulation of many brain neural networks, as well as in several neurologic disorders such as epilepsy, schizophrenia, anxiety, tardive dyskinesia, and so on. And as the pharmacology of GABAergic system becomes better understood, novel drugs might be developed.

It is described as in vivo anticonvulsant effect from denatured crude venom and partially fractions from *Scaptocosa raptoria* wolf spider venom. ICV injections of this venom and fraction SrTx1 abolished rat conclusive tonic-clonic seizures induced by picrotoxin, bicuculline, and pentilenetetrazole, and also, inhibited GABA uptake in synaptosomes of the rat cerebral cortex.[45] The SrTx1 was chromatographed and produced three molecules, SrTx1.1., SrTx1.2., and SrTx1.3., and they were injected into the substantia nigra at doses of 100, 200, and 400 ng/0.2 μL, respectively. SrTx1.3 protected 50%, 85.7%, and 100% of the rats, respectively, against the seizures elicited by bicuculline injected into area tempestas. This suggests that *S. raptoria* venom as well as its SrTx1.3 may be potential sources of new anticonvulsant drugs.[46]

As described earlier, several neuroactive compounds might be found in the *P. bistiata* venom. Another neurotoxin has been isolated from *P. bistriata* venom; FrPbAII inhibits synaptosomal GABA uptake in a dose-dependent manner and probably does not act on Na^+, K^+, and Ca^{2+} channels, $GABA_B$ receptors, or γ-aminobutyrate: α-ketoglutarate aminotransferase enzyme. Therefore, it is not directly dependent on these structures for its action. A direct increase of GABA release and reverse transport are also ruled out as mechanisms of FrPbAII activities as well as unspecific actions on pore membrane formation. FrPbAII is selective for GABA and glycine transporters, having slight or no effect on monoamines or glutamate transporters. According to experimental glaucoma data in rat retina, FrPbAII is able to cross the blood-retina barrier and promote effective protection of retinal layers submitted to ischemic conditions.[47]

Considering that FrPbAII inhibits high-affinity GABAergic uptake in a dose-dependent manner, studies in vivo have been performed. Injection of FrPbAII in the Wistar rat hippocampus induced a marked anxiolytic effect, increasing the occupancy in the open arms of the elevated plus maze (EPM) ($EC_{50}=0.09$ µg/µL) and increasing the time spent in the lit area of the light-dark apparatus ($EC_{50}=0.03$ µg/µL). Anxiolytic effects were also observed considering the number of entries in the open arms of the EPM and in the lit compartment of the light-dark box. When microinjected bilaterally in the SNPr of freely moving rats, FrPbAII (0.6 µg/µL) effectively prevented seizures induced by the unilateral GABAergic blockade of Area tempestas (bicuculline). This anticonvulsant effect was similar to that evoked by muscimol (0.1 µg/µL) and baclofen (0.6 µg/µL) but differed from that of the specific GAT1 inhibitor nipecotic acid (0.7 µg/µL). This difference could be accounted either for the parallel action of FrPbAII over glycinergic transporters or to an unspecific activity on GABAergic transporters.[48]

FrPbAII was effective against seizures induced by the ICV injection of pilocarpine, picrotoxin, and kainic acid, and the systemic administration of pentylenetetrazole (PTZ) in rats. The anticonvulsant effect of FrPbAII differed from that of nipecotic acid in potency, because the doses needed to block the seizures were more than 10-fold lower. Toxicity assays revealed that in the rotarod, the toxic dose of the FrPbAII is 1.33 µg/rat, and the therapeutic indexes were calculated for each convulsant. Furthermore, the spontaneous locomotor activity of treated animals was not altered when compared with control animals but differed from the animals treated

with nipecotic acid. Still, FrPbAII did not induce changes in any of the behavioral parameters analyzed. Finally, when tested for cognitive impairments in the Morris water maze, the ICV injection of FrPbAII did not alter escape latencies of treated animals.[49]

These studies are relevant by providing a better understanding of neurochemical mechanisms involved in brain function for possible development of new neuropharmacologic and therapeutic tools, and having a GABA neurotransmission as the main target.

WASP NEUROTOXINS

Phylantotoxins are polyamines that were isolated from *Philanthus triangulum* Egypt solitary wasp. These polyamines act irreversibly on open ionic channels on neuromuscular locust junction inhibiting L-Glu high-affinity uptake in synaptic terminal and glial cells. Triflouro-methyl-PTX-4.3.3 phylanthotoxin analog showed the highest potency of uptake blockade. Thirty-tree structural analogs from PhTx-4.3.3 were assayed on neuromuscular junctions of fly larvae, and the potency was increased when the polyamine chain was elongated by iodination of aromatic and aliphatic groups, or aromatic elongation was performed using butanoic acid. The main activity of PhTx4.3.3. is inhibition of NMDA transmission in the rat hippocampus. On the other hand, dideaza-PTX-12 antagonized calcium currents, and in the CA1 layer neurons reduced calcium currents to 40% at nM doses. Moreover, potassium rectifier current A are also affected.[50]

From *Polistes rothneyi iwatai* Japanese paper wasp were isolated mastoparans like (polystes-mastoparan-R1,2,3 and polytes-protonectin). They released histamine and had higher potency than mastoparan, and showed the highest hemolytic activity when compared with the other four peptides and mastoparan.[51]

Four synthetic analogs of vespulacinin1 isolated from *Vespula maculifrons* yellow jacket were studied on mammal smooth muscle preparation and in the cockroach cercal nerve giant neuron. All analogs showed potent effects such as bradykinin. At first, specific and reversible blocking of nicotinic excitatory transmission and concomitant activation of GABAergic system were observed. Next, a delayed irreversible block of transmission was observed, like threonin6-bradykin (Thr6-BK) and bradykinin (BK) blockers. Cyclization or partial cyclization of the analogs of vespulacin1 showed significant diminution of potency than alyphatics.[52]

Catalepsy is a state of immobility that is commonly experienced by patients with chronic use of many antiparkinsonism and neuroleptic drugs. Following this idea, fractions from *Agelaia vicina* Brazilian wasp venom were assayed into rat brain. Rodents showed ataxia and catalepsy within 10 minutes. The cataleptic effects were antagonized by the peripheral pretreatment with theophylline and ketamine. Moreover, these central effects were compared with those elicited by the neuroleptic drug haloperidol. These findings suggest that *A. vicina* venom may affect neural substrates involved with catalepsy in the central nervous system.[53]

The effects of the crude and boiled venom of the Brazilian social wasp *A. vicina*, in rat cerebral cortex synaptosomes showed that it uncompetitively inhibited high- and low-affinity GABA uptake by 91.2% and by 76%, respectively. This inhibition profile was also found to affect high- (99.6%) and low-affinity (905) uptake of L-Glu.[54]

Many investigations have provided information about defensive behaviors elicited by stimulation of deep layers of superior colliculus, which are subjected to inhibitory nigral modulation. This inhibition is made mainly through GABAergic neurons from substantia nigra, pars reticulata that sends output toward neural networks of the deep layers of the superior colliculus and dorsal periaquedutal gray matter involved with the organization of fear-like responses. Nigral microinjection of AvTx8 isolated from *Agelaia vicina* wasp venom in rats induced effects similar to those of baclofen, such as decreasing the intensity of behavioral defensive reactions caused by $GABA_A$ receptor blockade in the dorsal mesencephalon. These findings suggest that AvTx8 has some effects on GABAergic dynamics, increasing the activity of the inhibitory nigrocollicular pathways, causing antipanic (antiaversive) effect. Therefore, this neurotoxin is a novel pharmacologic tool used to study mode of actions of different types of GABAergic receptors and excitatory amino acid–mediated mechanisms in the brain and brainstem networks.[55]

From this same wasp venom was isolated another neurotoxin named AvTx7. AvTx7 inhibits L-Glu uptake in a dose-dependent and uncompetitive manner in the rat cerebral cortex synaptosomes. AvTx7 was found to stimulate the L-Glu release in the presence of calcium and sodium channel blockers, suggesting that its action is not mediated through these channels. Moreover, the AvTx7 potentiates L-Glu release in the presence of K^+ channel blockers tetraethylammonium and 4-aminopyridine, indicating that the neurotoxin may act through these drug-sensitive K^+ channels. Therefore, AvTx7 can be a valuable tool to enhance our understanding of K^+ channels involvement in the release of L-Glu.[6]

Two denatured venoms from social wasps *Polybia ignobilis* and *P. occidentalis* when injected by ICV in Wistar rats inhibited convulsive crisis elicited by bicuculline, pricrotoxin and kainic acid, but were not effective against convulsive crisis caused by pentilenetetrazole.[57,58] Several neurotoxins were isolated from *P. occidentalis* venom. The most active fraction contained Thr^6-bradikinin (Thr^6-BK) induced antinociceptive effects that were approximately twice as potent as either morphine or bradykinin, also given ICV. The antinociceptive activity of Thr^6-BK peaked at 30 minutes after injection and persisted for 2 hours, longer than bradykinin. The primary mode of action of Thr^6-BK involved the activation of B_2 bradykinin receptors because the antinociceptive effects of Thr6-BK were antagonized by a selective B_2 receptor antagonists. Therefore, this peptide could provide a novel tool in the investigation of kinin pathways involved with pain.[59] Although the role of the brain kallikrein-kinin system in the development of various diseases, such as edema formation following brain injury or induction of central hypertonia, has generated major interest, the possible role of this system in nociceptive processing has received little attention. The unknown underlying mechanism of this powerful antinociceptive effect reminds us that the supraspinal antinociceptive system is still a "black box" in many aspects and waits thorough investigation.[60]

CONCLUSIONS AND FUTURE PERSPECTIVES

Neurotoxins from venoms are evolutionary landmarks that act to immobilize prey and also are used in self-defense. Many toxins have shown high specificity and affinity for nervous tissue structures such as ion channels, receptors, and transporters in invertebrates and vertebrates. The study of neurotoxins has developed significantly over the past three decades. Therefore, neurotoxins represent a powerful source of probes useful for understanding synaptic dynamic events, identifying insecticide targets, and aiding in the design of novel drugs for the study and treatment of neurologic disorders.

Until now, very few compounds isolated from venoms have been used in clinical practice. However, with the use of novel methodologies for the purification and synthesis analog of natural compounds, it is to be expected that very soon, a novel generation of neuroactive compounds will become available for both basic use and for the development of new therapeutic alternatives.[3]

References

1. Fontana AC, Guizzo R, de Oliveira Beleboni R, Meirelles E, Silva AR, Coimbra NC, et al. Purification of a neuroprotective component of *Parawixia bistriata* spider venom that enhances glutamate uptake. *Br J Pharmacol*. 2003;139:1297-309.
2. Gao L, Feng W, Shan BE, Zhu BC. Inhibitory effect of the venom of spider *Macrothele raveni* on proliferation of human hepatocellular carcinoma cell line BEL-7402 and its mechanism. *Ai Zheng*. 2005;24:812-816.
3. Mortari MR, Cunha AOS, Ferreira LB, Santos WF. Neurotoxins from invertebrates as anticonvulsants: from basic research to therapeutic application. *Pharmacol Ther*. 2007;114:171-183.
4. Lewis RJ, Garcia ML. Therapeutic potential of venom peptides. *Nat Rev Drug Discov*. 2003;2:790-802.
5. Meinwald J. Eisner T. The chemistry of phyletic dominance. *Proc Natl Acad Sci U S A*. 1995;92:14-18.
6. Platnick, NI. *Advances in Spider Taxonomy, 1992-1995: With Redescriptions 1940-1980*. New York: New York Entomological Society & The Americam Museum of Natural History, 1997.
7. Peñalver E, Grimaldi DA, Delclòs X. Early cretaceus spider web with its prey. *Science*. 2006;312:1761.
8. Sollod BL, Wilson D, Zhaxybayeva O, Gogarten JP, Drinkwater R, King GF. Were arachnids the first to use combinatorial peptide libraries? *Peptides*. 2005;26:131-139.
9. Catterall WA. From ionic currents to molecular mechanisms: the structure and function of voltage-gated sodium channels. *Neuron*. 2000;26:13-25.
10. Yu FH, Catterall WA. Overview of the voltage-gated sodium channel family. *Genome Biol*. 2003;4:207.
11. Cestele S, Catterall WA. Molecular mechanisms of neurotoxin action on voltage-gated sodium channels. *Biochimie*. 2000;82:883-892.
12. Beleboni RO, Pizzo AB, Fontana AC, de O G Carolino R, Coutinho-Netto J, Dos Santos WF. Spider and wasp neurotoxins: pharmacological and biochemical aspects. *Eur J Pharmacol*. 2004;493:1-17.
13. Nicholson GM. Insect-selective spider toxins targeting voltage-gated sodium channels. *Toxicon*. 2007;49: 490-512.
14. Stapleton A, Blankenship DT, Ackermann BL, Chen TM, Gorder GW, Manley GD, et al. Curtatoxins. Neurotoxic insecticidal polypeptides isolated from the funnel-web spider *Hololena curta*. *J Biol Chem*. 1990;265:2054-2059.
15. Adams ME. Agatoxins: ion channel specific toxins from the American funnel web spider, *Agelenopsis aperta*. *Toxicon*. 2004;43:509-525.
16. Omecinsky DO, Holub KE, Adams ME, Reily MD. Three-dimensional structure analysis of mu-agatoxins: further evidence for common motifs among neurotoxins with diverse ion channel specificities. *Biochemistry*. 1996;35:2836-2844.
17. Bloomquist JR, Kinne LP, Deutsch V, Simpson SF. Mode of action of an insecticidal peptide toxin from the venom of a weaving spider (*Diguetia canities*). *Toxicon*. 1996;34:1072-1075.
18. Krapcho KJ, Kral RM Jr, Vanwagenen BC, Eppler KG, Morgan TK. Characterization and cloning of insecticidal peptides from the primitive weaving spider *Diguetia canities*. *Insect Biochem Mol Biol*. 1995;9:991-1000.
19. Bosmans F, Rash L, Zhu S, Diochot S, Lazdunski M, Escoubas P, Tytgat J. Four novel tarantula toxins as selective modulators of voltage-gated sodium channel subtypes. *Mol Pharmacol*. 2006;69:419-429.
20. Li D, Xiao Y, Xu X, Xiong X, Lu S, Liu Z, et al. Structure-activity relationships of hainantoxin-IV and structure determination of active and inactive sodium channel blockers. *J Biol Chem*. 2004;279:37734-37740.
21. Xiao Y, Liang S. Inhibition of neuronal tetrodotoxin-sensitive Na+ channels by two spider toxins: hainantoxin-III and hainantoxin-IV. *Eur J Pharmacol*. 2003;477:1-7.
22. Clement H, Odell G, Zamudio FZ, Redaelli E, Wanke E, Alagón A, et al. Isolation and characterization of a novel toxin from the venom of the spider *Grammostola rosea* that blocks sodium channels. *Toxicon*. 2007;50:65-74.
23. Smith JJ, Cummins TR, Alphy S, Blumenthal KM. Molecular interactions of the gating modifier toxin ProTx-II with NaV 1.5: implied existence of a novel toxin binding site coupled to activation. *J. Biol Chem*. 2007;282:12687-12697.
24. Diniz MR, Theakston RD, Crampton JM, Nascimento Cordeiro M, Pimenta AM, De Lima ME, et al. Functional expression and purification of recombinant Tx1, a sodium channel blocker neurotoxin from the venom of the Brazilian "armed" spider, *Phoneutria nigriventer*. *Protein Expr Purif*. 2006;50:18-24.
25. Martin-Moutot N, Mansuelle P, Alcaraz G, Dos Santos RG, Cordeiro MN, De Lima ME, et al. *Phoneutria nigriventer* toxin 1: a novel, state-dependent inhibitor of neuronal sodium channels that interacts with micro conotoxin binding sites. *Mol Pharmacol*. 2006;69:1931-1937.
26. Uchitel OD. Toxins affecting calcium channels in neurons. *Toxicon*. 1997;35:1161-1191.
27. Rash LD, Wayne CD. Pharmacology and biochemistry of spider venoms. *Toxicon*. 2002;40:225-254.
28. Llinas R, Sugimori M, Hillman DE, Cherksey B. Distribution and functional significance of the P-type, voltage-dependent Ca2+ channels in the mammalian central nervous system. *Trends Neurosci*. 1992;9:351-355.
29. Estrada G, Villegas E, Corzo G. Spider venoms: a rich source of acylpolyamines and peptides as new leads for CNS drugs. *Nat Prod Rep*. 2007;24:145-161.

30. Pinheiro AC, Gomez RS, Massensini AR, Cordeiro MN, Richardson M, Romano-Silva MA, Prado MA, De Marco L, Gomez MV. Neuroprotective effect on brain injury by neurotoxins from the spider *Phoneutria nigriventer*. *Neurochem Int*. 2006;49:543-547.

31. Martin-Moutot N, Haro L, Santos RG, Mori Y, Seagar M. *Phoneutria nigriventer* omega-Phonetoxin IIA: a new tool for anti-calcium channel autoantibody assays in Lambert-Eaton myasthenic syndrome. *Neurobiol Dis*. 2006;22:57-63.

32. Sutton KG, Siok C, Stea A, Zamponi GW, Heck SD, Volkmann RA, et al. Inhibition of neuronal calcium channels by a novel peptide spider toxin, DW13.3. *Mol Pharmacol*. 1998;54:407-418.

33. Newcomb R, Palma A, Fox J, Gaur S, Lau K, Chung D, et al. SNX-325, a novel calcium antagonist from the spider *Segestria florentina*. *Biochemistry*. 1995;34:8341-8347.

34. Hardie RC. Voltage-sensitive potassium channels in Drosophila photoreceptors. *J Neurosci*. 1991;11:3079-3095.

35. Sanguinetti MC, Johnson JH, Hammerland LG, Kelbaugh PR, Volkmann RA, Saccomano NA, et al. Heteropodatoxins: peptides isolated from spider venom that block Kv4.2 potassium channels. *Mol Pharmacol*. 1997;51:491-498.

36. Diochot S, Drici MD, Moinier D, Fink M, Lazdunski M. Effects of phrixotoxins on the Kv4 family of potassium channels and implications for the role of Ito1 in cardiac electrogenesis. *Br J Pharmacol*. 1999;126:251-263.

37. Lee CW, Kim S, Roh SH, Endoh H, Kodera Y, Maeda T, et al. Solution structure and functional characterization of SGTx1, a modifier of Kv2.1 channel gating. *Biochemistry*. 2004;43:890-897.

38. Wee CL, Bemporad D, Sands ZA, Gavaghan D, Sansom MS. SGTx1, a Kv channel gating-modifier toxin, binds to the interfacial region of lipid bilayers. *Biophys J*. 2007;92:L07-L09.

39. Kushmerick C, Kalapothakis E, Beirao PS, Penaforte CL, Prado VF, Cruz JS, et al. *Phoneutria nigriventer* toxin Tx3-1 blocks A-type K+ currents controlling Ca2+ oscillation frequency in GH3 cells. *J Neurochem*. 1999;72:1472-1481.

40. Lee JK, John SA, Weiss JN. Novel gating mechanism of polyamine block in the strong inward rectifier K channel Kir2.1. *J Gen Physiol*. 1999;113:555-564.

41. Usherwood PNR, Blagbrough IS. Spider toxins affecting glutamate receptors: polyamines in therapeutic neurochemistry. *Pharmacol Ther*. 1991;52:245-268.

42. Figueiredo SG, Garcia ME, Valentim AC, Cordeiro MN, Diniz CR, Richardson M. Purification and amino acid sequence of the insecticidal neurotoxin Tx4(6-1) from the venom of the 'armed' spider *Phoneutria nigriventer* (Keys). *Toxicon*. 1995;33:83-93.

43. Mafra RA, Figueiredo SG, Diniz CR, Cordeiro MN, Cruz JD, De Lima ME. PhTx4, a new class of toxins from *Phoneutria nigriventer* spider venom, inhibits the glutamate uptake in rat brain synaptosomes. *Brain Res*. 1999;831:297-300.

44. Fontana AC, Beleboni RO, Wojewodzic MW, Dos Santos WF, Coutinho-Netto J, Grutle NJ, et al. Enhancing glutamate transport: mechanism of action of Parawixin1, a neuroprotective compound from Parawixia bistriata spider venom. *Mol Pharmacol*. 2007;72:1228-1237.

45. Cairrão MAR, Ribeiro AM, Pizzo AB, Fontana ACK, Beleboni RO, Coutinho-Netto J, et al. Anticonvulsant and GABA uptake inhibition properties of venom fractions from the spiders *Parawixia bistriata* and *Scaptocosa raptoria*. *Pharm Biol*. 2002;40:472-477.

46. Mussi-Ribeiro A, Miranda A, Gobbo-Netto L, Peporine Lopes N, dos Santos WF. A anticonvulsive fraction from Scaptocosa raptoria (Araneae: Lycosidae) spider venom. *Neurosci Lett*. 2004;371:171-175.

47. Beleboni RO, Guizzo R, Fontana AC, Pizzo AB, Carolino RO, Gobbo-Neto L, et al. Neurochemical characterization of a neuroprotective compound from *Parawixia bistriata* spider venom that inhibits synaptosomal uptake of GABA and glycine. *Mol Pharmacol*. 2006;69:1998-2006.

48. Liberato JL, Cunha AO, Mortari MR, Gelfuso EA, Beleboni Rde O, Coutinho-Netto J, et al. Anticonvulsant and anxiolytic activity of FrPbAII, a novel GABA uptake inhibitor isolated from the venom of the social spider *Parawixia bistriata* (Araneidae: Araneae). *Brain Res*. 2006;1124:19-27.

49. Gelfuso EA, Cunha AO, Mortari MR, Liberato JL, Paraventi KH, Beleboni RO, et al. Neuropharmacological profile of FrPbAII, purified from the venom of the social spider *Parawixia bistriata* (Araneae, Araneidae), in Wistar rats. *Life Sci*. 2007;80:566-572.

50. Karst H, Piek T, Van Marle J, Lind A, Van Weeren-Kramer J. Structure-activity relationship of philanthotoxins-I Pre and postsynaptic inhibition of the locust neuromuscular transmission. *Comp Biochem Physiol C*. 1991;98:471-477.

51. Murata K, Shimada T, Ohfune Y, Hisada M, Yasuda A, Naoki H, et al. Novel biologically active peptides from the venom of Polistes rothneyi iwatai. *Biol Pharm Bull*. 2006;29,2493-2497.

52. Gobbo M, Biondi L, Filira F, Piek T, Rocchi R. Cyclic analogues of Thr6-bradykinin, N epsilon-Lys-bradykinin and endo-Lys8a-vespulakinin 1. *Int J Pept Prot Res*. 1995;45:459-465.

53. de Oliveira L, Cunha AO, Mortari MR, Coimbra NC, Dos Santos WF. Cataleptic activity of the denatured venom of the social wasp Agelaia vicina (Hymenoptera, Vespidae) in Rattus norvegicus (Rodentia, Muridae). *Prog Neuropsychopharmacol Biol Psychiatry*. 2006;30:198-203.

54. Pizzo AB, Fontana AC, Coutinho-Netto J, dos Santos WF. Effects of the crude venom of the social wasp Agelaia vicina on gamma-aminobutyric acid and glutamate uptake in synaptosomes from rat cerebral cortex. *J Biochem Mol Toxicol*. 2000;14:88-94.

55. de Oliveira L, Cunha AO, Mortari MR, Pizzo AB, Miranda A, Coimbra NC, et al. Effects of microinjections of neurotoxin AvTx8, isolated from the social wasp Agelaia vicina (Hymenoptera, Vespidae) venom, on GABAergic nigrotectal pathways. *Brain Res*. 2005;1031:74-81.

56. Pizzo AB, Beleboni RO, Fontana AC, Ribeiro AM, Miranda A, Coutinho-Netto J, et al. Characterization of the actions of AvTx 7 isolated from Agelaia vicina (Hymenoptera: Vespidae) wasp venom on synaptosomal glutamate uptake and release. *J Biochem Mol Toxicol*. 2004;18:61-68.

57. Cunha AO, Mortari MR, Oliveira L, Carolino RO, Coutinho-Netto J, dos Santos WF. Anticonvulsant effects of the wasp Polybia ignobilis venom on chemically induced seizures and action on GABA and glutamate receptors. *Brain Res*. 2006;1124:19-27.

58. Mortari MR, Cunha AO, de Oliveira L, Vieira EB, Gelfuso EA, Coutinho-Netto J, et al. Anticonvulsant

and behavioural effects of the denatured venom of the social wasp *Polybia occidentalis* (Polistinae, Vespidae). *Basic Clin Pharmacol Toxicol.* 2005;97:289-295.

59. Mortari MR, Cunha AO, Carolino RO, Coutinho-Netto J, Tomaz JC, Lopes NP, et al. Inhibition of acute nociceptive responses in rats after i.c.v. injection of Thr6-bradykinin, isolated from the venom of the social wasp, *Polybia occidentalis. Br J Pharmacol.* 2007;151:860-869.

60. Nagy I, Paule C, White J, Urban L. Taking the sting out of pain. *Br J Pharmacol.* 2007;151:721-722.

INDEX

Note: Page numbers followed by f refer to figures; those followed by t refer to tables.

485